Dermatology *and* Dermatological Therapy *of* Pigmented Skins

Dermatology *and* Dermatological Therapy *of* Pigmented Skins

Edited by
Rebat M. Halder

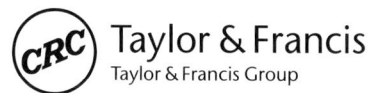
Taylor & Francis
Taylor & Francis Group

Boca Raton   London   New York

A CRC title, part of the Taylor & Francis imprint, a member of the
Taylor & Francis Group, the academic division of T&F Informa plc.

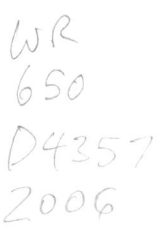

Published in 2006 by
CRC Press
Taylor & Francis Group
6000 Broken Sound Parkway NW, Suite 300
Boca Raton, FL 33487-2742

© 2006 by Taylor & Francis Group, LLC
CRC Press is an imprint of Taylor & Francis Group

No claim to original U.S. Government works
Printed in the United States of America on acid-free paper
10 9 8 7 6 5 4 3 2 1

International Standard Book Number-10: 0-8493-1402-X (Hardcover)
International Standard Book Number-13: 978-0-8493-1402-5 (Hardcover)
Library of Congress Card Number 2005044005

This book contains information obtained from authentic and highly regarded sources. Reprinted material is quoted with permission, and sources are indicated. A wide variety of references are listed. Reasonable efforts have been made to publish reliable data and information, but the author and the publisher cannot assume responsibility for the validity of all materials or for the consequences of their use.

No part of this book may be reprinted, reproduced, transmitted, or utilized in any form by any electronic, mechanical, or other means, now known or hereafter invented, including photocopying, microfilming, and recording, or in any information storage or retrieval system, without written permission from the publishers.

For permission to photocopy or use material electronically from this work, please access www.copyright.com (http://www.copyright.com/) or contact the Copyright Clearance Center, Inc. (CCC) 222 Rosewood Drive, Danvers, MA 01923, 978-750-8400. CCC is a not-for-profit organization that provides licenses and registration for a variety of users. For organizations that have been granted a photocopy license by the CCC, a separate system of payment has been arranged.

Trademark Notice: Product or corporate names may be trademarks or registered trademarks, and are used only for identification and explanation without intent to infringe.

Library of Congress Cataloging-in-Publication Data

Dermatology and dermatological therapy of pigmented skins / edited by Rebat Halder.
    p. ; cm.
  Includes bibliographical references and index.
  ISBN 0-8493-1402-X (alk. paper)
  1. Pigmentation disorder. 2. Dermatology--Cross-cultural studies. 3. Skin--Diseases--Diagnosis. I. Halder, Rebat M.
    [DNLM: 1. Skin Disease--therapy. 2. Ethnic Groups. 3. Skin Diseases--ethnology. 4. Skin Pigmentation. WR 650 D4356 2005]

RL790.D47 2005
616.5'06--dc22
                                             2005044005

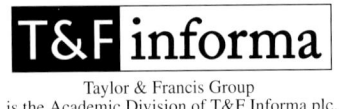

Taylor & Francis Group
is the Academic Division of T&F Informa plc.

Visit the Taylor & Francis Web site at
http://www.taylorandfrancis.com

and the CRC Press Web site at
http://www.crcpress.com

The L'Oreal Institute for Ethnic Hair and Skin Research, Chicago, Illinois is acknowledged for supporting the reproduction of the color plates in this book.

*This book is dedicated to the memory of my parents,
Ras M. Halder, Ph.D. and Sulekha Halder, who provided
great encouragement to me throughout their lives
and to the memory of John A. Kenney, Jr., M.D.,
mentor, teacher and friend and one of the founders
of the field of dermatology of pigmented skins.*

Table of Contents

About the Editor xxiii
Contributors xxv
Preface xxvii

PART I

Chapter 1 Structure and Function of Skin and Hair in Pigmented Races 3
Christian O. Oresajo, Sreekumar Pillai, and Georgianna M. Richards

Introduction 3
Biology, Structure, and Function of Pigmented Skin 3
    Racial Differences in Stratum Corneum Biology 3
    Racial Differences in Functional and Biophysical Properties of Stratum Corneum 4
    Racial Differences in Epidermal Structure 5
    Racial Differences in Melanocyte Biology and Function 6
        Melanocyte Biology 6
        Racial Differences 6
    Racial Differences in Dermal Structure 7
        Biology of Dermis 7
        Racial Differences 7
    Cutaneous Appendages 9
        Sebaceous Glands and Sweat Glands 9
        Racial Differences in Hair Follicles and Hair Structure 10
        Racial Differences 10
        Racial Differences in Nails 11
Racial Differences in Dermatological Conditions 11
    Scarring and Keloid Scars 11
    Irritation 12
    Allergic Contact Dermatitis 12
    Racial Differences in Skin Immunological Responses 13
References 14

Chapter 2 Common Dermatological Diseases in Pigmented Skins 17
Rebat M. Halder, Howard L. Brooks, and Juan Carlos Caballero

Common Dermatological Diseases 17
Acne Vulgaris and Related Disorders 17
    Acne Vulgaris 17
    Acne Conglobata 18
    Follicular Occlusion Triad 19
    Pomade Acne 20
    Rosacea 20

Treatment of Acne 21
    Benzoyl Peroxide 22
    Antibiotics 22
    Retinoids 23
    Oral Contraceptives 24
    Hydroquinone 24
    Azelaic Acid 25
    Chemical Peels and Microdermabrasion 25
Dermatitis in Pigmented Skin: Prevalence and Clinical Manifestations of Atopic and Contact
    Dermatitis 25
    Atopic Dermatitis 25
    Contact Dermatitis 28
Dermatophyte Infections in Ethnic Populations: Tinea Capitis 33
References 39

Chapter 3   Neonatal and Pediatric Dermatological Diseases in Pigmented Skins 43
Patricia A. Treadwell

Diseases with Increased Incidence 43
    Transient Neonatal Pustular Melanosis 43
    Mongolian Spots 43
    Dyspigmentation 44
    Acropustulosis of Infancy 45
    Traction Folliculitis and/or Alopecia 47
    Tinea Capitis 48
    Hypopigmented Mycosis Fungoides 49
    Lupus Erythematosus 50
    Neonatal Lupus Erythematosus 50
    Kawasaki Disease 51
Diseases with Different Clinical Presentations 53
    Erythema 53
    Atopic Dermatitis 53
    Nickel Contact Dermatitis 54
    Seborrheic Dermatitis 55
    Pityriasis Rosea 55
    Tinea Versicolor 56
    Polymorphous Light Eruption 58
    Lichen Striatus 58
    Lichen Planus 58
    Neurofibromatosis 1 59
Diseases with Decreased Incidence 60
References 60

Chapter 4   Hair and Scalp Disorders in Pigmented Skins 63
Amy J. McMichael and Valerie D. Callender

Introduction 63
Basic Principles 63
Inflammatory Scalp Disorders with Flaking 64

        Seborrheic Dermatitis 64
            Therapy 65
        Psoriasis Vulgaris 67
            Therapy 68
        Atopic Dermatitis 70
            Therapy 71
        Contact Dermatitis 71
            Irritant Contact Dermatitis 71
            Allergic Contact Dermatitis 72
        Tinea Capitis 72
            Therapy 74
        Lupus Erythematosus and Dermatomyositis 74
            Lupus Erythematosus 74
            Dermatomyositis 75
    Inflammatory Disorders with Pustules or Cysts 75
        Uncomplicated Folliculitis 76
            Treatment 76
        Folliculitis Decalvans 76
            Treatment 76
        Acne Keloidalis Nuchae 76
            Treatment 78
        Dissecting Cellulitis 78
            Treatment 78
    Scarring Hair Loss with Little or No Clinical Inflammation 80
        Traction Alopecia 80
            Treatment 80
        Central Centrifugal Cicatricial Alopecia 80
            Treatment 82
        Sarcoidosis 83
    Hair Shaft Disorders 84
        Trichorrhexis Nodosa 84
        Heat, Chemicals, and Other Drying Agents 85
            Heat 85
            Chemicals 85
            Other Drying Agents 87
    Summary 88
    References 88

Chapter 5 Pigmentary Disorders in Pigmented Skins 91
Rebat M. Halder, Maithily A. Nandedkar, and Kenneth W. Neal

Introduction 91
Disorders of Hypopigmentation 91
    Pityriasis Versicolor 91
    Pityriasis Alba 92
    Idiopathic Guttate Hypomelanosis 92
Disorders of Depigmentation 93
    Vitiligo 93
Postinflammatory Hyperpigmentation and Hypopigmentation 95

Disorders of Hyperpigmentation ... 100
    Linea Nigra ... 100
    Erythema Dyschromicum Perstans (Ashy Dermatosis) ... 100
    Melasma ... 101
    Familial Racial Periorbital Hyperpigmentation ... 103
The Management of Pigmentary Disorders ... 103
    Topical Corticosteroids ... 103
    Phenolic Agents ... 104
    Azelaic Acid ... 104
    Kojic Acid ... 105
    Arbutin ... 105
    Licorice Extract ... 105
    Topical Retinoids ... 105
    Combination Therapy ... 106
    Tars ... 106
    Topical Tacrolimus ... 106
    Other Treatments ... 106
Pigmented Nevi ... 107
    Nails ... 107
    Palmoplantar Racial Differences ... 107
    Nevus of Ota/Nevus of Ito ... 107
Genetic Diseases ... 107
    Piebaldism ... 107
    Albinism and Hermansky–Pudlak Syndrome ... 108
References ... 110

Chapter 6   Infectious Diseases of Pigmented Skins: Latinos ... 115
Miguel R. Sanchez

Introduction ... 115
Superficial Fungal Infections ... 115
Human Papilloma Virus (HPV) ... 117
Hepatitis ... 118
Syphilis ... 119
Onchocerciasis ... 119
Cysticercosis ... 120
Mycobacterium Infection ... 121
Chagas Disease ... 122
Dengue Fever ... 124
Paederus Dermatitis ... 124
Bartonellosis (Carrion's Disease) ... 125
Cutaneous Larva Migrans ... 126
Cutaneous Larva Currens ... 127
Gnathostomiasis ... 128
Myiasis ... 129
Leishmaniasis ... 130
Chromomycosis ... 132
Hansen's Disease ... 133
Rhinoscleroma ... 136
Paracoccidioidomycosis (South American Blastomycosis) ... 136
Sporotrichosis ... 137

Cutaneous *Balamuthia mandrillaris* Infection ... 138
Chronic Infective Lymphocytic Psoriaform Dermatitis ... 139
Lymphatic Filariasis ... 139
References ... 140

Chapter 7 Cutaneous Manifestations of Systemic Disease in Pigmented Skins ... 147
Yamini V. Saripalli and Sharon Bridgeman-Shah

Introduction ... 147
Sarcoidosis ... 147
Autoimmune Disease ... 149
    Scleroderma ... 149
    Lupus Erythematosus ... 151
    Dermatomyositis ... 157
Hematologic Disease ... 158
    Hermansky–Pudlak Syndrome ... 158
Endocrine Disease — Diabetes Mellitus ... 158
    Waxy Skin ... 159
    Dermopathy ... 159
    Acanthosis Nigricans ... 159
    Diabetic Foot Ulcers ... 160
    Necrobiosis Lipoidica Diabeticorum ... 160
    Diabetic Bullae ... 161
Hepatic Disease ... 162
    Lichen Planus ... 162
    Pruritus in Hepatic Disease ... 163
    Cryoglobulinemia and Hepatitis C ... 163
Renal Disease ... 164
    General ... 164
    Kyrle's Disease ... 164
    Pruritus in Renal Disease ... 164
Systemic Medication Reactions ... 165
Conclusion ... 169
References ... 169

Chapter 8 Skin Cancer in Pigmented Skins ... 181
Rebat M. Halder and Collette J. Ara

Introduction ... 181
African-Americans, Afro-Caribbeans, and Africans ... 181
Hispanics ... 189
Asians ... 191
Native Americans ... 193
Public Health Issues for Skin Cancer in Pigmented Skins ... 193
References ... 194

Chapter 9 Intrinsic Skin Aging in Pigmented Races ... 197
Monte O. Harris

Introduction ... 197
General Considerations ... 197

Anthropologic Considerations and Facial Characteristics 198
    Asian Morphology 198
    Latino Morphology 198
    African-American Morphology 198
Morphological Facial Aging 200
Ethnic Considerations — Facial Aging 202
    Upper Face 202
    Midface 202
    Lower Face 203
Rejuvenation Procedures 204
Conclusion 206
References 208

Chapter 10 Photoaging in Pigmented Skins 211
Rebat M. Halder and Georgianna M. Richards

Introduction 211
Photoaging in East and Southeast Asians 212
Photoaging in Blacks 214
Photoaging in Hispanics 216
Summary of Photoaging in Pigmented Skins 216
Therapy of Photoaging of Pigmented Skins 217
    Retinoids 217
        Topical Tretinoin 217
        Systemic Retinoid Therapy 218
    Bleaching Agents 218
    Chemical Peels 218
    Microdermabrasion 218
    Photorejuvenation 218
References 219

Chapter 11 Pharmacological Agents for Pigmented Skins 221
Pearl E. Grimes

Introduction 221
Retinoids 221
    Tretinoin 221
    Tazarotene 223
    Adapalene 224
Retinol 224
Niacinamide 224
Benzoyl Peroxide 225
Anti-Infective Therapy 225
    Topical Antibiotics 225
    Systemic Antibiotics 226
Topical Corticosteroids 226
Vitamin C 227
Hydroquinone 227
Topical Immunomodulators 228
References 228

Chapter 12 Cosmetic and Dermatologic Surgery for Pigmented Skins 233
Pearl E. Grimes and Brooke A. Jackson

Introduction 233
Rejuvenation in Ethnic Skin 233
Botulinum Toxin 233
Chemical Peels 234
    Peeling Agents 234
    Peeling Protocol 235
    Glycolic Acid 236
    Salicylic Acid 236
    Trichloroacetic Acid 237
    Jessner's Solution 237
    Medium and Deep Peels 238
Microdermabrasion 238
Injectable Filling Agents 238
    Collagen 240
    Hyaluronic Acid 240
    Hydroxylapatite 240
Body Image and Body-Contouring Procedures 240
    Tumescent Liposuction 241
References 241

Chapter 13 Hair Transplantation for Pigmented Skins 245
Valerie D. Callender

Introduction 245
Racial Variations in Hair Morphology 246
Indications for Hair Transplantation in African-American Women 248
    Traction Alopecia 249
    Central Centrifugal Cicatricial Alopecia (CCCA) 249
Hair Transplantation: Special Considerations for Black Women 251
    Why Larger Grafts May Be Preferred in CCCA 251
    How to Reduce the Risk of Scarring 254
    The Importance of Physician–Patient Communication 255
Summary 255
References 256

Chapter 14 Laser Therapy for Pigmented Skins 259
Lori M. Hobbs and Eliot F. Battle

Introduction 259
    Historical Aspects of Laser Surgery 259
    Laser Principles 259
    Laser Principles in Pigmented Skin 261
Types of Lasers Commonly Used for Pigmented Skins 262
    Vascular Lasers and Light Sources 262
    The Intense Pulse Light Systems 264
    Lasers for Pigmented Lesions 264
Specific Pigmented Disorders Common to Ethnic Skin Types 265

  Melasma..265
  Postinflammatory Hyperpigmentation...266
  Lentigines...266
  Dermatosis Papulosis Nigra (DPN)...266
  Nevus of Ota..267
  Tattoos..267
 Miscellaneous Disorders...269
  Keloids and Hypertrophic Scars 269
  Psoriasis Vulgaris...269
 Newer Applications for Lasers 270
  Acne Vulgaris..270
  Vitiligo...270
  Laser-Assisted Hair Removal..270
  Acne Keloidalis Nuchae..273
  Nonablative Lasers 273
Conclusion...274
References...274

Chapter 15 Cosmetics, Hair Care Products, and Personal Care Products for Pigmented
    Skins 277

Victoria L. Holloway

Introduction 277
Hair Care..277
 Unique Characteristics of Ethnic Hair...277
 Hair Relaxers..278
  History 278
  Chemistry..278
  Proper Use...278
  Adverse Events...279
 Thioglycolates for Permanent Waves, "Curls," and Thermal Reconditioning....................279
 Hair Bleach and Hair Color 280
 Shampoos, Conditioners, and Styling Products..280
 Depilatories..281
Skin Care..281
 Skin Lightening and Brightening Products...281
 Sunscreens 282
Color Cosmetics...284
Conclusion..285
References..285

PART II

Chapter 16 Dermatologic Disease in Asians 289

Chai Sue Lee, Hiok-Hee Tan, Mark Boon-Yong Tang, Chee-Leok Goh, and Henry W. Lim

Dermatoses Common or Unique in Asians 289
 Acne Vulgaris 289
 Atopic Dermatitis 292

  Xerosis, Nummular Dermatitis, and Dyshidrotic Eczema 294
  Contact Dermatitis..295
  Pigmented Contact Dermatitis 299
  Prurigo Nodularis, Actinic Prurigo, and Prurigo Pigmentosa 301
  Primary Cutaneous Amyloidosis...304
  Melasma...307
  Mongolian Spot 310
  Nevus of Ota and Nevus of Ito 311
  Nonmelanoma Skin Cancer..313
  Melanoma 314
  Ofuji's Disease...316
Dermatoses Occurring in Asians 318
  Vitiligo 318
  Chronic Actinic Dermatitis 319
  Erythropoietic Protoporphyria..320
  Dermatoses Secondary to Asian Cultural Medical Practice...321
    Coin rubbing...322
    Cupping...323
    Moxibustion 323
Summary 323
References 324

Chapter 17 Dermatologic Disease in Blacks 331
Rebat M. Halder, Camille I. Roberts, Pavan K. Nootheti, and A. Paul Kelly

Basic Structure of Black Skin and Hair...331
Cultural Issues in Treating Blacks for Dermatologic Disease...331
Normal Variants of Black Skin..332
Common Skin and Hair Diseases...333
  Seborrheic Dermatitis of Skin..333
  Tinea (Pityriasis) Versicolor 334
  Contact Dermatitis..334
    Adverse Reactions to Hair-Coloring Products...334
  Trichorrhexis Nodosa 334
  Pseudofolliculitis Barbae..335
    Clinical Presentation...336
    Pseudofolliculitis Barbae in Women..337
    Acne Keloidalis Nuchae 337
    Treatment of Pseudofolliculitis Barbae..338
    Adjuvant Treatment Measures 339
    Electrolysis 339
    Surgical Therapy...339
    Summary — PFB 340
  Dermatosis Papulosa Nigra (DPN) 340
  Pigmentary Disorders 341
    Vitiligo 341
    Melasma..341
  Keloids 342
    Medical Therapies 343
    Surgical Therapies 345

Radiation Therapy 346
Physical Modalities for Treatment 346
Skin Diseases with Unusual Presentations in Blacks 347
Atopic Dermatitis 347
Pityriasis Rosea 348
Secondary Syphilis 348
Sarcoidosis 348
Discoid Lupus Erythematosus 349
Systemic Lupus Erythematosus 349
Scleroderma 350
Skin Cancer in the Black Races 350
Melanoma 350
Basal Cell Carcinoma 351
Squamous Cell Carcinoma 351
Mycosis Fungoides 351
Dermatofibrosarcoma Protuberans 351
References 351

Chapter 18 Dermatologic Disease in Hispanics/Latinos 357
Miguel Sanchez

Introduction 357
Cultural Aspects of Skin Disease 357
Skin Diseases 359
Pigmentary Disorders 359
Postinflammatory Hyperpigmentation 359
Erythema Dyschromicum Perstans 361
Lichen Planas Actinicos 362
Lichen Planas Pigmentosus 363
Prurigo Pigmentosa 363
Macular Amyloidosis 364
Drug-Induced Pigmentation 364
Melasma 365
Riehl's Melanosis 368
Poikiloderma of Civatte 369
Erythromelanosis Follicularis Facei 369
Linea Fusca 370
Arsenical Melanosis 370
Hermansky–Pudlak Syndrome 370
Pityriasis Alba 371
Idiopathic Guttate Hypomelanosis 371
Acne 371
Eczema 373
Actinic Prurigo 373
Capsaicin Dermatitis 375
Balanitis Xerotica Obliterans 375
Acanthosis Nigricans 376
Prayer Callouses 377

Skin Cancer 378
    Basal Cell and Squamous Cell Carcinomas 378
    Melanoma 379
References 381

Chapter 19 Dermatologic Diseases in Native Americans..385
Willie F. Richardson, Jr. and R. Steven Padilla

Background 385
Special Considerations 386
Basic Science of Native American Skin...386
Dermatoses in Native Americans: Unique Dermatoses 387
    Hereditary Polymorphous Light Eruption 387
        Clinical Presentation..387
    Neutropenic Poikiloderma (formerly known as Navajo Poikiloderma)..............387
Dermatoses in Native Americans: Common Dermatoses 389
    Oral Focal Epithelial Hyperplasia (Heck's Disease) 389
    Hereditary Benign Intraepithelial Dyskeratosis 389
    Acne Vulgaris 390
    Acne Rosacea 391
    Atopic Dermatitis 392
    Dermatophyte Infection..393
    Congenital Melanocytic Nevi, Pigmentary Anomalies, and Other Nevi 394
    Other Nevi 395
    Psoriasis Vulgaris..395
        Differential Diagnosis...396
    Seborrheic Dermatitis...397
    Lichen Planus 397
    Granuloma Annulare 398
Dermatoses in Native Americans: Uncommon Dermatoses 400
    Nonmelanoma Skin Cancer..400
    Melanoma 400
Conclusion...402
References 402

Index..405

About the Editor

Rebat M. Halder, M.D. is professor and chairman of the department of dermatology at Howard University College of Medicine, Washington, D.C. He is also director of the Ethnic Skin Research Institute within the department as well as director of the Vitiligo Center. He is director of the dermatology residency program at Howard University Hospital. Dr. Halder is an internationally recognized expert in the areas of ethnic skin diseases and pigmentary skin disorders. He has been active in both laboratory and clinical research studies in these areas. Dr. Halder received his medical education at Howard University and completed his residency in dermatology at Howard University Hospital. He is the author of numerous publications including book chapters, peer-reviewed journal articles, and editorships. He has been an invited lecturer throughout the United States as well as internationally. Dr. Halder is a member of many professional organizations including the American Academy of Dermatology, the Society for Investigative Dermatology, and the prestigious American Dermatological Association.

Contributors

Collette J. Ara
Private Practice
Chicago, Illinois

Eliot F. Battle
Department of Dermatology
Howard University College of Medicine
Washington, D.C.

Sharon Bridgeman-Shah
Department of Dermatology
Howard University College of Medicine
Washington, D.C.

Howard L. Brooks
Department of Dermatology
Howard University College of Medicine
Washington, D.C.

Juan Carlos Cabalerro
Department of Dermatology
Washington Hospital Center
Washington, D.C.

Valerie D. Callender
Department of Dermatology
Howard University College of Medicine
Washington, D.C.

Chee-Leok Goh
National Skin Centre
Singapore

Pearl E. Grimes
Vitiligo and Pigmentation Institute of Southern California
Los Angeles, California

Rebat M. Halder
Department of Dermatology
Howard University College of Medicine
Washington, D.C.

Monte O. Harris
Department of Dermatology
Howard University College of Medicine
Washington, D.C.

Lori M. Hobbs
Department of Dermatology
Howard University College of Medicine
Washington, D.C.

Victoria L. Holloway
L'Oreal Institute for Ethnic Hair and Skin Research
Chicago, Illinois

Brooke A. Jackson
Department of Dermatology
Northwestern University
Chicago, Illinois

A. Paul Kelly
Division of Dermatology
Charles R. Drew University of Medicine and Science
Los Angeles, California

Chai Sue Lee
Department of Dermatology
University of California–Davis
Sacramento, California

Henry W. Lim
Department of Dematology
Henry Ford Hospital
Detroit, Michigan

Amy J. McMichael
Department of Dermatology
Wake Forest University Medical Center
Winston-Salem, North Carolina

Maithily A. Nandedkar
Private Practice
Sterling, Virginia

Kenneth W. Neal
Department of Dermatology
University of Cincinnati
Cincinnati, Ohio

Pavan K. Nootheti
Department of Dermatology
Howard University College of Medicine
Washington, D.C.

Christian O. Oresajo
Engelhard Corporation
Stony Brook, New York

Steven R. Padilla
Department of Dermatology
University of New Mexico School of Medicine
Albuquerque, New Mexico

Sreekumar Pillai
Engelhard Corporation
Stony Brook, New York

Georgianna M. Richards
Department of Dermatology
Howard University College of Medicine
Washington, D.C.

Willie F. Richardson, Jr.
Department of Dermatology
University of New Mexico School of Medicine
Albuquerque, New Mexico

Camille I. Roberts
Private Practice
Worcester, Massachusetts

Miguel R. Sanchez
New York University School of Medicine
New York, N.Y.

Yamini V. Saripalli
Department of Dermatology
Howard University College of Medicine
Washington, D.C.

Hiok-Hee Tan
National Skin Centre
Singapore

Mark Book-Yong Tang
National Skin Centre
Singapore

Patricia A. Treadwell
Department of Dermatology
University of Indiana School of Medicine
Indianapolis, Indiana

Preface

The changing demographics of the United States have given a new face to North America. With current projections indicating that the majority of the United States population will be non-Caucasian by mid-century, there are already changes in the ethnic and racial groups seen in the dermatologist's office. This book is devoted to skin diseases in pigmented or non-Caucasian skins.

With approximately one third of the United States population now being non-Caucasian, changing demographics have occurred not only in metropolitan areas but also in pockets throughout the country. The contributing authors of this book have attempted to give a better understanding of skin and hair disorders seen in the major non-Caucasian ethnic groups in the United States. There are disorders that may be found frequently in some groups and some that may be found rarely. Furthermore, the presentation of common dermatological disorders may vary from one ethnic group to another.

Medical and surgical therapies may be different in non-Caucasian populations for diseases of skin and hair. Newer treatment modalities such as lasers require knowledge of proper parameters as well as knowledge of adverse reactions in darker skin. With the consumer market becoming much wider for ethnic populations, knowledge of unique cosmetics and personal care products becomes necessary. Another important aspect of treating non-Caucasian patients is an awareness of cultural issues specific to those populations.

One must realize that the majority of the world's population is composed of peoples with pigmented skins. Approximately 80% of the world's population is pigmented; however, there has not yet been published a comprehensive textbook on dermatology and dermatological therapy of pigmented skins. This book includes chapters concerning particular dermatological disorders or related disorders occurring in pigmented skins, as well as chapters concerning dermatological diseases found in specific racial groups.

Rebat M. Halder, M.D.
Department of Dermatology
Howard University College of Medicine
Washington, D.C. 20060, USA

Part I

1 Structure and Function of Skin and Hair in Pigmented Races

Christian O. Oresajo, Sreekumar Pillai, and Georgianna M. Richards

INTRODUCTION

There are many racial and ethnic groups that may be categorized as people with skin of color. These include Asians, African-Americans, Afro-Caribbeans and Africans, as well as Hispanics and Native Americans. Within each of these ethnic and racial groups, there are subgroups. Although obvious differences exist among human populations, little data exists in defining ethnic and racial differences in skin and hair structure and physiology.

There are various observed racial and ethnic differences in the structure, function, and physiology of skin and hair. These differences are important in considering how skin and hair disorders vary between races as well as how cultural practices may influence the presentation of these disorders.

Obvious physical differences exist among human populations, in hair color, texture, skin color, and facial features. Although all humans are members of the same species, understanding the causes of skin diseases may hinge on the structural and physiologic variations that exist among different ethnic groups in skin and hair.

The demographics of the United States reflect a constantly changing mixture of people of various ethnic and racial groups. Although the majority of Americans are currently white-skinned, it has been projected that in the mid-21st century people with dark skin will constitute the majority of the American and international populations.[1] This change necessitates the need to understand the differences in the structure and function of skin of color, the presentation of disease, and treatment management of disorders of the hair and skin.

BIOLOGY, STRUCTURE, AND FUNCTION OF PIGMENTED SKIN

RACIAL DIFFERENCES IN STRATUM CORNEUM BIOLOGY

The stratum corneum (SC) is the outermost layer of skin and is the principal barrier tissue preventing water loss from the body and providing mechanical protection. The cells of the SC, called corneocytes, are platelike structures that are approximately 50 μm across and 1 μm thick and are stacked in layers, the numbers of which vary between anatomical body sites and races. In various studies the SC of blacks has been found to consist of more layers when compared with that of Caucasians. The numbers of cell layers appear to be increased in black skin, although the mean thickness of SC is the same in both races.[2] There are 20 cell layers in black skin as compared to 16 cell layers in comparable sites in white skin. The fact that the total thickness is similar suggests that the SC of black skin is more compact than that of white skin.[3] Investigators have also observed higher lipid content in black epidermis, greater cellular cohesion, less permeability to certain chemicals, and more difficulty in stripping off the black skin SC. The number of cellophane tape strippings required to remove the SC has been reported in 25 Caucasians and 21 blacks in a comparative study.[2] A greater number of strippings was required for removal of SC in blacks than was required in Caucasians; black subjects were also found to have a greater variance in the thickness of SC layers as well as with SC stripping. A difference in the pH gradient has also been reported between black and white skin.[4] The initial 3–6 tape strippings showed significantly increased water loss and decrease in pH in black skin as compared to white skin. However, this difference disappeared with subsequent tape strippings. These data suggest that the superficial SC pH is lower in black skin. Within black individuals, the degree of pigmentation has no correlation with the number of cell layers seen.[5] An increase in spontaneous desquamation in blacks as compared to other races has also been reported. This was attributed to a difference in the composition of the intercellular cement of the SC. In a study by Sugino et al.,[6] blacks were found to have the lowest levels of ceramides in the SC compared with Caucasians, Hispanics, and Asians. This study also showed an inverse correlation with the transepidermal water loss (TEWL) and the ceramide levels; water content, however, had a direct correlation with the ceramide levels.

Other studies could not find differences in the SC properties between black and white skin. Despite differences in age, anatomic areas of skin for skin roughness, scaliness, and SC hydration, there were no significant differences between black and white skin.[7] Skin hydration and roughness or scaliness were similar between different races.[7] Another study also found no differences in SC surface area between white and black skin.[8] However, the spontaneous desquamation rate was higher in black skin.

RACIAL DIFFERENCES IN FUNCTIONAL AND BIOPHYSICAL PROPERTIES OF STRATUM CORNEUM

In a study by Kompaore et al.,[9] a significantly higher TEWL after tape stripping of the SC was evident in Asians and blacks than observed in whites. In addition to showing the highest TEWL after stripping, Asians also showed greater skin permeability than other races. Other studies, however, although showing variation in the recovery of the barrier between skin types II–III and skin type IV, showed generally no difference between races. Darker skin types have faster barrier recovery and display more resistant barrier than the skin of lighter pigmentation.[10]

To investigate the racial differences in skin function, various biophysical parameters have been studied. TEWL, skin conductance, and skin thickness were studied in whites, Hispanics, and blacks under basal conditions.[5] The data showed no differences in TEWL between race or sites without tape stripping. In Hispanics, the water content was increased on the volar forearm compared with blacks. But in whites, the water content was decreased on the dorsal forearm compared with blacks. In a study on physiological differences in skin of different races, Berardesca et al.[11] found that marked differences between races exist in skin biophysical parameters. They concluded that these differences are mainly related to the protective role of melanin present in races with darker skin.

Skin conductance was higher in blacks and Hispanics than in whites.[12] In addition to skin water content, there are other factors in the SC (such as lipid content) that alter skin conductance measurement. A major determinant of the physical properties of SC (barrier properties) is the lipid content of the SC. It has been suggested that the lipid content of black skin may be higher than that of Caucasian skin.[3] There is also evidence that black skin is more prone to dryness, suggesting racial differences in lipid content of skin. The relationship between lipid content and skin dryness has been well established.[13] More than the total lipid content, the proper ratio of ceramide to cholesterol to fatty acids, the type of ceramides, and the type of sphingosine backbone play an important role in skin barrier properties and skin dryness. It remains to be established whether there are any differences in the barrier lipid profile between black and white skin in these specific aspects of lipid biochemistry. Studies from Elias's group[10] suggest that there may be lipid differences in the dark vs. lighter skin. The darkly pigmented skin showed a more resistant barrier and recovered more quickly after perturbation by tape strippings than skin of individuals with lighter pigmentation. This would suggest a higher rate of lipid synthesis in darker skin. In summary, although several studies tend to suggest differences in barrier properties and lipid composition between black and white skin, conclusive evidence for these differences have not been demonstrated.

RACIAL DIFFERENCES IN EPIDERMAL STRUCTURE

The epidermis is subdivided into: (a) a basal cell layer of keratinocytes, which is the germinative layer of the epidermis; (b) the stratum spinosum, which comprises several layers of polyhedral cells lying above the germinal layer; (c) the stratum granulosum, which is a layer of flattened cells containing distinctive cytoplasmic inclusions, keratohyalin granules; and (d) the stratum corneum. The SC is generated from the basal layers in a process of vectorial differentiation. The time lag for a basal cell to form a corneocyte is about 24–40 days in normal epidermis. The SC is desquamated into the environment as they are continuously replaced from below. The time of transit of a cell from the lower portion of SC to desquamation is approximately 14 days.

Overall, the morphology and structure of epidermis is similar between different skin types, although some racial differences in epidermal structure have been demonstrated (see Table 1.1). Among those differences is the variation in the thickness of the epidermis occurring between black (6-5 μm) and Caucasian groups (7.2 μm), although individual variations were also evident.[14] The stratum lucidum consists of 1–2 layers in the non-sun-exposed skins in both black and Caucasian groups. In blacks the stratum lucidum is compact and unaltered in sun-exposed skin, whereas in white individuals the stratum lucidum appears thicker. In both groups the stratum granulosum consists of up to three layers.[14]

The hair follicle is a major component of the epidermal structure. The hair follicle is composed of epithelial (epidermal) and dermal components interacting with each other in an autonomous way. This is a self-renewing organ where interactions between epithelial and mesothelial components take place. Each of the follicular compartments is endowed with a specific differentiation pathway under the control of an intricate network of growth factors, cytokines, and hormones. Major differences in the hair follicle that determine the shape of hair exist between different races. This is discussed in the section on hair in this chapter.

TABLE 1.1
Comparison of Epidermis of Different Racial Groups

	White	Black	Asians
Stratum corneum thickness	7.2 μm	6.5 μm	
Stratum corneum layers	17 layers	22 layers	
Stratum lucidum	1–2 layers. On exposure to sun becomes swollen and distinctly cellular	Remains compact and unaltered with sun exposure	
Water barrier	High	Low	
Melanosomes	Small. Group melanosomes in keratinocytes less dense, more numerous in SC than basal layer	Larger. Individually dispersed melanosomes in keratinocytes more numerous in basal layer	Mainly aggregated melanosomes; nonaggregated in sunlight-exposed areas
Stratum corneum lipids	Low	High	
Vitamin D production	High	Low	
MED	Low	High	
Photodamage	Significant changes in the epidermis	Marginal changes in the epidermis	Significant changes in the epidermis
Melanin	Has greater protective capability in the stratum corneum	Has less protective capability in the stratum corneum	
Mast cell morphology	Smaller granules. Less cathepsin G	Larger granules. Greater amount of cathepsin G	

Racial Differences in Melanocyte Biology and Function

Melanocyte Biology

The major color determinant in the skin is the pigment melanin, a product of specialized cells known as melanocytes. Within the melanocytes, melanin is synthesized in specialized organelles called melanosomes, which are subsequently transferred (along with their melanin) to adjacent keratinocytes in the basal epidermal layer, giving rise to skin pigmentation. The type and quantity of melanin produced and the distribution of the melanosomes in basal epidermal keratinocytes affect the final color of the individual's skin. Fitzpatrick and Szabo indicate the association of one melanocyte and 30–35 keratinocytes in skin as the epidermal melanin unit.[15] The function of melanin is to absorb UV light and block free radical generation, acting as a protective mechanism against sun damage and skin aging.

Human melanin is composed of two distinct polymers, dark brown/black eumelanin and yellow/red pheomelanin.[16] Eumelanin and pheomelanin are produced in the eumelanosomes and pheomelanosomes, respectively. Both of these types of melanosomes undergo four stages of maturation, resulting in synthesis and deposition of melanin. The two types of melanin differ in their composition and physical properties. Due to the incorporation of sulfur containing the amino acid cysteine, pheomelanin has higher sulfur content than eumelainin. Eumelanin is made and deposited in ellipsoidal melanosomes that contain a fibrillar internal structure, whereas pheomelanin is synthesized in spherical melanosomes and is associated with microvesicles.[17] The final melanin composition and, therefore, its color depend on the relative rates of pheo- and eumelanogenesis occurring in the melanocyte. Whereas eumelanogenesis is increased after UV exposure (tanning), the constitutive levels of pheo- and eumelanin are believed to be genetically determined. Black-skinned people have a higher content and synthesis of eumelanin than pheomelanin. Eumelanin and pheomelanin are both derived from the common substrate tyrosine. The hydroxylation of tyrosine to dihydroxyphenylalanine (DOPA) and the oxidation of DOPA to dopaquinone are both reactions catalyzed by the tyrosinase enzyme. Other enzymes involved in melanogenesis include tyrosinase-related protein-1 and -2 (TRP-1 and -2). Recent studies also indicate the importance of melanosomal P-protein that is involved in the acidification of melanosomes in melanogenesis.[18]

Racial Differences

A darkly pigmented person has a similar number of melanocytes as a more lightly pigmented person, but the melanocytes are much more active. The morphology, content, and distribution of melanosomes also differ between races. Black skin contains more eumelanin; melanosomes are uniformly distributed throughout the epidermis, do not appear to have a limiting membrane, and are stuck closely together. Caucasian skin melanin also contains pheomelanin (the ratio of eu- to pheo- depends on the particular skin color); the melanosomes are smaller, round, contain limiting membrane, and are distributed in clusters with spaces between them, giving a lighter color. In lighter-skinned individuals the melanin content is much less in the upper layers of SC due to increased breakdown of the melanosomes. In summary, in black skin melanocytes are more active in making melanin, and melanosomes are packed, distributed, and broken down differently than in white skin.

Keratinocytes also play a role in regulating the distribution pattern of recipient melanosomes. Melanosomes inside the keratinocytes of black skin are larger and distributed individually, whereas those within the keratinocytes of Caucasian skin are smaller and distributed in clusters.[19] *In vitro* coculture studies using keratinocytes and melanocytes of black and white individuals indicate that irrespective of the melanocytes, the recipient keratinocytes determine the melanosomal behavior. Melanosomes are distributed individually by keratinocytes in dark skin, whereas they are distributed in membrane-bound clusters by keratinocytes in white individuals.[19] These results suggest that regulatory factors within the keratinocytes determine recipient melanosome distribution patterns.

Although the actual number of melanocytes may vary in different individuals from one anatomic site to another, there has been no evidence of major differences in the number of melanocytes between races.[20] Although gene expression of tyrosinase is similar between black and white subjects, other genes related to melanin synthesis show some differences. Human genes involved in melanin synthesis, such as MSH cell surface receptor gene and gene for melanosomal p-protein, may show differences between races or skins of different color.[21] These genes may in turn regulate the levels and activities of melanogenic enzymes tyrosinase, TRP-1 and TRP-2. In addition to the activity of the tyrosinase enzyme, other differences exist between races. The variations in the number, size, and aggregation of melanosomes within the melanocyte and keratinocyte result in the racial and ethnic differences in skin color that are seen.[20,22] Melanosomes occur in groups or aggregates, and it has been demonstrated that the different groupings have a correlation to the lightness or darkness of an individual's skin. Blacks with dark skin have large, nonaggregated melanosomes, whereas light-skinned blacks have a combination of large nonaggregated and smaller aggregated melanosomes.[23] There is also a correlation between melanosome groupings and sun exposure. Dark-skinned white subjects, when exposed to sunlight, have nonaggregated melanosomes, and those with light skin without sun exposure have aggregated melanosomes. Similarly in Asian skin, on the non-sun-exposed areas of the body, there are mainly aggregated melanosomes, and the sun-exposed areas have predominantly nonaggregated melanosomes.[20,24,25] Individuals with skin type VI, when compared to those with types I and II, have a higher total melanin content of the skin.[20,26] Differences in the epidermal distribution of melanosomes between races have also been documented. In white-skinned individuals, melanosomes are more numerous in the SC, whereas in dark-skinned individuals (blacks) melanosomes are more numerous in the basal layer. This correlates with the differences in photoprotection offered by Caucasian vs. black skin. In Caucasian skin, the main site of UV filtration is reported to be the SC, whereas in blacks it is the Malpighian layers (basal and spinous layers).[27] The distribution of melanosomes and skin tone appears to be correlated.[28] This is supported by the finding that dark Caucasian skin resembles the melanosome distribution observed in black skin.[24]

RACIAL DIFFERENCES IN DERMAL STRUCTURE

Biology of Dermis

The dermis is a dense fibroelastic connective tissue, composed of collagen fibers, elastic fibers, and an interfibrillar gel of glycosaminoglycans, salt, and water. The structural elements of the dermis are synthesized by the fibroblasts, the major cell type of the dermis. Collagen, constituting 77% of the fat-free dry weight of skin, accounts for the tensile strength of the dermal fabric. Type I is the major collagen subtype, followed by type III and types V and VI. The ratio of type I to III changes with age. Interwoven between the collagen bundles is the elastic fiber network, comprising other fibrillar proteins such as fibrilin. The outermost dermis is called the papillary dermis, where the dermal connective tissue is molded against the overlying epidermis. The bulk of the dermis below the papillary dermis is called the reticular dermis. This is relatively avascular, dense, collagenous, elastic tissue and other matrix components that hold water in the dermis (glycosaminoglycans).

Racial Differences

In general, because of the high melanin content of black skin, the amount of photodamage observed in older Caucasian skin is usually less apparent in black skin. However, despite the common perception that black skin shows less chronological aging than white skin, a detailed study suggests that black skin shows similar chronological changes as white skin with age.[29] Similar to white skin, the dermo-epidermal junction becomes flattened with multiple zones of basal lamina and anchoring fibril reduplication; microfibrils in papillary dermis become disoriented, and elastic fibers show

TABLE 1.2
Comparison of Dermal Structure between Black and White Skin

	White	Black
Dermis	Thinner and less compact	Thick and compact
Papillary and reticular layer	More distinct	Less distinct
Collagen fiber bundles	Bigger	Smaller. Close stacking and surrounded by ground substance
Fiber fragments	Sparse	Prominent and numerous
Melanophages (macrophages that phagocytize). Melanosomes that spill into the dermis)	Many	Numerous and larger
Lymphatic vessels	Moderate, dilated	Many dilated, empty lymph channels, usually surrounded by masses of elastic fibers
Fibroblasts	Not as numerous. Some binucleated cells	Numerous and large. Many binucleated and multinucleated cells
Elastic fibers	More. In photodamage, only fibers in papillary and reticular dermis stain pink; the others stain lilac or deep blue	Less. All dermal elastic fibers stain pink, just like in sun-protected skin. Elastosis is uncommon
Superficial blood vessels	Sparse to moderate	More numerous, mostly dilated
Glycoprotein molecules	Variable	Numerous in the dermis

cystic changes. Despite a decrease in the number of melanocytes with age (similar to white skin), the melanin granule density in aged black skin remained dense. Some subtle differences have been reported in the literature between the dermal structures of black and white skin. Black dermis is generally thick and compact when compared to white dermis, which is thinner and less compact.[30] The papillary and reticular layers are more distinct in white skin. They also contain larger collagen fiber bundles and the fiber fragments are sparse. Smaller collagen fiber bundles are present in blacks, with close stacking and a surrounding ground substance. Fiber fragments are more prominent and numerous in black skin. Both black and white skin have numerous melanophages; however, they are larger in blacks. Fibroblasts and lymphatic vessels are more numerous in black skin; they are dilated, empty lymph channels usually surrounded by masses of elastic fibers.[30] This same group has also reported differences in fibroblast size and structure between black and fair-skinned people. Fibroblasts are more numerous, are larger, have more biosynthetic organelles, and are more multinucleated in black skin than white skin.[14] In photodamaged white skin, only elastic fibers in the papillary and reticular dermis stain pink, whereas the others stain lilac or deep blue. In blacks, on the other hand, all the dermal elastic fibers stain pink, similar to that seen in sun-protected skin.[30] No racial differences in the epidermal nerve fiber network has been observed using laser-scanning confocal microscopy,[31] suggesting that there is no difference between races in terms of sensory perception, as suggested by the capsaicin response to C-fiber activation.

Biomechanical properties related to elasticity of the skin, such as skin extensibility, skin elastic recovery, and skin elastic modulus showed more marked variability between races. Differences were observed between the races in dorsal (sun-exposed) and volar (non-sun-exposed) sites on the forearm. Skin extensibility differed significantly between both sites in whites and Hispanics but not in blacks. On the dorsal forearm blacks had greater skin extensibility than whites but were similar to Hispanics.[5] The results were similar for elastic recovery. The exposed and unexposed sites were the same in blacks but different in whites and Hispanics. Elastic recovery was slightly higher in black than Hispanic and white skin.[5] All groups had the same skin elastic modulus on the volar forearm, but on the dorsal forearm, it was lowest in blacks and greater in Hispanics than whites.[5] These results may be due to the different degrees of solar exposure between the volar and dorsal sides of the forearm.

CUTANEOUS APPENDAGES (TABLE 1.3)

Sebaceous Glands and Sweat Glands

The cutaneous appendages include the pilosebaceous unit, which comprises the hair and sebaceous glands, the nails, eccrine sweat glands, and apocrine sweat glands (sweat glands are also referred to as sudoriferous glands). Some early studies suggest that there may be racial differences in the cutaneous appendages.[32] The ratio of sebaceous gland to sweat glands is believed to be higher in blacks and the sweat glands in darker skin are believed to be larger, providing better tolerance to hot climates.[32] The apocrine sweat glands found in axilla, pubic, and perianal areas are greater in number, and darker skin has more sebaceous glands and higher sebum secretion. However, carefully controlled clinical studies suggest no significant differences between black and white skin with regard to the amount of sweat and sebaceous glands.[3] It has been suggested that black subjects withstand humid heat better, whereas whites cope better with dry heat.[3] Other indirect evidence indicates similarities between black and white skin with regard to sebum and sweat secretion. If there is a racial difference in the sebum levels, then one can assume a racial difference in the control of bacterial, viral, and other infections (because sebum and sweat contribute to the "acid-protective mantle" of the skin). Both blacks and whites have a similar rate of cutaneous infection,[33] suggesting that there may not be a racial difference in sebum and sweat secretion between these two racial groups.

In a study of black and white female subjects, the appendages such as sweat glands and hair follicles in blacks were found to be generally similar to those of white subjects but contained more pigment. In black skin, the bulbs of vellus hair follicles are frequently pigmented, whereas in white skin they do not contain any melanin.[14]

The variation in eccrine sweat gland quantity, structure, and function between different racial or ethnic groups is controversial. No significant differences have been found.[20] Apocrine glands in different groups show interindividual variation, but one study has shown that these glands are found more frequently in female black facial skin than in female white facial skin. Apocrine glands are also found on all levels of the dermis in black skin.[14] Some studies have suggested racial differences in sebaceous glands size and activity;[32] however, no significant difference has been shown in sebum production between black and white skin. In another study of black and white subjects, blacks were found to have much larger sebaceous glands than whites.[34] A comparison of 649 male and female subjects of different races found no consistent differences in sebaceous gland activity between black and white skin. These findings are consistent with the clinical impression and epidemiological data that the incidence of acne is similar between blacks and whites.[35]

TABLE 1.3
Differences in Skin Appendages among Different Groups

	White	Asian	Black
Sweat glands	Few apocrine–eccrine mixed glands		More epocrine–eccrine glands
Hair follicles	Anchored by more elastic fibers, ovoid	Round	Flat and elliptical
Hair appearance	Wavy	Straight	Spiral
Hair diameter	Intermediate	Largest	Smallest

Racial Differences in Hair Follicles and Hair Structure

Hairs are keratinous fibers growing from epithelial follicles distributed universally over the skin surface, except for palms and soles. There are two types of hair: terminal hair, which populates the scalp and constitutes 95% of the trunk hair in males but only 35% of the body hair of females, and a fine body hair called vellus hair, rarely achieving lengths greater than 1 cm and often shorter and softer than terminal hair. The hair fiber is produced by the mitotic activity of the hair follicle, which is one of the most proliferative cell types in the human body. Hair growth follows a recurring pattern of active growth (anagen), regression (catagen), or rest (telogen). These cycles are not synchronized, each follicle maintaining an independent rhythm of growth and rest. Structurally, hair consists of an outer cortex and a central medulla. Enclosing the hair shaft is a layer of overlapping keratinized scales, the hair cuticle, that serves as protective layers. The hair follicle is a unique composite organ, composed of epithelial and dermal compartments interacting with each other in a surprisingly autonomous way. This is a self-renewing organ that seems to be a true paradigm of epithelial and mesenchymal interactions. Each of the follicular compartments is endowed with a specific differentiation pathway under the control of an intricate network of growth factors, cytokines, and hormones.

Racial Differences

Hair can be classified into four types, based on the physical characteristics. Of the four hair types, the majority of blacks have spiral hair. The hair of blacks is naturally more brittle and more susceptible to breakage and spontaneous knotting than that of whites. The kinky or wooly structure of black hair, the weak intercellular cohesion between cortical cells, and the specific hair-grooming practices among black people account for these effects.[3] The difference in the shape of the hair shaft is intrinsically programmed from the bulb, indicating a genetic difference in hair follicle structure.[8] Some characteristics observed on cross-sectional evaluation of black hair include a longer major axis and flattened elliptical shape; they also have curved follicles. Asian hair type has the largest cross-sectional area, and that of Western Europeans has the smallest area.[36,37] In a comparative study of different racial and ethnic groups, there were no significant differences in the thickness of the cuticle, scale size and shape, and cortical cells of whites compared with those of blacks. Black hair has an elliptical shape, whereas Asians have round-shaped, straight hair, and Caucasian hair is intermediate. The length and degree of curliness is determined genetically. The curly nature of black hair is believed to result from the shape of the hair follicle.[38]

A relationship exists between the cross-sectional shape of the hair shaft and the form of the hair. By serial sectioning of hair follicles and computer-aided reconstruction from people of different races, Lindelof et al.[39] concluded that the black hair follicle has a helical form, whereas the Asian follicle is completely straight. The Caucasian hair follicle represents variation between these extremes.[39] In studies of the hair follicles, blacks were found to have fewer elastic fibers anchoring the hair follicles to the dermis when compared to white subjects. Melanosomes were found to be in both the outer root sheath and in the bulb of vellus hairs in blacks but not in whites. Black hair also has more pigment and on microscopy has larger melanin granules, in comparison to hair from light-skinned and Asian individuals. Members of all races share similar structural characteristics of hair, although several differences have been identified.[20] There is no difference in keratin types between hair from different races, and no difference has been found in the amino acid composition of hair from different races,[40] although one study found variation in the levels of some amino acids between black and white hair.[41] Black subjects had significantly greater levels of tyrosine, phenylalanine, and ammonia in the hair but were deficient in serine and threonine.[41]

In an unpublished study the morphologic features of African hair were examined using the transmission and scanning electron microscopic (SEM) techniques. The cuticle cells of African hair were compared with those of Caucasian hair.[42] Two different electronic density layers were shown. The denser exocuticle is derived from the aggregation of protein granules that first appear when the scale cells leave the bulb region. The endocuticle is derived from the zone that contains the nucleus and cellular organites. The cuticle of Caucasian hair is usually 6 to 8 layers thick and constant in the hair perimeter, covering the entire length of each fiber. Black hair, on the other hand, has variable thickness; the ends of the minor axis of fibers are 6 to 8 layers thick, and the thickness diminishes to 1 or 2 layers at the ends of the major axis. The loss of several layers of cuticle cells revealing the cortex is usually seen on SEM micrographs of this area. The weakened endocuticle is subject to numerous fractures.[42]

The investigation of the growth and morphology of black hair follicles has shown that in contrast to Caucasian type, the dermal implantation of African-American hair follicles is curved. Thibaut et al.[43] observed that the bulb itself was bent in the shape of a golf club and the outer root sheath was asymmetric along the follicle. They also found that the *in vitro* growth rate, at 0.25 mm/day, was slightly slower than that of Caucasian follicles, which was 0.30 mm/day.

Black hair has a tight-curl pattern, which makes it particularly susceptible to breakage when manipulated mechanically.[44] In order to obtain the widest variety of styles, people with excessively curly hair, as do blacks, often straighten the hair by either pressing or use of a chemical relaxer.[44] This is among the many cultural practices that may impact the disorders of the skin and hair that are experienced by people of different ethnic groups.

Racial Differences in Nails

The nail, a hard and durable epidermal appendage, is derived from special epidermal cells. Nail grows out from the nail plate that rests on the nail bed, produces a cornified layer without the keratohyalin granules, and contains no sebaceous or pilosebaceous glands. The cells that constitute nails are dead corneocytes without nuclei or organelles, but the bottom of the nail plate is rich in microvasculature. The keratins and structural proteins of hair, nails, and SC are similar but not identical.[45]

Racial differences in nail conditions have been described. Hyperpigmentation of nail plate has been reported in darker races.[46] Blacks are reported to have lower nail nitrogen content, suggesting an inherent difference in the nail composition between different races.[47] Pigmented longitudinal bands of the nail are a common condition associated with dark-skinned individuals. The cause of this is due to increased melanotic macule of the nail matrix, consisting of increased pigmentation of the epidermis with no apparent increase in the number of melanocytes.[48]

RACIAL DIFFERENCES IN DERMATOLOGICAL CONDITIONS

Many differences exist between races in skin conditions, reactions to agents, and skin disorders. Although this chapter does not try to cover these areas in detail, some differences are worth mentioning. Pigmentation disorders, reaction to light and heat, and inflammatory reactions to scarring are some common differences between white and pigmented skin. There have also been suggestions that skin sensitivity to chemicals, irritation response, and dermatitis disorders are different in pigmented skin compared with Caucasian skin.

Scarring and Keloid Scars

A keloid is an overgrowth of fibrous tissue on the skin following trauma (e.g., acne, vaccination, ear piercing, insect bite, or surgical incision). It can be due to the overproduction of collagen or the deficiency of metalloproteases. The tissue response is abnormal to the normal process of wound healing or repair. The result is a raised, firm, thickened red/brown scar that may grow for a prolonged period and develop claw-like projections. The increase in scar size is due to the abnormal amount of collagen in the tissue, causing it to be itchy or tender. Genetics and age play a role in keloid development. Although more prevalent in dark skins, East Indians and Polynesians represent large proportions of patients with keloids as compared to African Americans with the same condition.[49]

IRRITATION

Differences in the response to irritants in different ethnic groups have been reported in several studies. Although there is a clinical consensus that blacks are least reactive and Asians are most reactive compared with Caucasians, the data supporting this hypothesis are sketchy. A review comparing irritant contact dermatitis (ICD) of different ethnic groups concluded that race could be a factor, but not the major factor.[50] A difference between Asian and Caucasian subjects to irritation patch testing was reported.[51,52] Similar results were also reported for acute skin irritation. Japanese subjects were more sensitive than Caucasian subjects. Cutaneous reactions to 1% dichloroethylsulfide showed erythema in 58% of white subjects but in only 15% of black subjects.[53,54] Another study,[53] using o-chlorobenzylidene malonitrile to elicit patch test reactions, showed that blacks had decreased susceptibility to cutaneous irritants and required much longer exposure to develop an irritant reaction.[54] Blacks were found to be less susceptible to cutaneous irritants before the SC was removed by tape stripping.[2] Sensory irritation has also been reported after application of an irritant; it is described as a stinging sensation occurring in the nasolabial folds and on cheeks.[27,55] It was reported as occurring more often in light-complexioned persons who tanned poorly and burned easily. However, later studies showed that there was no skin-type association with "stinging."[56]

ALLERGIC CONTACT DERMATITIS

This condition may be affected by differences in genetic and environmental factors. A study comparing patch test results from black and white individuals found no statistical differences between the two races in 41 different allergens tested.[57] However, white patients revealed slightly higher rates of sensitization to formaldehyde, glutaraldehyde, and a number of formaldehyde-releasing preservatives. Black patients exhibited higher rates of sensitization to paraphenylenediamine, cobalt chloride, thiourease, and p-tert butyl phenol formaldehyde resin. They concluded that although there were no differences in the overall responses, there were some differences between white and black patients in their responses to specific allergens.[57] Another study comparing patch test results between white and black ethnic groups concluded that there were ethnic differences. These differences may be reflecting variations in the rate of allergen exposure (differences in the barrier properties, for example) or due to the variations in the N-acetylation capacities of human skin (inactivation of the allergens) among various ethnic groups.[58] Other reports on the incidence of allergic contact dermatitis have been conflicting. In several studies, the incidence was found to be less in blacks.[59] Darkly pigmented South African blacks were found to have a lower incidence of industrial contact dermatitis.[60] On the other hand, after testing many topical materials on both black and white subjects, there was no significant difference in the two races.[61] Fisher[62] reported approximately equal incidence of contact dermatitis, most commonly to p-phenylenediamine, nickel, and potassium bichromate in blacks and whites. The clinical presentation of acute contact dermatitis is usually different in blacks and whites; blacks tend to develop disorders of pigmentation and lichenification more commonly. Contact dermatitis with exudation, vesiculation, or bullae occurs more commonly in whites. Racial and sex-related differences in sensitization were identified using transdermal clonidine. When an occlusive patch was applied to the skin for one week, the results showed significant differences between both the races and sexes, with sensitization of white women 34%, white men 18%, black women 14%, and black men 8%.[63] Cultural practices may also play a role in the racial differences observed in chemical sensitivity. The higher incidence of contact dermatitis seen in blacks among users of hair dye may be explained by the higher levels of paraphenylenediamine contained in darker shades of hair dyes that are used by blacks.[20] Black persons may also have cross-sensitization to other chemically related substances that are more frequently used by blacks, thus causing a higher sensitivity to paraphenylenediamine.[20]

RACIAL DIFFERENCES IN SKIN IMMUNOLOGICAL RESPONSES

Irritant responses and contact dermatitis are multifactorial diseases whose onset and modulation depend on both endogenous and exogenous factors. Endogenous factors include age, race site, sex, and history of dermatitis. The exogenous factor includes the type of irritant, the type of cytokine or mediators released by the skin keratinocytes and other cell types to the irritant, and the barrier properties of the SC at the site of contact. Furthermore, differences in the mechanism of inflammation between acute and chronic irritants may also exist. These differences maybe further complicated by the differences in the hyperproliferation and hyperkeratosis following initial inflammation. All these variables make it difficult to predict differences in irritant or contact sensitivity between populations.[64]

A difference in the cutaneous cell–mediated immunity between fair-skinned and dark-skinned people has been described.[65] Fair-skinned people (skin type I/II who are sun sensitive and tan poorly) are more sensitive to UVR (typically 1 h noonday exposure to sun) in protection from erythema and suppression of contact hypersensitivity than skin type III/IV individuals. This 2–3-fold difference in sensitivity to sunburn may play a role in the greater incidence of skin cancer in fair-skinned individuals. Another study compared the immunological responses of white- and black-skinned people to UVB radiation.[66] Whole-body irradiation with a low dose of UVB on lymphocyte activation was studied. In white subjects, UVB increased the number of CD 19 (B cells) and CD 4/29 (inducer of helper T cells) that infiltrated the skin. In black subjects UVB caused a slight decrease in CD 3 (subset of T cells). Natural killer T-cell activity was increased in black subjects and was not affected in white subjects. This race-specific immune response to UVB appears to be mediated by skin and may partly explain the resistance of blacks to photodependent skin cancer.

An ultrastructural difference in the mast cell morphology has been reported.[67] Mast cells in black skin contain larger granules than those in white skin due to increased fusion of smaller granules. Black skin mast cell granules appear to contain a higher amount of cathepsin G reactivity than white skin. There are more granules in the cytoplasm of mast cells in white skin than black skin, but, although the mast cells of blacks contain more amorphous electron-dense cores, they do not fully meet the criteria for immaturity. The morphological criteria of immaturity include a high nuclear/cytoplasmic ratio, presence of few granules, small cell size, and one or more amorphous electron-dense cores.[67]

The presence of a larger percentage of parallel–linear striations and a smaller percentage of curved lamellae of black skin in comparison to white skin is evident, but the significance remains unclear. Mast cell granules contain histamine, proteoglycans, cytokines, and proteinases. The subgranular distribution of histamine and serine proteases has been characterized by recent immuno-electron microscopy studies using Immunogold labeling. These include tryptase, which is localized over the less electron-dense crystalline regions, and chymase and cathepsin G, which are in the more electron-armorphous granule region. There has been some evidence suggesting that mast cells participate in aberrant fibrosis in diseases such as keloid, scleroderma, hypertrophic scar, and chronic graft-vs.-host disease. The likely mast cell mediators in this process are fibroblast growth factor, histamine, and tryptase.[68–70] Tryptase-positive mast cells are distributed throughout the dermis and among the collagen bundles in keloids. A greater number of total mast cells under a given epidermal area is suggested by the much thicker dermis in a keloid; the density of tryptase-positive mast cells, however, was not significantly different from that in normal skin.[71] In general, the size and density, subgranular structures and localization differ between mast cells of white and black skin, as demonstrated qualitatively in the study by Sueki et al.[67]

These observations may have implications for explaining why blacks have a higher incidence of fibrosing skin diseases such as keloids or hypertrophic scars.

REFERENCES

1. Washington DC, Populations Projections Program, Population Division, US Census Bureau. Projections of the resident population by race, Hispanic origin, and nationality: Middle series 2050–2070.
2. Weigand DA, Haygood C, Gaylor JR. Cell layers and density of Negro and Caucasian stratum corneum. *J Invest Dermatol* 1974; 62: 563–567.
3. La Ruche G, Cesarini JP. Histology and physiology of black skin. *Ann Dermatol Venereol* 1992; 119: 567–574.
4. Beradesca E, Pirot F, Singh M, Maibach H. Differences in stratum corneum pH gradient when comparing white Caucasian and black African-American skin. *Br J Dermatol* 1998; 139: 855–857.
5. Berardesca E, De Rigal J, Leveque JL, Maibach HI. *In vivo* biophysical characterization of skin physiological differences in races. *Dermatologica* 1991; 182: 89–93.
6. Sugino K, Imokawa G, Maibach FF. Ethnic difference of stratum corneum lipid in relation to stratum corneum function (Abstract). *J Invest Dermatol* 1993; 100: 597.
7. Manuskiatti W, Schwindt DA, Maibach HI. Influence of age, anatomic site and race on skin roughness and scaliness. *Dermatology* 1998; 196: 401–407.
8. Courcuff P, Lotte C, Rougier A, Maibach HI. Racial differences in corneocytes — a comparison between black, white and Oriental skin. *Acta Dermatol Venereol* 1991; 71: 146–148.
9. Kompaore F, Marty JP, Dupont C. *In vivo* evaluation of the stratum corneum barrier function in blacks, caucasians and Asians with two noninvasive methods. *Skin Pharmacol* 1993; 63: 200–207.
10. Reed JT, Ghadially R, Elias PM. Skin type, but neither race nor gender, influence epidermal permeability barrier function. *Arch Dermatol* 1995; 131: 1134–1138.
11. Berardesca F, do Rigal I, Leveque X, Maibach HI. *In vivo* biophysical differences in races. *Dermatologica* 1991; 182: 89–93.
12. Berardesca E, Maibach H. Racial differences in skin pathophysiology. *J Am Acad Dermatol* 1996; 34: 667–671.
13. Rawlings AV. Trends in stratum corneum research and management of dry skin conditions. *Int J Cosmet Sci* 2003; 25: 63–95.
14. Montagna W, Carlisle K. The architecture of black and white facial skin. *J Am Acad Dermatol* 1991; 24: 929–937.
15. Fitzpatrick TB, Szabo G. The melanocyte: cytology and cytochemistry. *J Invest Dermatol* 1959; 32: 197–209.
16. Jimbow K, Fitzpatrick TB, Wick MM. Biochemistry and physiology of melanin pigmentation. In: Goldsmith LA (Ed) *Physiology, Biochemistry and Molecular Biology of the Skin*. Oxford University Press, New York, 1991; 893.
17. Jimbow K, Oikawa O, Sugiyama S, Takeuchi T. Comparison of eumelanogenesis and pheomelanogenesis in retinal and follicular melanocytes: role of vesiculo-globular bodies in melanosome differentiation. *J Invest Dermatol* 1979; 73: 278–284.
18. Sturm RA, Teasdale RD, Box NF. Human pigmentation genes: identification, structure and consequences of polymorphic variation. *Gene* 2001; 277(1–2): 49–62.
19. Minwalla L, Zhao Y, Le Poole IC, Wickett RR, Boissy RE. Keratinocytes play a role in regulating distribution patterns of recipient melanosomes *in vitro*. *J Invest Dermatol* 2001; 117: 341–347.
20. Taylor SC. Skin of color; biology, structure, function, and implications for dermatologic disease. *J Am Acad Dermatol* 2002; 46: S41–S62.
21. Sturm RA, Box NF, Ramsay M. Human pigmentation genetics: the difference is only skin deep. *Bioessays* 1998; 20: 712–721.
22. Starkoo RS, Pinkush. Quantitative and qualitative data on the pigment cell of adult human epidermis. *J Invest Dermatol* 1957; 28: 33.
23. Olson RL, Gaylor J, Everett MA. Skin color, melanin, and erythema. *Arch Dermatol* 1973; 108: 541–544.
24. Toda K, Fatnak MK, Parrish A, Fitzpatrick TB. Alteration of racial differences in melanosome distribution in human epidermis after exposure to ultraviolet light. *Nat New Biol* 1972; 236: 143–144.
25. Jimbow M, Jimbow K. Pigmentary disorders in Oriental skin. *Clin Dermatol* 1989; 7: 11–27.

26. Smit WPM, Kolb RM, Lentjes EGWM, Noz KC, Van der Meulaen H, Koarten HK, et al. Variations in melanin formation by cultured melanocytes from different skin types. *Arch Dermatol Res* 1998; 290: 342–349.
27. Kaidbey KH, Agin PP, Sayre RM, Kligman AM. Photoprotection by melanin — a comparison of black and Caucasian skin. *J Am Acad Dermatol* 1979; 1: 249–260.
28. Kotrajaras R, Kligman AM. The effect of topical tretinoin on photodamaged facial skin: the Thai experience. *Br J Dermatol* 1993; 129: 302–309.
29. Herzberg AJ. Dinehart SM. Chronological aging in black skin. *Am J Dermatopathol* 1989; 11: 319–328.
30. Montagna W, Giusseppe P, Kenney JA. The structure of black skin. In: Montagna W, Giusseppe P, Kenney JA (Eds) *Black Skin Structure and Function*. Academic Press, 1993; 37–49.
31. Reilly DM, Ferdinando D, Johnston C, Shaw C, Buchanan KD, Green MR. The epidermal nerve fiber network: characterization of nerve fibers in human skin by confocal microscopy and assessment of racial variations. *Br J Dermatol* 1997; 137: 163–170.
32. Nicolaides N, Rothman S. Studies on the chemical composition of human hair fat: the overall composition with regard to age, sex and race. *J Invest Dermatol* 1952; 21: 90.
33. McDonald CJ. Structure and function of the skin — are there differences between black and white skin. *Dermatol Clin* 1988; 6: 343–347.
34. Kligman AM, Shelley WB. An investigation of the biology of the sebaceous gland. *J Invest Dermatol* 1958; 30: 99–125,
35. Pochi PE, Strauss JS. Sebaceous gland activity in black skin. *Dermatol Clin* 1988; 6: 349–351.
36. Bernard BA. Hair shape of curly hair. *J Am Acad Dermatol* 2003; 48(6 Suppl): S120–S126.
37. Vernall DO. Study of the size and shape of hair from four races of men. *Am J Phys Anthropol* 1961; 19: 345.
38. Brooks O, Lewis A. Treatment regimens for "styled" black hair. *Cosmetics Toiletries* 1983; 98: 59–68.
39. Lindelof B, Froslind B, Hedblad MA, Kaveus U. Human hair form: morphology revealed by light and scanning electron microscopy and computer aided three dimensional reconstruction. *Arch Dermatol* 1988; 124: 1359–1363.
40. Gold RJM, Schriver CH. The amino acid composition of hair from different racial origins. *Clin Chim Acta* 1971; 33: 465–466.
41. Menkart J, Wolfram L, Mao I. Caucasian hair, Negro hair and wool: similarities and differences. *J Soc Cosmet Chem* 1966; 17: 769–787.
42. Hadjur C, Fiat, Huart M, Tang D, Leroy F. Morphology of the cuticle of African hair. Unpublished data.
43. Thaibut S, Gaillard O, Nsangou E, Bernard E. The form of African American hair is programmed from the hair bulb: a functional and immunohistological study. Unpublished data.
44. Syed AN. Ethnic hair care: history, trends and formulation. *Cosmetics Toiletries* 1993; 108: 99–107.
45. Baden HP, Kvedar JC. The nail. In: Goldsmith LA (Ed) *Physiology, Biochemistry and Molecular Biology of the Skin*. Oxford University Press, New York, 1991; 697.
46. Henderson AL. Skin variations in blacks. *Cutis* 1983; 32: 376–377.
47. Hein K, Cohen MI, McNamara H. Racial differences in nitrogen content of nails among adolescents. *Am J Clin Nutr* 1977; 30: 496–498.
48. Molina D, Sanchez JL. Pigmented longitudinal bands of the nail. A clinicopathologic study. *Am J Dermatopathol* 1995; 17: 539–541.
49. Inalsingh CH. An experience in treating five hundred and one patients with keloids. *Johns Hopkins Med J* 1974; 134(5): 284–290.
50. Modjtahedi SP, Maibach HI. Ethnicity as a possible endogenous factor in irritant contact dermatitis: comparing the irritant response among Caucasians, blacks and Asians. *Contact Dermatitis* 2002; 47: 272–278.
51. Robinson MK. Population differences in acute skin irritation responses — race, sex, age, sensitive skin and repeat subject comparisons. *Contact Dermatitis* 2002; 46: 86–93.
52. Foy V, Weinkauf R, Whittle E, Basketter DA. Ethnic variation in the skin irritation response. *Contact Dermatitis* 2001; 45: 346–349.
53. Marshall EK, Lynch V, Smith HV. Variation in susceptibility of the skin to dichloroethylsulfide. *J Pharmacol Exp Ther* 1919; 12: 291–301.

54. Weigand DA, Mershon MM. The cutaneous irritant reaction to agent o-chlorbenzylidene malonitrile. (ca) (1) Quantitation and racial influence in human subjects. Edgewood Arsenal Technical Report 4332, February 1970.
55. Frosch RJ, Kligman AM. The chamber scarification test for assessing irritancy of topically applied substances. In: Drill VA, Lazar P (Eds) *Cutaneous Toxicity*. Academic Press, New York, 1977; 127–154.
56. Grove OL, Soschin DM, Kligman AM. Adverse subjective reactions to topical agents. In: Drill VA, Lazar P (Eds) *Cutaneous Toxicology*. Raven Press, New York, 1984.
57. Deleo VA, Taylor SC, Belsito DV, Fowler JF Jr, Fransway AF, Maibach HI, et al. The effect of race and ethnicity on patch test results. *J Am Acad Dermatol* 2002; 46: S107–S112.
58. Dickel H, Taylor JS, Evey P, Merk HF. Comparison of patch test results with a standard series among white and black racial groups. *Am J Contact Dermatol* 2001; 12: 77–82.
59. Kenney J. Dermatoses seen in American Negroes. *Int J Dermatol* 1970; 9: 110–113.
60. Mushall I, Heyl T. Skin diseases in the Western Cape Province. *S Afr Mod J* 1963; 37: 1308.
61. Epstein W, Kligman AM. The interference phenomenon on allergic contact dermatitis. *J Invest Dermatol* 1958; 31: 175.
62. Fisher AA. Contact dermatitis in black patients. *Cutis* 1977; 20: 905–922.
63. Berardesca E, Maibach H. Ethnic skin: overview of structure and function. *J Am Acad Dermatol* 2003; 48: S139–S142.
64. Berardesca E, Distante F. The modulation of skin irritation. *Contact Dermatitis* 1994; 31: 281–287.
65. Kelly DA, Young AR, McGregor JM, Seed PT, Potten CS, Walker SL. Sensitivity to sunburn is associated with susceptibility to UV radiation–induced suppression of cutaneous cell–mediated immunity. *J Exp Med* 2000; 191: 561 566.
66. Matsuoka LY, McConnachie P, Wortsman J, Holick MF. Immunological responses to UVB radiation in black individuals. *Life Sci* 1999; 64: 1563–1569.
67. Sueki H, Whitaker-Menezes D, Kligman AM. Structural diversity of mast cell granules in black and white skin. *Br J Dermatol* 2001; 144: 85–93.
68. Russel JD, Russell SB, Trupin KM. The effect of histamine on the growth of cultured fibroblasts isolated from normal and keloid tissue. *J Cell Physiol* 1977; 93(3): 389–393.
69. Reed JA, Albino AP, MacNutt NS. Human cutaneous mast cells express basic fibroblast growth factor. *Lab Invest* 1995; 72(2): 215–222.
70. Ruoss SJ, Hartman T, Caughey GH. Mast cell tryptase is a mitogen for cultured fibroblasts. *J Clin Invest* 1991; 88: 493–439.
71. Craig SS, Schecter NM, Schwartz LB. Ultrastructural analysis of maturing human T and TC mast cells *in situ*. *Lab Invest* 1989; 60: 147–157.

2 Common Dermatological Diseases in Pigmented Skins

Rebat M. Halder, Howard L. Brooks, and Juan Carlos Caballero

COMMON DERMATOLOGICAL DISEASES

ACNE VULGARIS AND RELATED DISORDERS

Although acne occurs in all races and ethnicities, there are differences in presentation between each group. A recent survey found that papules were the most frequent presentation of acne in African-Americans (70.7%) and Hispanics (74.5%), with Asians and other races having similar presentations.[1] The same survey also found that postinflammatory hyperpigmentation was a frequent complaint; in fact, it is often the chief complaint for acne in patients of darker races with acne.

Wilkins and Voorhees found that the nodulocystic variant of acne occurs less frequently in African-Americans than in Caucasians.[2] That study also found that nodulocystic acne occurred at a similar rate in Hispanics and Caucasians.

Some studies have shown that Caucasians have more inflammation with acne than blacks.[2] This was thought to occur because follicles of blacks were much less likely to rupture and thus less likely to cause an inflammatory reaction. Follicles of blacks were more likely to keratinize and form comedones. Also, the follicular epithelium of the pilosebaceous unit is thicker in blacks. This is likely why blacks do not present with the clinically apparent inflammatory and cystic acne that is seen in whites. It is important to note that although African-American patients do not seem to clinically have as much inflammatory acne as whites, if one of their acne lesions is biopsied, a histologically significant inflammatory process is seen.[3] An abundance of polymorphonuclear leukocytes was found in areas of acne that appeared to be clinically mild. This marked histological inflammation is usually not seen in other races. That study of 30 black female patients with a variety of clinical acne lesions showed marked inflammation histologically in all lesions including comedones. This "hidden" inflammation may account for the high prevalence of postinflammatory pigmented macules seen commonly with acne in darker-skinned races.

ACNE VULGARIS

Acne vulgaris is the most common dermatosis encountered in the general population as well as in ethnic groups.[4] It accounts for approximately 27% of the dermatoses seen in black individuals.[5] It is also the most common dermatologic disease in the Latino population[6] and the second most common dermatologic disease in the Asian population[7] (Figure 2.1). Clinically, the disease has predilection for the face and to a lesser degree the upper chest, back, and shoulders. A variety of lesions can be seen. The inflammatory lesions consist of papules, pustules, nodules, and cysts. The noninflammatory lesions are comedones, both open and closed (Figure 2.2).

African-American patients with acne vulgaris rarely present with the nodulocystic variant.[5] The course of the disease in this patient population is usually mild. Papules, hyperpigmented macules, pustules, and comedones (both open and closed) are the most common lesions seen in African-Americans; rarely, nodules and cysts are seen. When nodules and cysts are present, they often heal

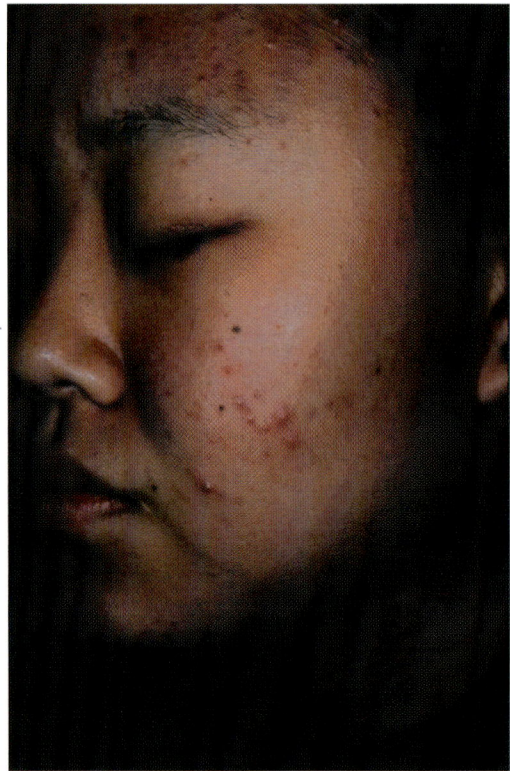

FIGURE 2.1 Asian female with inflammatory lesions of acne. (Reproduced from Halder, R.M., *Dermatol. Clin.,* 2003: 21:609–615. With permission from Elsevier.)

with hypertrophic scarring and keloids.[5] Although nodulocystic acne is seen infrequently in the African-American population, a study reports that cystic lesions occur in 10.5% of Asians, 18% of African-Americans, and 25.5% of Hispanics with acne[1] (Figure 2.3).

In all darker-skinned races, postinflammatory hyperpigmentation is commonly seen in patients with acne vulgaris and can be a prominent feature. Often, this is of greater concern to the patient than the acute acne lesions themselves[8] (Figure 2.4).

ACNE CONGLOBATA

This type of acne is rare in African-Americans and Africans. It consists of multiple comedones, cysts, nodules, and often sinus and abscess formation and suppuration. The lesions typically occur on the forehead, cheeks, and anterior neck but can be seen on the shoulders, back, and chest as well. Most lesions heal with severe scarring and keloid formation, especially if lesions occur in an African-American patient. This type of acne is most frequent in males. It has a later age of onset than acne vulgaris; it usually develops in the second or third decade. A report has shown, however, that cystic acne in association with filiform and keratotic lesions can be a presenting sign of HIV infection,[9] which may be important to remember when evaluating patients of skin of color.

Cystic acne is the mildest form of acne conglobata. This milder variant does not have sinus or abscess formation. It has the same distribution as the more severe forms. This type of acne conglobata tends to respond better to treatment than the more severe form.

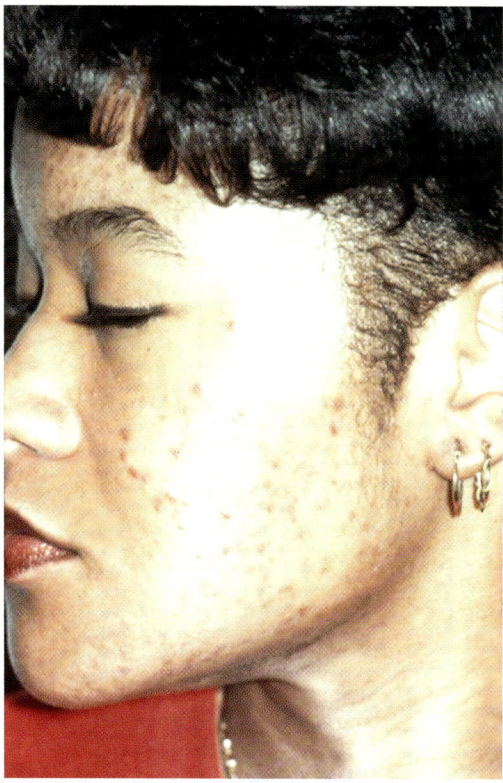

FIGURE 2.2 African-American female with a variety of inflammatory and noninflammatory lesions of acne. (Reproduced from Halder, R.M., *Dermatol. Clin.,* 2003: 21:609–615. With permission from Elsevier.)

FOLLICULAR OCCLUSION TRIAD

The disorders acne conglobata, hidradenitis suppurativa, and dissecting cellulitis can be seen in the same patient. This triad is more common in the African-American population. Hidradenitis suppurativa is a chronic inflammatory disease of the apocrine gland–bearing areas of the skin, mainly the axilla, buttocks, and groin, characterized by tender, erythematous nodules and abscesses that eventually become fluctuant and extremely painful. As the disease progresses, the abscesses increase in size and eventually discharge a malodorous material if untreated. Sinus tract and fistula formation often occur with secondary bacterial infection.

The most common site is in the axilla of women. When it occurs in males, the most common site is the groin. The lesions are thought to occur because of follicular keratinization and blockage of the apocrine duct and resulting inflammation of the apocrine gland. There has been an association with nonmelanoma skin malignancies in patients with hidradenitis suppurativa.[10]

Dissecting cellulitis, also known as perifolliculitis capitis abscedens et suffodiens, is a disease of the scalp that occurs most frequently on the vertex of African-American men.[1] Inflammatory follicular and perifollicular nodules that coalesce to form sinus tracts characterize this disease. The initial lesions resemble folliculitis; abscess and sinus tract formation then begin, resulting in a scarring alopecia. The histologic picture is similar to acne conglobata and hidradenitis suppurativa. There is follicular occlusion, resulting in follicular and perifollicular inflammation.

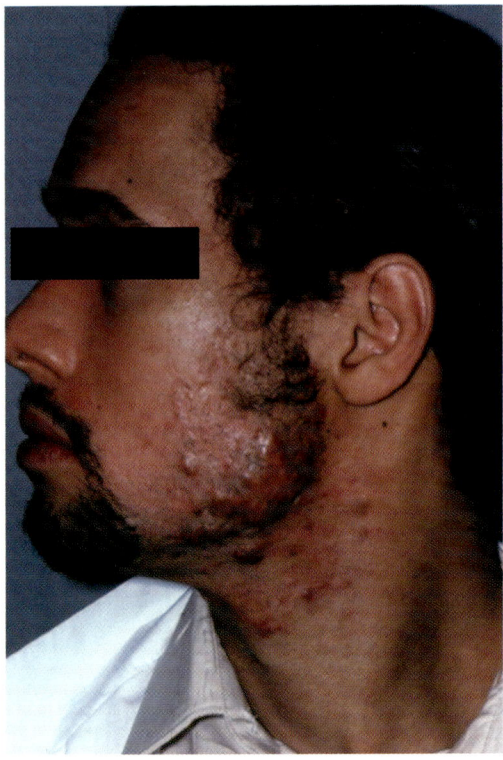

FIGURE 2.3 African-American male with nodulocystic acne and resultant keloid formation. (Reproduced from Halder, R.M., *Dermatol. Clin.*, 2003: 21:609–615. With permission from Elsevier.)

POMADE ACNE

This is a type of acne that occurs primarily in African-Americans. The lesions most commonly associated with this type are multiple closed comedones along the patient's hairline and temples. It results from pomades and other comedogenic oils and waxes used as hair lubricants. These products induce the follicular response seen in acne and thus lead to the formation of the comedone. Because of the use of other grooming techniques, pomade acne is not seen as frequently in African-Americans as in the past.

Although usually seen in African-Americans, Latinos also can be affected with pomade acne. In the Latino population, pomade acne usually affects males who use oils and other lubricating products on their scalp and facial hair.[12]

ROSACEA

Rosacea, an inflammatory disease that is seen relatively frequently in Caucasians, is less frequent in other ethnic groups. Some reports state that approximately 4% of rosacea patients are of African, Latino, or Asian descent.[13] The disease is characterized by flushing, erythematous papules and pustules, telangectasias, and often rhinophyma (Figures 2.5 and 2.6). The typical sites of predilection are the chin, nose, and cheeks and glabella. It can also be seen on the ears and the anterior upper chest. The lesions appear in the same distribution in persons with darker skin types; however, because of the pigment, they may not appear as erythematous (Figures 2.5 and 2.6). The trigger factors for rosacea include cold weather, wind, spicy foods, hot and alcoholic beverages, and caffeine.

The eye may also be involved. Ocular involvement may vary from symptoms of burning, grittiness, and redness to findings of blepharitis, corneal thinning, ulceration, and perforation.[3]

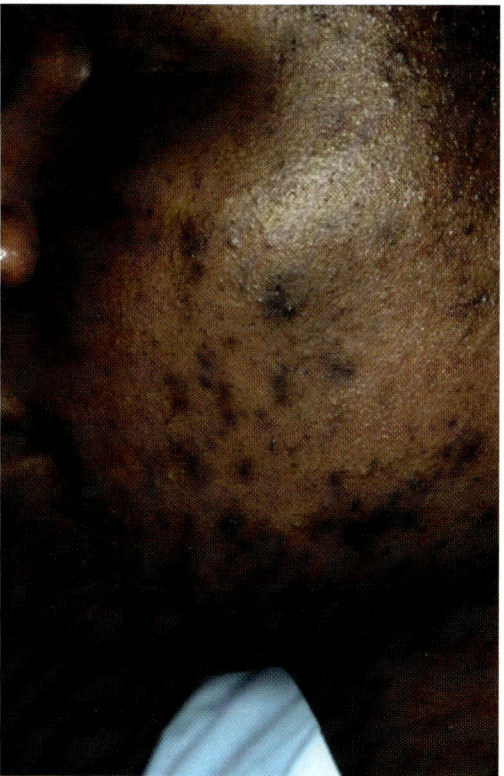

FIGURE 2.4 Lesions of postinflammatory hyperpigmentation from acne in a darkly pigmented person. (Reproduced from Halder, R.M., *Dermatol. Clin.*, 2003: 21:609–615. With permission from Elsevier.)

Because of the latter complications, it is important to consider ocular rosacea in the differential diagnosis of these problems. Moreover, because rosacea is relatively rare in darker-skinned individuals and because the cutaneous lesions appear differently or may be obscured by the darker pigment,[14] it is important to examine the skin in darker-pigmented patients presenting with the above ocular findings.

Granulomatous rosacea is another variant of this disease. This type of rosacea is more prevalent in African-Americans and Afro-Caribbeans. It usually presents as yellowish brown nodules and papules in the malar, perioral, and periocular regions. Histologically, there are perifollicular inflammation and noncaseating granulomas. Because of the presentation and histologic findings, sarcoidosis and lupus miliaris disseminatus faciei are in the differential diagnosis. FACE syndrome (facial Afro-Caribbean childhood eruption) is now considered a variant of granulomatous rosacea. It presents as grouped papules in the perinasal and perioral location with a histologic picture similar to granulomatous rosacea. African-American and Afro-Caribbean children are usually affected.[15]

TREATMENT OF ACNE

An important goal of treatment for acne patients with darker skin is the prevention of postinflammatory hyperpigmentation; this is achieved by starting treatment early in the course of the disease. When selecting topical acne treatment agents, one should consider the patient's propensity for developing irritation and whether the skin is oily or dry.[16] Irritation from topical acne agents such as retinoids and benzoyl peroxide is also a concern in treating pigmented skin, because the irritation itself can lead to hyperpigmentation.

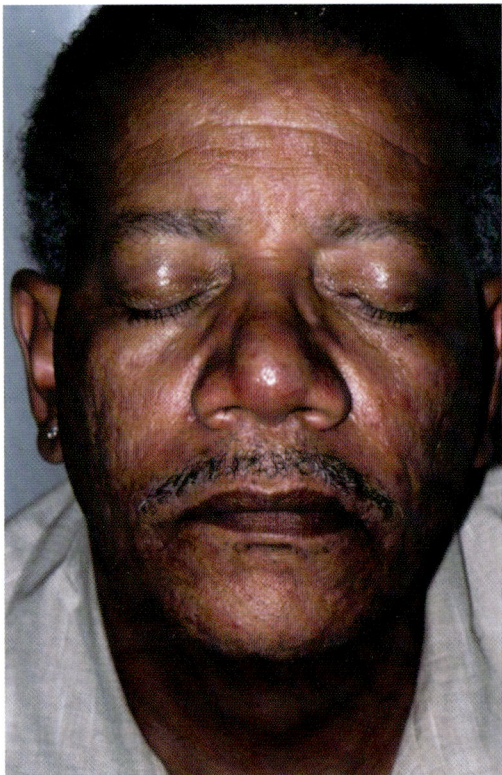

FIGURE 2.5 Rosacea in a fair-skinned African-American male. (Reproduced from Halder, R.M., *Dermatol. Clin.*, 2003: 21:609–615. With permission from Elsevier.)

Monotherapy is often ineffective for most cases of acne. Combination therapy is usually indicated; however, two agents that dry the skin should not be used in patients with darker skin types. Topical retinoids or benzoyl peroxide agents can be used in combination with systemic or topical antibiotics.

Benzoyl Peroxide

Although studies have not been conducted, it appears that darker skin may be more susceptible to the irritating effects of benzoyl peroxide. Not only does benzoyl peroxide irritate but it also has a drying effect which, however, can be beneficial to the patient who complains of oily skin. It has been shown that a 2.5% concentration of benzoyl peroxide is as effective in lowering the inflammatory lesion count as 5% and 10% concentrations, while producing less erythema and desquamation.[17] Therefore, lower concentrations of benzoyl peroxides should be used initially in treating acne in patients with skin of color to decrease potential irritation and resultant postinflammatory hyperpigmentation. Not only is the concentration an important factor when using benzoyl peroxide, but the vehicle in which it is delivered can also affect the drying and irritating effects. As with other topical agents, benzoyl peroxides are available in a variety of formulations (creams, cream-based washes, lotions, water-based and alcohol-based gels). The alcohol-based gels seem to be the most irritating to acne patients with darker complexions, so the cream or water-based gels should be used initially.

Antibiotics

For milder cases of acne, benzoyl peroxide can be used in combination with a topical antibiotic. Clindamycin and erythromycin are the two most commonly used topical antibiotics for acne, both

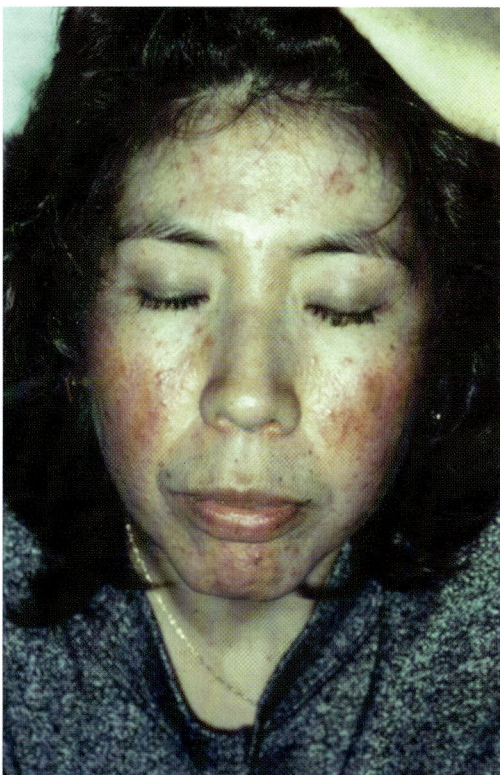

FIGURE 2.6 Rosacea in a Hispanic female with flushing and telangiectasiae.

of which are effective in reducing the amount of *Propionibacterium acnes* from the follicles. They both also have anti-inflammatory effects, which can help reduce development of scarring and hyperpigmentation in skin of color. A major concern is developing resistance with long-term use of topical antibiotics. This resistance can be reduced by using these topical agents in combination with benzoyl peroxides.[18]

Often oral antibiotics are indicated for more moderate cases of acne. They are also effective in reducing *P. acnes* in the follicles and have anti-inflammatory effects, which is important in treating skin of color in preventing postinflammatory hyperpigmentation. The most commonly used oral antibiotics for acne are tetracycline, doxycycline, and minocycline. Caution must be taken when using minocycline. It has been associated with a lupus-like syndrome,[10] which can occur at an increased rate in young, otherwise healthy, acne patients. It has not been observed whether members of any specific ethnic group may be more likely to develop this syndrome. A bluish-gray pigmentation of the skin can develop from the use of minocycline, particularly in scars and lower legs, but can be generalized as well.[20] This minocycline-induced pigmentation is darker in skin of color.

RETINOIDS

For mild to moderate cases of acne in skin of color, a topical retinoid may be indicated. Retinoids provide several benefits in treating acne; they decrease comedones, papules, and pustules as well as combat postinflammatory hyperpigmentation. Besides normalizing follicular keratinization, it has been shown that retinoids and retinoid analogues also have an anti-inflammatory effect.[21] In an 8-week, double-blind, vehicle-controlled study, Halder showed that there was a decrease in the number of papules and pustules and in hyperpigmented macules in 83% of 12 African-American patients treated with tretinoin 0.025% cream.[5] Another study showed that adapalene gel 0.1% and

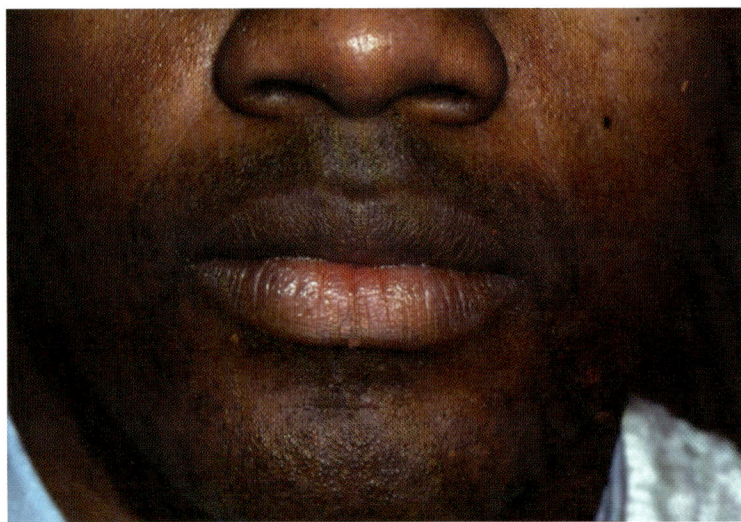

FIGURE 2.7 Hyperpigmentation in an African-American male as a result of irritation from the use of topical retinoid for acne in an African-American male.

tretinoin gel 0.025% decreased the number of inflammatory and noninflammatory lesions in Chinese patients with acne.[22]

Retinoids cause melanin granule dispersion; therefore, less pigmentation is seen clinically. A study of African patients with acne treated with adapalene gel 0.1% reported that there was an improvement not only in the lesion count but also in the degree of postinflammatory hyperpigmentation seen.[23] Irritation associated with retinoids can be lessened with vehicle choice. A cream is preferred over gel in skin of color, because it is less dry. However, hyperpigmentation from topical retinoids can occur without the clinical signs of irritation being present in darker-skinned persons[24] (Figure 2.7). It could be that the erythema is not as easily seen in darker-skinned patients. A microsponge delivery of tretinoin is now available in 1% and 0.04% concentrations, which are less irritating to the skin; this is of particular significance when treating skin of color. Proper instructions must be given to patients with darker skin when prescribing topical retinoids. Patients should be told to apply the retinoid every other night for 2 weeks, then every night thereafter if tolerated. Taylor reports that African-Americans, Hispanics, and Asians tolerate adapalene well.[16] This third-generation retinoid is available in a cream vehicle, which is less irritating to the skin and therefore less likely to produce postinflammatory hyperpigmentation.

Isotretinoin can be used to treat nodulocystic acne in African-American patients.[25] Two conditions, dissecting cellulitis of the scalp and hidradenitis suppurativa, are related to nodulocystic acne but have a different pathogeneses. Some reports state that they also respond to isotretinoin.[26,27]

ORAL CONTRACEPTIVES

Oral contraceptives, sometimes used in the treatment of acne in women, can cause melasma. The resulting pigmentation may be more of a concern to the patient than the acne itself in women of color.

HYDROQUINONE

The major complaint of patients of darker races with acne is often the hyperpigmented macules. The presence of these lesions can have a psychological impact on the patient's self-esteem; therefore, it is essential to treat the hyperpigmentation. Hydroquinone-based agents are the mainstay for treating these lesions. Hydroquinone actively blocks melanocyte pigment production. It accomplishes this through oxidation of melanin and tyrosinase into oxygen radicals that prevent melanin production. When using a hydroquinone, a halo can form when the hydroquinone is in contact with the adjacent normal skin,[16] but this usually fades after the medication is discontinued.

Azelaic Acid

Azelaic acid is a naturally occurring dicarboxylic acid. Topical application of 20% cream has been shown to be effective in treating comedonal, inflammatory, and hyperpigmented macules of acne.[28] Hyperpigmentation is improved by azelaic acid's ability to reversibly inhibit tyrosinase. Theoretically, azelaic acid specifically targets hyperactive melanocytes and, therefore, should not lighten the normal skin.

Chemical Peels and Microdermabrasion

Other options for treating the postinflammatory changes of acne in ethnic skin are chemical peels and microdermabrasion. Grimes[29] studied the efficacy and safety of salicylic acid peels on patients with Fitzpatrick's skin types V and VI. In that study, patients were pretreated for 2 weeks with hydroquinone 4% and then treated with salicylic acid 20% or 30% at 2-week intervals. A moderate to significant improvement was noted in 83% of the 25 patients. Nine of these patients had acne vulgaris and five had postinflammatory hyperpigmentation.

Microdermabrasion utilizes aluminum oxide crystals for superficial peeling and resultant improvement in hyperpigmented macules of acne. However, postinflammatory hyperpigmentation is itself a major concern when treating darker skin types with microdermabrasion.[24]

DERMATITIS IN PIGMENTED SKIN: PREVALENCE AND CLINICAL MANIFESTATIONS OF ATOPIC AND CONTACT DERMATITIS

Dermatitis is one of the most common skin disorders found in pigmented skin.[30] Given the changes in the demographics of the population and the incidence of these skin conditions in these populations, it is necessary to establish clinical guidelines to accurately identify and treat this common condition. Current literature identifies different clinical manifestations, morphology, and time response of irritation and severity of inflammatory reaction in these populations, as compared to Caucasian skin. Also, it is important to clarify that some of these populations may be at higher risk of experiencing problems, due to certain cultural practices and environmental exposure, rendering individuals in certain ethnic communities more susceptible to dermatitis.

Atopic Dermatitis

The prevalence of atopic dermatitis (AD) in ethnic populations has been a topic of intense scrutiny during the last few years. Little was known about the prevalence of AD outside Northern Europe; as such, it was largely believed that it was a skin condition predominantly affecting Caucasians, especially those of Scandinavian origin. The ISAAC study (International Study of Asthma and Allergies in Childhood) phase I was designed to investigate the magnitude and geographic distribution of atopic eczema, asthma, and hay fever in many countries of the world by making use of a standardized questionnaire. This study revealed that the highest prevalence values for AD symptoms (above 15%) were found in urban Africa, the Baltics, Australasia, and Northern and Western Europe. Lowest prevalence values (under 5%) were present in China, Eastern Europe, and Central Asia. Very high values were observed in developed countries, such as Scandinavia, the United Kingdom, Japan, Australia, and New Zealand. Latin America and the Asia Pacific yielded intermediate values of prevalence.[31] Other studies have demonstrated that AD and other eczemas are common in non-Caucasians. Dunwell and Rose[32] demonstrated that the prevalence of AD and other eczemas in Afro-Caribbean populations corresponds to the rates normally seen in other countries of the western world. Halder and Nootheti[30] demonstrated that the most frequent dermatoses among blacks in Washington, D.C. were acne vulgaris and dermatitis. Similar patterns were noted in a southeast London black patient population studied by Child et al.[33] and Williams et al.,[34] who reported a two-fold difference in the prevalence of AD between black Caribbean children and white children born in London, England. Although these population-based studies suggest that indeed there is an increase, prevalence of AD among black and/or Asian children, the possibility of overutilization of resources, as well as differing referral patterns, has been questioned by others. Neame et al. suggests that the higher prevalence of AD seen in Asians as compared to non-Asians in a study by Sladden et al. is artifactual and could be explained by either difference in methodology or differing referral patterns.[35] In a study conducted to assess whether health care utilization for AD differs among different ethnic groups in the United States, Janumpally et al.[36] concluded that blacks and Asian/Pacific Islanders were more likely to make office visits for AD than whites. Blacks are three times more likely and Asian/Pacific Islanders are almost seven times more likely to report AD than whites.[36] We must bear in mind that differences in health care utilization do not necessarily represent higher prevalence rates. In general, although there is lower health care utilization among blacks and other ethnic groups, this striking observation in terms of increased consultation rates for AD may be due in part to postinflammatory pigmentary changes in these groups. These studies, however, have implications for differences in incidence, prevalence, and/or severity of AD among different ethnic groups. On the other hand, a relatively large epidemiological survey conducted in the San Francisco area interviewed women from four different ethnic groups (African-Americans, Asians, Euro-Americans, and Hispanics) and found that the only statistically significant difference among these races was the actual incidence of current eczema in these populations. The researchers found that eczema was less frequent in the Hispanic population (6%) than in the population as a whole (11%). Although not statistically significant, the survey also observed that the incidence for past and current eczema was higher in the African-American group.[37]

Although several studies have been conducted to determine the prevalence of skin disease in people of color, little is known about the relationships between dark skin and severity of disease. Many severity scales are available to assist the clinician in the diagnosis and assessment of severity of disease. The SCORAD (SCORe Atopic Dermatitis); Six Area, Six Sign AD (SASSAD) severity score; and Nottingham Eczema Severity Score (NESS) use erythema almost uniformly to determine extent of disease. In a study by Ben-Gashir et al.,[38] black children with AD were found to have more severe disease than their white counterparts and that this difference tended to be masked by reliance on erythema scores.[38] Erythema can be difficult to assess in black or pigmented skin and reliance on erythema alone may have underestimated severe disease in children of color. The authors suggest that perhaps lichenification and papule formation, which can be easily scored in pigmented skin as well as white skin, may be a more accurate measure to determine severity of disease in this population. In the study by Ben-Gashir et al., conducted in south London and mid-Wales, the authors noted that the difference in disease severity could not be easily explained by environmental factors such as urbanization and suggested that the difference in severity between black and white children who were born and lived in the same area could be perhaps attributed to genetic factors.

Atopic dermatitis is usually diagnosed on clinical grounds by its typical clinical presentation. Hanifin and Rajka[39] characterized major and minor criteria for the diagnosis of AD, and these guidelines have become accepted somewhat universally. Since then, several questions have been raised, mainly about the different clinical and morphological manifestations of AD in different racial or ethnic populations. Nevertheless, few clinicians dispute the signs and symptoms that seem to be accepted as universal in making the diagnosis of AD, namely, atopy, pruritus, eczema, and altered vascular reactivity. So how is it that AD manifests itself differently in blacks, Asians, or Hispanics?

Although dermatitis occurs in all races, there are differences in its presentation. A study reported that although there are guidelines for the diagnosis of AD, the diagnostic significance of the "minor features" of AD described by Hanifin and Rajka have not been clearly explored, especially when these minor features may be significantly dependent upon the ethnic and genetic background of a population.[40] It seems that although there may be little dispute about the major manifestations of AD, some minor features may actually represent specific ethnic-dependent markers. Lee et al.,[41] for instance, found that some characteristic minor features not previously described in the literature were present in Asian (South Korean) patients, namely, sandpaper-like skin lesions on elbow/knee/lateral malleolus, hangnail, ventral wrist dermatitis, itchy hyperkeratotic papules on dorsum of the hands, oily skin, fissured heel, and palmar erythema. Few data are available on the different clinical presentations of AD in non-Caucasian populations, and the relatively high incidence of ichthyosis and perifollicular accentuation in dark-skinned people exemplifies these variations. The prevalence of ichthyosis vulgaris in AD patients was about 30% in the Japanese and Chinese populations, in contrast to 2%–6% in the Caucasian population.[41] Another study established that the presence of a prominent infraorbital crease (Morgan–Denne line) was much more common in black children, regardless of AD status. In the study 24% of white children had a prominent crease, compared with 47% of black children.[40] Furthermore, the increased prevalence of infraorbital crease was consistent within each of the black ethnic subgroups (Afro-Caribbean, black African, and black other). Although the results of the study suggest that a prominent infraorbital crease may be a common finding in some ethnic groups regardless of AD status, it is possible nevertheless that with more objective methods of recording this sign, it could become one of the ethnic-specific markers discussed.

As mentioned earlier, the manifestations of AD in skin of color may present with distinctive lesions. Everyday observations from clinical dermatologists concur that African-American children, for instance, may present with fine papules occurring in the typical atopic areas such as posterior neck, antecubital fossae, and popliteal fossae. Occasionally, these children may also present with discrete, circumscribed areas of marked follicular accentuation. Postinflammatory pigmentation (pytiriasis alba) after AD and seborrheic dermatitis may cause significant concern to patients.[42] Pytiriasis alba consists of variable hypopigmented patches with predilection for the face, neck, and shoulders (Figure 2.8). It has been regarded as postinflammatory hypopigmentation following eczema. Most clinicians agree that AD is relatively common yet surprisingly difficult to diagnose given the numerous and varied presentations, especially because of its tendency for certain morphologic features to cluster in specific racial groups. In the views of one particular dermatologist, AD had at least six distinct morphologic presentations in African-American children: (1) perifollicular/follicular AD, (2) lichen planus-like AD, (3) localized or regionalized nummular or psoriasiform AD with virtually normally intervening skin, (4) pityriasis alba, (5) generalized xerotic AD with scalp involvement (Figure 2.9), and (6) classic flexural AD (Figure 2.10).[42] The perifollicular accentuation and folliculocentric dermatitis is perhaps the most racially specific variation of AD in African-American children (Figure 2.11). Some other children demonstrate a predominant papular eruption, with violaceous, flat-topped polygonal papules that clinically may resemble lichen planus; most also have other unequivocal signs and symptoms of AD, and biopsy usually confirms this diagnosis. Some other patients have a nummular-psoriasiform plaquelike form of AD with intervening normal skin. The lesions are often present in the extremities. Also, it is worth mentioning that many African-American children may suffer from striking hypopigmentation associated with the dermatitis. This may occur *de novo* or as a postinflammatory event after a bout of eczematous dermatitis. In any event this may cause tremendous anxiety for affected children and parents. Some Hispanic patients may also present with a predominant follicular pattern of AD, with irregular patches of follicular papules on the trunk and extremities in addition to other major or minor features of the disorder.

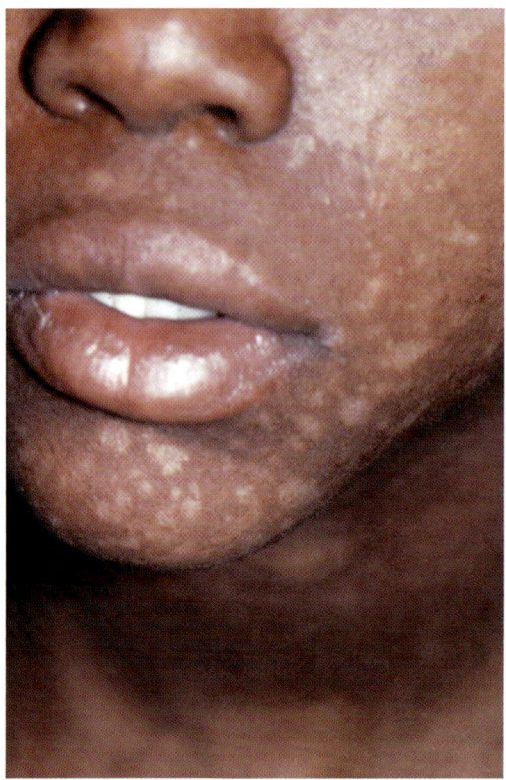

FIGURE 2.8 Pityriasis alba.

CONTACT DERMATITIS

Irritant contact dermatitis (ICD) is the most common form of dermatitis and is loosely defined as nonspecific damage to the skin after exposure to an irritant. This disorder can be further subdivided into several classes depending on the nature of the exposure and the resulting clinical presentation. Clinical manifestations are obviously influenced by a variety of factors such as concentration of chemicals, duration of exposure, temperature, humidity, and anatomic location, to name a few. Acute contact dermatitis presents with the classic symptoms of localized and superficial erythema, edema, and chemosis; it may occur as a result of a single exposure to an acute irritant. Cumulative contact dermatitis, on the other hand, presents with similar symptoms but occurs when exposure to a less potent irritant is repeated until symptoms develop over weeks or months.[43]

Several studies attempting to examine the differences in susceptibility between black and white skin to irritation point toward a reduced susceptibility to irritant contact dermatitis among participants with black skin and relate this to apparently stronger skin barrier properties in blacks.[44] Earlier studies by Marshal et al.[45] investigated cutaneous reactions to 1% dichloroethylsulfide in whites and blacks; a drop on the forearm elicited erythema in 58% of whites but in only 15% of blacks, again suggesting a decreased susceptibility to cutaneous irritants in blacks. Similar studies by Weigand and Gaylor[46] indicated again that blacks were more resistant and required a significantly longer exposure to develop an irritant reaction. This seemingly decreased susceptibility was believed to be due to structural differences of the stratum corneum of blacks. Studies suggested that the stratum corneum of blacks had increased intercellular cohesiveness, possibly creating a denser, more compact stratum corneum. Others demonstrated higher lipid content in the stratum corneum of people with black skin, again attributing this to be the reason for a better functional barrier. Weigand et al.[47] showed that if the stratum corneum of black and Caucasian subjects was removed,

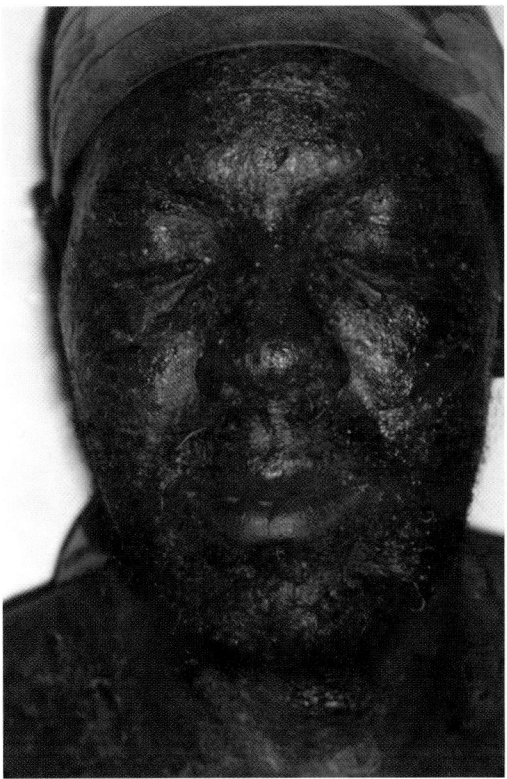

FIGURE 2.9 Xerotic atopic dermatitis.

there was no significant difference in irritation as measured by erythema between the two groups. Again, they concluded that there might be structural differences in the stratum corneum that provided more protection to black skin. As we know, however, it is difficult to conclude that black skin is less susceptible to cutaneous irritation based only on studies using visual scoring of erythema. Older studies, then, using erythema as the only indicator for irritation, may have been misleading. More recent studies using objective bioengineering techniques by Berardesca and Maibach[48] and Gean et al.[49] did not show statistically significant differences in the irritation response between these two groups. In fact, findings by Berardesca et al. contradict the hypothesis that blacks are less reactive than Caucasians. Adding to the controversy, the most recent study by Hicks et al.,[50] using reflectance confocal microscopy (RCM), transepidermal water loss (TEWL) measurement, and laser Doppler velocimetry (LDV), found that participants with white skin did tend to have more intense clinical reactions to irritants than did participants with black skin. By using RCM, which is a novel imaging tool that permits real-time qualitative and quantitative study of human skin, the researchers used a near-infrared laser beam, which enables a type of "virtual sectioning" of live tissue with high resolution, almost comparable with routine histology. The morphometric epidermal changes as measured by RCM and TEWL conclusively showed that, as evidenced by earlier studies, white skin showed a more severe clinical reaction and supported the concept that the stratum corneum of black skin provides better barrier function.

Similar studies were conducted by Robinson et al.[51] to substantiate a historical notion that Asians, specifically Japanese, were more sensitive to irritants than Caucasians. Robinson compared Caucasian and Japanese subject skin irritation responses and found that in both the acute and cumulative irritation tests, the Japanese subjects showed a tendency to respond faster than the Caucasian subjects. A repeat of this exact study protocol was then conducted among Caucasian, Japanese, and Chinese subjects. In this second study, however, Robinson did not find any differences

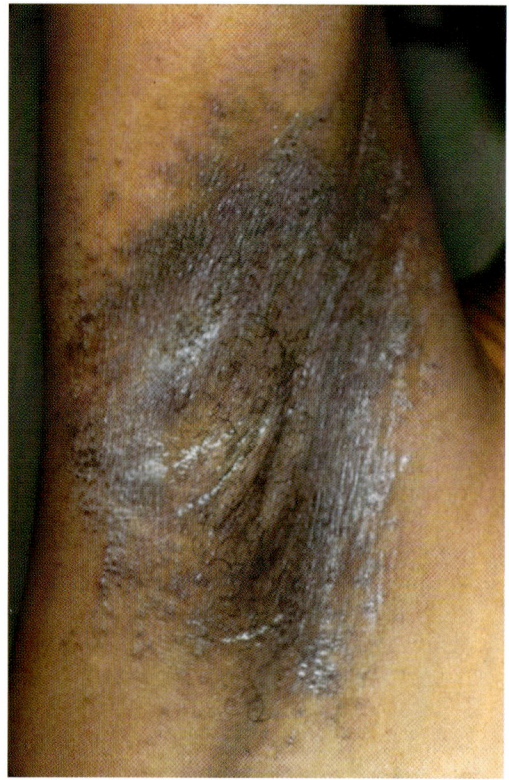

FIGURE 2.10 Eczema of flexural region.

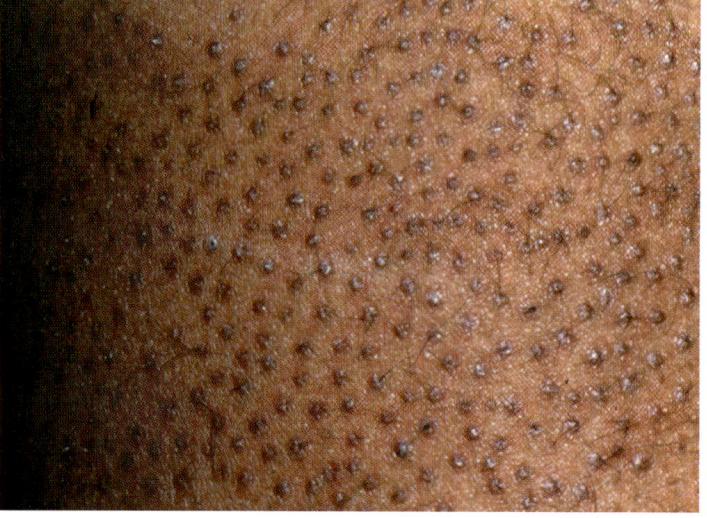

FIGURE 2.11 Follicular atopic dermatitis.

in irritation responses between the Japanese and Caucasian subjects. Another study by Foy et al.[52] compared new Japanese migrants to the United States and compared these to a matched group of Caucasians in an attempt to eliminate variables such as using groups whose ethnic origin is clear but who are no longer in their original ethnic environments, such as the case was with the earlier study by Robinson. The results indicated that the acute irritant response tended to be greater in the Japanese group. Whereas the acute irritant response to highly concentrated irritants was significantly different between the Japanese and Caucasian subjects, the cumulative irritant response rarely reached statistical significance. Newer studies by Aramaki et al.,[53] using more objective bioengineering methods, found no significant differences of the barrier function in the stratum corneum between Japanese and German women. The study did find, however, significant subjective sensory differences between these two groups. The researchers concluded that the stronger sensations of the Japanese women perhaps reflect a different cultural behavior rather than measurable differences in skin physiology. The lack of statistical significance as well as reproducibility in these studies lead us to believe that there is perhaps no fundamental difference between Asian and Caucasian cutaneous irritant response. There appears to be no consensus on whether race is indeed an endogenous factor in ICD.[54] Intuitively, it is suspected that ethnic differences exist in skin function but other more subjective factors need to be taken into consideration, such as cultural behavior and attitudes. Other studies speculate that although there are no significant differences in overall response rate to allergens, there are some differences to specific allergens that are possibly related to genetic factors based on race but more likely represent differences in allergen exposure determined by ethnicity.[55] This was illustrated in a brief study by Hsu et al.,[55] which documented allergic contact dermatitis in the beard area of Arabic men as a result of their propensity to dye their beards.

Despite the interest in studying the different irritation responses among ethnic groups and the seemingly conflicting findings, little is known about specific clinical manifestations in ethnic groups and how these manifestations vary from the pathology observed in Caucasian skin. Clinically, it seems acute contact dermatitis with exudation, vesiculation, or frank bullae formation is more commonly observed in whites, whereas blacks, for instance, more commonly have disorders of pigmentation and lichenification.[56] More studies are needed to objectively compare not only the different responses to irritants between ethnic groups but, specifically, the clinical manifestations of ICD. Whether Asian skin is more sensitive than Caucasian skin and black skin is more resistant than Caucasian skin, clinicians need to determine whether these differences could account for diagnostic problems, differences in treatment modalities, and differences in the presentation and manifestation of disease.

As mentioned earlier, perhaps the diagnostic criteria for AD need to be revised to incorporate the different clinical manifestation or lack thereof in ethnic skin or skin of color. Based on Williams et al.[57] and The U.K. Working Party's diagnostic criteria for AD, an individual must have an itchy skin condition (or parental report in a child) plus three or more of the following: (1) a history of flexural involvement (including cheeks in children younger than 10 years), (2) a personal history of asthma or hay fever (or a history of atopic disease in a first-degree relative of children younger than 4 years), (3) a history of generalized dry skin in the past year, (4) visible flexural eczema (including the cheeks, forehead and outer limbs in children younger than 4 years), and (5) onset of rash at younger than 2 years (not used if child is younger than 4 years). A study by Firooz et al.[58] was conducted in Iran to validate these criteria in another population with a different ethnic background, different environmental factors, and a different health care system. The study concluded that the diagnostic criteria proposed by the U.K. Working Party for the diagnosis of AD seemed to be highly specific, which made it particularly useful for clinical trials; however, they were not believed to achieve high sensitivity in other communities with different genetic backgrounds, environmental factors, or access to healthcare.[58] Ensuring some international consistency in the criterion standard for diagnosing AD is thus a major concern and a goal for the future. Attention should also be diverted to examining the statistical significance of the 30 or so minor features of AD, many of which may be considered to vary considerably according to ethnicity, as illustrated above. One option is perhaps to agree on one objective criterion, such as visible flexural dermatitis, as a working standard until better, more uniform criteria are developed. This is the approach currently used in phase II of the International Study of Asthma and Allergies in Childhood.[59]

Patients with AD essentially have a lower threshold of irritant responsiveness; in addition, dysregulation of epidermal barrier function invariably results in dry skin and consequently in pruritus, scratching, eczema, and superinfection. The skin of patients suffering from AD demonstrates reduced water-binding capacity, higher transepidermal water loss, and decreased water content. It is no surprise, then, that skin care is the cornerstone of treatment. Dermatologic treatment is based on the care of xerotic skin; avoidance of irritants such as detergents, soaps, and chemicals; and disruption of the itch–scratch cycle. Rehydrating the skin is often accomplished by bathing or soaking affected areas for approximately 15–20 minutes in warm water; the number of baths can be increased to several times a day during flares of AD. The use of emollients or moisturizers, however, is highly encouraged and should be applied within 3 minutes after bathing to retain hydration (3-minute rule). Moisturizers are available in lotions, oils, creams, and ointments. In general, ointments have the least number of additives and are the most occlusive. Lotions and creams may be irritating because of added preservatives or fragrances. In addition, lotions contain more water than creams and may have a drying effect due to evaporation.

Topical corticosteroids are generally regarded as the mainstay of treatment for AD. Topical corticosteroids are available in potencies ranging from extremely high (class 1) to low (class 7); also, the vehicle in which the product is formulated can alter its potency. The choice of topical corticosteroid must consider the required potency and the vehicle and must be adapted to the skin condition, severity, and distribution of the eczematous lesion. In general, the most effective but least potent corticosteroid should be used. The most common side effect seen with topical steroids is thinning of the skin; early changes are usually reversible, but after extended periods of application, especially with the more potent topical steroids, collagen and elastin synthesis are decreased, which can result in skin fragility, dermal atrophy, striae, telangiectasia, purpura, and poor wound healing.[60] Hypopigmentation is another side effect that is especially relevant to patients with darker skin. Contact leukoderma has been reported with the use of topical corticosteroids as well as with intralesional and intra-articular injections of corticosteroids.[61] Patients should be informed regarding the potential side effects of corticosteroid use.

Pruritus is a cardinal symptom of AD, and the associated scratching can contribute to open, superinfected lesions, bleeding, lichenification, or nodular changes. Antihistamines are often used as adjuvant treatment in the management of AD, as they afford symptomatic improvement of pruritus and in this way they help to interrupt the vicious cycle "pruritus–scratch–eczema–pruritus." Systemic antihistamines may be most useful through their tranquilizing and sedative effects and can be taken primarily in the evening to avoid daytime drowsiness. Patients with AD have an increased tendency to develop skin infections; these infections, often caused by staphylococci, have to be treated with penicillinase-resistant antibiotics topically twice a day or systemically, especially if impetiginization is clinically evident. Oral antibiotic treatment should last for about 2 weeks, and topical treatment should not exceed 4 weeks. There is ample clinical evidence that patients without superinfection show clinical improvement when treated with a combination of antistaphylococcal antibiotics and topical corticosteroids.

New and developing therapies for the management of AD have emerged during the last few years. Immunomodulatory agents such as cyclosporine, which acts by altering cytokine gene transcription, thereby modulating the cell-mediated immune response, is reserved for short-term treatment of adults with severe disease. Significant adverse effects, including nephrotoxicity and hypertension and the potential increase in risk of cutaneous and possibly internal malignancies, limit the use of cyclosporine to patients with severe, refractory disease. Topical cyclosporine has not been effective in treating AD. However, another member of the macrolide immunosuppressive family has shown extremely positive results in a topical formulation: Tacrolimus, with a mechanism of action similar to cyclosporine, exhibits greater potency and improved skin penetration. Tacrolimus has established itself as a safer alternative to the use of topical steroids, especially for vulnerable areas such as the face and eyelids, where glucocorticosteroids should not be given for more than

3 weeks due to glucocorticosteroid withdrawal dermatitis, atrophy, or telangiectasia. Tacrolimus quickly clears eczematous skin lesions and pruritus and provides excellent long-term control with no rebound effect.

Ultraviolet light can also be helpful as a steroid-sparing therapy. Light therapy should ideally be used when skin disease is stabilized and should supplement topical maintenance therapies. For patients with mild AD, standard UV-B regimens may be adequate, but patients with moderate to severe disease do better with combined UV-A/UV-B therapy. Its use must be carefully regulated to avoid photocarcinogenesis. In severe cases, PUVA (psoralen ultraviolet A) treatment represents another therapeutic option. However, its use is less acceptable because of slow onset of effect, frequent inflammatory flares after dosing, and long-term aging and carcinogenic effects. Several alternative regimens involving ultraviolet light have been described in the current literature but are beyond the scope of this chapter.

DERMATOPHYTE INFECTIONS IN ETHNIC POPULATIONS: TINEA CAPITIS

Tinea capitis is a fungal infection of the skin and hair with involvement of the hair shaft and the pilosebaceous unit (Figure 2.12). It probably represents the most common of all cutaneous mycoses in children. There appears to be a disproportionate infection rate in the African-American urban population. The reason for this phenomenon is not known; some of the theories that attempt to explain this racial predilection will be discussed here. Several studies have been conducted in different urban populations and similar patterns of infection appear to emerge worldwide. A shift in the geographic predominance of some of the infective agents has also taken place during the

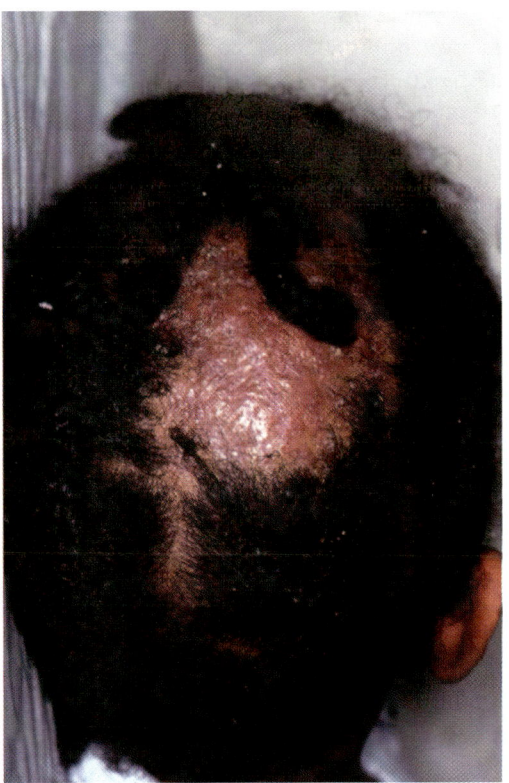

FIGURE 2.12 Tinea capitis with hair loss.

last few decades; whether this is related to the current epidemic in African-American children is a matter that deserves further research. The fact remains, however, that, as mentioned earlier, similar patterns of infection have been reported in the current literature in different parts of the world. Last, some of the common clinical manifestations of tinea capitis, and the different types of infections as well as the current therapeutic recommendations for its treatment, will be reviewed.

The epidemiology of tinea capitis in the United States has changed quite remarkably in the last century. During the last 50 years or so, *Trichophyton tonsurans* has replaced *Microsporum audouinii* and *Microsporum canis* as the dominant causative organism of tinea capitis in the United States. In fact, this dermatophyte accounts for more than 90% of ringworm infections of the scalp in the United States. *Trichophyton tonsurans* is an anthropophilic organism producing endothrix invasion of the hair shaft that does not fluoresce on Wood's light examination. In a study by Laude et al.,[62] it was noted that the chief cause of tinea capitis was predominantly due to infections with *T. tonsuras*. In fact, 89% of culture-proved cases encountered were caused by *T. tonsurans* and only 11% were caused by *Microsporum* organisms. This represented a complete reversal of preponderance of the causative fungal organism. Twenty years earlier all the cases of tinea capitis in New York City were due to *Microsporum* organisms.[63] The aforementioned study by Laude et al. was conducted in The Kings County Hospital Pediatric Ambulatory Service, which is a large municipal hospital facility serving an inner-city population of black people and Puerto Ricans in Brooklyn, New York. Similar reports had been noted by researchers in other American cities, suggesting that the emergence of this organism was a nationwide phenomenon rather than a regional one.[64] Dermatologists, pediatricians, epidemiologists and mycologists cannot explain this phenomenon; in a period of only 20 to 30 years almost a total disappearance of microsporosis has occurred in most areas of the United States. One of the main theories to explain this almost complete reversal argues that *T. tonsurans* may have been introduced into this country from Mexico, Puerto Rico, and Central and South America, where infections with *T. tonsurans* are more common.[62] Perhaps this change represents the migratory patterns recently observed and the subsequent change in demographics in all major American cities. The arrival of new immigrants carrying dermatophytes endemic to their country of origin may have contributed to, but does not completely explain, the rise in the incidence of infection with *T. tonsurans*. It is interesting to note, however, that tinea capitis currently represents approximately 4%–10% of all dermatophyte infections in Mexico, and its prevalence in schoolchildren is between 69% and 90%. *Microsporum canis* causes approximately 80% of these infections and *T. tonsurans* only 15%; *T. tonsurans*, however, has been noted to be the predominant agent in some rural areas of the country and mostly in the northern borders of Mexico.[65]

Another observation previously reported in the literature was that *T. tonsurans* seemed to affect black children much more than their Caucasian counterparts. Microsporosis, on the other hand, seemed to affect Caucasian children more commonly. Laude et al.[62] could not confirm this observation, given that the general population in their study was 85% black, 14.5% Hispanic, and only 0.5% white. A survey conducted among 92 medical mycology laboratories across 19 European countries showed an overall increase in the number of cases caused by anthropophilic infections, which in 1997 were the dominant causes of scalp infection; the greatest increase was seen in laboratories covering urban populations and in African-Caribbean children living in Europe.[66] In a study by Hay et al.,[67] it was confirmed that the main cause of tinea capitis in London was caused by anthropophilic fungi, mainly *T. tonsurans*. This particular study was conducted using 514 (49%) girls and 543 (51%) boys. Of these, a total of 42% had Caucasoid and 42% had Afro-Caribbean hair types. This is important from the point of view that the majority of those infected and a significant number of carriers had Afro-Caribbean hair type. There appears to be a racial predilection in disease susceptibility, most cases occurring in children of African or West Indian extraction. The reason for the disparity in infection and carriage rate was not understood; however, the study concluded that there was a higher risk of infection in children with Afro-Caribbean hair. Some researchers have suggested that hairstyling practices may be a factor in acquisition of the disease. Sharp and blunt trauma have been shown to contribute to dermatophyte infections. Hair oils and pomades may also promote the transmission of the disease. Compounding matters in African-Americans is the practice of less frequent shampooing, which has some spore-removal benefits, traction hair styling; and the plaiting of hair into tight rows, which can also allow easier fungal access to the impaired hair shaft. These theories lead researchers to believe that the higher rates of infection in African-Americans are the result of culturally dictated grooming practices. The aim of most hair-styling products and techniques is to create more manageable hair. However, careless technique, excessive use, and improper maintenance can lead to considerable damage to the hair. In one of the few studies of its kind, however, Sharma et al.[68] concluded that hair-grooming practices, such as the use of oils, gels, and specific hairstyles, were not associated with tinea capitis infections, as suggested by some researchers. Others have speculated that improved personal hygiene alone may play a role in the control of tinea capitis. Sharma et al. did not find the frequency of shampooing to be associated with tinea capitis infection. In conclusion, the study failed to find an association with hairstyling practices but did find a possible protective effect for the use of conditioners.[68]

The prevalence of tinea capitis infections in African-American children in the United States is reaching epidemic proportions. Data obtained from the National Ambulatory Medical Survey (NAMCS) were analyzed based on age, gender, and race. They showed that in 1996, 207,000 cases of tinea capitis were reported nationwide. Children between the ages of 5 and 18 years represented 77.1% of the cases. Males accounted for 57.5% of the cases, whereas females accounted for only 42.5%. African-Americans represented 80.9% of the cases reported. Based on these data alone, the relative risk for African-Americans acquiring tinea capitis is 29.4 times higher that the general population! These data demonstrate the male predominance, high relative risk in African-Americans, and school-age distribution.[69] In a study by Lobato et al.[70] among California children to determine subpopulations at increased risk for tinea capitis infections, the authors used prescriptions for griseofulvin suspension as a "surrogate marker" for tinea capitis infection in the California Medicaid (Medi-Cal) population. The study was conducted among Medi-Cal-enrolled children under 10 years of age; 48.5% were Hispanic, 24.9% were white, 13.1% were African-American, 9.2% were Asian or Pacific Islander, and 0.6% were Native American or Native Alaskan. Lobato et al.[70] found that the annual incidence rate for African-American children in 1984 was 5.8 times the mean rate for all other children, and in 1993, it was 13.9 times the mean rate. Since 1984, the rate of griseofulvin suspension usage increased among African-American children 209.7% and among white children 140.4%. Hispanic children had a stable incidence rate that peaked at 21.1 per 10,000 enrolled in 1985. In 1993, incidence rates (per 10,000 enrolled) were 251.1 claimants for African-American children, 23.1 for white, 17.5 for Hispanic, and 14.3 for Asian/Pacific Islander.[70] Again, the authors could not explain the disproportionate incidence of tinea capitis in African-Americans. Historical data seem to indicate that epidemics of tinea capitis have always been more common in poorer communities and that the accompanying increased population density certainly plays a role. The data also showed increased griseofulvin use in other racial groups, suggesting that the epidemic is not confined to African-American children.

There is, however, another trend that deserves further investigation. Although the majority of the research focuses on tinea capitis as an epidemic in the school-age population, there has been an increase in the incidence of adult infections as well. In fact, a gender differential in adults for active tinea capitis as well as carrier states has been observed. In the 1980s, Bronson et al.[71] evaluated nine adults with tinea capitis, six of whom were women. In the 1990s, Aeste et al.[72] reported 17 adult tinea capitis cases from Italy, all women between the ages of 17 and 76. Similarly, a study done in Taiwan in the early 1990s found that the occurrence of tinea capitis infection in adult patients, particularly middle-aged and elderly, was striking. Adults accounted for 63% of patients and all patients affected were women. The majority of infections were caused by *Trichophyton violaceum*.[73] It was not known why adult women were preferentially affected. Another recent French study revealed that 11% of patients with positive cultures were adults, 75% of whom were female.[74] Several investigators have suggested that endothrix fungi are more likely to invade the hair shaft and thus become chronic and persistent from childhood into adulthood. This theory fails to explain the phenomenon completely because most of the adult female patients acquired the infection as adults. It is important, however, to specify that tinea capitis appears to be increasing in African-American women in the United States. A study by Silverberg et al.[75] showed that 11.4% of tinea capitis patients were adult African-Americans, and 77% of these adults were women aged 25 to 67. The role of the woman as the primary caretaker of children in the household is likely to be a factor in this phenomenon or at least contribute to the rise of the disease in women. Women are most likely to manage and style their children's hair, giving them a high level of exposure to spores on the scalp. Most likely, however, the higher incidence of infection in women worldwide is related to a combination of factors, namely, being the primary caretakers of children infected with the disease, high-level exposure from the background population, and hair care practices.[75]

The issue of asymptomatic carriers is also a factor to consider. A study to determine the prevalence of the carrier state in household contacts in children with tinea capitis was conducted by Pomeranz et al.,[76] who found that at least one carrier was present in 32% of households that had a child with tinea capitis. The population studied was almost entirely African-American (96%). Several other studies have demonstrated a remarkable occurrence of either previously undetected clinical disease or asymptomatic carriage in family members of index cases. Vargo and Cohen[77] reported a carrier rate of 28% in family members of index cases, and Babel and Baughman[78] found that 34% of adult family members (parents and grandparents) of children with clinically apparent tinea capitis were actually carriers. What is significant about this is the possibility that a cycle of infection and reinfection could be taking place between index cases and asymptomatic carriers. Contagion is most likely bidirectional; i.e., untreated adult parents with the disease can infect children, and untreated children with the disease can infect parents. Asymptomatic adult carriers could be acting as reservoirs of the disease while children manifest the acute infectious phase. This geometric progression of infectivity represents a true public health issue. Furthermore, this pattern of infection is consistent with the shift observed in the causative organism from predominantly a zoophilic fungus to an anthropophilic one like *T. tonsurans*; in fact the common denominator was *T. tonsurans* as the only pathogen identified in both studies. Co-sleeping (whether with the index case or among other family members) and comb sharing were common practices among all contacts and occurred in 75% and 78%, respectively; but the study by Pomeranz et al. did not find these practices statistically associated with the carrier state. Similarly, in a report from Ethiopia,[79] no relationship was found between household overcrowding and either clinical infection or carriage where *T. violaceum* was the primary pathogen. Whether co-sleeping, comb sharing, and overcrowding play a role in the establishment of the carrier state and whether this in turn plays a role in the development or spread of disease have not been adequately determined. We cannot ignore, however, that certain cultural practices as well as socioeconomic status may predispose certain individuals to tinea capitis infection or at least provide more favorable conditions for the establishment of infections. Surveys within the United States suggest that, indeed, large family size, crowded living conditions, and low socioeconomic situations may contribute to the increased incidence of tinea capitis caused by *T. tonsurans* in some urban populations.[80]

The geographic distribution of dermatophyte infections varies and is perhaps related to changes in the living conditions of affected communities, or perhaps it represents fungal adaptation. For instance, tinea capitis is endemic in many African countries; its prevalence has been estimated to be between 10% and 30%, and it is estimated that there are approximately 20 million active infections, with an even higher carriage rate.[79] In fact, more recently there has been a rise in the overall adult incidence of tinea capitis on the African continent and in tinea capitis cases in adult immigrants from Africa;[75] whether these observations are related to the HIV epidemic is unknown. The predominant organism in North Africa, as well as South Africa, India, Jordan and the Far East, is *T. violaceum.* In Mexico, tinea capitis represents 4%–10% of dermatophyte infections, with *M. canis* causing 80% of all infections and *T. tonsurans* responsible for approximately 15%. As we have mentioned before, major etiological agents of tinea capitis in a given geographic region can also change over time. During the late 19th and early 20th centuries, *M. audouinii* and *M. canis* were the predominant etiologic agents of tinea capitis in Western and Mediterranean Europe, whereas *Trichophyton schoenleinii* predominated in Eastern Europe.[80] Current cases of anthropophilic tinea capitis in Western Europe are now due predominantly to *T. tonsurans*, whereas *T. violaceum* is currently the dominant agent in Eastern Europe. Similarly, in the United States *T. tonsurans* has surpassed *M. audouinii* and *M. canis* as the primary etiologic agent, as elucidated before. The overall prevalence in the United States is generally estimated to be between 3% and 8% of the pediatric population, with carriers occurring in as many as 34% of household contacts or infected persons.[80]

There are different clinical patterns of tinea capitis infection, making diagnosis somewhat difficult as presentations are wide-ranging and variable. Tinea capitis can be inflammatory or noninflammatory. When the presentation is noninflammatory, it may manifest in several ways. Some clinical appearances of scalp ringworm are the following:

1. The gray type which presents mainly with patches of alopecia with marked scaling.
2. The black dot type, which refers to the breakage of hairs at the scalp; the swollen stubs of broken-off hairs are visible within the patch of alopecia as "black dots." The dermatophytes invade the inside of the hair shaft, making it fragile and vulnerable to fracture.
3. Seborrheic dermatitis-like pattern.
4. Alopecia areata-like pattern.
5. Diffuse scale type; this form looks like dandruff, with widespread scaling throughout the scalp that can be masked with hair oils.
6. Moth-eaten type; hair loss is patchy and the underlying scalp may be generally scaly.

The kerion, which is a boggy, localized swelling that occurs due to an aggressive inflammatory response to the organism, and the diffuse pustular pattern, with widespread scattered pustules on the scalp, are the two types of inflammatory infections. There may be associated pain lymphadenopathy, malaise, and fever. Favus characteristically exhibits scutula, that is, yellow cup-shaped crusts around a hair; it can also be accompanied by inflammation and scarring. The crusts may be confluent and form a large, yellow, hyperkeratotic mass. Clinically, childhood and adult tinea capitis infections are similarly polymorphic in appearance. A combination of alopecia, seborrhea, black dot, and inflammatory changes is generally expected with *T. tonsurans* infection. Because of this varied presentation, tinea capitis can often go unrecognized or be mistaken for clinical mimics. In a study by Silverberg et al.,[75] adult patients were diagnosed with seborrheic dermatitis, alopecia areata, and folliculitis before the correct diagnosis of tinea capitis was ever made.[75] This is of paramount importance for clinicians observing adult seborrhea, alopecia areata, and scalp folliculitis, as they should always include tinea capitis in their differential diagnosis.

There are no significant clinical differences in the manifestation of disease among ethnic groups. In a study by Laude et al.[62] in a predominantly African-American population of 96 culture-proved cases, 40% were clinically inflammatory (kerions) and 60% were not. Some patients with noninflammatory tinea had severe diffuse scaliness, crusting of the scalp, and minimal alopecia, whereas others had the typical "black dot" appearance.[62] Marked cervical adenopathy was present in those patients with predominantly inflammatory infection. "Id" reaction, a hypersensitivity reaction to the fungal antigen, was manifested as a generalized maculopapular rash by a fraction of patients with kerions. Scaling was the most common clinical lesion in a study by Figueroa et al.[79] in southwestern Ethiopia and was found in approximately 95% of the positive clinical diagnoses. Hair loss was identified in 48% of clinical diagnoses, crusting was identified in only 9% of confirmed cases, and black dots were identified in 3%; pustules, kerion, scutulum, and id reaction were not present in mycologically confirmed cases. Because *T. tonsurans* is by far the most common cause of hair loss in African-American children, any black child with patchy scaling in the scalp, especially of recent onset, must be evaluated for tinea capitis infection.

The principles of tinea capitis management consist of oral antifungal therapy, adjunctive therapy, and strategies to reduce reinfection. Tinea capitis requires systemic treatment because topical antifungal creams are unable to penetrate the hair shaft to clear infection and should never be given as sole therapy. Griseofulvin is the "gold standard" for the treatment of dermatophyte infections in children. It has been the drug of choice since the late 1950s and has become the standard therapy against which all other therapies are judged. Griseofulvin has shown great efficacy and an excellent safety profile. Although dosages of 10 mg/kg per day for 4 weeks were previously considered effective for the treatment of tinea capitis, most specialists now use doses of 20–25 mg/kg per day for 6–8 weeks. Longer treatment may be required, given the reports in the current literature about possible treatment failures and the development of resistance. Some reports about unresponsiveness to griseofulvin therapy may be attributed to the interpatient variability known to exist with griseofulvin kinetics, a true resistance to the organism, continued exposure to the pathogen, or variation in patient's immune response.[81] Ketoconazole is an imidazole that is currently used for the treatment of onychomycosis and other dermatophyte infections. Its mechanism of action is similar to that of other azoles. In fact, ketoconazole was the first orally administered broad-spectrum antifungal compound of the azole group with activity against anthropophilic dermatophytes. Comparative trials between griseofulvin and ketoconazole have not demonstrated a superiority of this imidazole. In several of the studies conducted, ketoconazole did not improve outcome or shortened the duration of treatment required. One of the main problems encountered with ketoconazole is a significant incidence of idiosyncratic hepatic toxicity and a rather lengthy list of drug interactions. Furthermore, there are virtually no data available regarding the biodisposition and metabolism of the drug in infants and in children. No liquid formulation is available, and no systematic evaluation of ketoconazole tablet preparations has been done with pediatric patients. In fact, ketoconazole is not specifically approved in the United States for the treatment of tinea capitis. Considering the higher cost of treatment as well as the potential for adverse effects, especially hepatotoxicity, and the availability of other agents with a much more favorable side effect profile, this azole is not currently considered the preferred agent for the treatment of tinea capitis.

The newer fungicidal drugs, such as oral terbinafine and itraconazole, are promising and appear to be effective in tinea capitis; however, there are few comparative studies as of yet, because due to their fungicidal action they would require shorter treatments than griseofulvin and ketoconazole. Itraconazole has been approved in the United States for the treatment of onychomycosis and some systemic mycoses only but not for the treatment of tinea capitis. Similarly, terbinafine, which was introduced in 1996 for the management of dermatophyte toenail onychomycosis, is not approved in the United States for the treatment of tinea capitis. A small randomized trial found that antifungal shampoo (selenium sulfide) increases the rate of eradication, which may reduce the transmissibility of the organism.[82] The value of other adjunctive measures, such as ketoconazole shampoo or povidone–iodine, may help reduce the shedding of fungal organisms (spores); however, their effectiveness has not been assessed by clinical trials. Preventive measures play a very important role in management and control of infection, especially in urban populations where infection rates appear to have reached epidemic proportions. Control of scalp ringworm is possible using measures such as class inspection, improving grooming practices, and counseling children against the sharing of objects that might help spread tinea capitis to others, e.g., caps and combs. It is also possible, as clarified earlier, that symptom-free adult carriers and siblings living at home may act as reservoirs for the infection; in fact, contacts and environment at home may be a greater source of infection than contacts in school.

REFERENCES

1. Taylor SC, Cook-Bolden F, Rahman Z, Strachan D. Acne vulgaris in skin of color. *J Am Acad Dermatol* 2002; 46(2) Suppl: S98–S103.
2. Wilkins JW, Voorhees JJ. Prevalence of nodulocystic acne. *Arch Dermatol* 1970; 102: 631–634.
3. Halder RM, Holmes YC, Bridgeman-Shah, S, Kligman AM. A clinicopathological study of acne vulgaris in black females. *J Invest Dermatol* 1996; 106: 888.
4. Halder RM, Grimes, PE, McLaurin CI, Kress MA, Kenney JA. Incidence of common dermatoses in a predominantly black dermatologic practice. *Cutis* 1983; 32: 388–390.
5. Halder RM. The role of retinoids in management of cutaneous conditions in blacks. *J Am Acad Dermatol* 1998; 39: S98–S103.
6. Sanchez MR. Cutaneous diseases in Latinos. *Dermatol Clin* 2003; 21: 689–697.
7. Goh CL, Akarapanth R. Epidemiology of skin disease among children in a referral skin clinic in Singapore. *Pediatr Dermatol* 1994; 11(2): 125–128.
8. Grimes PE, Stoktonm T. Pigmentary disorders in blacks. *Dermatol Clin* 1988; 6: 407–412.
9. Resnick SD, Murrell DF, Woosley JT. Pityriasis rubra pilaris, acne conglobata, and elongated follicular spines: an HIV-associated follicular syndrome? *J Am Acad Dermatol* 1993; 29(2 Pt 1): 283.
10. Lapins J, Ye W, Nyren O, Emtestam L. Incidence of cancer among patients with hidradenitis suppurativa. *Arch Dermatol* 2001; 137(6): 730–734.
11. Scerri L, Williams HC, Allen BR. Dissecting cellulites of the scalp: response to isotretinoin. *Br J Dermatol* 1996; 134: 1105–1108.
12. Halder RM, Nootheti PK, Richards GM. Dermatological disorders and cultural practices: understanding practices that cause skin conditions in non-Caucasian populations. *Skin Aging* 2002; Aug: 46–50.
13. Adler, M. Rosacea in patients with darker skin types. *Acne and Rosacea Briefs* 2002; 1(4).
14. Browning DJ, Rosenwasser G, Lugo M. Ocular rosacea in blacks. *Am J Ophthalmol* 1986; 101(4): 441–444.
15. Williams HC, Ashworth J, Pembroke AC, Breathnach SM. FACE: facial Afro-Caribbean childhood eruption. *Clin Exp Dermatol* 1990; 15: 163.
16. Taylor SC. Retinoids: an effective choice for treating skin of color. Acne and Rosacea. Academy 2001.
17. Mills OH, Kligman AM, Pocchi P, Comite H. Comparing 2.5%, 5% and 10% benzoyl peroxide on inflammatory acne vulgaris. *Int J Dermatol* 1986; 25(10): 664–667.
18. Leyden J, Levy S. The development of antibiotic resistance in *Propionibactrium acnes*. *Cutis* 2001; 67(2 suppl): 21–24.
19. Sturkenboom MC, Meier CR, Jick H, Stricker BH. Minocycline and lupus-like syndrome in acne patients. *Arch Intern Med* 1999; 159: 493–497.
20. Wasel NR, Schloss EH, Lin AN. Minocycline-induced cutaneous pigmentation. *J Cutan Med Surg* 1998; 3(2): 105–108.
21. Wolf JE. Potential anti-inflammatory effects of topical retinoids and retinoid analogues. *Adv Ther* 2002; 19(3): 109–118.
22. Zhu XJ, Tu P, Zhen J, Duan YO. Adapalene gel 0.1%: effective and well tolerated in the topical treatment of acne vulgaris in Chinese patients. *Cutis* 2001, 68(4 suppl): 55–59.
23. Jacyk WK, Mpofu P. Adapalene gel 0.1% for topical treatment of acne vulgaris in African patients. *Cutis* 2001; 68(4 suppl): 48–54.
24. Perez A, Sanchez JL. Treatment of acne vulgaris in skin of color. *Cosmet Dermatol* 2003; 4: 23–28.
25. Kelly AP, Sampson DD. Recalcitrant nodulocystic acne in black Americans: treatment with isotretinoin. *J Natl Med Assoc* 1987; 79: 266–270.
26. Bjellerup M, Wallengren J. Familial perfolliculitis capitis abscedens et suffodiens in two brothers successfully treated with isotretinoin. *J Am Acad Dermatol* 1990; 23: 752–753.
27. Dicken CH, Powell St, Spear KL. Evaluation of isotretinoin treatment of hidradenitis suppurativa. *J Am Acad Dermatol* 1984; 11: 500–502.
28. Fitton A, Goa KL. Azeleic acid. A review of its pharmacological properties and therapeutic efficacy in acne and hyperpigmentary skin disorders. *Drugs* 1991; 41(5): 780–798.
29. Grimes PE. The safety and efficacy of salicylic acid chemical peels in darker racial-ethnic groups. *Dermatol Surg* 1999; 25: 18–22.

30. Halder RM, Nootheti PK. Ethnic skin disorders overview. *J Am Acad Dermatol* 2003; 48: 143–148.
31. Williams H, Robertson C, Stewart A, Ait-Khaled N, Anabwani G, Anderson R, et al. Worldwide variations in the prevalence of symptoms of atopic eczema in the international study of asthma and allergies in childhood. *J Allergy Clin Immunol* 1999; 103(1 pt 1): 125–138.
32. Dunwell P, Rose A. Study of the skin disease spectrum occurring in an Afro-Caribbean population. *Int J Dermatol.* 2003; 42(4): 287–289.
33. Child FJ, Fuller LC, Higgins EM, DuVivier AWP. A study of the spectrum of skin disease occurring in a black population in south-east London. *Br J Dermatol* 1999; 141: 512–517.
34. Williams HC, Pembroke AC, Forsdyke H, Boodoo G, Hay RJ, Burney PGJ. London-born black Caribbean children are at increased risk of atopic dermatitis. *J Am Acad Dermatol* 1995; 32: 212–217.
35. Neame RL, Berth-Jones J, Kurinczuk JJ, Graham-Brown RAC. Prevalence of atopic dermatitis in Leicester: a study of methodology and examination of possible ethnic variation. *Br J Dermatol* 1995; 132: 772–777.
36. Janumpally SR, Feldman SR, Gupta AK, Fleischer AB. In the United States, blacks and Asian/Pacific Islanders are more likely than whites to seek medical care for atopic dermatitis. *Arch Dermatol* 2002; 138(5): 673–674.
37. Jourdain R, deLachariere O, Bastien P, Maibach HI. Ethnic variations in self-perceived sensitive skin: epidemiological survey. *Contact Dermatitis* 2002; 46(3): 162–169.
38. Ben-Gashir MA, Seed PT, Hay RJ. Reliance on erythema scores may mask severe atopic dermatitis in black children compared with their white counterparts. *Br J Dermatol* 2002; 147(5): 920–925.
39. Hanifin JM, Rajka G. Diagnostic features of atopic dermatitis. *Acta Derm Venereol* 1980; 92(suppl): 44–47.
40. Williams H, Pembroke AC. Infraorbital crease, ethnic group, and atopic dermatitis. *Arch Dermatol* 1996;132(1): 51–54.
41. Lee HJ, Cho SH, Ha SJ, Ahn WK, Park YM, Byun DG, Kim JW. Minor cutaneous features of atopic dermatitis in South Korea. *Int J Dermatol* 2000; 39 (5): 337–342.
42. Laude TA, Kenney JA Jr, Prose NS, Treadwell PA, Resnick SD, Gosain S, Levy ML. Skin manifestations in individuals of African or Asian descent. *Pediatr Dermatol* 1996; 13(2): 158–168.
43. Modjtahedi SP, Maibach HI. Ethnicity as a possible endogenous factor in irritant contact dermatitis: comparing the irritant response among Caucasians, blacks, and Asians. *Contact Dermatitis* 2002; 47(5): 272–278.
44. Robinson MK. Racial differences in acute and cumulative skin irritation response between Caucasian and Asian populations. *Contact Dermatitis* 2000; 42(3): 134–143.
45. Marshall EK, Lynch V, Smith HW. Variations in susceptibility of the skin to dichlorethylsulphide. *J Pharmacol Exp Ther* 1919; 12: 291–301.
46. Weigand DA, Gaylor JR. Irritant reaction in Negro and Caucasian skin. *South Med J.* 1974; 67: 548–551.
47. Weigand DA, Haygood C, Gaylor JR. Cell layers and density of Negro and Caucasian stratum corneum. *J Invest Dermatol* 1974; 62: 563–568.
48. Berardesca E, Maibach HI. Racial difference in sodium lauryl sulphate induced cutaneous irritation: black and white. *Contact Dermatitis* 1988; 18: 65–70.
49. Gean CJ, Tur E, Maibach HI, Guy RH. Cutaneous responses to topical methylnicotinate in black, Oriental, and Caucasian subjects. *Arch Dermatol Res* 1989; 281: 95–98.
50. Hicks SP, Swindells KJ, Middlekamp-Hup MA, Sifakis MA, Gonzales E, Gonzalez S. Concocal histopathology of irritant contact dermatitis *in vivo* and the impact of skin color (black vs. white). *J Am Dermatol* 2003; 48(5): 727–734.
51. Robinson MK. Population differences in acute skin irritation responses. Race, sex, age, sensitive skin and repeat subject comparisons. *Contact Dermatitis* 2002; 46(2): 86–93.
52. Foy V, Weinkauf R, Whittle E, Basketter DA. Ethnic variation in the skin irritation response. *Contact Dermatitis* 2001; 45(6): 346–349.
53. Aramaki J, Kawana S, Effendy, I, Happle R, Loffler H. Differences of skin irritation between Japanese and European women. *Br J Dermatol* 2002; 146(6): 1052–1056.
54. DeLeo VA, Taylor S, Belsito DV, Fowler J, Fransway A, Maibach HI, Marks JG, et al. The effect of race and ethnicity on patch test results. *J Am Acad Dermatol* 2002; 46: S107–S112.

55. Hsu TS, Davis MDP, el-Azhary R, Corbett JF, Gibson LE. Beard dermatitis due to para-phenylenediamine use in Arabic men. *J Am Dermatol* 2001; 44(5): 867–869.
56. Berardesca F, Maibach H. Racial differences in skin pathophysiology. *J Am Acad Dermatol* 1996; 34(4): 667–672.
57. Williams HC, Burney PGJ, Hay RJ, Archer CB, Shipley MH, Hunter JJ, et al. The U.K. Working Party's diagnostic criteria for atopic dermatitis, I: derivation of a minimum set of discriminators for atopic dermatitis. *Br J Dermatol* 1994; 131: 383–396.
58. Firooz A, Davoudi SM, Farahmand AN, Majdzadeh R, Kashani MN, Dowlati Y. Validation of the diagnostic criteria for atopic dermatitis. *Arch Dermatol* 1999; 135: 514–516.
59. *International Study of Asthma and Allergies in Childhood. Phase II modules.* University of Munster, Munster, Germany, 1998.
60. Boguniewicz M, Nicol N. Conventional therapy for atopic dermatitis. *Immunol Allergy Clin North Am* 2002; 22(1).
61. Ortone JP, Mosher DB, Fitzpatrick TB. Chemical hypomelanoses. In: *Vitiligo and Other Hypomelanoses of Hair and Skin.* Plenum, New York, 1983; 479–508.
62. Laude TA, Ahah BR, Lynfield Y. Tinea capitis in Brooklyn. *Am J Dis Child* 1982; 136(12): 1047–1050.
63. Behrman HT, Mandel EH, Morse JL. Modern treatment of ringworm of the scalp. *J Pediatr* 1962; 60: 252–258.
64. Prevost E. Nonfluorescent tinea capitis in Charleston, SC. *JAMA* 1979; 242: 1765–1767.
65. Arenas R. Dermatophytoses in Mexico. *Rev Iberoam Micol* 2002; 19(2): 63–67.
66. Hay RJ, Robles W, Midgley G, Moore MK. Tinea capitis in Europe: new perspective on an old problem. *J Eur Acad Dermatol Venereol* 2001; 15(3): 229–233.
67. Hay RJ, Clayton YM, De Silva N, Midgley G, Rosser E. Tinea capitis in Southeast London — a new pattern of infection with public health implications. *Br J Dermatol* 1996; 135: 955–958.
68. Sharma V, Silverberg NB, Howard R, Tran CT, Laude TA, Frieden IJ. Do hair care practices affect the acquisition of tinea capitis? A case control study. *Arch Pediatr Adolesc Med* 2001; 155: 818–821.
69. Tack DA, Fleischer A Jr, McMichael A, Feldman S. The epidemic of tinea capitis disproportionately affects school-aged African-Americans. *Pediatr Dermatol* 1999; 16(1): 75.
70. Lobato MN, Vugia DJ, Frieden IJ. Tinea capitis in California children: a population-based study of a growing epidemics. *Pediatrics* 1997; 99: 551–554.
71. Bronson DM, Desai DR, Barsky S, Foley SM. An epidemic of infection with *Trychophyton tonsurans* revealed in a 20-year survey of fungal infection in Chicago. *J Am Acad Dermatol* 1983; 8: 322–330.
72. Aste N, Pau M, Biffio P. Tinea capitis in adults. *Mycoses* 1996; 39: 299–301.
73. Lee JY-Y, Hsu M-L. Tinea capitis in adults in southern Taiwan. *Int J Dermatol* 1991; 30: 572–575.
74. Cremer G, Bournerias I, Vandemeleubroucke E, Houin R, Revuz J. Tinea capitis in adults: misdiagnosis or reappearance? *Dermatology* 1997; 194: 8–11.
75. Silverberg NB, Weinberg JM, DeLeo VA. Tinea capitis: Focus on African-American women. *J Am Acad Dermatol* 2002; 46(2 Suppl Understanding): S120–S124.
76. Pomeranz AJ, Sabnis SS, McGrath GJ, Esterly NB. Asymptomatic dermatophyte carriers in the households of children with tinea capitis. *Arch Pediatr Adolesc Med* 1999; 153(5): 483–486.
77. Vargo K, Cohen BA. Prevalence of undetected tinea capitis in household members of children with disease. *Pediatrics* 1993; 92: 155–157.
78. Babel DE, Baughman SA. Evaluation of the adult carrier state in juvenile tinea capitis caused by Trichophyton tonsurans. *J Am Acad Dermatol* 1989; 21: 1209–1212.
79. Figueroa JI, Hawranek T, Abraha A, Hay RJ. Tinea capitis in south-western Ethiopia: a study of risk factors for infection and carriage. *Int J Dermatol* 1997; 36: 661–666.
80. Elewski BE. Tinea capitis: a current perspective. *J Am Acad Dermatol* 2000; 42: 1–20.
81. Abdel-Rahman SM, Nahata MC. Treatment of tinea capitis. *Ann Pharmacother* 1997; 31: 338–348.
82. Allen HB, Honig PJ, Leyden JJ, McGinley KJ. Selenium sulfide: adjunctive therapy for tinea capitis. *Pediatrics* 1982; 69: 81–83.

Neonatal and Pediatric Dermatological Diseases in Pigmented Skins

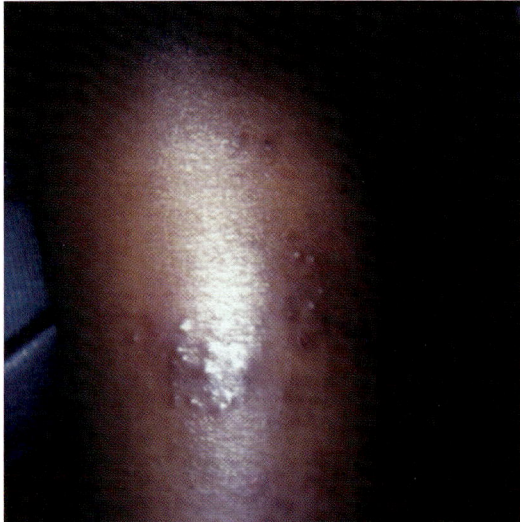

FIGURE 3.7 Papules and pustules of the lower leg in acropustulosis of infancy.

TRACTION FOLLICULITIS AND/OR ALOPECIA

This disorder occurs as a result of traction caused by cornrowing, tight braiding, ponytails, or weight from hair ornaments. Follicular-centered sterile pustules can be noted in the early stages (Figure 3.8). With prolonged traction, scarring alopecia can occur.[10] The most characteristically involved region of the scalp is the area above the ears, with sparing of shorter hairs of the hairline itself (Figure 3.9).

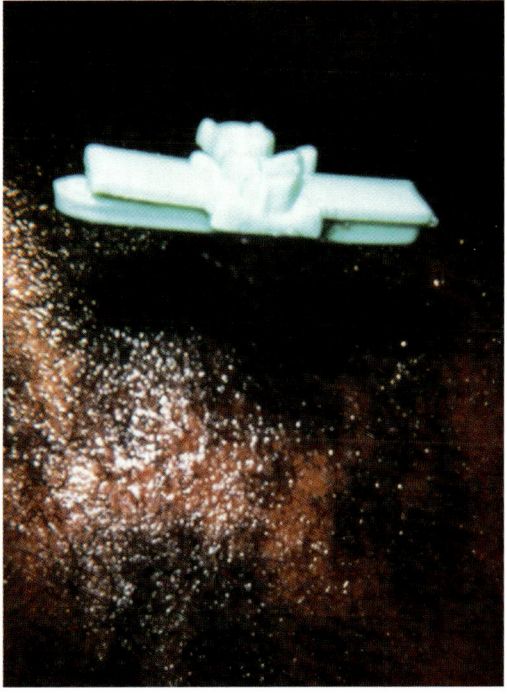

FIGURE 3.8 Pustular lesions of traction folliculitis.

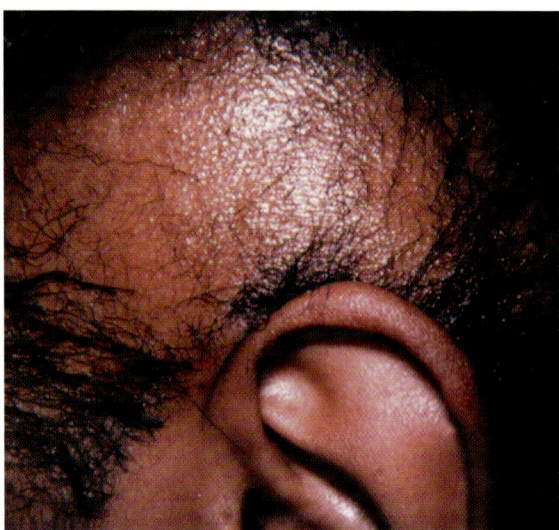

FIGURE 3.9 Scarring alopecia resulting from traction.

Histology of an early lesion can show a neutrophilic infiltrate in the follicles, whereas later histology may show a scarring alopecia. Differential diagnoses include bacterial folliculitis, tinea capitis, alopecia areata, trichotillomania, and syphilis.[11]

Recommended treatments involve avoiding practices that cause excessive traction on hair as well as utilizing varying hairstyles that redistribute traction. Traction folliculitis can also be treated with a topical antibiotic ointment.

TINEA CAPITIS

Tinea capitis occurs more frequently in African-American children as compared to Caucasian children. It occurs rarely in postpubertal individuals. The organisms are transferred from infected individuals, infected animals, or fomites to the patient. The most common causative dermatophyte is *Trichophyton tonsurans*,[12] although tinea capitis can also be caused by *Microsporum canis*, *Microsporum audouini*, or *Trichophyton violaceum*.

Characteristic clinical findings are patchy alopecia with scale, diffuse scalp scaling, and scattered crusts or papules. Often, occipital and/or posterior cervical lymphadenopathy are present (Figure 3.10). A kerion (an intensely inflammatory host response to the dermatophyte infection) may develop with edema, weeping, and/or thick crusting (Figure 3.11).

The diagnosis can be made on potassium hydroxide examination, which shows spores and hyphae in broken hairs. A Wood's light examination will show fluorescence of individual infected hairs when the etiologic agent is an ectothrix (e.g., *Microsporum* species) but will be negative when the etiologic agent is an endothrix (e.g., *Trichophyton* species). A fungal culture can confirm the diagnosis. Differential diagnoses include seborrheic dermatitis, bacterial folliculitis, traction folliculitis, trichotillomania, and alopecia areata.

Treatment is accomplished with oral antifungal agents. Griseofulvin is used as first-line therapy. Because there have been some bioavailability issues with the liquid preparations, microsized tablets are recommended in children more than 1 year of age. The dose of microsized griseofulvin is 15–20 mg/kg per day (maximum 1 g) for a 6–8 week course. The second-tier treatment group includes: fluconazole (6 mg/kg per day, 20-day course), itraconazole (3–5 mg/kg per day, 4–6-week course), and terbinafine 62.5 mg/day (10–20-kg body weight) *or* 125 mg/day (20–40-kg body weight) *or* 250 mg/day (>40 kg body weight) with a 14–21-day course. Selenium sulfide or ketoconazole shampoo is prescribed for weekly use as adjunctive therapy.[13] Oral antibiotics are

Neonatal and Pediatric Dermatological Diseases in Pigmented Skins

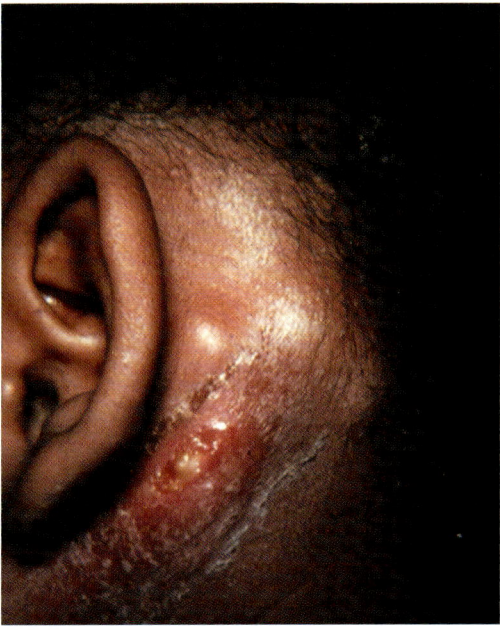

FIGURE 3.10 Retroauricular lymphadenopathy and a draining node in a patient with tinea capitis.

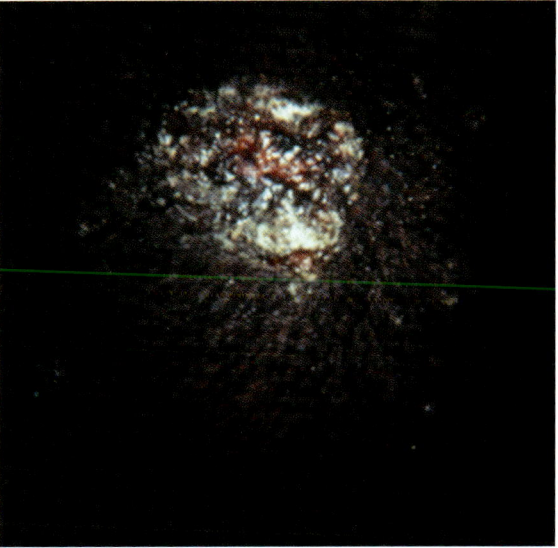

FIGURE 3.11 A kerion on the scalp.

prescribed if a secondary bacterial infection is present. A 3–5-day course of oral corticosteroids is prescribed if the kerion appears clinically destructive. If treatment is initiated in a timely fashion, most patients will experience hair regrowth.

HYPOPIGMENTED MYCOSIS FUNGOIDES

Hypopigmented mycosis fungoides is a rare variant of mycosis fungoides (MF) that typically has a predilection for young individuals with dark complexions. Lesions are noted initially in childhood or

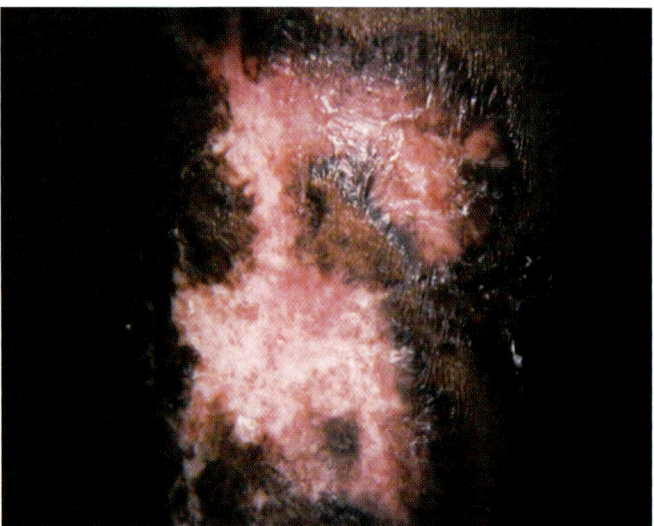

FIGURE 3.12 A discoid lupus lesion with hypopigmentation, scarring, and crusting.

adolescence (2–19 years of age); however, the histologic diagnosis tends to be delayed by 2–10 years.[14] Characteristic clinical findings are scattered hypopigmented macules or patches on the trunk and extremities. The lesions tend to lack scale and are nonpruritic.

Histologic examination reveals epidermotropism with abnormal lymphocytes and, occasionally, Pautrier microabscesses.[15] Usually T helper/inducer (CD4) cells are noted in the infiltrate. T-cell gene rearrangement has been variably reported.[16] Electron microscopy studies show a decreased number of melanosomes within keratinocytes and normal melanocytes in normal or decreased numbers. It is thought that the hypopigmentation may be postinflammatory, which occurs as a result of a nonspecific response to inflammation. Differential diagnoses include postinflammatory hypopigmentation, pityriasis alba, vitiligo, pityriasis lichenoides et varioliformis acuta, and sarcoidosis.

The exact course and prognosis are not known. Treatments have included topical corticosteroids, UVB, psoralen UVA (PUVA), and topical nitrogen mustard.

Lupus Erythematosus

Childhood lupus erythematosus is seen with an increased frequency among African-American, Hispanic, and Asian children as compared to Caucasian children.[17] Systemic lupus erythematosus (SLE), which has a predominance in female patients, has its initial presentation between the ages of 9 and 15 years of age in 15% of patients. Eighty percent of adolescents with SLE have cutaneous findings, and in 25%, the cutaneous findings are the presenting sign. Cutaneous findings in SLE include: "butterfly" malar eruption, discoid lesions[18] (Figure 3.12), telangiectasias, livedo reticularis, and Raynaud's phenomenon.

Histologic examination shows an interface dermatitis with vacuolar alteration and necrotic keratinocytes in the epidermis and adnexal structures.[15] Differential diagnoses include dermatomyositis, serum sickness, drug eruptions, rheumatic fever, and juvenile rheumatoid arthritis.

Treatment of the cutaneous manifestations includes sun avoidance and UVA protection, antimalarials, immunosuppressive therapy, and additional topical corticosteroid therapy.

Neonatal Lupus Erythematosus

Neonatal lupus erythematosus (NLE) occurs as a result of transplacental spread of maternal antibodies. The estimated frequency of occurrence is between 1 in 2500 to 1 in 20,000 births. The

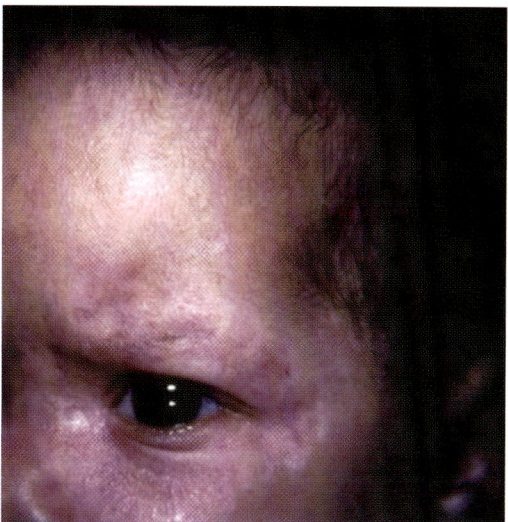

FIGURE 3.13 Atrophic lesions of the forehead and periorbital areas in an infant with NLE.

manifestations may be cardiac findings, cutaneous findings, or both. The cardiac abnormalities occur when the maternal antibodies are present at 9–10 weeks of gestational age. The antibodies bind selectively to fetal myocytes and cells of the conduction system. Varying degrees of congenital heart block or myocarditis can result. The cutaneous findings include annular lesions, discoid lesions, atrophic lesions (Figure 3.13), "raccoon eyes," and/or telangiectasias.[19] The lesions may worsen with sun exposure.

Histology shows vacuolar alteration of the epidermis and adnexal structures, necrotic keratinocytes, and papillary edema with a lymphohistiocytic dermal infiltrate.[15] The diagnosis is made by demonstrating the presence of anti-Ro (SS-A), anti-La (SS-B), or anti-RNP antibodies in the mother and infant. The antibodies are usually decreased at about 6 months of age. Third-degree heart block is typically diagnosed prenatally because of bradycardia. A baseline EKG after birth can rule out lesser degrees of heart block. Differential diagnoses include tinea corporis, annular erythema, and congenital infections.

Treatment includes sun avoidance and UVA protection. A Class 7 topical corticosteroid can be added as needed. Children who have had neonatal lupus may have some increased risk of developing an autoimmune disease in early childhood.[20]

Kawasaki Disease

Kawasaki disease (mucocutaneous lymph node syndrome) is an idiopathic multisystem disorder primarily affecting infants and young children. The highest incidence of Kawasaki disease is found among Japanese children and Korean children and the lowest incidence is Caucasian children, with an intermediate incidence in African-American, Hispanic, Chinese, Filipino, and Polynesian children.[21,22] The case definition is listed in Table 3.1.

Many authors theorize that the disorder is due to an infectious agent, possibly an agent that produces a superantigen. The evidence for an infectious cause includes the seasonal incidence, presence of geographic clusters, and increased incidence among siblings. Cutaneous clinical findings include conjunctival injection, erythema of the lips (Figure 3.14) and oral pharynx, strawberry tongue, fissures of the lips, swelling of the hands and feet, perineal desquamation (Figure 3.15), and, later, desquamation of the hands and feet.

Histologic examination of a punch biopsy specimen is nonspecific with dermal edema, dilated vessels, and lymphohistiocytic infiltrate. A deep surgical specimen can demonstrate the medium-sized

TABLE 3.1
Kawasaki Disease: Case Definition

Fever
Erythema and swelling of the palms and soles — later, desquamation
Polymorphous exanthema
Conjunctival injection
Erythema of the lips and oral pharynx, strawberry tongue
Lymphadenopathy

Source: Neuhaus IM, et al. *Pediatr Dermatol* 2000; 17: 403–406. With permission.

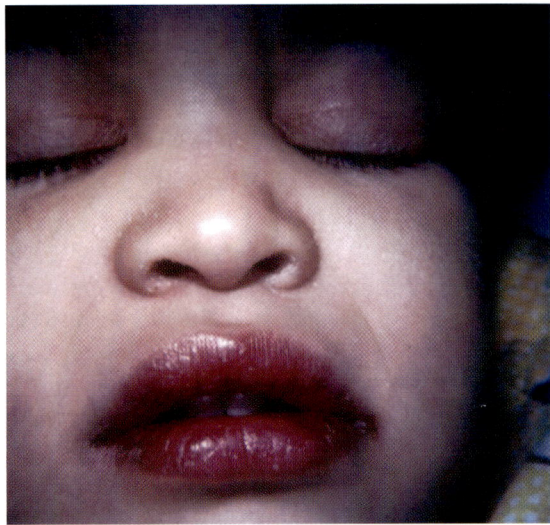

FIGURE 3.14 Erythema of the lips in a patient with Kawasaki syndrome.

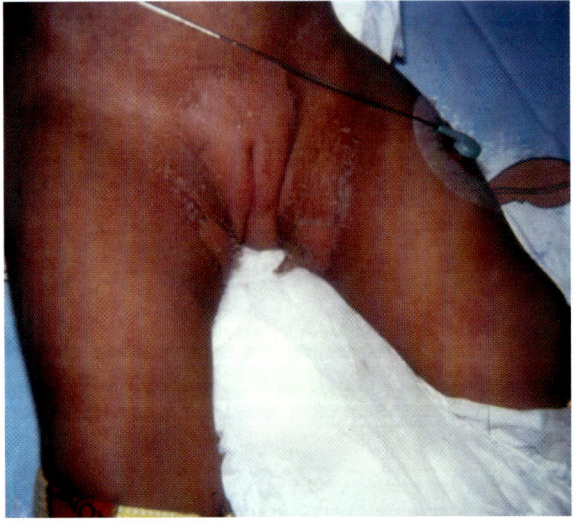

FIGURE 3.15 Perineal desquamation in a patient with Kawasaki syndrome.

arteritis that characterizes this disorder. Differential diagnoses include scarlet fever, toxic shock syndrome, erythema multiforme major, staphylococcal scalded skin syndrome, rubeola, and infantile periarteritis nodosa.

When the diagnosis has been made, a cardiac consultation is appropriate. Treatment with intravenous immunoglobulin (IVIG) and aspirin is recommended for patients at the highest risk for formation of coronary artery aneurysms.

DISEASES WITH DIFFERENT CLINICAL PRESENTATIONS

ERYTHEMA

Erythema in children of color often is more difficult to discern than in children with a lighter complexion (Figure 3.16). The degree of inflammation can be as severe while not as obvious. Thus, the severity of involvement can be underestimated if erythema is the primary measure. This difference will also affect some scoring measures in clinical studies.[23,24]

ATOPIC DERMATITIS

Atopic dermatitis occurs in approximately 3%–10% of the population. The atopic dermatitis patients have an increased prevalence of asthma and allergies. The family history (especially in the father) is often positive for atopic dermatitis, allergies, and asthma. Associated findings in children with atopic dermatitis include: (1) hyperlinear palms, (2) Morgan–Dennie folds (lower eyelid folds), (3) infra-auricular fissures, (4) xerosis, and (5) ichthyosis.

The clinical presentation of atopic dermatitis in African-American children tends be more papular and/or follicular-centered (Figure 3.17). Papular eczema and lichen spinulosus are seen more frequently than in Caucasian children. In papular eczema, the lesions are noted to be eczematous papules noted on the extremities and trunk. If extensive rubbing occurs, the papules may become thickened and may eventually resemble prurigo nodularis lesions. Lichen spinulosus is

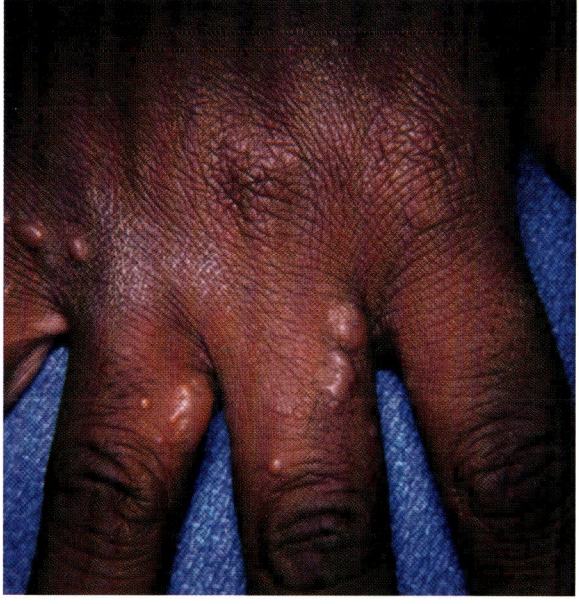

FIGURE 3.16 Allergic contact dermatitis in an African-American patient with only vesicles and no erythema present.

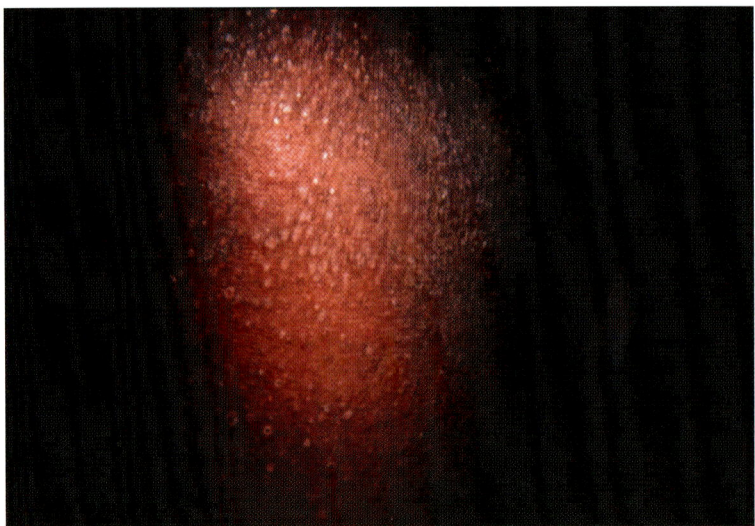

FIGURE 3.17 Papular lesions in a child with atopic dermatitis.

characterized by hyperkeratotic follicular-centered papules. Pityriasis alba is a common variant that presents as hypopigmented macules or patches with scale, most often involving the face.

Histologic findings of lichen spinulosus show a mild perifollicular infiltrate of lymphocytes. In addition, compact eosinophilic keratinous debris and hair shaft fragments are noted in dilated infundibulum.[25] Differential diagnoses include seborrheic dermatitis, keratosis pilaris, lichen nitidus, and contact dermatitis.

Treatment begins with education regarding gentle treatment of the skin, including 100% cotton clothing, mild soap for bathing, short baths, second rinse of laundry detergent, and avoidance of dryer fabric softeners. Liberal lubrication of the skin is recommended,[26] with ointments and creams being more effective than lotions. We recommend avoidance of individuals with herpetic lesions (to prevent eczema herpeticum) and frequent trimming of the fingernails. Low- to medium-potency topical corticosteroids (Classes 5–7) are prescribed for use twice daily. Topical immunomodulators (pimecrolimus or tacrolimus) can be used as steroid-sparing agents for maintenance or as initial treatment in areas of thin skin (e.g., eyelids). Antihistamines, especially hydroxyzine (2 mg/kg per day) are used to control the pruritus. Oral and topical antibiotics are prescribed to minimize overgrowth or frank secondary bacterial infection (usually with *Staphylococcus aureus*).

NICKEL CONTACT DERMATITIS

Allergic contact dermatitis occurs with the same frequency in children of color as other children. Nickel is the most common sensitizing metal. Nickel alloy or nickel plating can be found in identification bands, zippers, metal shoelace tips, metal clothing snaps, safety pins, metal toys, magnets, doorknobs, keys, scissors, bracelets, bra snaps, thimbles, jeans, snaps and studs, and jewelry.[27,28] Nickel contact dermatitis, especially that occurring in the periumbilical area, tends to be more papular in African-American children (Figure 3.18).

Differential diagnoses include atopic dermatitis, psoriasis, tinea corporis, sarcoid, and lichen planus.

Treatment consists of strict avoidance of nickel, topical corticosteroids (Classes 3–6), and antihistamines.

Neonatal and Pediatric Dermatological Diseases in Pigmented Skins

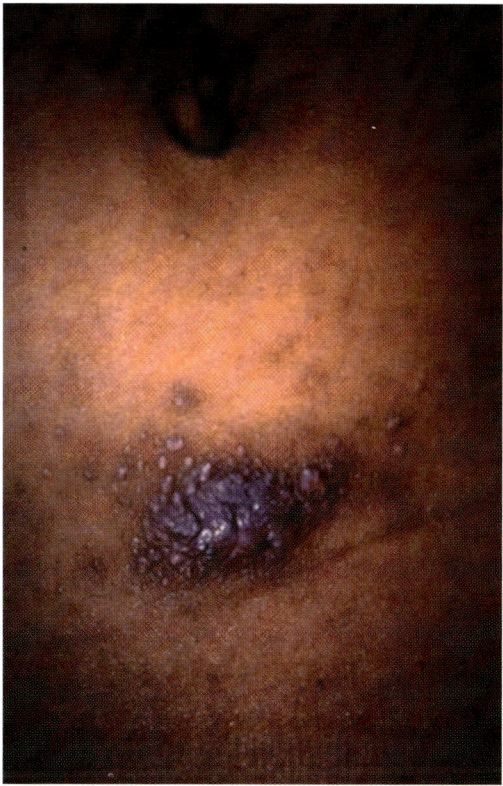

FIGURE 3.18 Allergic contact dermatitis from nickel with a papular appearance.

Seborrheic Dermatitis

Seborrheic dermatitis in adolescents has a predilection to involve areas with increased sebaceous glands.[29] The condition is subject to hormonal influences and action of the normal flora on the sebaceous gland secretions. African-American adolescents with a diagnosis of seborrheic dermatitis may have annular lesions, especially in the paranasal areas (Figure 3.19). The lesions are slightly raised with scale.

Differential diagnoses include tinea corporis and secondary syphilis.

Treatment is accomplished with ketoconazole shampoo 1–2 times weekly, topical antifungals and/or topical corticosteroids (Classes 6–7 for the facial lesions) twice daily. There have been reports of some success with the use of pimecrolimus.[30]

Pityriasis Rosea

Pityriasis rosea is a papulosquamous skin condition that is most likely to be caused by an infectious agent. In children of color, the lesions of pityriasis rosea have a tendency to be more inflammatory with crusting (Figure 3.20) and/or be more papular and follicular centered.[31]

Clinical findings in general include a herald patch 2–5 cm in diameter 5–7 days prior to the onset of multiple oval lesions, mainly on the trunk and proximal extremities. The truncal lesions often form a "Christmas-tree" pattern, whereas the lesions of the flank form a "school of minnows" pattern. Individual lesions have an erythema and scale, in some cases forming a "collarette" of scale (Figure 3.21).

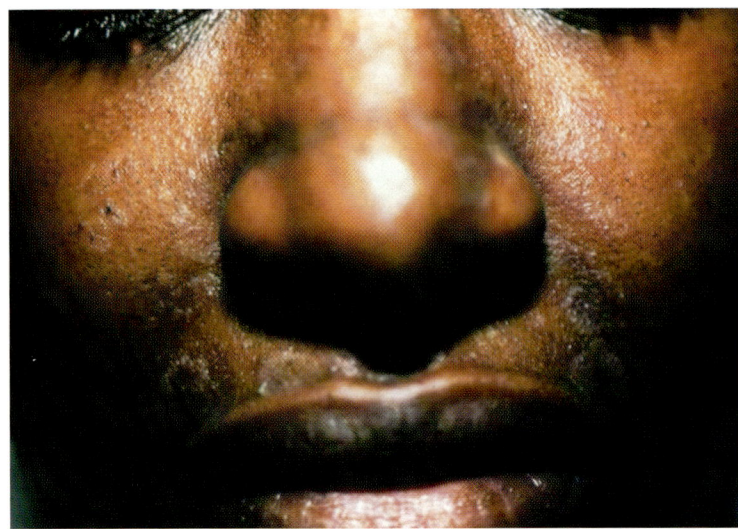

FIGURE 3.19 Annular seborrheic dermatitis. Patient had negative serology for syphilis.

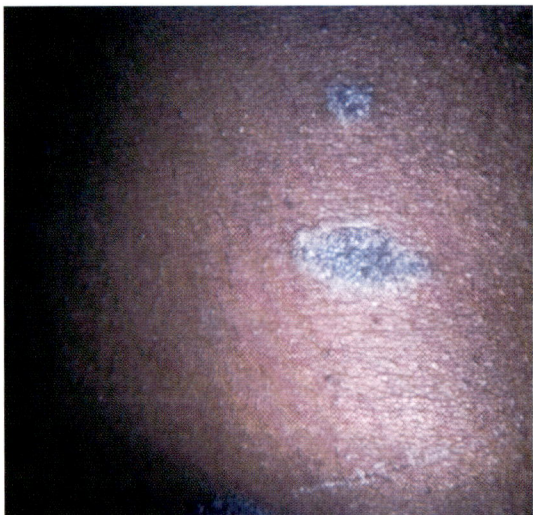

FIGURE 3.20 Crusted lesions of pityriasis rosea in an African-American patient.

Histologic findings show focal parakeratosis, a diminished granular layer, and spongiosis. Differential diagnoses include tinea corporis, psoriasis, and secondary syphilis.

Topical corticosteroids (Class 4–7) twice daily may be helpful if the lesions are pruritic. Oral antihistamines are prescribed if necessary. In 2000, a study showed some efficacy with the use of oral erythromycin.[32] In adolescents, obtaining a serologic test for syphilis should be considered.

TINEA VERSICOLOR

Tinea versicolor, a superficial fungal infection caused by *Pityrosporum orbiculare*, is primarily seen after adolescence but can be seen at any age. The incidence is increased in the summer and in tropical climates and also in settings of diabetes, pregnancy, and immunosuppression. The lesions are usually located on the upper back, chest, and proximal arms.[33] Facial involvement is noted

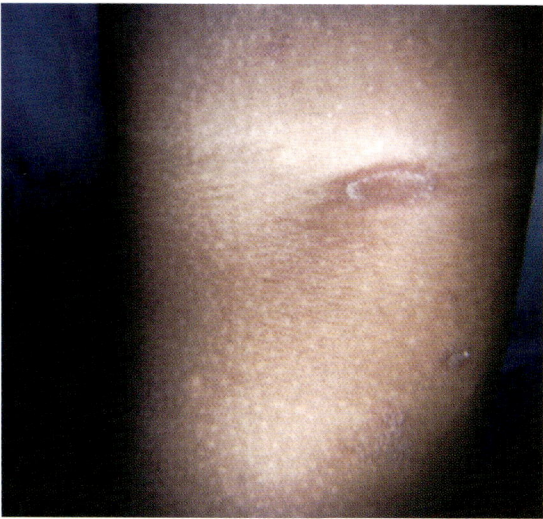

FIGURE 3.21 "Collarette "of scale in a pityriasis rosea lesion.

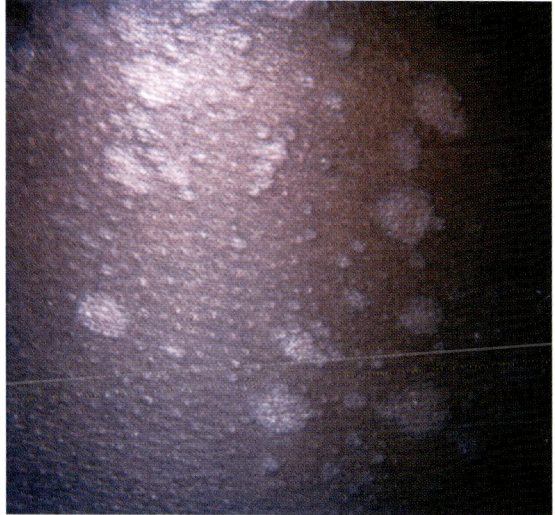

FIGURE 3.22 Hypopigmented tinea versicolor with follicular accentuation.

when it affects younger children. In persons of color, the color variations of the hyperpigmentation or hypopigmentation tend to be more significant. In addition, follicular accentuation may be present (Figure 3.22). Clinically, the lesions are flat or slightly raised with scale.

Microscopic examination (with potassium hydroxide and ink) of the scales shows short hyphae and spores. Examination with a Wood's light may reveal orange fluorescence. Differential diagnoses include tinea corporis, pityriasis alba, postinflammatory hypopigmentation or hyperpigmentation, hypopigmented MF, and vitiligo.

Treatment of limited lesions on the face in younger children can be accomplished with topical antifungal creams (e.g., clotrimazole, miconazole, ketoconazole) used twice a day for 2–3 weeks. For more extensive cases, selenium sulfide lotion 2.5% or ketoconazole shampoo 2% is applied nightly for a few weeks. Oral fluconazole or ketoconazole can be prescribed in older children and adolescents.[34]

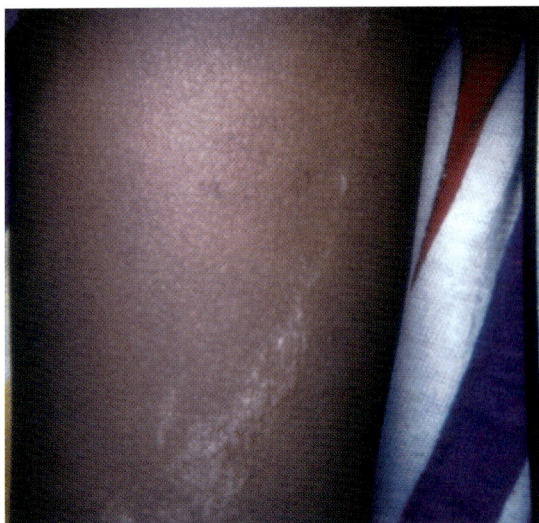

FIGURE 3.23 Hypopigmented grouped papules in a linear arrangement in a patient with lichen striatus.

Polymorphous Light Eruption

Polymorphous light eruption is the most common photodermatosis in children. The usual presentation is pruritic, skin-colored or erythematous papules and plaques present in a photosensitive distribution. In more darkly pigmented skin, a pinpoint papular variant may be seen.[35] Photoprovocation tests have shown pathologic reactions to both UVB and UVA, UVB alone, and UVA alone.[36]

Histologic examination has revealed two patterns: (1) a focal lichenoid and perivascular lymphohistiocytic infiltrate and (2) a superficial and deep interstitial lymphocytic infiltrate with papillary dermal edema. Differential diagnoses include systemic lupus erythematosus, porphyria, solar urticaria, and drug-induced photoeruptions.

Treatment consists of medium- to low-potency topical corticosteroids (Classes 5–7), antihistamines, and broad-spectrum sunscreens. With more severe and/or symptomatic cases, prophylactic treatment with UVB can be considered.

Lichen Striatus

Lichen striatus is a self-limited (typically lasting 2–4 years) skin condition that is characterized by grouped papules arranged in a linear pattern and often following Blaschko's lines[37] (Figure 3.23). The papules may be inflamed initially; however, postinflammatory hypopigmentation can develop. In darkly pigmented individuals, the erythema may not be easily appreciated, and there is a tendency for many of the lesions to be hypopigmented. When the lichen striatus involves a nail, dystrophic changes can be seen.[38]

Histologic findings are hyperkeratosis, necrotic keratinocytes, and vacuolar alteration of the epidermis and adnexa. A lichenoid lymphocytic infiltrate may be present.[15]

As stated above, the condition is self-limited, so no therapy is necessary. If inflammation or itching are prominent, therapy with topical corticosteroids (Classes 3–5 on nonfacial lesions) or oral antihistamines may be given.

Lichen Planus

Lichen planus (LP) is a pruritic dermatosis of unknown etiology (except in drug-induced cases) that affects the skin and mucous membranes.[39] It primarily affects individuals 30–60 years of age, with only 3%–6% of cases reported in persons under 20 years of age.

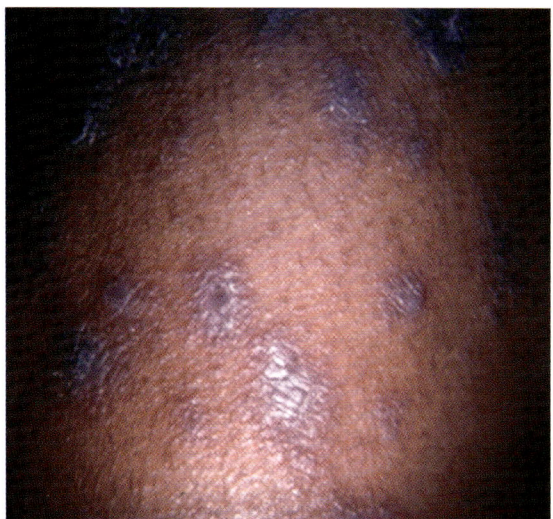

FIGURE 3.24 Hypertrophic lichen planus on the leg of a young girl.

Various patterns of clinical presentation have been noted, including classic form, actinic LP, linear LP, annular LP, mucosal LP, and hypertrophic LP. In African-Americans, the lesions have a more purple or gray color than the violaceous color that is typically described. The hypertrophic form (Figure 3.24) is somewhat more common and oral LP is less common than in Caucasian patients. Nail involvement in LP is estimated to occur in 10% of patients; however, it has been reported infrequently in children.

Clinical findings with the classic form of LP in children of color are grayish flat-topped papules of the extremities, especially inner aspects of the forearms. Patients with hypertrophic LP have verrucous lesions, usually located on the lower extremities.

Histology shows a dense lichenoid lymphohistiocytic infiltrate that obscures the dermoepidermal junction. The hypertrophic lesions show dilated, hyperplastic, and bulbous infundibula with the characteristic lichenoid lymphohistiocytic infiltrate.[15] The differential diagnoses are psoriasis, verrucae vulgaris, and aphthous ulcers (oral lesions).

Treatment options are many, each with only limited success. The options are topical and systemic corticosteroids, retinoids, azathioprine, dapsone, cyclosporine, hydroxychloroquine, oral and bath alpha interferon, PUVA, and narrow-band UVB.[40]

NEUROFIBROMATOSIS 1

Neurofibromatosis 1 (NF 1) is a neurocutaneous syndrome that is inherited in an autosomal dominant pattern. Its prevalence is approximately 1 in 4000 individuals.[41] One criterion (Table 3.2) for the diagnosis of Neurofibromatosis 1 is the presence of café-au-lait macules.[42] The lesions are flat with an even color. The term café-au-lait macules refers to the tan (coffee with cream) color of these lesions in Caucasian children. In children of color, the lesions are more darkly pigmented with a dark brown color (Figure 3.25). It is important to be aware of the differing presentation in order that the diagnosis can be made in a timely manner.

Histologic findings show increased melanin in the keratinocytes and in melanophages in the dermis. Increased macromelanosomes may be seen in the melanocytes; however, these are not diagnostic for NF 1. Differential diagnoses include junctional nevi, Mongolian spots, and McCune–Albright syndrome.

The café-au-lait macules are cutaneous markers of the disease and require no therapy.

TABLE 3.2
Neurofibromatosis 1: Diagnostic Criteria

1. Six or more café-au-lait macules >5 mm in diameter in prepubertal children, >1.5 cm in postpubertal children
2. Two or more neurofibromas *OR*
   One plexiform neuroma
3. Axillary or inguinal freckling (Crowe's sign)
4. Optic glioma
5. Two or more Lisch nodules (iris hamartomas)
6. A distinctive bony lesion — Dysplasia of the sphenoid bone
   Dysplasia or thinning of the long bone cortex
7. First-degree relative with Neurofibromatosis 1

Source: Lynch TM, Gutmann DH. *Neurol Clin* 2002; 20: 841–865. With permission.

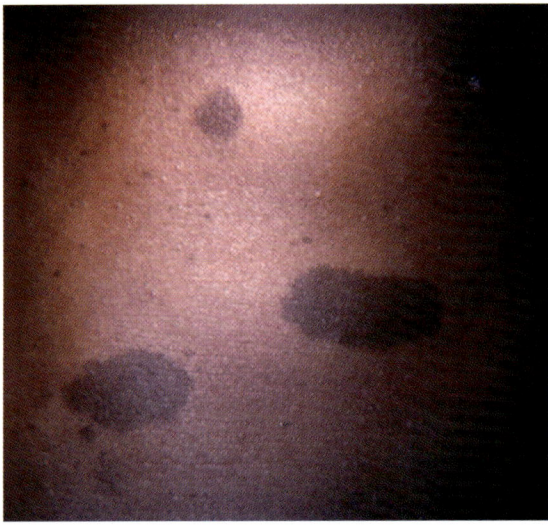

FIGURE 3.25 "Café-au-lait" macules in an African-American child with neurofibromatosis 1 show a dark brown color.

DISEASES WITH DECREASED INCIDENCE

There is a decreased incidence in African-American children noted for pediculosis capitis, scabies, acquired nevi, verrucae vulgaris, and Henoch–Schonlein purpura.[22,43,44] The reasons for the decreases in incidence are not well defined.

REFERENCES

1. Treadwell PA. Dermatoses in newborns. *Am Fam Physician* 1997; 56: 443–450.
2. Mengesha YM, Bennett ML. Pustular skin disorders: diagnosis and treatment. *Am J Clin Dermatol* 2002; 3: 389–400.
3. Buckley DA, Munn SE, Higgins EM. Neonatal eosinophilic pustular folliculitis. *Clin Exp Dermatol* 2001; 26: 251–255.
4. Leung AK, Kao CP. Extensive mongolian spots with involvement of the scalp. *Pediatr Dermatol* 1999; 16: 371–372.

5. Leung AK, Kao CP, Lee TK. Mongolian spots with involvement of the temporal area. *Int J Dermatol* 2001; 40: 288–289.
6. Grimes PE. The safety and efficacy of salicylic acid chemical peels in darker racial-ethnic groups. *Dermatol Surg* 1999; 25: 18–22.
7. Jacyk WK. Adapalene gel 0.1% for topical treatment of acne vulgaris in African patients. *Cutis* 2001; 68(Suppl): 48–54.
8. Truong AL, Esterly NB. Atypical acropustulosis in infancy. *Int J Dermatol* 1997; 36: 688–691.
9. Braun-Falco M, Stachowitz S, Schnopp C, Ring J, Abeck D. Infantile acropustulosis successfully controlled with topical corticosteroids under damp tubular retention bandages. *Acta Derm Venereol* 2001; 81: 140–141.
10. Mulinari-Brenner F, Bergfeld WF. Hair loss: an overview. *Dermatol Nurs* 2001; 13: 269–272, 277–278.
11. Shapiro J, Wiseman M, Lui H. Practical management of hair loss. *Can Fam Physician* 2000; 46: 1469–1477.
12. Ghannoum M, Isham N, Hajjeh R, Cano M, Al-Hasawi F, Yearick D, et al. Tinea capitis in Cleveland: survey of elementary school students. *J Am Acad Dermatol* 2003; 48: 189–193.
13. Sharma V, Silverberg NB, Howard R, Tran CT, Laude TA, Frieden IJ. Do hair care practices affect the acquisition of tinea capitis? A case-control study. *Arch Pediatr Adolesc Med* 2001; 155: 818–821.
14. Neuhaus IM, Ramos-Caro FA, Hassanein AM. Hypopigmented mycosis fungoides in childhood and adolescence. *Pediatr Dermatol* 2000; 17: 403–406.
15. Hurwitz RM, Hood AF. *Pathology of the Skin: Atlas of Clinical-Pathological Correlation*. Appleton and Lange, Connecticut, 1998.
16. Qari MS, Li N, Demierre MF. Hypopigmented mycosis fungoides: case reports and literature review. *J Cutan Med Surg* 2000; 4: 142–148.
17. Boon SJ, McCurdy D. Childhood systemic lupus erythematosus. *Pediatr Ann* 2002; 31: 407–417.
18. Van Gysel D, de Waard-van der Spek FB, Oranje AP. Childhood discoid lupus erythematosus: report of five new cases and review of the literature. *J Eur Acad Dermatol Venereol* 2002; 16: 143–147.
19. Burch JM, Lee LA, Weston WL. Neonatal lupus erythematosus. *Dermatol Nurs* 2002; 14: 157–160.
20. Martin V, Lee LA, Askanase AD, Katholi M, Buyon JP. Long-term followup of children with neonatal lupus and their unaffected siblings. *Arthritis Rheum* 2002; 46: 2377–2383.
21. Chang RK. Epidemiologic characteristics of children hospitalized for Kawasaki disease in California. *Pediatr Infect Dis J* 2002; 21: 1150–1155.
22. Gardner-Medwin JM, Dolezalova P, Cummins C, Southwood TR. Incidence of Henoch-Schonlein purpura, Kawasaki disease, and rare vasculitides in children of different ethnic origins. *Lancet* 2002; 360: 1197–1202.
23. Ben-Gashir MA, Hay RJ. Reliance on erythema scores may mask severe atopic dermatitis in black children compared with their white counterparts. *Br J Dermatol* 2002; 147: 920–925.
24. Connolly C, Bikowski J. *Dermatological Atlas of Black Skin*. Merit Publishing International, Florida, 1998.
25. Cheigh NH. Managing a common disorder in children: Atopic dermatitis. *J Pediatr Health Care* 2003; 17: 84–88.
26. Sator PG, Schmidt JB, Honigsmann H. Comparison of epidermal hydration and skin surface lipids in healthy individuals and in patients with atopic dermatitis. *J Am Acad Dermatol* 2003; 48: 352–358.
27. Sharma V, Beyer DJ, Paruthi S, Nopper AJ. Prominent pruritic periumbilical papules: allergic contact dermatitis to nickel. *Pediatr Dermatol* 2002; 19: 106–109.
28. Ehrlich A, Kucenic M, Belsito DV. Role of body piercing in the induction of metal allergies. *Am J Contact Dermatitis* 2001; 12: 151–155.
29. Lee DJ, Eichenfield LF. Atopic, contact, and seborrheic dermatitis in adolescents. *Adolesc Med* 2001; 12: vi, 269–283.
30. Crutchfield CE III. Pimecrolimus: a new treatment for seborrheic dermatitis. *Cutis* 2002; 70: 207–208.
31. Bernardin RM, Ritter SE, Murchland MR. Papular pityriasis rosea. *Cutis* 2002; 70: 51–55.
32. Sharma PK, Yadav TP, Gautam RK, Taneja N, Satyanarayana L. Erythromycin in pityriasis rosea: a double-blind, placebo-controlled clinical trial. *J Am Acad Dermatol* 2000; 42(Pt 1): 241–244.
33. Ritter SE, Bryan MG, Elston DM. Photo quiz. Trichrome tinea versicolor. *Cutis* 2002; 70: 92: 121–122.
34. Farschian M, Yaghoobi R, Samadi K. Fluconazole versus ketoconazole in the treatment of tinea versicolor. *J Dermatol Treat* 2002; 13: 73–76.

35. Kontos AP, Cusack CA, Chaffins M, Lim HW. Polymorphous light eruption in African Americans: pinpoint papular variant. *Photodermatol Photoimmunol Photomed* 2002; 18: 303–306.
36. Boonstra HE, van Weelden H, Toonstra J, van Vloten WA. Polymorphous light eruption: a clinical, photobiologic, and follow-up study of 110 patients. *J Am Acad Dermatol* 2000; 42: 199–207.
37. Ro YS, Shin YI. A case of lichen striatus following Blaschko lines. *Cutis* 2001; 67: 31–32, 34.
38. Kavak A, Kutluay L. Nail involvement in lichen striatus. *Pediatr Dermatol* 2002; 19: 136–138.
39. Handa S, Sahoo B. Childhood lichen planus: a study of 87 cases. *Int J Dermatol* 2002; 41: 423–427.
40. Taneja A, Taylor CR. Narrow-band UVB for lichen planus treatment. *Int J Dermatol* 2002; 41: 282–283.
41. Kandt RS. Tuberous sclerosis complex and neurofibromatosis type 1: the two most common neurocutaneous diseases. *Neurol Clin* 2002; 20: 941–964.
42. Lynch TM, Gutmann DH. Neurofibromatosis 1. *Neurol Clin* 2002; 20: 841–865.
43. Child FJ, Fuller LC, Higgins EM, Du Vivier AW. A study of the spectrum of skin disease occurring in a black population in south-east London. *Br J Dermatol* 1999; 141: 512–517.
44. Schachner LA, Hansen RC. *Pediatric Dermatology.* 2nd ed. Churchill Livingstone, New York, 1995.

4 Hair and Scalp Disorders in Pigmented Skins

Amy J. McMichael and Valerie D. Callender

INTRODUCTION

The African-American patient with a hair disorder is often a multifaceted enigma, even for the seasoned dermatologist. The chief complaint may be a problem with the hair, but the layers of hair care history leading up to the visit are complicated by the litany of attempts at self-treatment as well as the underlying coarse and curled nature of the hair. This chapter will attempt to uncover and explain each layer of the problems that may be encountered with patients of color who have coarse and tightly-curled hair. The composite parts of the hair disorder must be understood before a diagnosis can be rendered, but treatment of the total patient is always the goal of the dermatologist. Once the various parts of the hair disorder are clear, an overarching diagnosis and treatment plan should be offered.

Important structural characteristics of the African-American hair shaft include an elliptical or flattened shape in cross section and spiral or tight curls in its tertiary structure. Within the black race, significant variations are seen as well. In most African-Americans, the curled hair does not emanate from a straight follicle. Instead, the follicle where the hair is formed is just as curved as the hair itself.[1] Biochemical hair structures from different racial populations have been compared using various techniques and no biochemical differences have as yet been elucidated.[2] Hair density varies widely in patients of all races. One recent study suggests there is a decreased hair density on the scalp of adult African-Americans as compared to adult white Americans.[3] In a retrospective review of 4-mm scalp biopsies from healthy scalp skin, Sperling[3] compared the total number of follicles, terminal follicles, vellus follicles, terminal anagen hairs, and terminal telogen hairs in biopsies from 22 African-Americans and 12 whites and previously reported data on whites. He found significantly lower total hair density, total number of terminal follicles, and terminal anagen hairs in the biopsies from African-Americans as compared to those from the whites. Although this information is of interest, a larger sample size with inclusion of African-Americans of all ages and scalp locations would be necessary to prove that these density data are correct.

In this chapter, the inflammatory, nonscarring disorders will be discussed, and then scarring processes will be considered. The final disorders to be covered are the hair shaft abnormalities. Treatment options will be discussed for each entity with a therapeutic ladder offered, when possible, to help the reader choose the most appropriate option with progressively invasive therapies. Each entity will be discussed in terms of the clinical presentation, pathophysiology, differential diagnosis (Table 4.1), triggering factors, and, finally, treatment options.

BASIC PRINCIPLES

Relatively little is known about how the structure of African-American hair impacts function. Noted hair characteristics of African-American hair include the coiled shape of the hair fiber resembling a twisted rod.[4] Bernard has performed *in vitro* experiments comparing the growth of curly and straight hair.[5] He found that curled hairs dissected out of the scalp and placed into culture continued

TABLE 4.1
Differential Diagnosis of Scalp Disorders

Scalp flaking with little or no hair loss	Seborrheic dermatitis
	Psoriasis vulgaris
	Atopic dermatitis
	Allergic contact dermatitis
	Irritant contact dermatitis
	Tinea capitis
	Early chronic cutaneous lupus
	Dermatomyositis
Scalp pustules or cysts, no hair loss	Tinea capitis
	Uncomplicated folliculitis
Scalp pustules or cysts with hair loss	Folliculitis decalvans
	Acne keloidalis nuchae
	Dissecting cellulitis
	Tinea capitis
	Bacterial infection
Hair loss with scarring/little inflammation	Traction alopecia
	Central centrifugal cicatricial alopecia
	Folliculitis decalvans
	Sarcoidosis
Hair Breakage	Hair shaft defect
	Pruritus from seborrheic dermatitis, atopic dermatitis, etc.
	Tinea capitis
	Weathering/traumatic fragility of hair shaft

to grow in curled fashion, suggesting that the shape of the hair may be intrinsically programmed by the lower half of the hair follicle with or without the usual dermal environment. No true structural or chemical composition differences have been found in African-American hair vs. Caucasian and Asian hair, but there is an elliptical shape of African hair in diameter with a decreased combability and a decreased tensile strength as compared to Caucasian hair. There also appears to be less moisture in the hair shaft of African patients than in Caucasians. Franbourg et al. found that African hair shows the greatest percentage of cross-sectional variability compared with Caucasian and Asian hair.[6]

INFLAMMATORY SCALP DISORDERS WITH FLAKING

Many African-American patients present to the dermatologist with a chief complaint of itching and/or flaking of the scalp. There are many home remedies and alternative treatments utilized by lay persons to control pruritus and scale that may or may not be helpful symptomatically. The most common diagnoses causing these symptoms are seborrheic dermatitis, atopic dermatitis, and psoriasis. A few less common diagnoses are irritant contact dermatitis, allergic contact dermatitis, and tinea capitis. Very rarely, dermatomyositis or lupus erythematosus may cause flaking and pruritus of the scalp without a significant number of other skin or systemic signs.

SEBORRHEIC DERMATITIS

Seborrheic dermatitis is a common, chronic papulosquamous disorder that affects sebaceous-rich areas of the body, including specific areas of the scalp, face, and body. The condition affects approximately 2%–5% of the population and occurs in individuals of all ages, but the true incidence of seborrheic dermatitis of the scalp may be higher in African-American females due to the varying

Hair and Scalp Disorders in Pigmented Skins

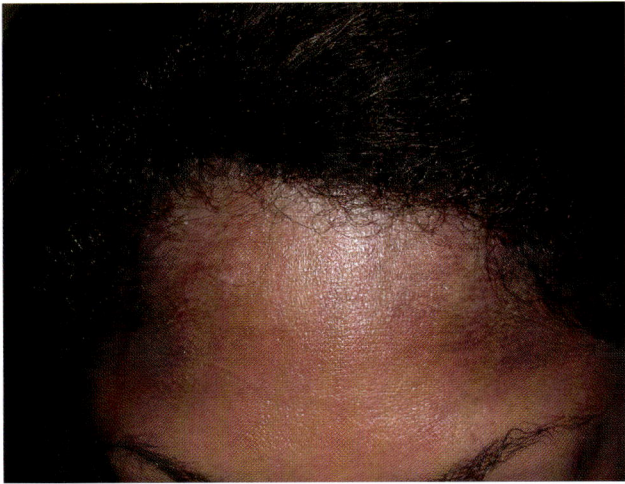

FIGURE 4.1 Young woman with mild, partially treated seborrheic dermatitis with hypopigmentation.

degree of hair-washing frequency in this population.[1] An increased incidence and severity of seborrheic dermatitis is often seen in patients with HIV disease. The etiology of seborrheic dermatitis is unknown; however, the yeast *Malassezia furfur* (*Pityrosporum ovale*) may play a role in the development of the disease.[7,8] Genetic, environmental, and immunological factors also play a role in the course and severity of this disease.

In infancy, seborrheic dermatitis is referred to as "cradle cap" and presents as thick, yellow, greasy adherent scales on the scalp. Other areas may be involved, such as the face and intertriginous areas, including the diaper area. The extent of involvement may be localized or generalized in this population. The skin eruption has been described as erythematous and scaly, but in pigmented skin erythema may not be present; rather, the skin lesions appear hypopigmented or hyperpigmented.

Adults with seborrheic dermatitis typically present with erythema, dyspigmentation, and diffuse scaling of the scalp (Figure 4.1). Common complaints include itching, dry scalp, hair breakage, and hair loss along the anterior hair line. When the disease state is severe, lichen simplex chronicus can ensue from chronic scratching. The lichen simplex chronicus may be localized with minimal skin thickening and hair breakage, or it may be diffuse with extreme thickening of the scalp skin and severe breakage of hair. Differential diagnosis includes psoriasis, contact dermatitis, and tinea capitis. Silverberg et al. performed a retrospective analysis of positive cases of tinea capitis and reported that 11.4% (9 patients) were adult African-Americans with tinea capitis.[9] The majority of these patients were women. The clinical presentations varied — all patients demonstrated mild alopecia, whereas seven presented with seborrheic-type scale, two with black dot, one with alopecia areata-type hair loss, and one with a kerion. This study demonstrates the importance of ruling out tinea capitis in African-American adult females who present with a scaly scalp.

Seborrheic dermatitis may also extend to nonscalp areas. Characteristic locations on the face include the hairline, forehead, eyebrows, eyelashes, and nasolabial folds. The ears and chest may be involved as well. Males with seborrheic dermatitis may have involvement of the mustache and beard areas. Hypopigmented or hyperpigmented annular lesions are common in pigmented skin, and must be differentiated from tinea versicolor, sarcoidosis, syphilis, and cutaneous T-cell lymphoma.

Therapy

One of the first therapies to consider in the treatment of seborrheic dermatitis is the selection of a shampoo. There are various shampoos available, both over the counter (OTC) and prescription strength. These include shampoos containing selenium sulfide, tar, salicylic acid, ketoconazole[10,11]

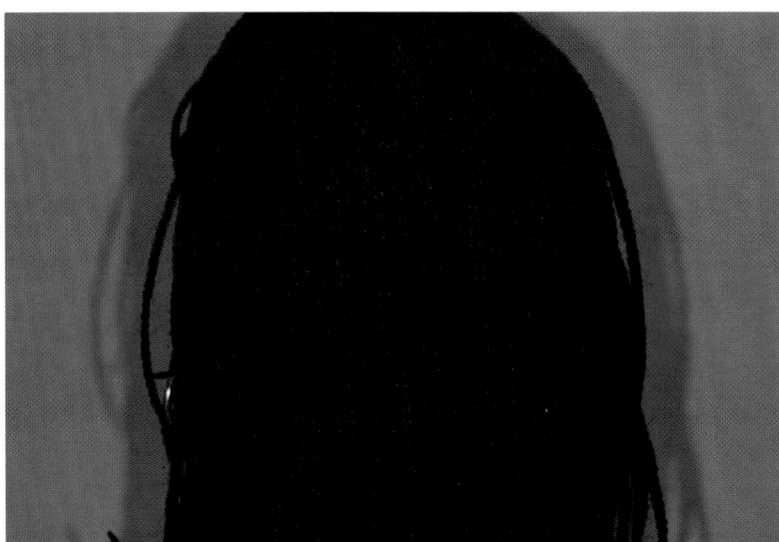

FIGURE 4.2 African-American woman with individual braids.

and zinc pyrithione,[12] fluocinolone acetonide, ciclopirox, and urea. Not all shampoos are appropriate for use with coarse and kinky hair. For example, OTC antidandruff shampoos containing tar, selenium sulfide, and salicylic acid may be too harsh on chemically treated hair. They can cause excessive dryness and hair breakage, especially if used daily as instructed on many OTC labels. Shampoos containing zinc pyrithione and mid-potency steroids are alternative agents for African-American women who chemically straighten their hair, and these appear to be well tolerated. Fluocinolone acetonide shampoo can be helpful, especially in the early inflammatory stages of seborrheic dermatitis. Hair-washing frequency differs greatly in patients of color. Males with short hair tend to wash their hair in the shower daily. In contrast, if the hair is braided or in dreadlocks (Figures 4.2–4.4), the frequency of shampooing may vary from every 2–3 days to once a week. Because many African-American women chemically straighten their hair, the frequency of hair washing may range from twice a week to every 2 weeks. Commonly the hair washing is performed weekly at the hair salon rather than at home. Therefore, a detailed history must be obtained from the patient prior to initiating therapy. The key to the successful management of seborrheic dermatitis in patients of color is understanding the diverse hairstyles and unique hair care practices of this population, including the frequency of hair washing for that particular patient and the incorporation of the appropriate therapeutic shampoo into the patient's normal routine.

Ethnic hair care products are also important in the management of seborrheic dermatitis and should be discussed with patients. Deep hair conditioning after shampooing and the daily use of a leave-in conditioner are both essential components, particularly in African-American females. These two steps can help to decrease hair dryness and fragility associated with the use of antidandruff and antiseborrheic shampoos. Conditioners that contain lanolin and its derivatives should be avoided because these additives have been associated with worsening seborrheic dermatitis as well as comedogenesis.

Topical corticosteroid therapy is commonly used for the treatment of moderate to severe seborrheic dermatitis of the scalp. There are multiple agents and formulations that are available.[13,14] George et al. demonstrated the cosmetic acceptability of the foam vehicle in an African-American population with various hairstyles and hair care practices.[15] For example, black women with chemically relaxed hair may prefer an oil- or foam-based topical corticosteroid vehicle rather than an ointment to allow a more cosmetically appealing hairstyle. However, natural hairstyles, such as an "afro" (Figure 4.5), or thermally straightened hair ("hot comb" styling) may benefit by the

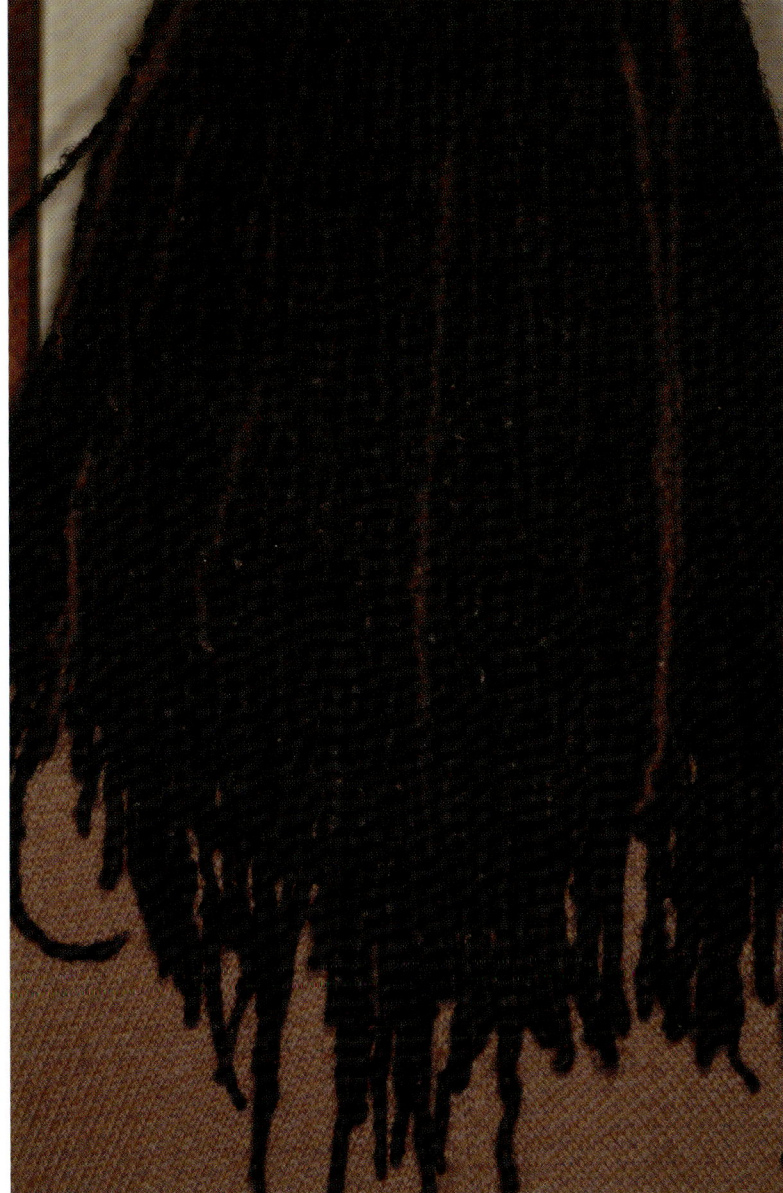

FIGURE 4.3 African-American woman with dreadlocks.

application of an oil or ointment-based vehicle rather than a solution, lotion, or foam-based vehicle, which contains water or alcohol. These latter agents may reverse hot comb–straightened hair to its natural curly state.

Psoriasis Vulgaris

Psoriasis is a chronic papulosquamous disease that commonly affects the scalp, extensor surfaces of the body, and nails. The true incidence of psoriasis in the black population is unknown, although Obasi reported an incidence of 0.8% of patients seen in a Nigerian clinic.[16] Scalp involvement occurs in approximately 50% of psoriasis patients and involvement increases with the duration of the disease.

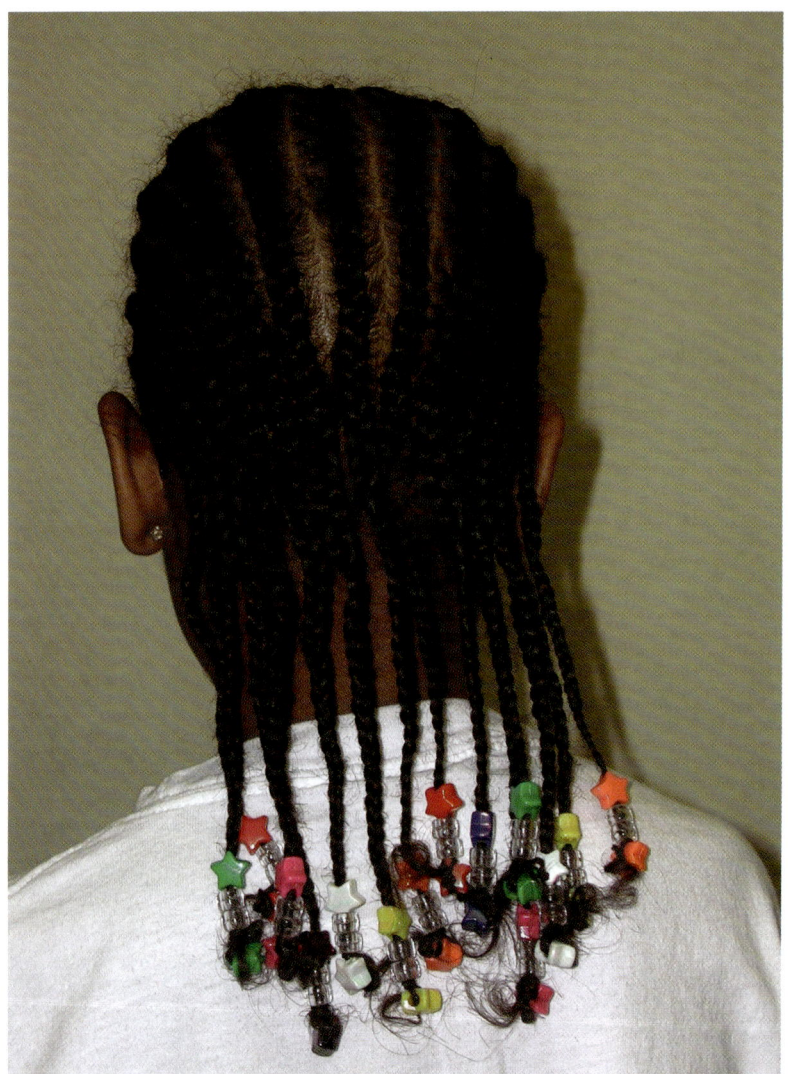

FIGURE 4.4 African-American girl with corn rows.

The characteristic lesion of scalp psoriasis is described as a well demarcated, circumscribed, scaly, erythematous plaque. The number may vary from one isolated lesion to several areas throughout the scalp. Similar to seborrheic dermatitis of the scalp, psoriatic plaques in pigmented skin may not appear erythematous but instead may appear violaceous, hyperpigmented, or hypopigmented (Figures 4.6 and 4.7). Common symptoms include itching, pain, and bleeding. In African-American patients, there may be significant lichenification with a lichen simplex chronicus appearance of the scalp lesions. Hair may be broken in the affected areas secondary to patient manipulation of the inflamed plaques (Figure 4.8).

Therapy

The shampoos used for the treatment of scalp psoriasis usually contain keratolytic agents, such as salicylic acid and tar derivatives, which may cause excessive dryness and subsequent hair breakage in patients with coarse and curly hair. Similar to seborrheic dermatitis of the scalp, special attention

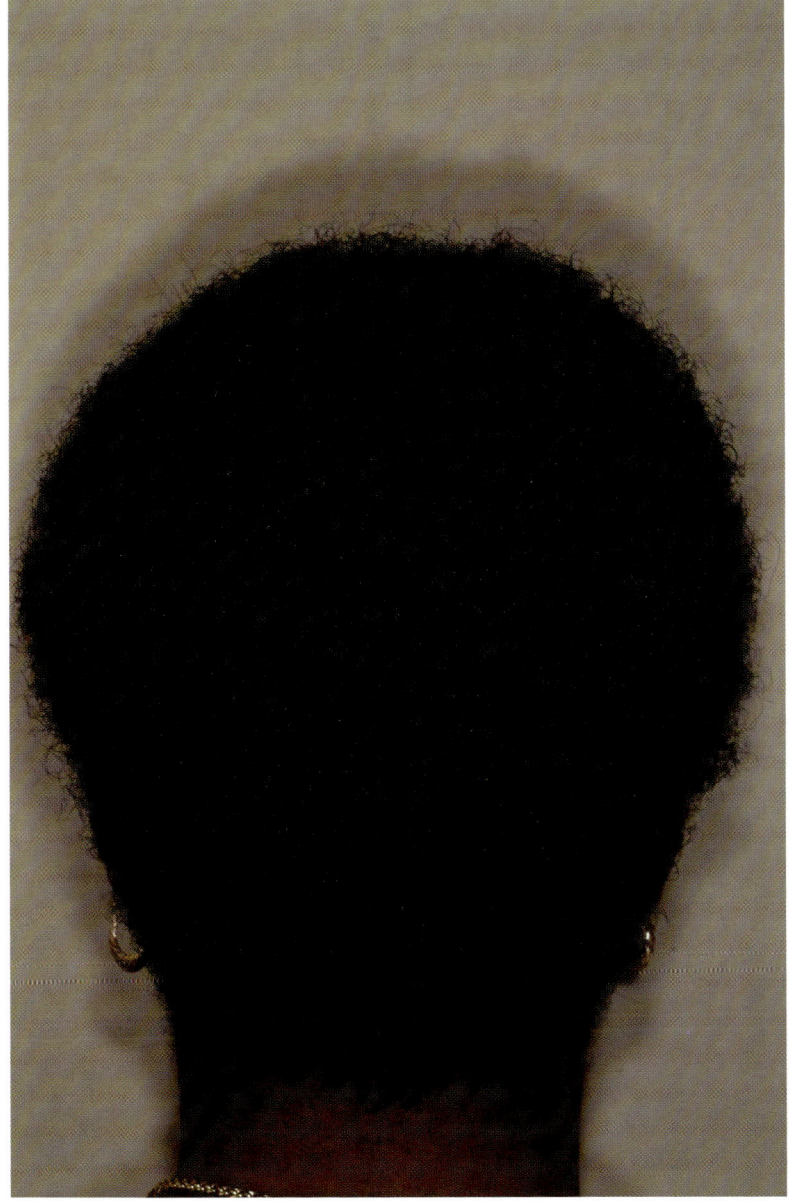

FIGURE 4.5 African-American woman with untreated hairstyle known as an "afro."

must be given to the appropriate selection of the shampoo, the frequency of hair washing, and the hair style of the patient.

The management and treatment of psoriasis of the scalp in the male patient with coarse and curly hair is essentially the same as in Caucasians. The treatment in black women is more complex and can pose a challenge to the physician. Topical treatment options for scalp psoriasis include corticosteroids, salicylic acid, tar derivatives, calcipotriene, tazarotene, and urea. The use of topical immunomodulators such as tacrolimus and pimecrolimus in psoriasis has been reported,[17,18] but their use in the scalp has yet to be determined. Intralesional corticosteroid therapy administered every 2–4 weeks for resistant plaques may be highly therapeutic in some patients. Much like the treatment for seborrheic dermatitis, treatment with alternating shampoos should be offered, keeping

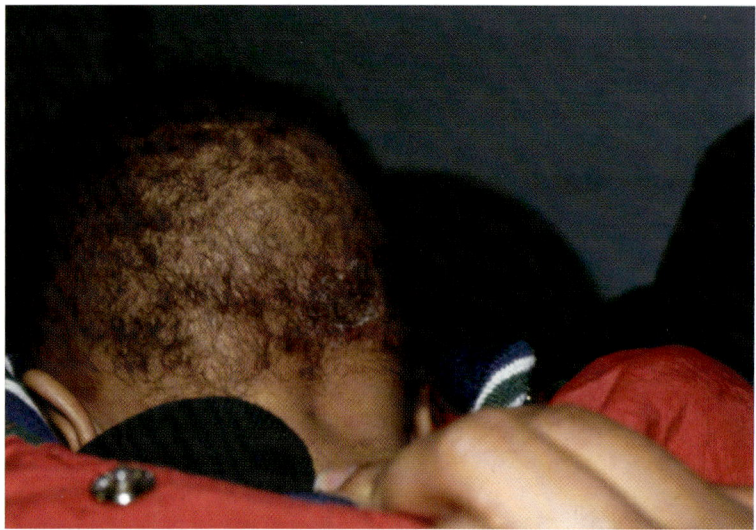

FIGURE 4.6 Sebo-psoriasis in an erythematous, scaling plaque in a toddler.

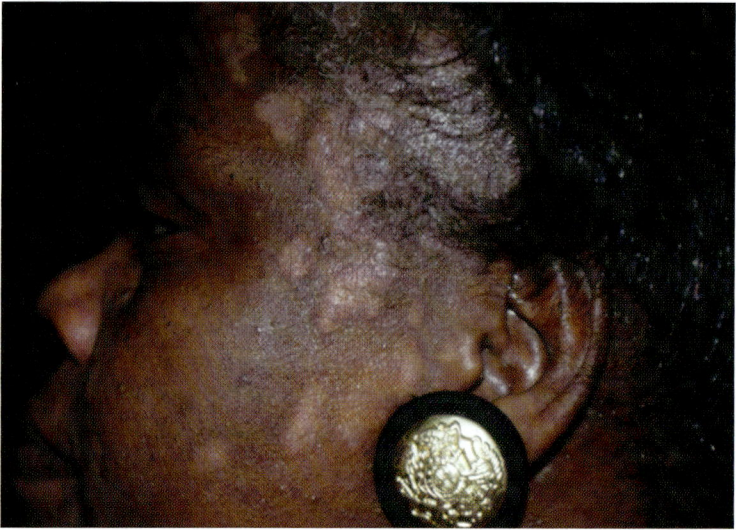

FIGURE 4.7 Young woman with sebo-psoriasis plaques in scalp extending to face with hypopigmentation.

a once- or twice-weekly washing regimen. All patients should be instructed to use moisturizing conditioners because the antidandruff shampoos are often drying to the hair shaft. The patient should be consulted regarding the choice of vehicle for all topical treatments because some patients will prefer an oil base, whereas others will prefer an ointment or lotion.

Atopic Dermatitis

Atopic dermatitis is a genetic eczematous condition of the skin, commonly seen in all ages. Although more clinically apparent on the face and body, scalp involvement may occur. There are certain clinical implications of atopic dermatitis of the scalp in black female patients with chemically straightened hair. Scalp pruritus and chemical burns to the scalp can be presenting complaints to the dermatologist, primarily due to the decreased barrier function in active lesions.

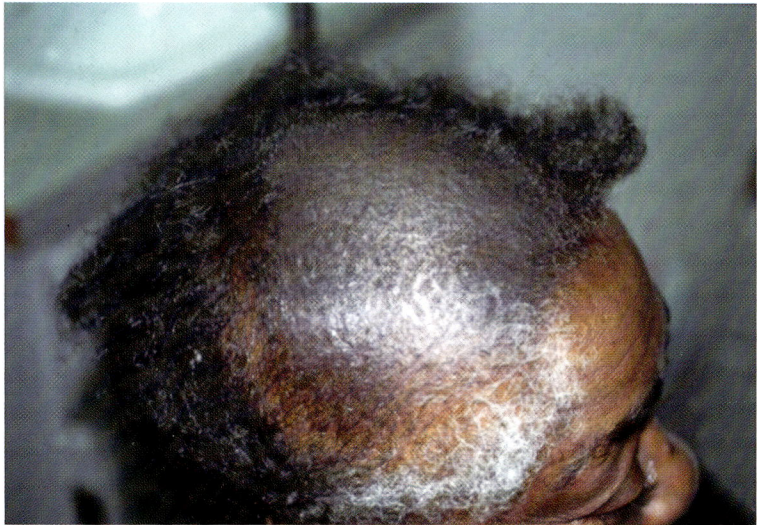

FIGURE 4.8 Lichen simplex chronicus in an elderly woman who has pruritus of the scalp.

The scalp lesions of atopic dermatitis are similar to the other areas of the body and present as scaly, erythematous or hyperpigmented, ill-defined patches of skin. In children, these patches frequently occur on the occipital area of the scalp and posterior neck. Because of the scalp involvement, a fungal culture should be obtained in these patients in order to distinguish atopic dermatitis from a fungal infection of the scalp. In adults, the lesions may present as lichenified plaques with scale and excoriation around the periphery of the hair line. Differential diagnosis may include tinea capitis, psoriasis, seborrheic dermatitis, or allergic contact dermatitis. Often, the easiest way to diagnose atopic dermatitis in the scalp is by the classic lichenified, symmetric lesions on the face, antecubital, and popliteal fossa.

Therapy

Mild shampoos that are fragrance free and/or preservative free and topical corticosteroids are the recommended treatment for atopic dermatitis of the scalp. Oral antihistamines are recommended for pruritus. The topical immunomodulators (tacrolimus or pimecrolimus) may also be used as steroid-sparing agents in the treatment of atopic dermatitis. African-American females with scalp involvement should avoid hair chemicals until active skin lesions resolve. The use of nonirritating, occlusive agents such as petrolatum should be recommended in these patients to protect the scalp prior to the application of any hair chemicals.

CONTACT DERMATITIS

Contact dermatitis of the scalp may be either irritant or allergic in nature. The etiology is usually associated with the use of hair cosmetics. This form of dermatitis occurs more commonly in adult females whose frequency of use of hair care products may influence the incidence of this condition.[19]

Irritant Contact Dermatitis

Hair relaxers used to chemically straighten black hair may result in a chemical burn on the scalp, ears, neck, or face (Figure 4.9). If left on the skin for an extended period of time, an irritant contact dermatitis may occur. These hair relaxers are alkaline products with a pH of 10–13 and are thus extremely caustic to the skin. Other reported complications of relaxer use include a primary irritant

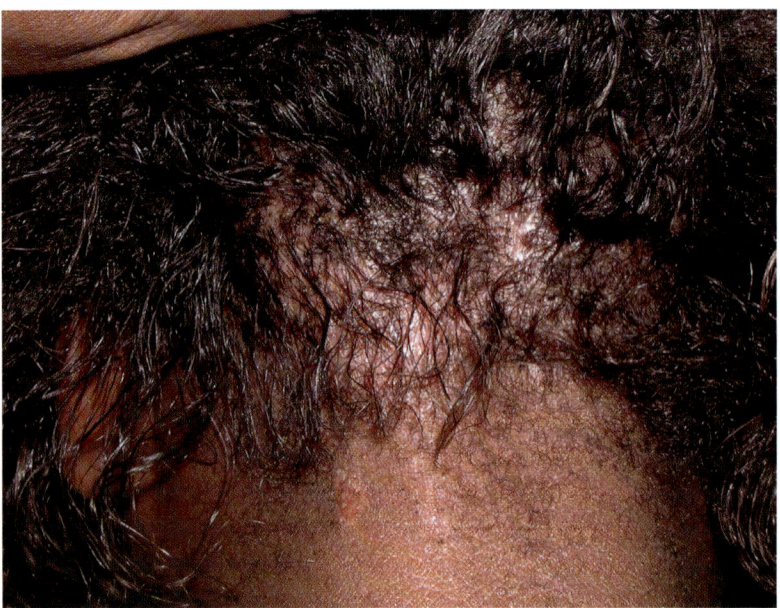

FIGURE 4.9 Irritant contact dermatitis in the occiput with diffuse hair breakage.

contact dermatitis of the skin to relaxers[20] and fibrosis and inflammation of the scalp associated with alopecia.[21]

If irritant contact dermatitis is suspected, it is imperative for the patient to stop all unnecessary hair cosmetics. Fragrance- and preservative-free shampoo and conditioner should be recommended until the culprit is found. Eliciting historical information regarding the use of all products is important because many patients do not report the many over-the-counter products that they use regularly.

Allergic Contact Dermatitis

Allergic contact dermatitis involving the scalp is frequently associated with the use of hair dyes, which contain para-phenylene diamine. Clinical examinations in African-Americans reveal hyperpigmented, lichenified plaques and, rarely, vesicles, in contrast to Caucasian patients, who often have more vesicular changes (Figure 4.10). There are likely many products in addition to para-phenylene diamine that can cause allergic reactions of the scalp in all populations, including African-Americans. Other than reactions to hair dye, little has been written on the subject of allergic contact reactions in the scalp. Because it is well known that allergic contact dermatitis can be fairly easily induced for treatment of alopecia areata,[22] more thought should be given to allergic responses to other products used on the scalp. There are reports of contact reactions to hair glue,[23] zinc pyrithione,[24] and minoxidil,[25] but few other scalp allergens are described. Part of the reason for few allergen reports may be that it is uncommon for other agents to cause a contact allergic reaction or that this reaction goes undiagnosed because of low suspicion. It is important to suspect contact allergy when a patient with typical scaling and pruritus of the scalp does not respond to typical anti-inflammatory treatment. A detailed history of hair care products and/or patch-testing may be warranted in recalcitrant patients.

Tinea Capitis

Tinea capitis is a major problem for school-aged children, especially African-Americans. The disease clinically can appear as delicate scaling of the scalp with or without alopecia, frank circular

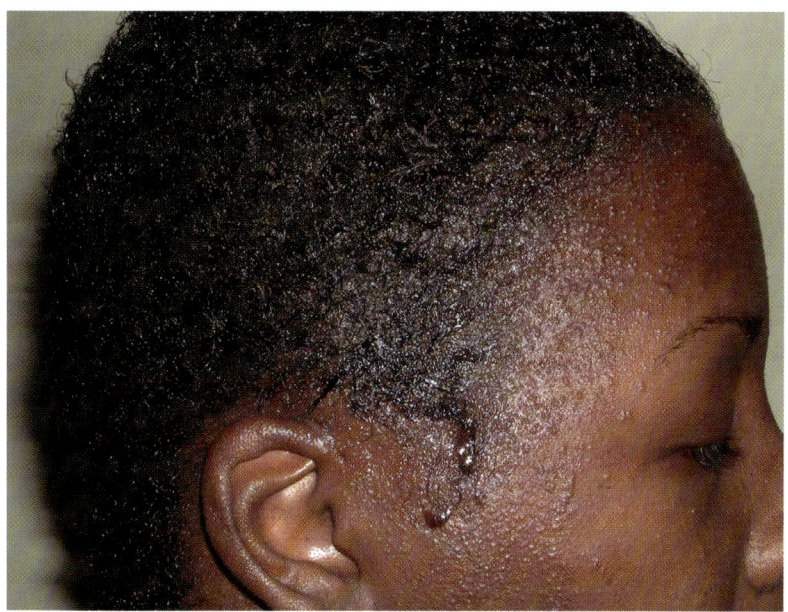

FIGURE 4.10 Severe allergic contact dermatitis in a young woman.

areas of alopecia with hair broken at the level of the scalp, and kerions (Figures 4.11 and 4.12). In general, the disease process is less common in adults, but there is an increased prevalence of tinea capitis in African-American adults. Silverberg et al. found that of nine adults with tinea capitis, seven were African-American.[9] According to data from the National Ambulatory Medical Care Survey (NAMCS), a sample survey of hospital-based offices, tinea capitis occurs twice as often in males as in females and is 23 times more common in African-Americans than in non-African-Americans.[26] The reason for the increased incidence in the black adult population has not been

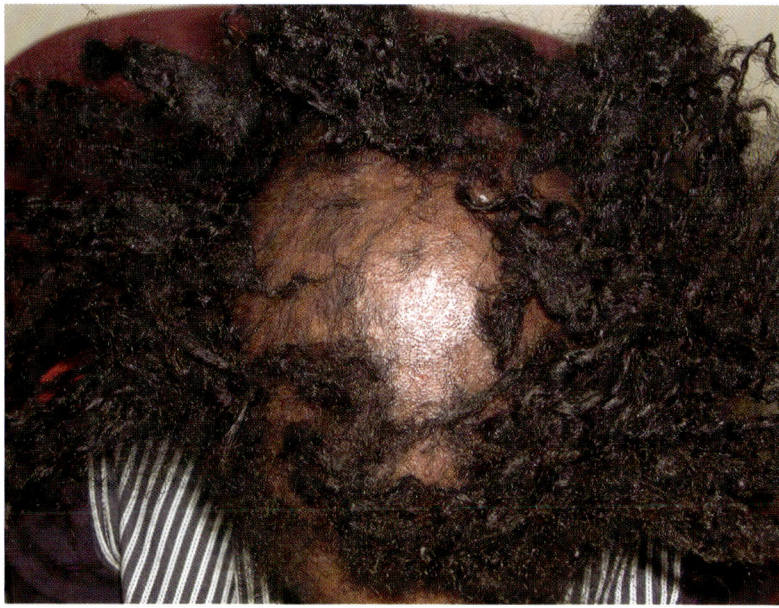

FIGURE 4.11 Tinea capitis with severe hair loss in a child.

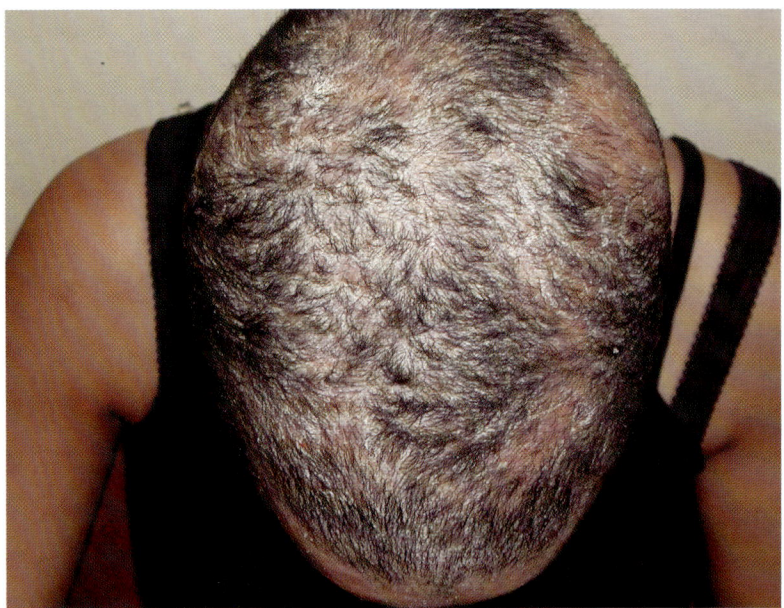

FIGURE 4.12 Severe tinea capitis with hair loss and breakage and diffuse scale.

explained by any epidemiologic data so far.[27] Sharma et al. have shown that hair products are not related to the development of tinea capitis.[28] This group performed a case-control study of 66 pediatric patients with and without tinea capitis to determine the association of hair care practices with tinea capitis in children. Hairstyling, frequency of washing, use of oils or grease, and other hair care practices were shown not to be associated with the presence of tinea capitis in this study.

The diagnosis of tinea capitis in adults is difficult unless the dermatologist has a high index of suspicion when patients present with scaling and hair breakage and there is no response to typical anti-inflammatory treatments. The diagnosis of tinea capitis can be made by potassium hydroxide (KOH) prep or fungal culture. Wood's lamp is less helpful for diagnosis in recent times because of the pathogen shift in the United States from *Microsporum canis* to *Trichophyton tonsurans*, which does not fluoresce. Differential diagnosis includes alopecia areata, in which exclamation point hairs can be confused with the broken hairs of tinea capitis, and trichotillomania, in which the broken hairs from compulsive pulling resemble the infected hairs of tinea. The KOH and culture help to distinguish tinea capitis from these two entities. If these tests are negative and tinea is still suspected, a scalp biopsy should be performed.

Therapy

Treatment of tinea capitis in children has not changed for many years. The standard of care for this population is oral griseofulvin for 2 months in uncomplicated cases. In adults, other choices include oral terbinafine, itraconazole, or fluconazole, but dosage regimens are not well worked out for these medications in tinea capitis.

LUPUS ERYTHEMATOSUS AND DERMATOMYOSITIS

Lupus Erythematosus

The importance of lupus in the African-American population is demonstrated by the increased incidence of the disease in this population. In one study, crude incidence rates of systemic lupus erythematosus were 0.4 for white males, 3.5 for white females, 0.7 for African-American males, and 9.2 for African-American females.[29] Hair loss that occurs with systemic lupus erythematosus (SLE) can be alopecia areata, telogen effluvium, or scarring in nature. It has been reported that between 24% and 70% of patients with SLE have some form of alopecia.[30] The best way to diagnose the type or types of hair loss occurring in patients with lupus of any kind is to perform a biopsy of the affected scalp area, because more than one type of hair loss may occur in the same area of the scalp.

Cicatricial alopecia is the usual presentation of scalp lesions in chronic cutaneous lupus erythematosus (CCLE), but there can be an overlap of discoid lesions in patients with systemic lupus. One study found 34% of 89 patients with CCLE suffered from scarring alopecia.[31] In the case of CCLE, hair stem cell failure is due to the inflammation associated with the disease and destruction of the follicular stem cells. Approximately one quarter of SLE patients will develop CCLE lesions at some point in the course of their disease, and it was shown in one study that 60% of 80 patients with discoid lesions developed lesions of the scalp, which usually resulted in scarring alopecia.[32,33] This may mean that up to 15% of patients with SLE may develop scarring alopecia. Treatment usually consists of topical and intralesional corticosteroids for localized disease. Antimalarial agents, dapsone, and methotrexate can be added for more extensive disease.[34] Rarely, thalidomide can be used to abate progression of severe scarring disease.[35]

Dermatomyositis

Although there is no increased prevalence of dermatomyositis in African-Americans, this is an important scalp diagnosis that should not be overlooked in the discussion of scalp disorders that can appear scaly. Dermatomyositis with scalp involvement is not rare, but it is uncommon to have significant dermatomyositis in the scalp without other systemic or skin signs. Even if the skin and systemic signs are subtle, one may still note diffuse scaling in the scalp associated with erythema and, occasionally, associated hair loss. When dermatomyositis does occur in the scalp, there is usually significant pruritus as well as pain associated with a fine, loose, and adherent scale, erythematous plaques, and alopecia. The diagnosis is made clinically from the association with other signs of cutaneous dermatomyositis or by biopsy of the scalp in association with diagnostic skin and systemic findings. In patients with intractable scalp discomfort out of proportion to what is seen clinically, the diagnosis of dermatomyositis should be suspected. Callen and Kasteler reported on a case series of 14 patients with scalp involvement of their dermatomyositis.[36] Five of these patients were diagnosed with seborrheic dermatitis or scalp psoriasis before progression of their disease or before tissue diagnosis of dermatomyositis, suggesting that scalp symptoms may be the presenting complaint in patients with dermatomyositis.

The treatment of scalp dermatomyositis is symptomatic. Often, the scalp improves with systemic treatment of the muscle involvement of the disease. When systemic corticosteroids are not employed (as with the lack of muscle involvement), topical agents may be offered. Topical steroid solutions, foams, or shampoos can improve symptoms in male patients and patients with thin, fine, or straight hair. In patients with thick or coarse hair, topical ointments, lotions, or oils may be preferred. If there is significant adherent scale, urea or salicylic acid–based treatments may be necessary to thin scalp scales enough for other treatments to be efficacious.

INFLAMMATORY DISORDERS WITH PUSTULES OR CYSTS

Both African-American men and women seek dermatologic management of many scalp disorders that are painful and/or pruritic because of the involvement of pustules or cysts. Even young children are noted to have pustules as part of scalp conditions that must be managed by a dermatologist. The most common scalp disorders that present with these symptoms include uncomplicated folliculitis, folliculitis decalvans, dissecting cellulitis, and acne keloidalis nuchae. These disorders can occur alone or be complicated by significant hair loss and/or hypertrophic and keloidal scarring.

Uncomplicated Folliculitis

Most patients with uncomplicated folliculitis complain of small pustules over the vertex scalp, though any area may be affected. There may be associated pain and purulent drainage, but there may also be only pruritus. The patient may also have acne vulgaris on the face, neck, or back. Differential diagnosis includes acne keloidalis nuchae, folliculitis decalvans, early dissecting cellulitis, and tinea capitis. Biopsy and/or KOH may be necessary to rule out the aforementioned diagnoses. Most patients have tried several OTC regimens prior to reaching the dermatologist, and many may have tried several prescription topical and oral agents. Others may report decades of the problem without relief. In any case, the first step to the appropriate treatment is finding out what the patient has used on the scalp and hair in the last 6 months. If the condition is acute, this information should be gathered from the onset of the pustules. The history must include shampoo, conditioner, and any topical agents, even if the patient has used the agent for many years. Even if these agents are not causing the condition, they may be exacerbating the folliculitis.

Treatment

Very little has been written about this form of folliculitis in African-Americans, so most of the therapies discussed here are anecdotal or standard therapies for any patient with folliculitis. First-line therapy for folliculitis should include topical antibiotics, such as clindamycin for localized disease. This is easily accomplished in men, but in women it is often difficult because of the density of hair on the scalp. In women or difficult-to-treat cases, it may be necessary to move early to oral antibiotics for control of the inflammatory component of the folliculitis. Another helpful treatment is an anti-inflammatory shampooing regimen, such as that utilized for seborrheic dermatitis. Often, an added topical corticosteroid used 2–3 times weekly can help, but care must be taken in choosing the corticosteroid vehicle, as ointments may be too occlusive in many patients and solutions may be too drying for the hair.

Folliculitis Decalvans

Folliculitis decalvans is a subtle scarring form of folliculitis that is likely on a continuum between uncomplicated folliculitis and dissecting cellulitis. This form of scarring hair loss is characterized by hair follicles that become inflamed with pustules, accompanied by progressive scarring alopecia. Infective agents are usually absent, though nonpathogenic skin bacteria may be isolated from affected areas. Etiology is not known, but the anecdotal prevalence of this disease appears increased in the black population. In one review of cicatricial alopecias, Whiting found that 8.9% of 358 patients biopsied for cicatricial alopecia had folliculitis decalvans, the third most common diagnosed scarring form of hair loss.[34] Diagnosis of this disorder is made by clinicopathologic correlation when there are pustules with more scarring than would be expected and no evidence of other diagnoses on biopsy.[37] The differential diagnosis includes central centrifugal cicatricial alopecia and tinea capitis.

Treatment

Treatment of folliculitis decalvans includes antibacterial and anti-inflammatory shampoos. Topical and oral antibiotics are often helpful. For more severe disease, dapsone or isotretinoin can be utilized. Topical steroids may be of help calming symptoms of pruritus, but caution should be used in choosing a vehicle that is not too occlusive.

Acne Keloidalis Nuchae

Also called keloidal folliculitis and dermatitis papillaris capillitii, acne keloidalis is a chronic condition most often seen in African-American men (Figures 4.13 and 4.14), although there are

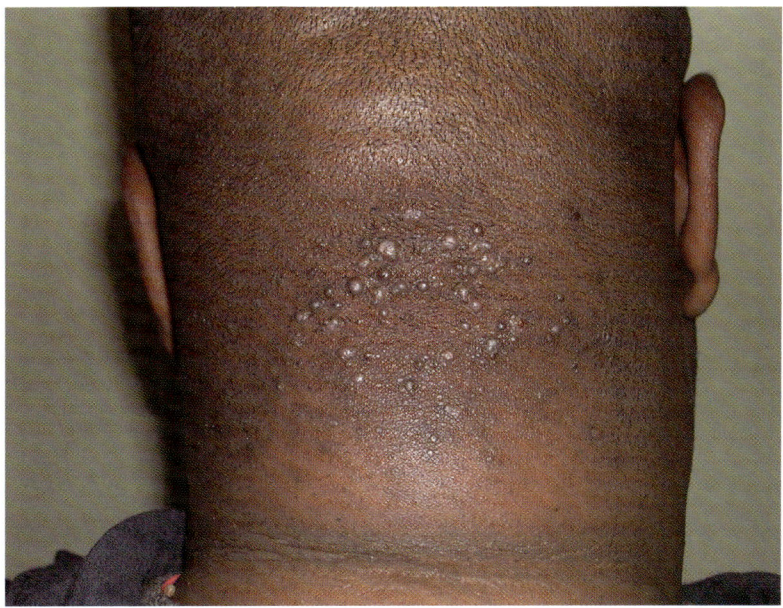

FIGURE 4.13 Mild keloidal nodules in the occiput in a young man.

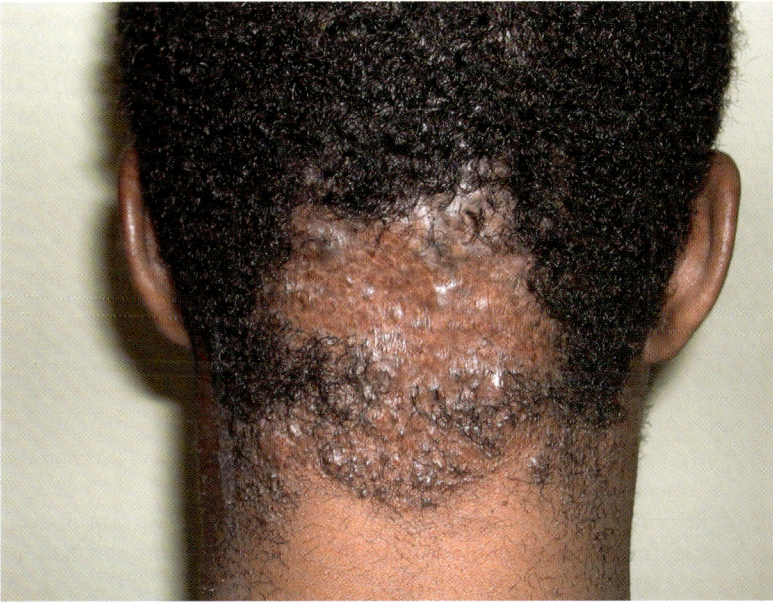

FIGURE 4.14 Diffuse keloid formation at the nape of the neck in acne keloidalis.

reported cases among African-American women[38,39] (Figure 4.15) and Caucasian men. Clinical examination reveals skin-colored to hyperpigmented, follicularly based papules on the nape of the neck and occipital scalp. Pustule formation at the follicular os and follicularly based keloidal papules are often observed. In some patients, the keloids become severe and disfiguring. Etiology of the disease is not known, but the curvature of the hair and follicle may play a role,[20] along with the coarse nature of the hair shaft.

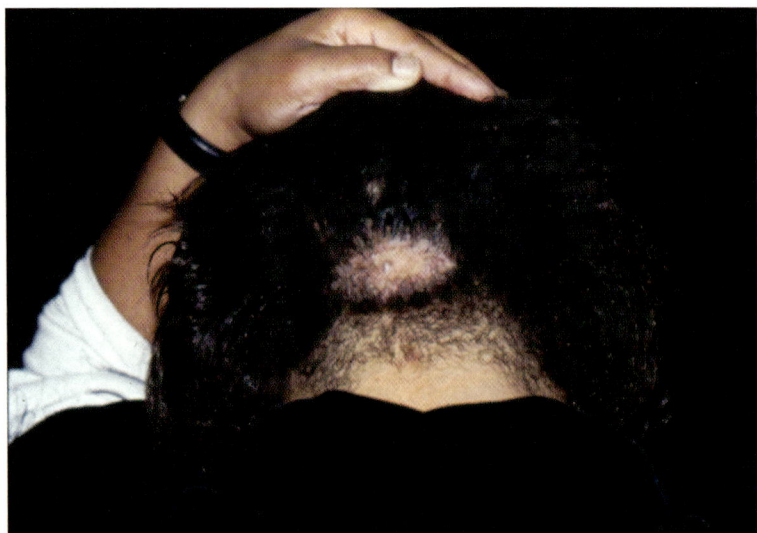

FIGURE 4.15 Keloidal plaque at the nape of the neck in a young woman.

Treatment

The mainstay of treatment in this disorder is to decrease inflammation. Topical and/or oral antibiotics coupled with intralesional steroids placed directly into papules works well to quiet the inflammation. High concentrations of intralesional corticosteroids at a level of 20 to 40 mg/cc of triamcinolone acetonide solution must be used to flatten the papules and plaques. Care must be taken to warn patients of the hypopigmentation that may result from intralesional steroid treatments, but most patients prefer to flatten the papules and incur some mild and usually temporary hypopigmentation rather than allow the disease process to continue. For severe involvement, local excision[40,41] and carbon dioxide laser[42] have been used with success. Laser hair ablation could be used as a mechanism to remove the hair from the posterior neck, thereby removing the source of follicular inflammation. Because permanent hair reduction will be the inevitable outcome, this option is best utilized in severe cases of acne keloidalis.

DISSECTING CELLULITIS

Perifolliculitis capitis abscedens et suffodiens, also known as dissecting cellulitis, is a common, chronic inflammatory disorder of the scalp. It occurs most commonly in African-American men but can be seen in women. Characterized by large, tender, and fluctuant cysts, dissecting cellulitis can form deep and painful sinus tracts on the vertex and occipital scalp that dissect through the subcutaneous tissue (Figures 4.16 and 4.17). The end result is often permanent hair loss secondary to the severity and chronicity of the process. Keloids may also form over the scalp in association with the active eruption. The pathogenesis of this disorder is unknown, as skin samples taken from the affected site are usually sterile,[43] but follicular plugging with ensuing reactive granulomatous inflammation is postulated to contribute to disease expression.[44]

Treatment

Acutely, treatment regimens can include oral antibiotics, short courses of oral corticosteroid tapers,[45] intralesional corticosteroids, and incision and drainage of specific fluctuant nodules.[46] Other reported successful treatments include oral zinc therapy,[46] oral isotretinoin,[47] and wide local

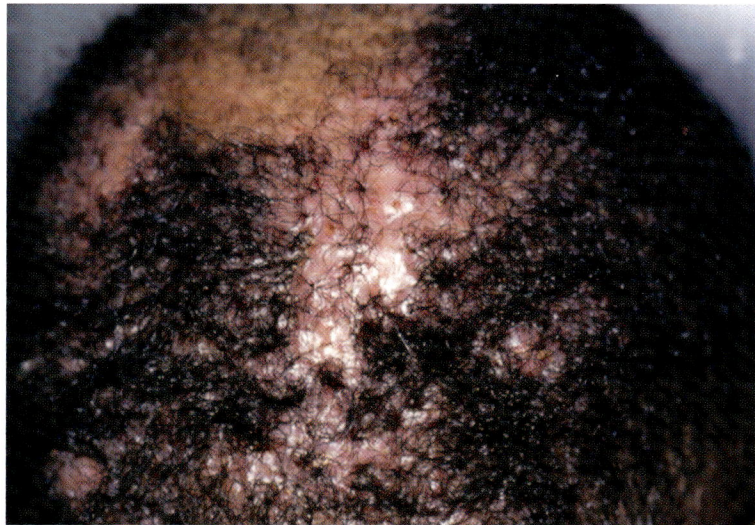

FIGURE 4.16 Pustules and keloidal nodules in the vertex and parietal scalp with hair loss.

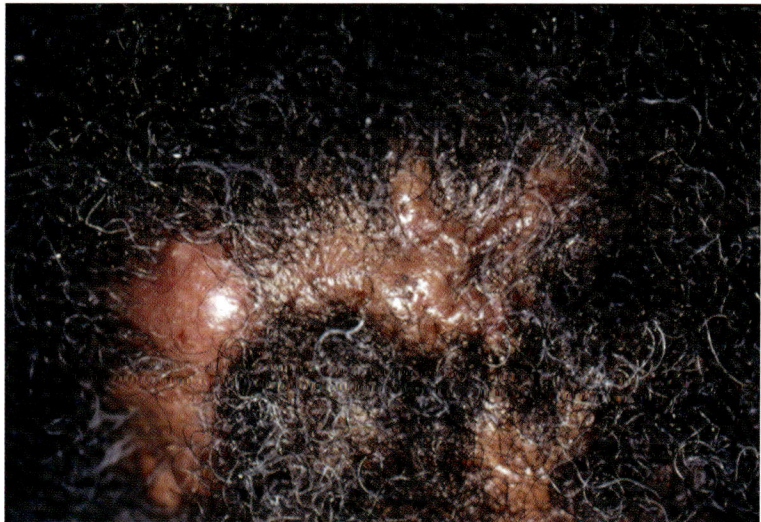

FIGURE 4.17 Large sinus tracts on the vertex scalp in dissecting cellulitis.

resection of the involved scalp followed by split-thickness grafting.[43] When isotretinoin is used, the treatment course must be longer than that for standard cystic acne. The maximum tolerated dose should be used to decrease the inflammation and improve the keratinization process. Treatment of the scalp with x-ray epilation has also been tried with success,[38,48] but several authors have questioned the use of x-ray treatment because there has been a report of *de novo* cancer in a patient at the site of dissecting cellulitis.[43] Laser hair removal may play a role in improving severe dissecting cellulitis,[49] but there may be technical difficulty in performing laser treatments if cystic and keloidal nodules are large and obstructive. Often, the natural history of the cellulitis is dissipation after several years, but treatment should always be undertaken to avoid unnecessary suffering and scarring. Because treatment is often begun after significant scarring has already occurred, it may be necessary to discuss expectations of permanent scarring with the patient prior to treatment.

SCARRING HAIR LOSS WITH LITTLE OR NO CLINICAL INFLAMMATION

TRACTION ALOPECIA

Traction alopecia is a common form of hair loss seen in black females. It occurs in both adults and children. This type of hair loss has been associated with the chronic use of tight braids,[50] pony tails, hair rollers,[51] and hair weaves.[23,52] The etiology of traction alopecia is thought to be secondary to a mechanical loosening of the hairs from the follicle and perifolliculitis.[38]

The areas of hair loss are usually symmetrical and occur commonly along the frontotemporal hairline (Figure 4.18). Involvement of the occipital area of scalp may occur but is less common. There is usually sparing of the vellus hairs and scattered broken hairs are usually seen within the areas of hair loss.[53] In acute cases, perifollicular papules and pustules may be seen.

Treatment

The treatment of traction alopecia is the discontinuance of any hairstyle that produces tension or pulling of the hair. Oral and topical antibiotics are used if folliculitis is present, and topical or intralesional corticosteroids are used if inflammation is present loss.[53] Topical minoxidil as a treatment for traction alopecia has also been reported. Surgical treatment of traction alopecia has been reported to be a successful option. Earles reported the use of punch grafting and rotation flaps in the correction of hair loss.[54] More recently, follicular unit transplantation in the treatment of traction alopecia has shown effective results (Valerie Callender, personal communication).

CENTRAL CENTRIFUGAL CICATRICIAL ALOPECIA

Central centrifugal cicatricial alopecia (CCCA) is the term used to describe the frontal-vertex scarring forms of alopecia that primarily affect women. Previously referred to as hot comb alopecia and follicular degeneration when the entity occurred in African-American women, the CCCA term was coined to be inclusive of patients of all races.[55] Clinically, CCCA develops in a roughly circular

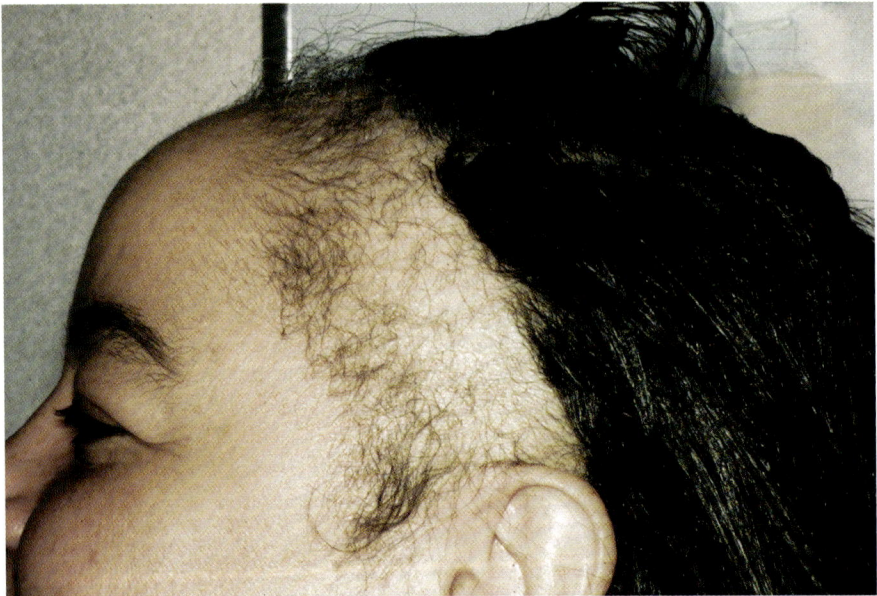

FIGURE 4.18 Classic traction alopecia in the temporal and preauricular scalp.

patch on the frontal-vertex region of the scalp. A circumferential increase in size of the scarred area is the natural progression of the process. The scalp is often smooth and shiny, with decreased hair density in the affected area (Figures 4.19 and 4.20). Usually the hair remaining in the scarred area is shorter, more brittle, and more fragile than hair remaining in the posterior scalp. Accompanying symptoms may include scaling, occasional pustules, and/or pruritus. The etiology of the disorder is unknown. Despite multiple associations with heat and chemical styling processes, no statistically significant associations between hair care practices and the development of the scarring have been published. LoPresti et al. described a scarring alopecia that was thought to occur from oils heated during the hot comb straightening process that were thought to drip onto the scalp and cause permanent damage.[56] There were no data to suggest true associations in this report.

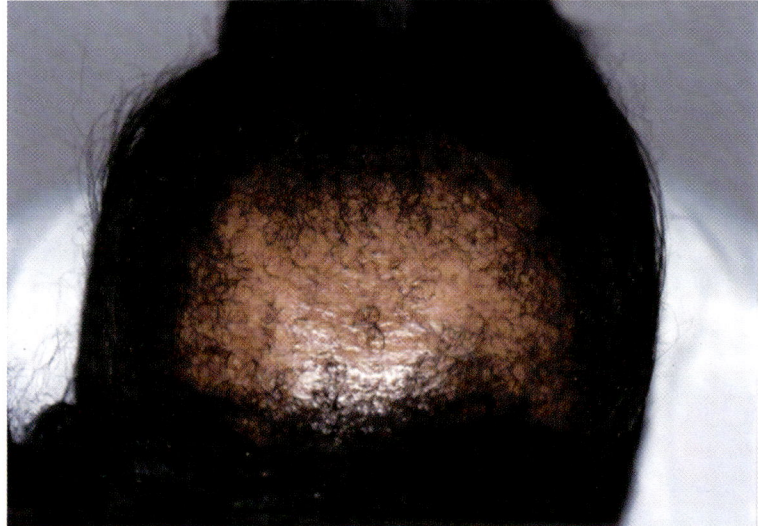

FIGURE 4.19 Scarring alopecia over the fronto-vertex scalp in central centrifugal cicatricial alopecia.

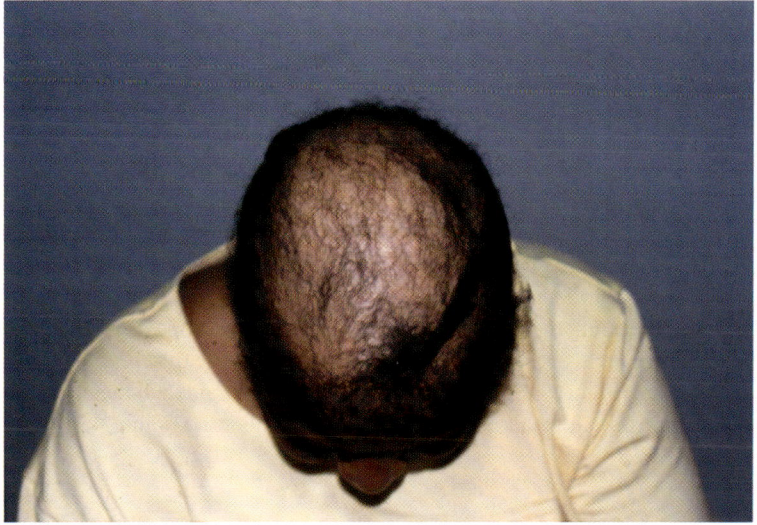

FIGURE 4.20 Extensive scarring in central centrifugal cicatricial alopecia.

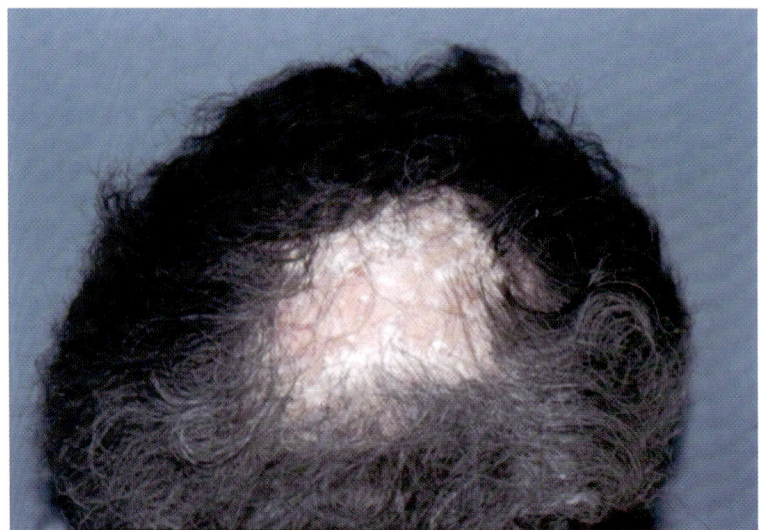

FIGURE 4.21 Central centrifugal cicatricial alopecia in a Caucasian woman.

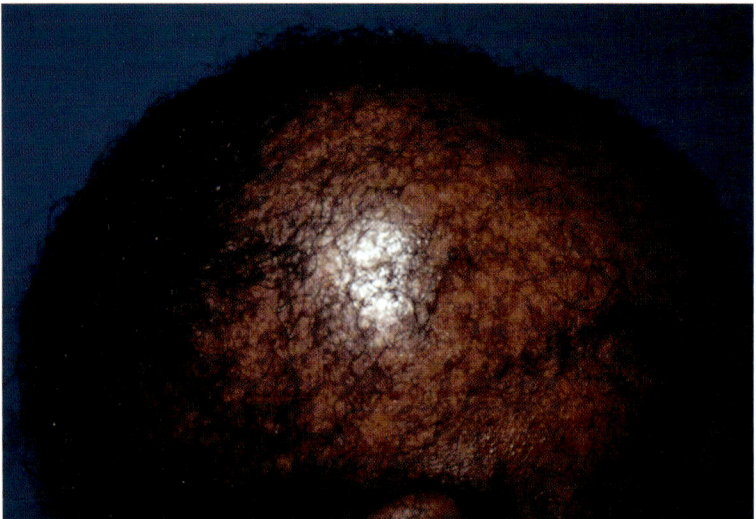

FIGURE 4.22 Alopecia areata mimicking central centrifugal cicatricial alopecia.

Sperling examined a small group of patients with CCCA, which he termed follicular degeneration syndrome. This research found poor correlation between scarring alopecia and hot comb use.[57,58] Because of confusion in nomenclature, the scarring clinical entity that is so recognizable in women of color has been renamed central centrifugal cicatricial alopecia by the Scarring Alopecia Work Group[55] to be more inclusive of other races (Figure 4.21). The differential diagnosis of CCCA includes alopecia areata (Figure 4.22), chronic cutaneous lupus, and lichen planopilaris, though other rare forms of scarring alopecia may occur in this population (Figure 4.23).

Treatment

Treatment should be approached symptomatically in patients with CCCA. There are no clinical trials examining effective treatments for this process, so treatment successes have been anecdotal

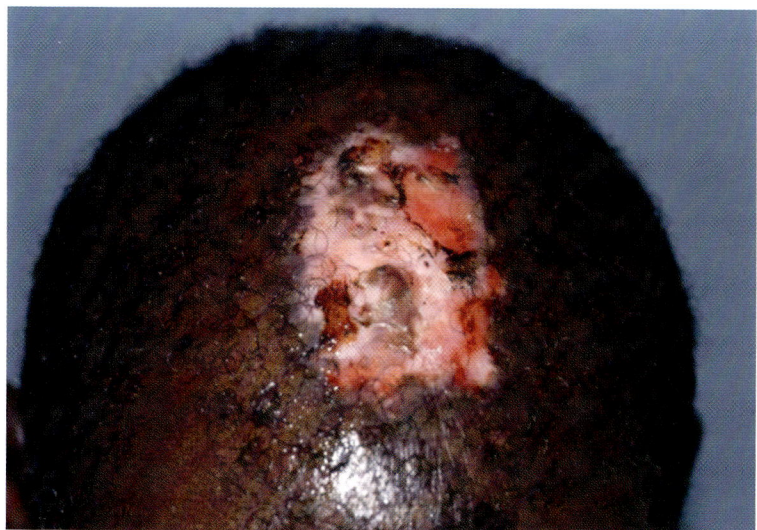

FIGURE 4.23 Cicatricial bullous pemphigoid in an African-American man.

at best. Pruritus and scaling can be treated with intralesional corticosteroids, topical corticosteroids, and increasing hair washing to at least once weekly. Often a seborrheic dermatitis regimen is helpful in decreasing inflammation. Removal of all potentially damaging hair care practices should be suggested, including increased duration between chemical relaxer applications, decreased use of heat to the scalp, and decreased use of hardening gels and sprays.[53]

Sarcoid

Sarcoidosis is a multisystem granulomatous disease that occurs more frequently in African-American women than other groups in the United States,[59] with a 5.3:1 annual ratio of newly diagnosed cases in African-Americans vs. whites.[60] Several epidemiologic studies of the disease have reported earlier age at diagnosis for African-Americans as compared to whites,[60,61] though case fatality rates have been comparable.[60] The diagnosis of cutaneous sarcoid is usually made by skin biopsy showing noncaseating granulomas that have been cultured and stained to rule out the presence of infection. Cutaneous involvement occurs in approximately 10%–46% of patients with sarcoidosis,[61] but to date there are no data documenting the incidence of scalp involvement. The clinical exam of scalp lesions usually reveals solitary or multiple erythematous, translucent plaques with little to no hair growth in the lesion (Figure 4.24). The plaques are usually smooth but may have scale and range in size.

The cause of sarcoid is not known, but there is evidence that the disease may be a reaction pattern to some infectious agent or allergen.[62] Once the diagnosis of the cutaneous sarcoidosis of the scalp is confirmed, the workup should include a complete review of systems as well as a chest x-ray because most patients have pulmonary involvement. Pulmonary function tests (PFTs) may be helpful for following pulmonary progression of disease, but they usually add little to diagnosis if review of systems and chest x-ray are within normal limits. Workup of other organ systems should be guided by patient symptomatology. Laboratory tests such as those for angiotensin-converting enzyme, serum protein electrophoresis, and calcium levels may show elevated levels in active sarcoid, but none of these findings is pathognomonic of the disease.

The mainstay of treatment for systemic sarcoidosis is oral glucocorticoid, which can improve the appearance of cutaneous lesions as well. When only skin disease is present, oral corticosteroids should be avoided, because topical or intralesional corticosteroids can be effective in flattening the sarcoid

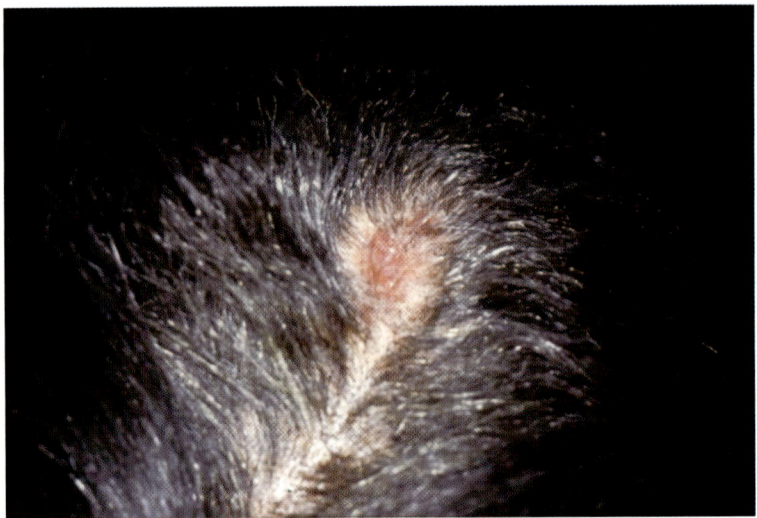

FIGURE 4.24 Smooth nodule of sarcoidosis in the scalp.

lesions and decreasing symptoms of pruritus. Tacrolimus ointment may have a role as a steroid-sparing agent in the treatment of scalp sarcoid.

Hydroxychloroquine has also been shown to be effective in the treatment of chronic cutaneous disease,[63] with a dose of 200 mg every other day.[64] The usual precautions for eye toxicity on this medication must be taken. Other immunosuppressive agents such as azathioprine, chlorambucil, and cyclophosphamide have all been used as adjunctive treatment with corticosteroids with some success,[64,65] but methotrexate may prove to be a safer and more efficacious agent than other immunosuppressant agents.[65]

HAIR SHAFT DISORDERS

A great concern of many African-American women is hair breakage. Many women mistakenly assume that increased shedding of hair during washing and styling is always from the root. In reality, there are many hair abnormalities that cause fragility of the hair shaft followed by significant breakage. African-American women are particularly at risk of hair breakage due to the various hair care practices that weaken the hair shaft as well as the dry nature of the hair. Another problem that the dermatologist may encounter is that many patients with hair breakage attempt to improve the problem with OTC products and hairstyles that can worsen the breakage over time. In this case, the history of hair care practices is of paramount importance in determining etiology of hair breakage.

TRICHORRHEXIS NODOSA

One of the most common, identifiable forms of hair shaft damage is trichorrhexis nodosa. Hair shafts demonstrating this damage are typified clinically by easily broken hairs upon minimal manipulation of the hair shaft. For instance, a pull test may cause a significant number of hairs to break off mid-shaft. Microscopically, these hair shafts demonstrate uneven breakages that resemble broomsticklike projections of cuticular material. This form of fragility can be seen frequently in African-American patients, especially in those who chemically or heat-treat their hair.[38]

TABLE 4.2
Guidelines for Hair Care in African-American Patients

1. If possible, choose a style close to your natural texture and curl pattern.
2. Choose a stylist who is able to explain hair care and treatments to you.
3. Wash hair at least every 1–2 weeks.
4. Use shampoos and conditioners that are specially formulated for dry or coarse hair.
5. Apply chemical relaxer every 6–8 weeks at most.
6. Use emollients for hair shafts only.
7. Remove and replace braids monthly.
8. Do not wear styles that put tension/traction on the hair in any way.
9. Trim hair shaft ends every 6–8 weeks.
10. Become familiar with all the products used on your hair at the salon.

HEAT, CHEMICALS, AND OTHER DRYING AGENTS

The major hair care practices that cause hair breakage include heat-related straightening of the hair, chemical straightening agents, hair color, and drying agents used to keep the hair in place (Tables 4.2 and 4.3).

Heat

Heat is most often used by African-American women who want to thermally straighten the hair without a permanent straightening process. In this form of straightening, a metal comb is heated to high temperatures (150–500° Fahrenheit) by a heat source such as a small electric warmer, gas burner, or hot flame. Washed and dried hair is treated with an ointment-based lubricant and the hot comb is slowly pulled through small sections of hair. This process temporarily rearranges hydrogen and disulfide bonds within the hair shaft.[20,38,66] The hair remains straight until it is exposed to moisture. Usually, after straightening, the hair may be curled with a curling iron for style. Upon rewetting, all signs of the hot combing effect are lost and the hair reverts back to its original state.

Thermal straightening of the hair is not as popular as it once was, because the more convenient and longer-lasting option of chemical straightening has become widespread. Common problems with thermal straightening include moderate to severe burns from accidental contact with the hot comb[67] and overheating of the hair shaft, causing weakening and breakage.[20,38] To avoid hair shaft damage, a well-trained professional should perform the procedure. Keeping hot comb treatment to a maximum of once weekly, only hot combing clean, dry hair, and obtaining regular trims of split ends will help to prevent damage from the procedure. If damage does ensue, the patient should suspend thermal straightening, cut the damaged hair, and used moisturizing shampoos and conditioners.

Chemicals

In the 1960s, the crude forerunners of chemical straighteners became more refined and less damaging to the hair and scalp. With this progress, African-American women began to utilize chemical relaxers (Figure 4.25), which are likely the most common method of hair straightening used by African-American women currently. Most chemical relaxers used on the hair in African-Americans contain sodium, potassium or guanine hydroxides, sulfites, or thioglycolates. All of these chemicals work to produce a straight appearance by affecting the cysteine disulfide bonds of the hair. The chemicals are applied first to virgin hair from the scalp to the ends of the hair shaft. The scalp is coated with a protective thick emollient prior to the application of the relaxer. The

TABLE 4.3
Hair Care Products Commonly Used by African-Americans

Product	Patient Use	Physician Utility
Solid emollients	Treat scalp scale Decrease pruritus Lubricate hair shafts Increase manageability	Dry hair shaft lubrication in natural, thermally straightened hair
Liquid emollients	Treat scale Lubricate hair shafts	Dry hair shaft lubrication in chemically straightened hair
Oil emollients	Lubricate hair shafts Decrease pruritus	Good for dry hair shafts
Conditioning shampoo	Decrease hair breakage Restore manageability to hair shaft	Coats hair shaft to decrease breakage
Conditioner for dry or chemically treated hair and leave-in conditioner	Decrease hair breakage Restore manageability to hair shaft	Coats hair shaft to decrease breakage
Styling gel, spritz	Increase styling options Decrease frequency of hair styling	Best avoided due to hair shaft dryness, breakage
Hot combing	Straighten the hair for increased management	Straighten hair instead without chemical relaxer Minimize when hair shafts damaged
Chemical relaxer	Straighten hair for long term	Avoid if hair and scalp damaged
Hair weave with glue (artificial hair glued to scalp)	Cover alopecia area Increase hair density Increase styling options	Best avoided due to traction from glue and contact dermatitis to scalp
Hair weave sewn (hair braided, then artificial hair connected to patient head with sewing technique)	Cover alopecia area Increase hair density	Used for short-term alopecia coverage Can cause traction if tight
Hair extensions (artificial or human hair braided into the patients' hair)	Cover alopecia Increase hair density	May cause traction Remove every 4 weeks
Dreadlocks/twists (twisted locks of natural hair)	Natural hair style Low maintenance	No traction or chemicals needed
Microbraids (small braids attached to the hair close to scale level allowing braided or curled styles)	Cover alopecia Increase styling options Ease of styling	Possible traction Need to keep frequency of shampoo

relaxer is kept on the hair for 15–20 minutes and then removed by rinsing, followed by a neutralizing shampoo. After shampooing, the hair is either set on rollers and dried under a hood dryer or blown dry and curled with a curling iron. Some African-Americans (men and women) use chemical relaxers to loosen the curl of the hair and then wear the hair in a natural style. As the hair grows, the chemical relaxer is applied only to the new growth to minimize overlap of the chemical onto previously treated hair. The reapplication of chemical to new growth is usually performed every 6–12 weeks and can prevent texture differences that may cause breakage during grooming.[67]

The damage that occurs with the thioglycolate chemicals is similar to that of the relaxing agents. Overprocessing with the thioglycolate agents can lead to significant hair breakage because tensile strength loss can be as high as 56%.[68] A form of verrucal alopecia has been described by Bulengo-Ransby, who reported this alopecia occurring after thioglycolate use.[69]

To avoid the side effects of chemical relaxers, patients should seek out professionals to apply the chemical if this is the preferred hair care regimen. Using a thick, protective emollient on the scalp during relaxer application may lessen relaxer-associated skin irritation. Maintenance of hair trims every 6 to 8 weeks, relaxer applications no more frequent than 6 to 8 weeks apart, and minimizing the application of other drying agents can make a large difference in the appearance of the hair shaft.

Hair and Scalp Disorders in Pigmented Skins

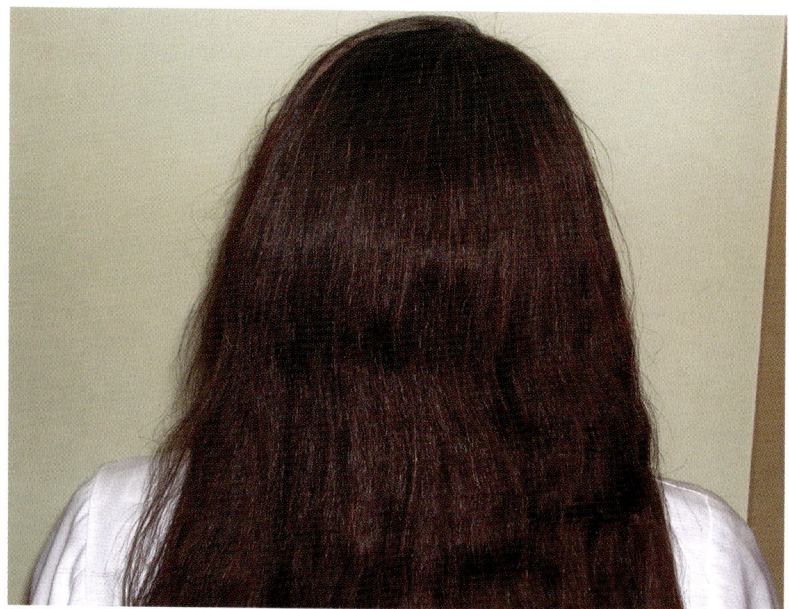

FIGURE 4.25 African-American woman with relaxed hair.

Other Drying Agents

Hairstyles that are sculpted to the scalp are very popular with many black women. Usually, the sculpted styles are used to minimize styling time, decrease weather-related hair frizzing, and restrain the hair in a neat fashion. Unfortunately, these styles are achieved with the use of gels (Figure 4.26), sprays, and spritzes, all of which may be drying to the hair shaft. A careful history of hair care products is important, but discussion of avoidance of these products must be undertaken with care.

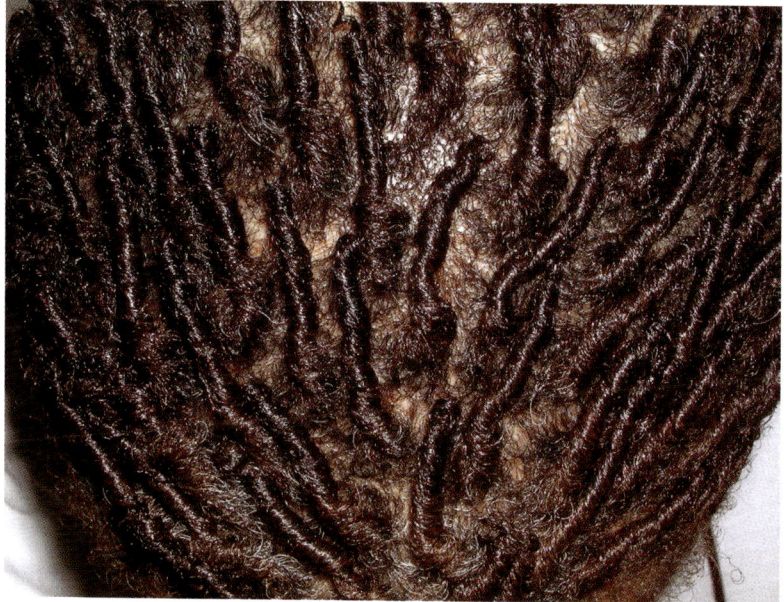

FIGURE 4.26 African-American woman with gel twists.

Many patients are unaware of how damaging these products can be and will not easily stop their use. Recommendations of less damaging hairstyles and products should be made to replace the sculpted styles. These options may include natural styles, wigs, or new hair styles.

SUMMARY

Disorders of hair and scalp are challenging dermatologic conditions. The added combination of pigmentation and unique scar and keloid formation in patients of color can test even the well-informed dermatologist. In this chapter, we have outlined the common disorders seen in the African-Americans, clinical appearance, pearls for treatment, and pitfalls of hair care practices. Also important to remember is that hair products and styles are constantly changing, so it will be important to continue to add new information to this lexicon.

REFERENCES

1. Lindelof B, Forslind B, Hedblad M, Kaveus U. Human hair form. *Arch Dermatol* 1988; 124: 1359–1363.
2. Rook A. Racial and other genetic variations in hair form. *Br J Dermatol* 1975; 92: 599–600.
3. Sperling LC. Hair density in African-Americans. *Arch Dermatol* 1999; 135(6):656–658.
4. Syed A, Kuhajda A, Ayoub H, Ahmad K, Frank EM. African-American hair: its physical properties and differences relative to Caucasian hair. *Cosmetics Toiletries* 1995; 110: 39–48.
5. Bernard BA. *J Am Acad Dermatol* 2003: 48: S120–S126.
6. Franbourg A, Hallegot P, Baltenneck F, Toutain C, Leroy F. Current research on ethnic hair. *J Am Acad Dermatol* 2003; 48: S115–S119.
7. Plewig G, Jansen T. Seborrheic dermatitis. In: Fitzpatrick TB, Eisen AZ, Wolf K, Freedberg IM, Austen KE (Eds) *Dermatology in General Medicine*, 4th ed. McGraw-Hill, New York, 1993; 1569–1574.
8. Faergemann JF, Jones TC, Hettler O, Loria Y. *Pityrosporum ovale* (*Malassezia furfur*) as the causative agent of seborrheic dermatitis: new treatment options. *Br J Dermatol* 1996; 134(Suppl 46): 12–15.
9. Silverberg NB, Weinberg JM, DeLo VA. Tinea capitis: focus on African-American women. *J Am Acad Dermatol* 2002; 46: S120–S124.
10. Brown M, Evans TW, Poyner T, Tooley PJH. The role of ketoconazole 2% shampoo in the treatment and prophylaxic management of dandruff. *J Dermatol Treat* 1990; 1: 177–179.
11. Danby FW, Maddin S, Margesson LJ, Rosenthal D. A randomized, double-blind placebo controlled trial of ketoconazole 2% shampoo versus selenium sulfide 2.5% shampoo in the treatment of moderate to severe dandruff. *J Am Acad Dermatol* 1993; 29: 1008–1012.
12. Warner RR, Schwartz JR, Boissy Y, Dawson TL. Dandruff has an altered stratum corneum ultrastructure that is improved with zinc pyrithione shampoo. *J Am Acad Dermatol* 2001; 45: 897–903.
13. McMichael A, Feldman SR. How to treat common scalp dermatoses. *Skin Aging* 1999; 7: 44–52.
14. Feldman SR, Sangha ND, Setaluri V. Topical corticosteroids in foam vehicle offers comparable coverage compared with traditional vehicles. *J Am Acad Dermatol* 2000; 42: 1017–1020.
15. George YA, Ravis SM, Gottlieb J, Hall S, Woods W, Callender V, et al. Betamethasone valerate 0.12% in foam vehicle for scalp seborrheic dermatitis in African-Americans. *Cosmet Dermatol* 2002; 15: 25–29.
16. Obasi OE. Psoriasis vulgaris in the Guinea Savannah region of Nigeria. *Int J Dermatol* 1986; 25: 181–183.
17. Freeman AK, Linowski GJ, Brady C, Lind L, Vandveldhuisen P, Singer G, Lebwohl M. Tacrolimus ointment for the treatment of psoriasis on the face and intertriginous areas. *J Am Acad Dermatol* 2003; 48(4): 564–568.
18. Rappersberger K, Komar M, Ebelin ME, Scott G, Burtin P, Greig G, Kehren J, et al. Pimecrolimus identifies a common genomic anti-inflammatory profile, is clinically highly effective in psoriasis and is well tolerated. *J Invest Dermatol* 2002; 119(4): 876–887.

19. Swee W, Klontz KC, Lambert LA. A nationwide outbreak of alopecia associated with the use of a hair-relaxing formulation. *Arch Dermatol* 2000; 136: 1104–1108.
20. Halder RM. Hair and scalp disorders in blacks. *Cutis* 1983; 32: 378–380.
21. Nicholson AG, Harland CC, Bull RH, Mortimer PS, Cook MG. Chemically induced cosmetic alopecia. *Br J Dermatol* 1993; 128: 537–541.
22. Pardasani AG, Turner E, McMichael AF. Squaric acid dibutylester: indications for use and efficacy in alopecia areata. *Arch Dermatol* 2001; 137: 970–972.
23. Cogen FC, Beezhold DH. Hair glue anaphylaxis: a hidden latex allergy. *Ann Allergy Asthma Immunol* 2002; 88: 61–63.
24. Nielsen NH, Menne T. Allergic contact dermatitis caused by zinc pyrithione associated with pustular psoriasis. *Am J Contact Dermatol* 1997; 8: 170–171.
25. Sinclair RD, Mallari RS, Tate B. Sensitization to saw palmetto and minoxidil in separate topical extemporaneous treatments for androgenetic alopecia. *Australas J Dermatol* 2002; 43(4): 311–312.
26. Lobato MN, Vugia DJ, Freiden IJ. Tinea capitis in California children: A population-based study of a growing epidemic. *Pediatrics* 1997; 99: 551.
27. Pomeranz AJ, Sabris SS, McGrath GJ, Easterly NB. Asymptomatic dermatophyte carriers in the households of children with tinea capitis. *Arch Pediatr Adolesc Med* 1999; 153: 483.
28. Sharma V, Silverberg NB, Howard R, Tran CT, Laude T, Frieden IJ. Do hair care practices affect the acquisition of tinea capitis? *Arch Pediatr Adolesc Med* 2001; 155: 818–821.
29. McCarty DJ, Manzi S, Medsger TA, Ramsey-Goldman R, LaPorte RE, Kwoth CK. Incidence of systemic lupus erythematosus. Race and gender differences. *Arthritis Rheum* 1995; 38(9): 1260–1270.
30. Wysenbeek AJ, Leibovici L, Amit M, Weinberger A. Alopecia in systemic lupus erythematosus: relation to disease manifestations. *J Rheumatol* 1991; 18(8): 1185–1186.
31. Wilson CL, Burge SM, Dean D, Dawber RPR. Scarring alopecia in discoid lupus erythematosus. *Br J Dermatol* 1992; 126: 307–314.
32. Sontheimer RD, Provost TT. *Cutaneous Manifestations of Rheumatic Diseases*. Williams and Wilkins, Baltimore, 1996.
33. Prystowsky SD, Herndon JH, Gilliam JN. Chronic cutaneous lupus erythematosus (CCLE) — A clinical and laboratory investigation of 80 patients. *Medicine* 1976; 55(2): 183–191.
34. Whiting DA. Cicatricial alopecia: Clinico-pathologic findings and treatment. *Clin Dermatol* 2001; 19: 211–225.
35. Holm AL, Bowers KE, McMeekin TO, Gaspari AA. Chronic cutaneous lupus erythematosus treated with thalidomide. *Arch Dermatol* 1993; 129(12): 1548–1550.
36. Kasteler JS, Callen JP. Scalp involvement in dermatomyositis. Often overlooked or misdiagnosed. *JAMA* 1994; 272(24): 1939–1941.
37. Templeton SF, Solomon AR. Scarring alopecia: a classification bases on microscopic criteria. *J Cutan Pathol* 1993; 21: 97–109.
38. Scott DA. Disorders of the hair and scalp in blacks. *Dermatol Clin* 1988; 6: 387–395.
39. Dinehart SM, Tanner L, Mallory SB, Herzberg AJ. Acne keloidalis in women. *Cutis* 1989; 44: 250–252.
40. Glenn MJ, Bennett RG, Kelly AP: Acne keloidalis nuchae: treatment with excision and second-intension healing. *J Am Acad Dermatol* 1995; 33: 243–246.
41. Sattler ME. Folliculitis keloidalis nuchae. *World Med J* 2001; 100(1): 37–38.
42. Kantor GR, Ratz JL, Wheeland RG. Treatment of acne keloidalis nuchae with carbon dioxide laser. *J Am Acad Dermatol* 1986; 14: 263–267.
43. Williams CN, Cohen M, Ronan SG, Lewandowski CA. Dissecting cellulitis of the scalp. *Plast Reconstr Surg* 1986; 77: 378–382.
44. Moyer DG. Perifolliculitis capitis abscedens et suffodiens. *Arch Dermatol* 1962; 85: 580–584.
45. Adrian RM, Arndt KA. Perifolliculitis capitis: successful control with alternate day corticosteroids. *Ann Plast Surg* 1980; 4: 166–169.
46. Berne B, Venge P, Ohman S. Perifolliculitis capitis abscedens et suffodiens (Hoffman). *Arch Dermatol* 1985; 121: 1028–1030.
47. Schewach-Millet M, Ziv R, Shapira D. Perifolliculitis capitis abscedens et suffodiens treated with isotretinoin (letter). *J Am Acad Dermatol* 1986; 15: 1291–1292.
48. McMullan FH, Zeligman I. Perifolliculitis capitis abscedens et suffodiens. *Arch Dermatol* 1956; 73: 259.

49. Chui CT, Berger TG, Price VH, Zachary CB. Recalcitrant scarring follicular disorders treated by laser-assisted hair removal: a preliminary report. *Dermatol Surg* 1999; 2599(1):34–7.
50. Rudolph RI, Klein AW, Decherd JW. Cornrow alopecia (letter). *Arch Dermatol* 1973; 108: 134.
51. Lipnik MJ. Traumatic alopecia from brush rollers. *Arch Dermatol* 1961; 84: 183–185.
52. Wakelin SH. Contact anaphylaxis from natural latex used as an adhesive for hair extensions. *Br J Dermatol* 14; 146(2): 340–341.
53. McMichael A. Scalp and hair diseases in the black patient. In: Johnson BL, Moy RL, White GM (Eds) *Ethnic Skin*. Mosby, St. Louis, 1998; 214–230.
54. Earles M. Surgical correction of traumatic alopecia marginalis or traction alopecia in black women. *J Dermatol Surg Oncol* 1986; 12: 78–82.
55. Olsen EA, Bergfeld WF, Cotsarelis G, Price VH, Shapiro J, Sinclair R, et al. Summary of North American Hair Research Society (NAHRS) — sponsored workshop on cicatricial alopecia, Duke University Medical Center, February 10 and 11, 2001. *J Am Acad Dermatol* 2003; 48: 103–110.
56. LoPresti P, Papa CM, Kligman AM. Hot comb alopecia. *Arch Dermatol* 1968; 98: 234–238.
57. Sperling LC. The follicular degeneration syndrome in black patients. *Arch Dermatol* 1992; 128: 68–74.
58. Sperling LC, Skelton HG, Smith KJ, Sau P, Friedman K. Follicular degeneration syndrome in men. *Arch Dermatol* 1994; 130: 763–769.
59. Abeles H, Roluns AB, Chaves AD. Sarcoidosis in New York City. *Am Rev Resp Dis* 1961; 84: 120.
60. Keller AZ. Hospital, age, racial, occupational, geographical, clinical and survivorship characteristics in the epidemiology of sarcoidosis. *Am J Epidemiol* 1971; 94: 222–230.
61. Takemura T, Shishiba T, Akiyama O, Oritsu M, Matsul Y, Eishi Y. Vascular involvement in cutaneous sarcoidosis. *Pathol Int* 1997; 47: 84–89.
62. Kerdel FA, Moschella SL. Sarcoidosis: an updated review. *J Am Acad Dermatol* 1984; 11: 1–19.
63. Mathur A, Kremer JM. Immunopathology, musculoskeletal features, and treatment of sarcoidosis. *Curr Opin Rheumatol* 1993; 5: 90–94.
64. Selroos O. Treatment of sarcoidosis. *Sarcoidosis* 1994; 11: 80–83.
65. Baughman RP, Lower E. The effect of corticosteroid or methotrexate therapy on lung lymphocytes and macrophages in sarcoidosis. *Am Rev Resp Dis* 1990; 142: 1268–1271.
66. DeVillez RL. Infectious, physical, and inflammatory causes of hair and scalp abnormalities. In: Olsen EA (Ed) *Disorders of Hair Growth*. McGraw-Hill, New York, 1994; 83.
67. Joyner M. Hair care in the black patient. *J Pediatr Health Care* 1988; 2: 281–287.
68. Khalil EN. Cosmetic and hair treatments for the black consumer. *Cosmetics Toiletries* 1986; 101: 51–58.
69. Bulengo-Ransby SM. Chemical and traumatic alopecia from thioglycolate in a black woman. *Cutis* 1992; 49: 99–103.

5 Pigmentary Disorders in Pigmented Skins

Rebat M. Halder, Maithily A. Nandedkar, and Kenneth W. Neal

INTRODUCTION

Pigmentary disorders are a global problem. Dyspigmentation, from hyperpigmentation to hypopigmentation, is often psychologically devastating to patients with darker skin.[1] There is marked contrast in skin of color between normally pigmented and hypopigmented or depigmented skin. Also, persons of color tend to have more intense pigmentation than others when hyperpigmentation occurs. Because skin is conspicuous, variations from the norm are noticeable. However, objective measures of the deleterious psychological effects of color alteration are difficult to assess because it is subjective from patient to patient.[2] Indeed, disorders of pigmentation are among the most common reasons for patients with skin of color to seek dermatological treatment.[3] Despite being common, pigmentary disorders remain difficult to treat.

DISORDERS OF HYPOPIGMENTATION

PITYRIASIS VERSICOLOR

This disease, also known as tinea versicolor, is a superficial fungal infection most commonly affecting the seborrheic areas of the trunk. However, in tropical climates the infection can extend to the face, arms, and lower back. It has no racial or sexual preference. It seems to prefer hot, humid weather, which accounts for its prevalence in tropical climates or the summer season in temperate climates.[4] It is more common in adults, whose sebaceous glands are more active than those of children. It has a distinctive clinical appearance.[8]

Classically, the disease presents as hypopigmented, dull white to tan scaly macules that are a few millimeters in diameter. Patches up to several centimeters in diameter are not unusual. Although clinically the acute eruption is unmistakable, a Wood's lamp examination is sometimes necessary to distinguish this from vitiligo. Vitiliginous skin will appear stark white, whereas pityriasis versicolor–induced hypopigmented skin will have a slightly greenish hue.[5] Microscopic examination of scales with potassium hydroxide reveals the classic appearance of hyphae and spores.[6]

The hypopigmentation resulting from the acute infection is the most distressing aspect of the disease in pigmented skins. The causative agent for the pigmentary disorder is a lipophilic yeast that has been given several names. Currently, it is known as *Pityrosporum ovale* and is synonymous with *Microsporon furfur*, *Malassazia furfur*, and *Pityrosporum orbiculare*.[4] To date, a satisfactory explanation for the pathogenesis of the hypopigmentation remains elusive. UV light was thought to play a role but does not explain consistently the hypopigmentation seen in non-sun-exposed areas.

In the past, the most compelling explanation for this disease was that the organism *P. ovale* has lipooxygenases that act on surface lipids, leading to the oxidization of oleic acid to azeleic acid.[7] Azeleic acid was thought to block melanogenesis via competitive inhibition of tyrosinase. This was found to be erroneous as investigators discovered that the diacid had no depigmenting effect on normal skin.[8] Although the enzymatic activity of the lipooxygenases is not in question, their effect currently is. *Pityrosporum ovale*'s activity on the unsaturated fatty acids found in sebum leads to the formation of lipoperoxidases. These enzymes are toxic only to abnormally active melanocytes. Their presence is thought to reduce DNA synthesis only in these melanocytes via mitochondrial damage, with subsequent depigmentation as an end result rather than direct prohibition of melanogenesis via hindrance of tyrosinase, as previously thought.[9]

Treatment of the acute disease consists of topical antifungal shampoos, creams, and lotions or systemic pulse antifungal therapy. After systemic or topical antifungal therapy, repigmentation is slow and recurrences are common.[10] Chronic postinflammatory hypopigmentation can respond to topical or oral psoralen UVA (PUVA) therapy or tar emulsion therapy, all of which may stimulate melanogenesis.

PITYRIASIS ALBA

This common eczematous disorder occurs most often in black children and children of Hispanic or Asian origin, presenting as hypopigmented, slightly scaly patches usually evident on the face, neck, and trunk.[11] Associated with atopic dermatitis, the disease is usually self-limiting.[12] Tar emulsions stimulate melanogenesis, thereby minimizing the contrast between light and dark skin. Likewise, topical steroids, topical PUVA, and oral PUVA may be beneficial.[13] Currently, topical steroid alternatives such as pimecrolimus or tacrolimus that work via the calcineurin pathway are used off label for treatment of severe disease.[14] Controlled trials have yet to prove the effectiveness of these agents.

IDIOPATHIC GUTTATE HYPOMELANOSIS

Idiopathic guttate hypomelanosis is an acquired leukoderma found in all races and has an unknown etiology, but it is very apparent in persons of color.[15] It is characterized by multiple, discrete, circumscribed, depigmented macules that occur on the extensor surfaces of arms and legs.[16] It can sometimes become generalized. Lesions occur on both sun-exposed as well as non-sun-exposed skin (Figure 5.1). Hairs within the lesions are not depigmented.[17] The number of lesions increases with age, and the lesions more common in individuals over the age of 70 years.[18]

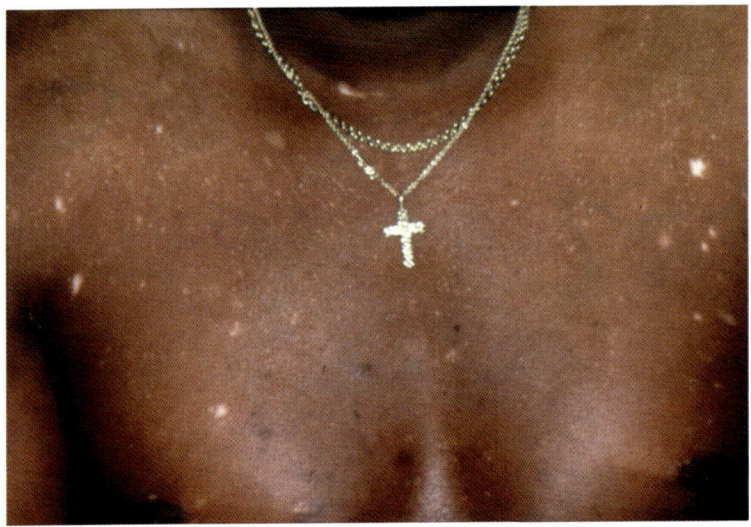

FIGURE 5.1 Idiopathic guttate hypomelanosis (IGH) on the chest of an African-American man. (Reproduced from Halder, R.M., *Dermatola Clin* 2003; 21: 617–628. With permission from Elsevier.)

No treatment is necessary, but patients with pigmented skin will request treatment because of the psychological impact. No effective treatments are available, although published treatment options include intralesional corticosteroids, topical and oral PUVA, liquid nitrogen, and skin grafts, all of which usually have unsuccessful results.[19,20]

DISORDERS OF DEPIGMENTATION

VITILIGO

Vitiligo is a disease that causes destruction of melanocytes not only in skin but also in mucous membranes, eyes, hair bulbs, and in the ears, leading to alterations in both structure and function of these organs.[21] It is seen clinically as depigmented, well-demarcated macules with variable progression. It can occur at any age, but it usually occurs before the age of 20 years in nearly 50% of patients and affects nearly 1%–2% of the world population.[22] The distribution is equal regardless of race, ethnicity, or gender[23,24] (Figure 5.2).

A person's physical appearance is the personal characteristic most obvious and most accessible to others in social interaction.[25] For this reason, vitiligo can be more psychologically devastating in people of color due to the marked contrast between normal and affected skin.[26] The etiology is as yet unknown; however, vitiligo has been associated with genetic disorders and endocrine disorders most commonly of the thyroid, and an autoimmune pathogenesis is preferred.[21]

Diagnosis of vitiligo is based almost exclusively on the clinical examination. Lesions may be found anywhere on the body. However, initial lesions are most frequently found on the hands, forearms, feet, face, and lips.[27]

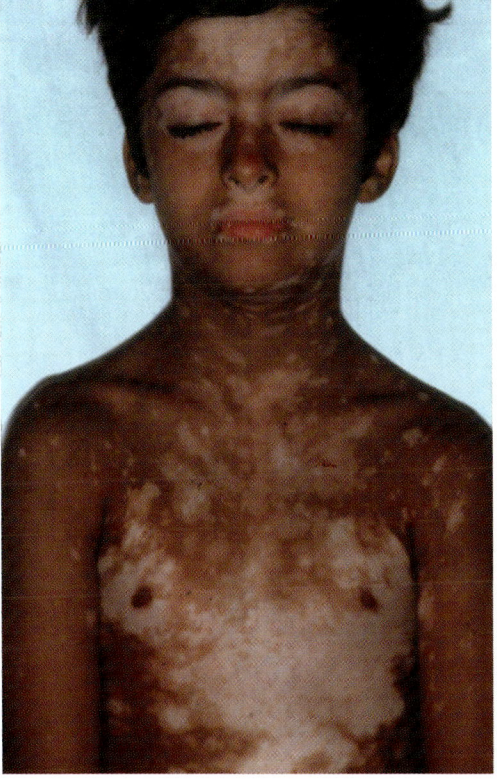

FIGURE 5.2 Generalized vitiligo in a Hispanic child. (Reproduced from Halder, R.M., *Dermatola Clin* 2003; 21: 617–628. With permission from Elsevier.)

There are four main types of vitiligo: generalized, acrofacial, segmental, and universal. Generalized is the most common type. Patients present with bilaterally symmetric lesions involving the peri-orofacial areas, neck, torso, bony prominences of hands, wrists, and legs, extensor surfaces, orifices, axillae, and mucosal areas.[21] Acrofacial vitiligo presents with lesions on distal fingers and on the facial orifices. Segmental vitiligo presents in an asymmetric dermatomal distribution. It has an earlier age of onset and is not associated with autoimmune diseases. Universal vitiligo, which has been associated with multiple endocrinopathies, presents with depigmented macules and patches involving almost the entire body.[21]

There are various modalities for treating vitiligo.[22] They include, but are not limited to, PUVA (oral/topical), PUVASOL (PUVA using natural sunlight), UVB, narrow-band UVB, topical/intralesional steroid, 308-nm excimer laser, topical tacrolimus, skin grafts, and cosmetics.[28–34] Color matching with cosmetics may not be ideal for darker-skinned individuals (Figure 5.3A,B). The areas that respond most favorably to PUVA are the face and trunk.[35] The mechanism by which PUVA acts to repigment is via stimulation of melanocytes in the outer root sheath of the hair follicle through the action of immune cytokines and inflammatory mediators released by keratinocytes.[32,36,37] Narrow-band UVB is a new alternative to PUVA without the adverse effects associated with PUVA.[32]

There are also surgical treatments for vitiligo; however, they should be used on patients in which vitiligo has been stable for approximately 4–6 months.[30] Autologous minigrafts involve harvesting 1.2–2.0-mm punch grafts from a donor site on the lower back below the waistline and placing them 3–4 mm apart on the recipient site, which has been prepared with a similar-sized punch (Figure 5.4A–C). Another technique termed autologous thin Thiersch grafting allows grafting of large areas in a relatively short time, prepared by a process similar to dermabrasion, with minimal scarring in treated areas.[38] However, the disadvantage of this technique is that it requires general

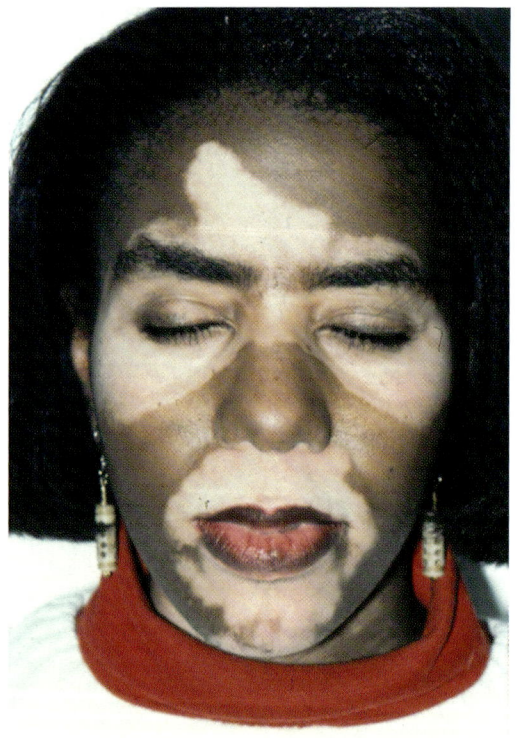

FIGURE 5.3 (A) Disfiguring facial vitiligo in an African-American woman.

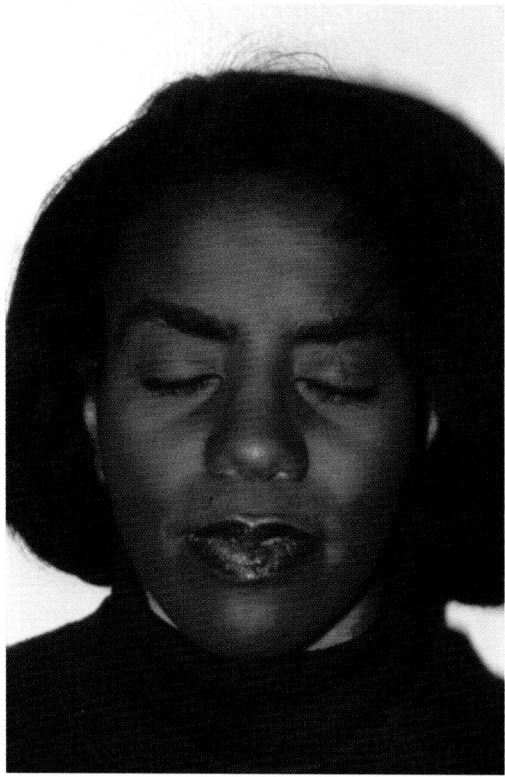

FIGURE 5.3 (B) Same woman as in A following the application of prosthetic cosmetics.

anesthesia. Last, the technique of suction-blister grafting is used to cover depigmented areas prepared by denuding them with liquid nitrogen blisters or dermabrasion.[28] Suction-blister grafts are obtained using negative pressure at 200 mmHg for nearly 4 h. The tops of the donor blisters are harvested and applied directly to the depigmented areas in a mosaic pattern, taking approximately 3–6 months for the depigmented areas to pigment.[28]

Melanocyte transplantation is another technique that theoretically has the potential to treat large areas of depigmented skin. However, the major disadvantages are the technical complexities and cost as well as its being impractical for most dermatologists.[30]

Depigmentation is sometimes considered when patients have greater than 50% cutaneous and have shown recalcitrance to repigmentation from various treatment modalities. Depigmentation is accomplished with the use of monobenzylether of hydroquinone[22] and can be considered for disfiguring or extensive disease in skin of color (Figure 5.5A, B) (see also the section on medications in this chapter).

POSTINFLAMMATORY HYPERPIGMENTATION AND HYPOPIGMENTATION

Postinflammatory hyperpigmentation and hypopigmentation are frequent end results of inflammatory cutaneous disorders, especially in darker-skinned individuals, or of irritation from therapeutic interventions such as topical retinoids or benzoyl peroxide. They are a normal biological response in human skin.[39] Postinflammatory hyperpigmentation and hypopigmentation can result from papulosquamous diseases such as allergic contact dermatitis and lichen planus or vesiculobullous diseases such as bullous pemphigoid and herpes zoster and commonly inflammatory diseases such

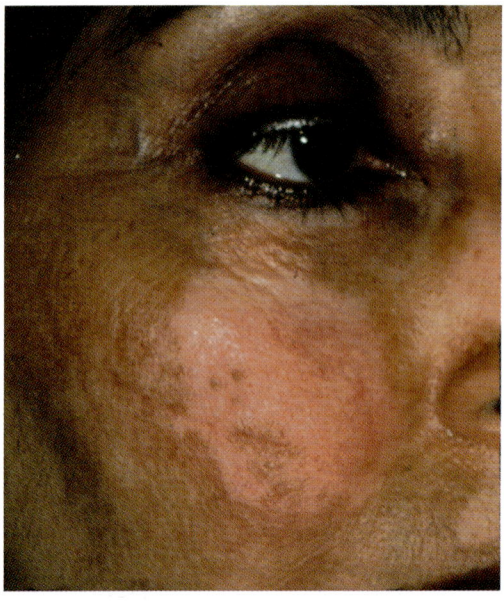

(A)

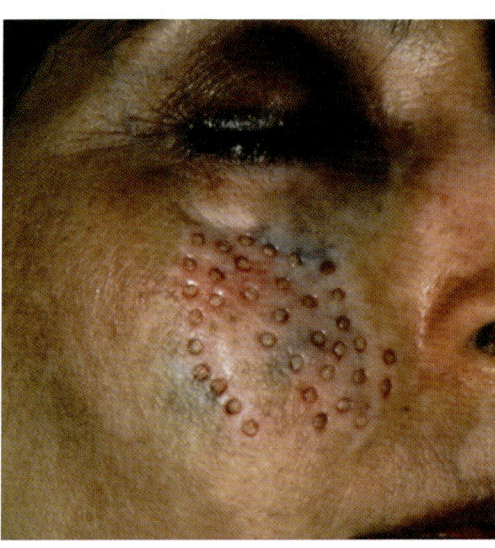

(B)

FIGURE 5.4 (A) East Indian woman with localized facial vitiligo. (B) Same woman as in A immediately after placement of epidermal punch grafts.

as acne vulgaris[40] (Figures 5.6–5.8). Indeed, the postinflammatory hyperpigmented macules of acne are often more distressing to the darker-skinned individual than are the acute lesions (Figure 5.9). Both postinflammatory hyperpigmentation and hypopigmentation are clinical entities that are of major concern to patients with pigmented skin and account for a significant number of visits to dermatologists.

Postinflammatory hyperpigmentation is due to an increase in melanin production and/or an abnormal distribution of melanin pigment.[41] In postinflammatory hypopigmentation there is a decrease in melanin production, resulting in clinically apparent light areas.[39] The skin color of the hyperpigmentation is related to the location of the melanin.[42] It appears brown when it is in the

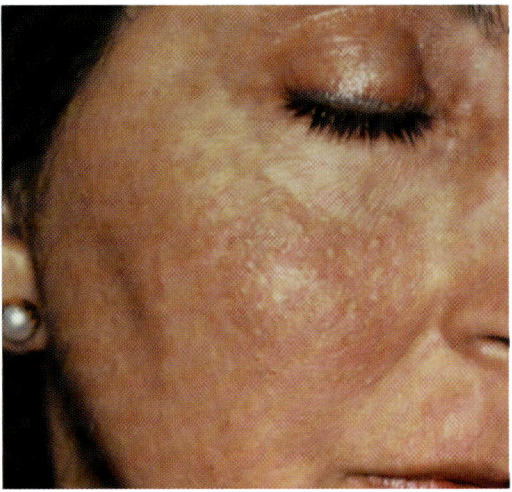

FIGURE 5.4 (C) Final result in woman shown in A, 4 months after treatment with grafts and topical PUVA.

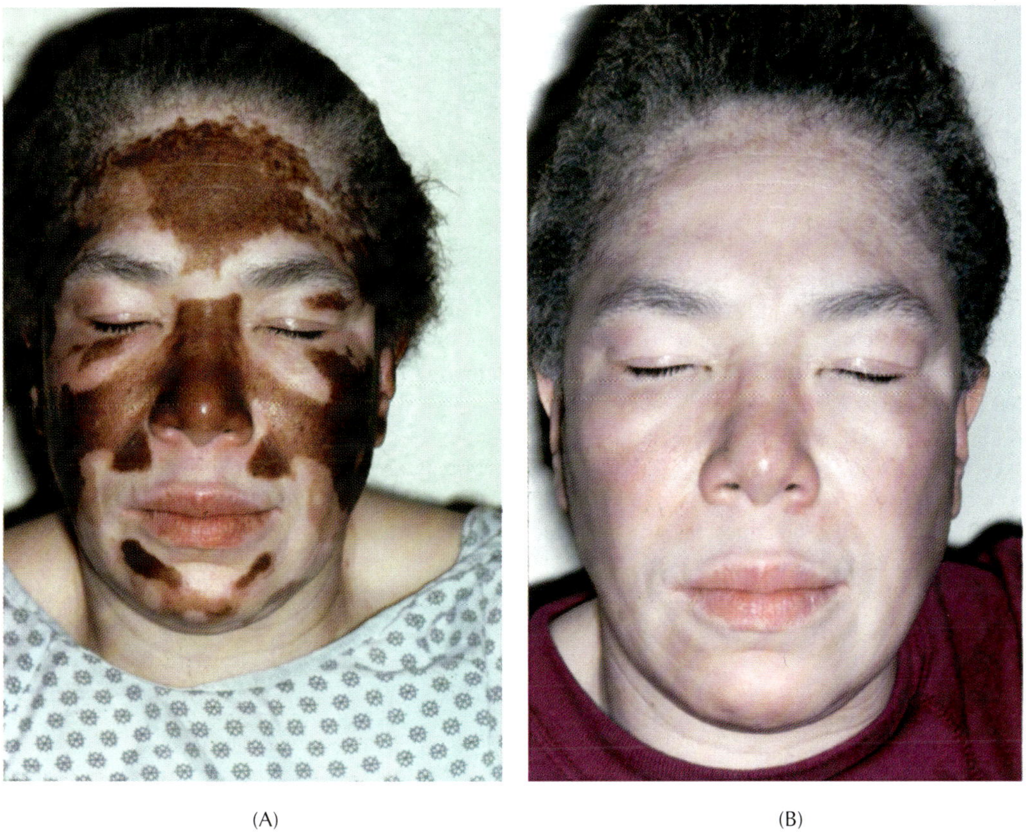

(A)   (B)

FIGURE 5.5 (A) Disfiguring facial vitiligo in Afro-Caribbean woman. (B) Same woman following depigmentation with monobenzoyl ether of hydroquinone (MBEH) used for 8 months.

epidermis whereas blue to bluish-gray if it is in the dermis. With the use of a Wood's lamp, the location of the increased melanin can be determined. The epidermal component is enhanced, whereas the dermal component becomes unapparent in hyperpigmentation.[42] Hypopigmentation is

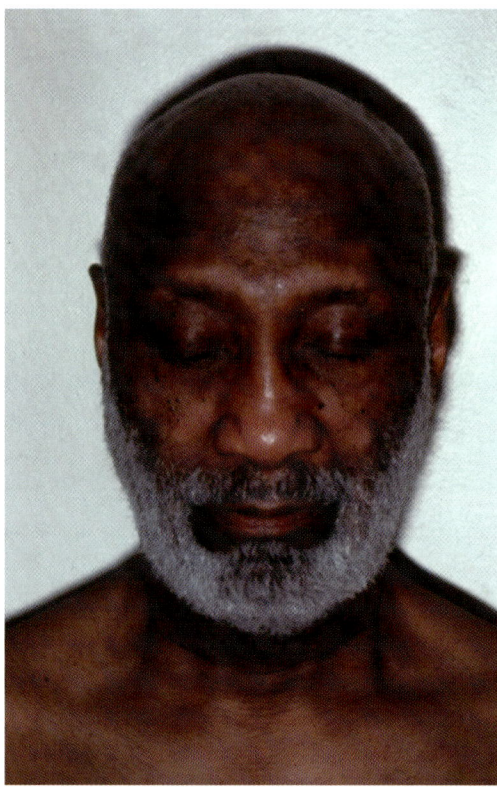

FIGURE 5.6 Postinflammatory hypopigmentation secondary to seborrheic dermatitis. (Reproduced from Halder, R.M., *Dermatola Clin* 2003; 21: 617–628. With permission from Elsevier.)

accentuated with Wood's lamp when it is due to melanocytopenic conditions such as vitiligo and piebaldism, in contrast to melanopenic conditions such as postinflammatory hypopigmentation. It should be noted, however, that the Wood's lamp technique is sometimes not helpful in persons of color because of optical factors.[42]

After cutaneous trauma or inflammation, melanocytes can react with normal, increased, or decreased production of melanin. Although the actual pathogenesis is unknown, it is thought that both hyperpigmentation and hypopigmentation result from cytokines and inflammatory mediators from keratinocytes, melanocytes, and inflammatory cells that are released in an inflammatory process in the skin. These include leukotriene (LT), prostaglandins (PG), and thromboxane (TXB).[43]

In vitro studies have shown that LT-C4, in addition to LT-D4, PG-E2, and TXB-2, stimulate human melanocyte enlargement and dendrocyte proliferation.[41] Also, LT-C4 significantly increases tyrosinase activity in cultured melanocytes and also increases mitogenic activity of melanocytes.[41] *In vitro* studies have also shown that transforming growth factor-alpha and LT-C4 stimulate movement of melanocytes. These mediators and cytokines are thought to play an important role in the pathogenesis of postinflammatory hyperpigmentation.[41]

The pathogenesis of postinflammatory hypopigmentation is believed to be secondary to melanocyte cell-surface expression of intercellular adhesion molecule (ICAM)-1 induced by inflammatory mediators such as interferon-gamma, tumor necrosis factor (TNF)-alpha, TNF-beta, interleukin (IL)-6 and IL-7.[44] The theory is that this may lead to leukocyte–melanocyte attachments, with the final result being innocent bystander destruction of melanocytes.

Treatment modalities for postinflammatory hyperpigmentation include cosmetic cover-ups, hydroquinones, kojic acid, topical steroids, topical retinoids, chemical peels, and Q-switched ruby and Nd:YAG lasers.[45–47] For postinflammatory hypopigmentation, treatment modalities include

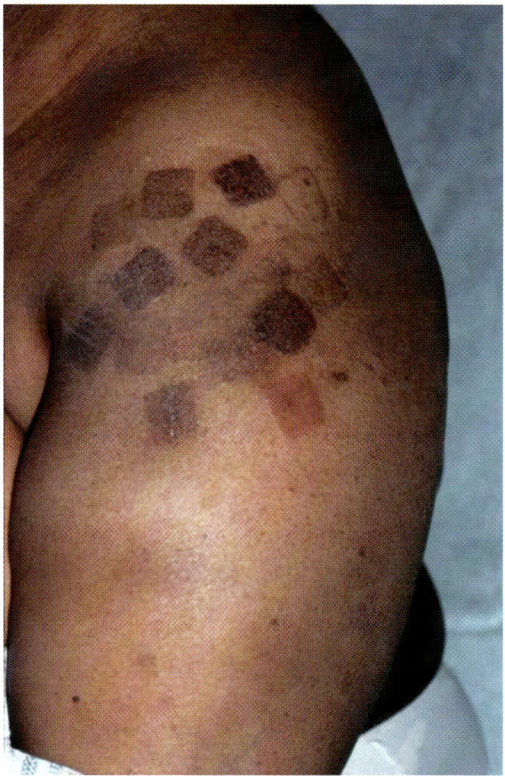

FIGURE 5.7 Postinflammatory hyperpigmentation from drug patch allergy. Note erythema in an acute lesion.

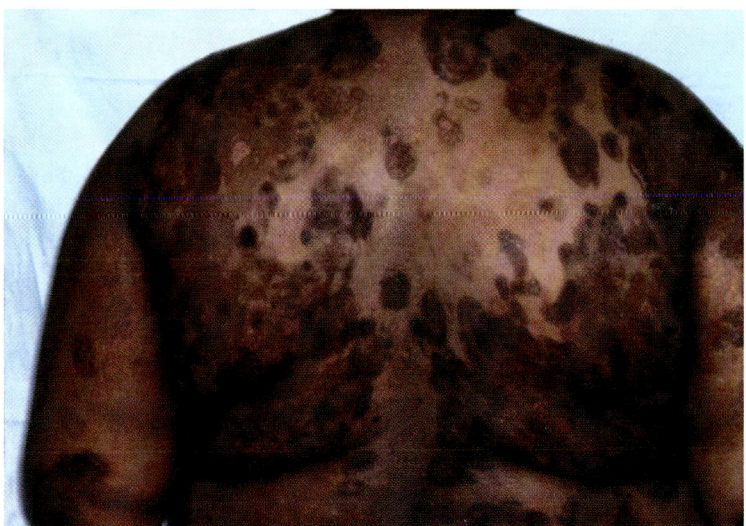

FIGURE 5.8 Extensive postinflammatory hyperpigmentation secondary to recurrent episodes of pemphigus vulgaris.

cosmetic cover-ups, topical or oral PUVA therapy, narrow-band UVB phototherapy, topical steroids, and skin grafts.[43] Treating the underlying cause of postinflammatory hyper- and hypopigmentation is an important aspect of preventing further dyschromia. The efficacies of previously mentioned treatment modalities are variable.

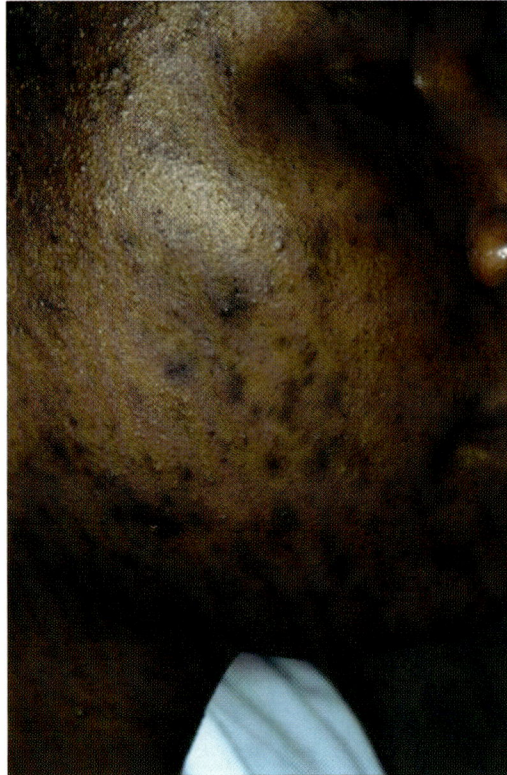

FIGURE 5.9 Postinflammatory hyperpigmentation secondary to acne vulgaris.

DISORDERS OF HYPERPIGMENTATION

Linea Nigra

This phenomenon is observed during pregnancy.[48] Normally, women appear to have a pale line on the abdomen that extends from the xyphoid process through the umbilicus to the symphysis pubis. It is called the linea alba. During pregnancy, this line darkens and is then called the linea nigra.[48,49] The exact mechanism for darkening is unclear and is attributed to the same hormonal mechanisms that likely contribute to melasma (see above discussion). The same darkening is also noticed around the nipples, areola, perineum, vulva, and inner thighs.[50] It is a benign and common condition that may be seen in up to 90% of pregnant women; however, the pigmentation is more intense in skin of color. Gestational pigment darkening usually resolves within several months postpartum.[51]

Erythema Dyschromicum Perstans (Ashy Dermatosis)

This disorder was first described in Central America in 1957 in the Hispanic literature as "Los Cenicientos," which means "the ashen ones" in Spanish.[52] Although the disease has been reported worldwide, it is most commonly seen and reported in young patients from Central America. Erythema dyschromicum perstans is also prevalent in blacks and Asians (particularly South Asians). It clinically manifests as asymptomatic ashy, blue-black hyperpigmented macules and patches on the face, back, arms, and legs (Figure 5.10). The palms and soles are typically spared. As the pigment is dermal in origin, there is no accentuation with Wood's lamp. There is usually no associated systemic disease.[52]

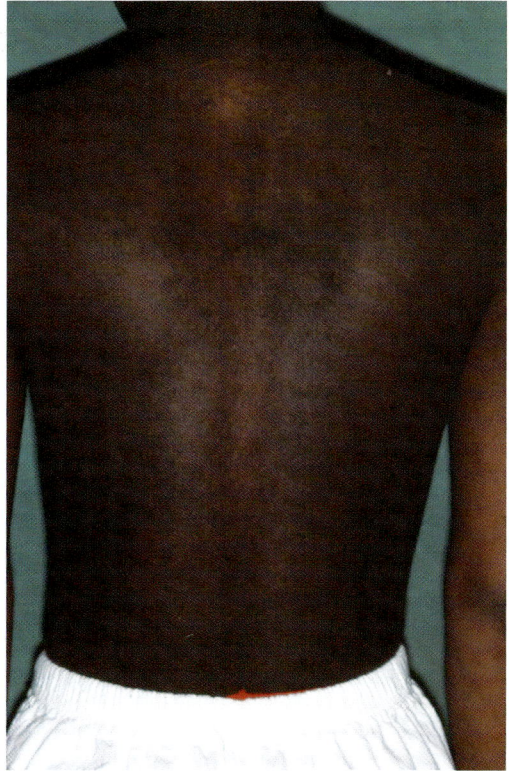

FIGURE 5.10 Erythema dyschromicum perstans of the back. There are extensive areas of blue-gray pigmentation.

Histologically, there is an increase in dermal melanophages with an overlying increase in epidermal melanin. There is epidermal spongiosis and basal layer vacuolization with dermal perivascular infiltrate in early lesions. Active lesions reveal colloid bodies that have dropped into the dermis.[53] This resolves with time, leaving dermal hyperpigmentation. As in dermal melasma, there is a blue appearance clinically secondary to the Tyndall effect.

The disease has no known cause. Some investigators believe that given the histological similarities to lichen planus, it is possibly a variant.[53–55] It is not responsive to topical corticosteroids, however, unlike lichen planus. Treatments have included systemic therapy with clofazamine, with mild to moderate success, respectively.[56] Given the dermal location of the pigment, lasers such as the 694-nm Q-switched ruby may be beneficial in treating the disorder. Further studies are necessary for determination of therapeutic efficacy.[47,57]

MELASMA

This disorder is characterized by arcuate or polycyclic, hyperpigmented macules and patches usually presenting on the face, but it can also be evident on the neck or forearms. It is most commonly seen in pregnant women or in women taking oral contraceptive pills (OCP), accounting for the colloquialism "the mask of pregnancy."[48] The term "mask" also implies the other key feature of the disease, namely its restriction to sun-exposed skin. Melasma of the upper lip is a marker for OCP use.[58]

While melasma is not exclusively a disorder of ethnic populations, studies of the epidemiology of melasma reveal it to be a common disorder among darker-skinned races (Figure 5.11). It is frequent among Latinos, African-Americans and Africans (particularly Ethiopians) as well as Asians

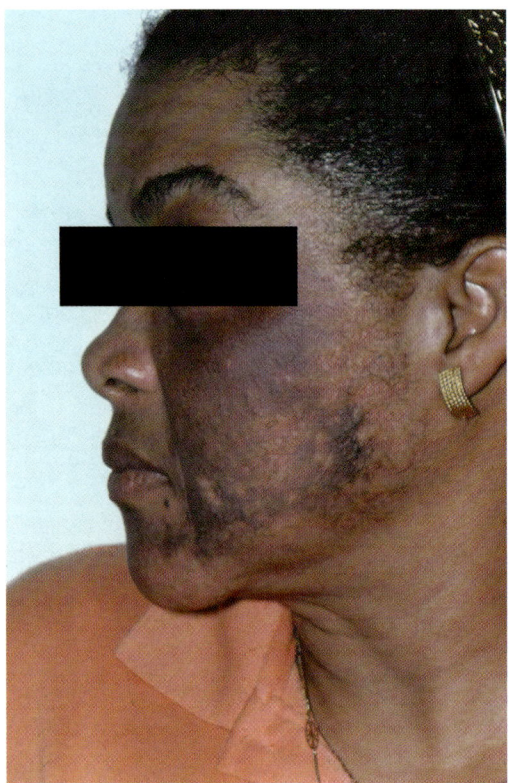

FIGURE 5.11 Facial melasma.

and Pacific islanders.[59] Clearly, there is a genetic predisposition to the development of melasma, as it can be seen in mothers of the same family as well as in twins.[58,60]

The pathogenesis of melasma is unclear. Some investigators have suggested that beta-lipotropin secreted by the pituitary gland may induce melasma. It is a known melanotropic peptide. However, this has yet to be proven, as levels of the protein are not altered between those affected and controls.[61] Melasma is clearly affected in some way by estrogen or progesterone, given the temporal relationship of onset to pregnancy and ingestion of birth control pills.[48,50,62,63] Studies of melasma in men have also implicated subtle hormonal imbalances as a possible mechanism for its pathogenesis.[64] Interestingly, women who are postmenopausal and on estrogen therapy do not usually have melasma.[60] However, if the woman is given hormone replacement therapy (HRT) that contains progesterone, she is likely to get melasma.[58] This implicates progesterone as a key mediating hormone in melasma induction. Another curious phenomenon is the entity of melasma isolated to the forearms, which is seen in both women receiving progesterone HRT and Native American women not receiving HRT[44] (Figure 5.12).

Melasma may appear brown or blue depending on the depth of the pigmentation, either epidermal or dermal, respectively. The so-called Tyndall effect accounts for the blue appearance of dermal melasma. This is due to melanin's absorption of light and the refractile properties of light itself, which lead to its subsequent dispersion and re-emergence with a perceived blue hue.[42]

Determining whether the patient has dermal vs. epidermal melasma will affect therapy, as the dermal form is not likely to respond to bleaching agents.[65,66] The color of dermal melasma is not enhanced when viewed with a Wood's light. By comparison, epidermal melasma will show marked contrast between normal skin and skin with melasma. That is to say, the melasma-affected skin will appear markedly darker than the normal surrounding skin.[67] If a Wood's lamp examination is

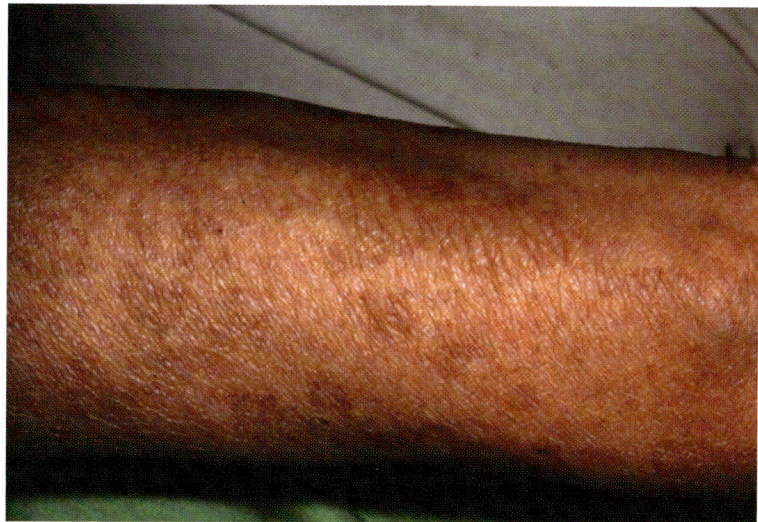

FIGURE 5.12 Forearm melasma secondary to hormone replacement therapy (HRT) in a Hispanic woman.

equivocal, then a biopsy may be necessary to distinguish the two. The epidermal type characteristically has increased melanin in the basal and suprabasal layers, with some basal-layer vacuolization. This is the most common as well as the most treatable type of melasma.[42]

FAMILIAL RACIAL PERIORBITAL HYPERPIGMENTATION

This is a relatively common condition in pigmented races particularly in South Asian (Indians, Pakistanis), Afro-Caribbeans, and African-Americans. It may be inherited in an autosomal-dominant manner.[68] Characterized by diffuse hyperpigmented patches in the periorbital area, this condition can give a raccoon-eye-like appearance, with patients complaining of dark circles around the eyes. However, the infraorbital area is more often affected. This condition is often blamed in many cultures as due to fatigue, worry, or anxiety.[69] Histologically, there is increased melanin in the basal cell layer of the epidermis and melanophages in the upper dermis.[70] Treatment with bleaching agents is usually ineffective. There are reports of successful lightening with Q-switched ruby laser and CO_2 laser.[71] These lasers should be used with caution in dark skin. Cosmetic cover up may be sufficient therapy for some patients.

THE MANAGEMENT OF PIGMENTARY DISORDERS

TOPICAL CORTICOSTEROIDS

Topical corticosteroids can be used to treat hyperpigmentation of the skin either alone or in combination with other topical agents. Kligman and Willis hypothesized that topical corticosteroids suppress melanin production without destroying melanocytes by suppressing biosynthetic and secretory functions within the melanocyte.[72] Hypopigmentation is a well-recognized side effect of extended topical corticosteroid use. However, topical corticosteroids can be used to treat disorders such as postinflammatory hyperpigmentation with variable effect. They have also been used to treat melasma as monotherapy or in combination with other agents.[73]

Because of the known effects of topical corticosteroids in lightening skin color, they have been abused in some ethnic populations to lighten and bleach the skin. In fact, high-potency topical corticosteroids (classes 1 and 2) are available against FDA regulations, over the counter, in ethnic stores in large metropolitan areas such as Washington, DC, New York City, Los Angeles, and Miami.

Phenolic Agents

Hydroquinone, which is a hydroxyphenolic chemical, has been the gold standard for treatment of hyperpigmentation for more than 50 years. It acts by inhibiting the enzyme tyrosinase, thereby reducing the conversion of DOPA to melanin. Some of the other possible mechanisms of action are the destruction of melanocytes, degradation of melanosomes, and the inhibition the synthesis of DNA and RNA.[58]

Hydroquinone can be compounded into 5%–10% concentrations, but at these strengths they may be irritating and unstable. The 2% concentrations of hydroquinone available over the counter in the U.S. and Canada are not as efficacious as the 3% and 4% prescription formulations, as their onset of action is later than with the higher concentrations. Antioxidants, such as vitamin C and retinoids, and alpha-hydroxy acids may be used as additives to increase penetration and enhance efficacy. Exogenous ochronosis with the use of hydroquinone has been reported in dark-skinned patients, in particular South African women who frequently use very high concentrations of hydroquinone over large surface areas. Although hydroquinone is used frequently in North America, there have only been about 45 reported cases of exogenous ochronosis from hydroquinone use there.

The use of hydroquinone products in women of pigmented races is extensive throughout the world. This has led to the abuse of hydroquinone products in darker races. The use of products with high concentrations of hydroquinone that are obtained illegally continues to rise. This no doubt will cause the number of cases of exogenous hydroquinone-induced ochronosis to increase throughout the world and in the United States. These illegal products are available over the counter in ethnic stores in metropolitan areas such as Washington, DC, New York City, Los Angeles, and Miami.

Adverse reactions from hydroquinone use include irritant and allergic contact dermatitis and nail discoloration. Postinflammatory hyperpigmentation may occur from the contact dermatitis. Hypopigmentation of the normal skin surrounding the treated areas may also occur. These usually resolve with the discontinuation of the hydroquinone treatment.[58]

Monobenzone, the monobenzyl ether of hydroquinone, is a special topical phenolic agent that is indicated only for the final depigmentation of disfiguring or extensive vitiligo. It is applied topically to permanently depigment normal skin surrounding vitiliginous areas in patients with extensive vitiligo (greater than 50% body surface area). The cream is applied in a thin layer and rubbed into the normally pigmented areas two or three times daily. Depigmentation is usually achieved after 6–12 months with 20% monobenzone treatment. It should then be applied only as often as required to maintain depigmentation. Monobenzone cream can produce satellite depigmentation at sites distant from the site of initial application. Direct skin contact with others should be avoided for at least 4 h following application. Most patients who are depigmented for vitiligo with monobenzone are pleased with the final result, regardless of their racial or ethnic background.

N-acetyl-4-cysteaminylphenol (NCAP) is another phenolic agent that is currently being developed and is not yet available in North America. NCAP acts to decrease intracellular glutathione by stimulating pheomelanin rather than eumelanin.[74] It also inhibits tyrosinase activity and has been found to be more stable and cause less irritation than hydroquinone. In a retrospective study of 12 patients with melasma using 4% NCAP, 66% showed marked improvement and 8% showed complete loss of melasma lesions. Changes of melanoderma were evident after 2–4 weeks of daily topical application of NCAP.[75]

Azelaic Acid

Azelaic acid is a naturally occurring nonphenolic, saturated nine-carbon dicarboxylic acid. Its use originated from the findings that *Pityrosporum* species can oxidize unsaturated fatty acids to dicarboxylic acids, which competitively inhibit tyrosinase. Azelaic acid was initially developed as a topical drug with therapeutic effects for the treatment of acne. However, because of its effect on tyrosinase, it has also been used to treat melasma, lentigo maligna, and other disorders of hyperpigmentation.[29,65] Azelaic acid has been reported to be effective for hypermelanosis caused by physical or photochemical agents and lentigo maligna melanoma as well as other disorders characterized by abnormal proliferation of melanocytes. Its mechanism of action is to inhibit DNA synthesis and mitochondrial enzymes, thereby inducing direct cytoxic effects toward the melanocyte.[65] Topical azelaic acid has no depigmentation effect on normally pigmented skin, freckles, senile lentigines, and nevi. This specificity may be attributed to its selective effects on abnormal melanocytes.

Azelaic acid can be used for postinflammatory hyperpigmentation in acne.[62] Free radicals are believed to contribute to hyperpigmentation, and azelaic acid acts by reducing free radical production.[76] Azelaic acid 15–20% is currently available in the U.S. and is indicated only for the treatment of acne, although it has off-label use for hyperpigmentation. In the treatment of melasma, a 24-week study in South America found that a 20% concentration of azelaic acid was equivlaent to 2% hydroquinone.[77] In the Philippines, a study found that a 20% concentration of azelaic acid was better that 2% hydroquinone.[66]

Kojic Acid

Kojic acid (5-hydroxy-2-(hydroxy methyl)-4-pyrone) is a naturally occurring hydrophilic fungal derivative evolved from certain species of *Acetobacter*, *Aspergillus*, and *Penicillium* and used in the treatment of hyperpigmentation disorders.[78] It acts by inhibiting the production of free tyrosinase, with efficacy similar to hydroquinone. In Japan, kojic acid has been increasingly used in skin care products. This is because, until recently, topically applied kojic acid at 1% concentration had not exhibited any sensitizing activity.[79] However, more recent long-term Japanese studies have shown that kojic acid has the potential for causing contact dermatitis and erythema.[79]

Arbutin

Arbutin, which is the β-D-glucopyranoside derivative of hydroquinone, is a naturally occurring plant-derived compound that has been used for postinflammatory hyperpigmentation.[80] It is effective in the treatment of disorders of hyperpigmentation characterized by hyperactive melanocytes.[80] The action of arbutin is dependent on its concentration. Higher concentrations are more efficacious than lower concentrations, but they may also result in a paradoxical hyperpigmentation.[80] In comparative *in vitro* studies of various compounds used to improve the appearance of disorders of hyperpigmentation, arbutin was found to be less toxic than hydroquinone. A dose-dependent reduction in tyrosinase activity and melanin content in melanocytes was also demonstrated.

Licorice Extract

Licorice extract is not yet available in North America but has been used in other parts of the world, particularly in Egypt. Its mechanism of action is similar to that of kojic acid. The main component of the hydrophobic fraction of licorice extract, with an effect on the skin, is glabridin. Studies investigating the inhibitory effects of glabridin on melanogenesis and inflammation have shown that it inhibits tyrosinase activity of these cells. No effect on DNA synthesis was detectable.[81]

Topical Retinoids

The efficacy of topical tretinoin 0.05%–0.1% as monotherapy for postinflammatory hyperpigmentation has been reported.[82] Tretinoin was also used as monotherapy in a study of 38 African-American patients with melasma, and 68%–73% of patients improved. In 88% of the patients, moderate side effects of desquamation and erythema were observed.[83,84] Darker-skinned patients who develop a dermatitis from tretinoin may develop postinflammatory hyperpigmentation secondary to the dermatitis.

The mechanism of action of tretinoin in the treatment of melasma is poorly understood. Clinical improvement has been found to be associated with a reduction in epidermal melanin, possibly as a result of the inhibition of tyrosinase by the action of tretinoin.[42] Although tretinoin can be effective as monotherapy for hyperpigmentation and melasma, it requires treatment periods of 20–40 weeks.

In a randomized clinical trial, the efficacy of adapalene 0.1% was found to be comparable to that of tretinoin 0.05% cream in the treatment of melasma (mainly epidermal type). The results showed fewer side effects and greater acceptability among patients using adapalene.[86]

COMBINATION THERAPY

Tretinoin can also be used in conjunction with hydroquinone or other depigmenting agents to improve efficacy. The first published study of combination therapy used tretinoin 0.1%, hydroquinone 5%, and dexamethasone 0.1% for postinflammatory hyperpigmentation.[85] Tretinoin was shown to reduce the atrophy of the corticosteroid and facilitated the epidermal penetration of the hydroquinone. The tretinoin-induced irritation was reduced by the corticosteroid. The first triple-combination topical therapy approved by the U.S. FDA for melasma is a modified formulation comprising fluocinolone acetonide, hydroquinone 4%, and tretinoin 0.05%. In studies of patients with melasma, 78% had complete or near-complete clearance after 8 weeks of therapy. Similar results and a favorable safety profile were seen in a 12-month study.

TARS

Topical tar has both anti-inflammatory and melanogenic properties. Although the melanogenic property is usually associated with a photodynamic mechanism, there is evidence that cutaneous melanogenesis can occur without the action of light.[87] Tar can be used to treat pigmentary disorders such as postinflammatory hypopigmentation and vitiligo.

TOPICAL TACROLIMUS

Tacrolimus is a macrolide immunosuppressant that is derived from the fungus *Streptomyces tsukubaensis*. It inhibits T-lymphocyte activation by binding to an immunophilin, FK-binding protein, found in the cytoplasm of T lymphocytes. The complex that is formed inhibits the phosphatase calcineurin. This inhibition prevents signal transduction pathways from occurring, which ultimately halts the transcription of cytokines such as IL-2, IL-3, IL-4, IL-5, IL-8, TFN, and interferon-gamma.

Topical tacrolimus can be used to treat vitiligo and may be effective because it suppresses autoantibody recognition of cell-surface melanocyte antigens and inhibits subsequent cytotoxic T-lymphocyte reactions. It has been used as ointment in concentrations of 0.03% and 0.1% to treat vitiligo. There are numerous reports of the efficacy of topical tacrolimus in treating vitiligo.[88,89]

OTHER TREATMENTS

Other treatments for hyperpigmentation include chemical peels[61] and are discussed in detail in Chapter 12. Newer depigmenting modalities are continually being investigated.[74,75] Lasers, most notably the 694-nm Q-switched ruby laser, have been tried and thus far appear to be ineffective for treating melasma but can be effective for nevus of Ota or postinflammatory hyperpigmentation. The successful treatment of diseases of skin hyperpigmentation in patients with pigmented skins can involve a combination of several modalities including topical agents, chemical peels, microdermabrasion, and laser (see also Chapters 12 and 14). All of these should be used judiciously in pigmented skins. One should be aware of potential adverse effects of all of these modalities in skin of color.

PIGMENTED NEVI

NAILS

Longitudinal melanonychia are common in darker-skinned populations. Indeed, all nails may have a pigment stripe.[90] These are hyperpigmented streaks seen in the nail plate but originate from melanocytes in the matrix. In Caucasians, this same stripe would be cause for alarm. This is due to the fact that, normally, nail matrix melanocytes are quiescent in Caucasians. When they suddenly become visible, it is a marker for a more ominous pathology malignant melanoma.[5] The key difference between normal nail and skin melanocytes, regardless of race, is their location in the skin. There are single melanocytes between keratinocytes in the basal layer.[91] In the nail matrix, melanocytes are found in small clusters above the basal layer. They are concentrated on the distal portion of the matrix. This may be visible through a transparent cuticle and proximal nail fold and is called "pseudo-Hutchinson's sign."[91] It is not associated with melanoma but must be differentiated from one.[5, 90]

PALMOPLANTAR RACIAL DIFFERENCES

The major palmoplantar difference between Caucasians and ethnic populations is the anatomical location of nevi that have potential for malignant transformation.[92] All races can have nevi that undergo spontaneous transformation to malignant melanoma. However, in darker-skinned races these nevi are usually seen on the palms, soles, and buccal mucosa.[93] Therefore, when doing full skin examinations, a thorough inspection of the oral cavity as well as acral sites is necessary, particularly in pigmented races.

NEVUS OF OTA/NEVUS OF ITO

Although these nevi are seen in all races, they are more common in Asians.[15] They are considered congenital rather than hereditary. Nevus of Ota and nevus of Ito differ clinically by location but are histologically similar. Nevus of Ota is characterized by blue-black macules or patches around the eye within the distribution of the first and second branch of the trigeminal nerve (Figure 5.13). There are four separate types based on the extent and location of the pigment present, having the potential for malignant transformation. Nevus of Ito is usually seen on the shoulder in the supraclavicular area.[71] Both nevus of Ito and Ota have been reported to respond well to laser therapy, particularly the Q-switched ruby laser.[82,94,95]

GENETIC DISEASES

PIEBALDISM

Piebaldism, also known as partial albinism, is a rare autosomal dominant congenital disorder caused by a defect in the c-kit gene that encodes the stem cell factor surface receptor.[17] It is characterized by a white forelock with skin-colored to hyperpigmented macules within the well-circumscribed white patches found characteristically on the forehead, ventral aspect of the trunk, and the midregions of the upper and lower extremities[96] (Figure 5.14) Piebaldism, like vitiligo, can be psychologically devastating, especially in people of color, due to the marked contrast between normal and affected skin.[25]

Two hypotheses have been proposed for the lesions associated with piebaldism. The first hypothesis proposes a defect in the migration of melanoblasts from the neural crest to the ventral

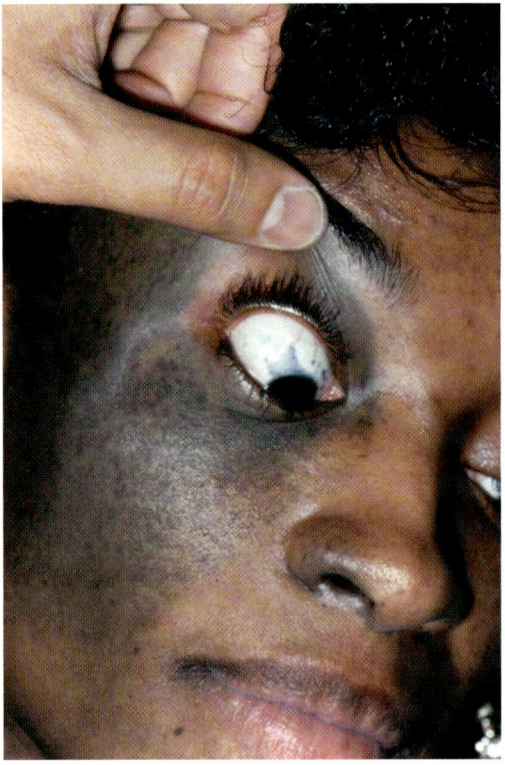

FIGURE 5.13 Nevus of Ota with conjunctival involvement.

aspect of the skin. The second proposes a failure of melanoblasts to survive or differentiate into melanocytes once they reach the ventral aspect of the skin.[17]

Piebaldism has been seen in association with mental retardation, cerebellar ataxia and Hirschsprung's disease. Two variants of piebaldism are Waardenburg syndrome and Woolf syndrome. Waardenburg syndrome is an autosomal-dominant disorder with variable expression.[17] It is characterized by lateral displacement of the inner canthi in the presence of normal interpupillary distance, broad nasal root, iris heterochromia, congenital sensorineural hearing loss, and a white forelock. The various types are due to a defect in several different genes: PAX3, MITF gene (PAX3 promoter), or SOX10.[17] Woolf syndrome is an autosomal-recessive form of piebaldism characterized by congenital sensorineural deafness.[97]

Treatment options for piebaldism include some of the same options as vitiligo, such as skin grafts and cosmetic cover-ups.[98] PUVA and narrow-band UVB, although not reported to be effective for piebaldism, have been successful in some patients in our experience.

ALBINISM AND HERMANSKY–PUDLAK SYNDROME

Albinism refers to a set of distinct genetic disorders characterized by either a lack of pigment or pigment dilution. There are a number of characteristic phenotypic expressions as a result of hundreds of distinct gene mutations.[99] The key feature of albinism is that there is a normal number of melanocytes but there is a defect in the synthesis of melanin. Oculocutaneous albinism (OCA) Type I is divided into two subtypes, A and B. Both are due to varying defects in the tyrosinase gene, leading to mild phenotypic variations in the disorder.[100] OCA 1A is more severe than OCA 1B in that there is a complete lack of tyrosinase.[101] This manifests as a congenital absence of pigment

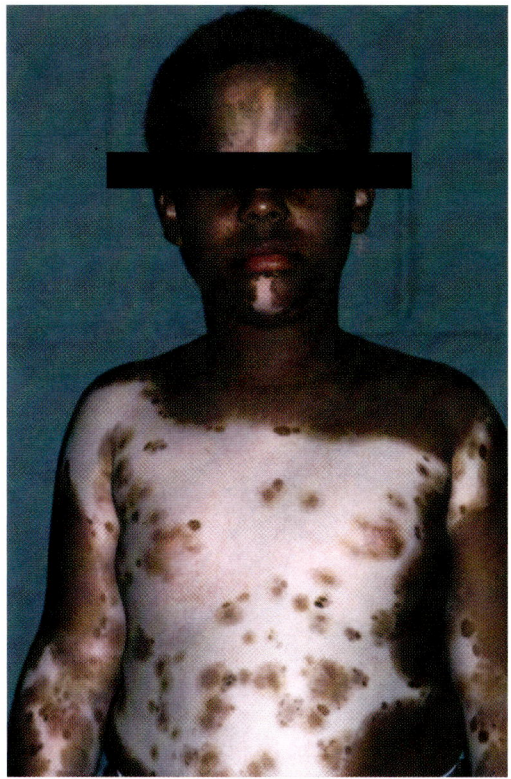

FIGURE 5.14 Piebaldism with central trunk and facial involvement.

of the skin and eyes, which leads to impaired visual acuity as well as other neurological abnormalities. OCA 1B differs in that markedly reduced tyrosinase activity is present, accounting for the visible amount of pigment that develops in the skin, hair, and eyes after birth (Figure 5.15).[100,102] Thus, these patients are able to tan. OCA 2 is due to mutations in the P gene and can vary from a strikingly albino appearance to nearly normal pigmentation.[103]

OCA 3 is interesting in that it has been described only in ethnic populations, particularly blacks. Patients present with brown skin, brown hair, and blue or brown eyes. They commonly have decreased visual acuity and nystagmus as in other forms of oculocutaneous albinism. The defect has been localized to the tyrosinase related protein 1 (TRP-1) gene, whose function as yet remains poorly characterized.[99,101] Studies suggest that a malfunction of this protein results in brown rather than black pigment formation, leading to its characteristic phenotype.[99,101]

Hermansky–Pudlak syndrome is a form of oculocutaneous albinism seen almost exclusively in Puerto Ricans, but has also been reported in Japanese individuals.[104] It is distinguished from the other types by its concomitant bleeding diathesis and ceroid storage in the aerodigestive tract[105] (see also Chapters 3 and 7).

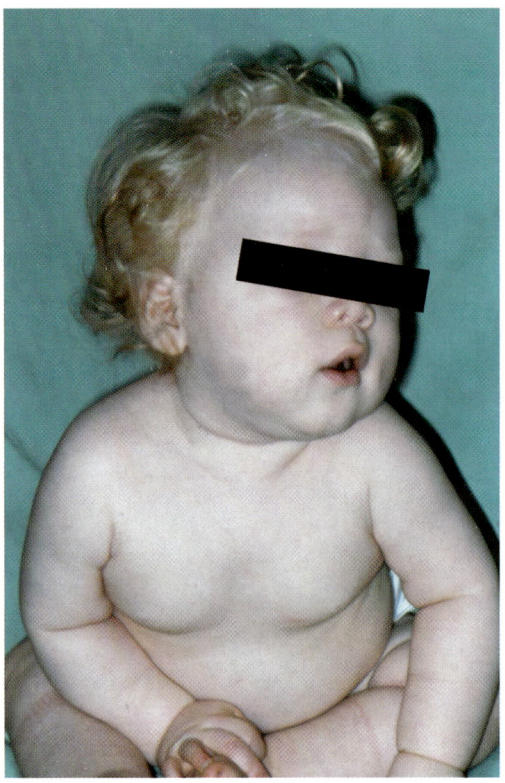

FIGURE 5.15 Albinism in an African-American infant. Hair color is blonde with dilution of skin pigmentation.

REFERENCES

1. Porter JR, Beuf AH, Lerner AB, Nordlund JJ. Psychosocial effects of vitiligo: a comparison of vitiligo with "normal" control subjects, with psoriasis patients, and with patients with other pigment disorders. *J Am Acad Dermatol* 1986; 15: 220.
2. Nordlund JJ, Ortonne J. The normal color of human skin. In: Nordlund JJ, Boissy RE, Hearing VJ, King RA,Ortonne J (Eds) *The Pigmentary System. Physiology and Pathophysiology.* Oxford University Press, New York, 1988; 475–484.
3. Halder RM, Nootheti, PK. Ethnic skin disorders overview. *J Am Acad Dermatol* 2003; 48: 143–148.
4. Lacour JP. Infectious melanosis. In: Nordlund JJ, Boissy RE, Hearing VJ, King RA,Ortonne J (Eds) *The Pigmentary System. Physiology and Pathophysiology.* Oxford University Press, New York, 1988; 634–639.
5. Lateur N, André J. Melanonychia: diagnosis and treatment. *Dermatol Ther* 2002; 15(2): 131–141.
6. Charles, CR. Hypopigmentation in tinea versicolor: histochemical and electomicroscopic study. *Int J Dermatol* 1973; 12: 48–58.
7. El Gothamy, Z. Tinea versicolor hypopigmentation: histochemical and therapeutic studies. *Int J Dermatol* 1975; 14: 510–516.
8. Karaoui R, Bou-Resli M, Al0Zaid NS, Mousa A. Tinea versicolor: ultrastructural studies on hypopigmented and hyperpigmented skin. *Dermatologica* 1981; 162: 69–71.
9. Ito K, Tanaka, T. Amino acid metabolism of fungi: decomposition of L-tyrosine by fungi. In: Nordlund JJ, Boissy RE, Hearing VJ, King RA,Ortonne J (Eds) *The Pigmentary System. Physiology and Pathophysiology.* Oxford University Press, New York, 1988; 634–639.
10. Borelli D, Jacobs PH, and Nall, L. Tinea versicolor: epidemiologic, clinical and therapeutic aspects. *J Am Acad Dermatol* 1991; 25: 300–305.

11. O'Farrell MM. Pityriasis alba. *Arch Dermatol* 1956; 73: 376–378.
12. Shah AS, Supapannachart N, Nordlund JJ. Acquired hypomelanotic disorders. In: Levine N (Ed) *Pigmentation and Pigmentary Disorders*. CRC Press, Boca Raton, FL, 1993; 352–353,
13. Zaynoun ST, Aftimos BG, Tenekjian, KK, Bahuth N, Kurban AK. Extensive pityriasis alba: a histological, histochemical and ultrastructural study. *Br J Dermatol* 1983; 108: 83–86.
14. Lin A. Topical immunotherapy. In: Wolverton SE (Ed) *Comprehensive Dermatological Therapy*. Saunders, Philadelphia, 2001; 617–619.
15. Falabella R. Idiopathic guttate hypomelanosis. *Dermatologic Clin* 1988; 6(2): 241–247.
16. Wilson P, Lavker R, Kligman A. On the nature of idiopathic guttate hypomelanosis. *Acta Derm Venereol* 1982; 62(4): 301–306.
17. Bolognia J, Pawelek J. Biology of hypopigmentation. *J Am Acad Dermatol* 1988; 19: 217–255.
18. Falabella R, Escobar C, Giraldo N, Rovetto P, Gil J, Barona MI, Acosta F, Alzate A. On the pathogenesis of idiopathic guttate hypomelanosis. *J Am Acad Dermatol* 1987; 16(pt 1): 35–44.
19. Golhar A, Pillar T, Eidelman S, Etzioni A. Vitiligo and idiopathic guttate hypomelanosis. Repigmentation of skin following engraftment onto nude mice. *Arch Dermatol* 1989; 125(10): 1363–1366.
20. Ploysangam T, Dee-Ananlap S, Suvanprakorn P. Treatment of idiopathic guttate hypomelanosis with liquid nitrogen: light and electron microscopic studies. *J Am Acad Dermatol* 1990; 23(4 Pt 1): 681–684.
21. Kovac, S. Vitiligo. *J Am Acad Dermatol* 1998; 38: 647–666.
22. Halder RM, Brooks HL. Medical therapies for vitiligo. *Dermatol Ther* 2001; 14: 1–6.
23. Boisseau-Garsaud A, Garsaud P, Cales-Quist D, Helenon R, Queneherve C, Claire RC. Epidemiology of vitiligo in the French West Indies (Isle of Martinique). *Int J Dermatol* 2000; 39: 18–20.
24. Falabella R, Barona M, Escobar C, Borrero I, Arrunategui A. Surgical combination therapy for vitiligo and piebaldism. *Dermatol Surg* 1995; 21: 852–857.
25. Hautmann G, Panconesi E. Vitiligo: a psychologically influenced and influencing disease. *Clin Dermatol* 1997; 15: 879–890.
26. Kent G, Al'Abadie M. Psychologic effects of vitiligo. *J Am Acad Dermatol* 1996; 35(6): 895–898.
27. Nordlund JJ, Halder RM, Grimes P. Management of vitiligo. *Dermatol Clin* 1993; 11(1): 27–33.
28. Falabella R. Surgical therapies for vitiligo. *Clin Dermatol* 1997; 15: 927–939
29. Grimes PE. Melasma: etiologic and therapeutic considerations. *Arch Dermatol* 1995; 131: 1453–1457.
30. Halder RM, Young CM. New and emerging therapies for vitiligo. *Dermatol Clin* 2000; 18(1): 79–89.
31. Jimbow K. Vitiligo: therapeutic advances. *Dermatol Clin* 1998; 16(2): 399–407.
32. Scherschun L, Kim JJ, Lim H. Narrow-band UVB is a useful and well-tolerated treatment for vitiligo. *J Am Acad Dermatol* 2001; 44: 999–1003.
33. Spencer JM, Nossa R, Ajmeri J. Treatment of vitiligo with the 308nm excimer laser: a pilot study. *J Am Acad Dermatol* 2002; 46(5): 727–731.
34. Westerhof W, Nieuweber-Krobotova L. Treatment of vitiligo with UVB radiation vs. topical psoralen plus UVA. *Arch Dermatol* 1997; 133: 1525–1528.
35. Halder RM. Topical PUVA therapy for vitiligo. *Dermatol Nurs* 1991; 3 (3): 178–180.
36. Arrunategue A, Arroyo C, Garcia L, Covelli C, Escobar C, Carrascal E, Falabella R. Melanocyte reservoir in vitiligo. *Int J Dermatol* 1994; 33: 484–487
37. Halder RM, Grimes PE, McLaurin CI, Kress MA, Kenney JA Jr. Incidence of common dermatoses in a predominantly black dermatologic practice. *Cutis* 1983; 32: 378–380. Bose S. Modified Thiersch grafting in stable vitiligo. *J Dermatol* 1996; 23: 362–364.
38. Ruiz-Maldonado R, Orozco-Covarrubias M. Postinflammatory hypopigmentation and hyperpigmentation. *Semin Cutan Med Surg* 1997; 16(1): 36–43.
39. Morelli JG, Norris DA. Influence of inflammatory mediators and cytokines on human melanocyte function (Review). *J Invest Dermatol* 1993; 100(2 Suppl): 191S-195S.
40. Tomita Y, Maeda K, Tagami H. Melanocyte-stimulating properties of arachidonic acid metabolites: possible role in postinflammatory pigmentation. *Pigment Cell Res* 1992; 5(5 Pt 2): 357–361.
41. Gilchrest BA. Localization of melanin pigmentation in skin with Wood's lamp. *Br J Dermatol* 1977; 96: 245–247.
42. Grover R, Morgan BDG. Management of hypopigmentation following burn injury. *Burns* 1996; 22(8): 727–630.
43. Johnston GA, Svukabd KS, McLelland J. Melasma of the arms associated with hormone replacement therapy (letter). *Br J Dermatol* 1998; 139: 932.

44. Ellis D, Tan A. How we do it: management of facial hyperpigmentation. *J Otolaryngol* 1997; 26(4): 286–289.
45. Katsambas AD, Stratigos AJ. Depigmenting and bleaching agents: coping with hyperpigmentation. *Clin Dermatol* 2001; 19: 483–488.
46. Tse Y, Levine VJ, McClain SA, Ashinoff R. The removal of cutaneous pigmented lesions with the Q-switched ruby laser and the Q-switched neodymium:yttrium–aluminum–garnet laser. A comparative study. *J Dermatol Surg Oncol* 1994; 20(12): 795–800.
47. Winton GB, Lewis CV. Dermatoses of pregnancy. *J Am Acad Dermatol* 1982; 6: 997–978.
48. Beischer NA, Wein P. Linea alba pigmentation and umbilical deviation in nulliparous pregnancy: the ligamentous sign. *Obstet Gynecol* 1996; 87(2): 254–256.
49. Kroumpouzos G, Cohen LM. Dermatoses of pregnancy. *J Am Acad Dermatol* 2001; 45: 1–19.
50. Lawley TJ, Yancey K. Skin changes and diseases in pregnancy, In: Freedberg IM et al. (Eds) *Dermatology in General Medicine*, 5th ed. McGraw-Hill, New York, 1999; 1963.
51. Byrne DA, Berger RS. Erythema dyschromicun perstans. *Acta Derm Venereol* 1974; 54: 65–68.
52. Berger RS, Hayes TJ, Dixon SL. Erthema dyschomicum perstans and lichen planus: are they related? *J Am Acad Dermatol* 1989; 21: 438–442
53. Kark EC, Litt RL. Ashy dermatosis-a variant of lichen planus? *Cutis* 1980; 25: 631–633.
54. Person JR, Rogers RL. Ashy dermatosis: an apoptotic disease? *Arch Dermatol* 1981; 117: 701–704.
55. Piquero-Martin J, Perez-Alfonzo R, Abrusci V. Clinical trial with clofazamine for treating erythema dyschromicum perstans. *Int J Dermatol* 1989; 28: 198–200.
56. Taylor CR, Anderson RR. Ineffective treatment of refractory melasma and postinflammatory hyperpigmentation by Q switched ruby laser. *J Dermatol Surg Oncol* 1994; 20: 592–597.
57. Grimes PE. Melasma: etiologic and therapeutic considerations. *Arch Dermatol* 1995; 131: 1453–1457.
58. Perez M, Sanchez JL, Aguilo F. Endocrinologic profile of patients with idiopathic melasma. *J Invest Dermatol* 1983; 81: 543–545.
59. Grimes PE, Stockton T. Pigmentary disorders in blacks. *Dermatol Clin* 1988; 6: 271–281.
60. Taylor, SC. Skin of color: biology, structure, function and implications for dermatologic disease. *J Am Acad Dermatol* 2002 Suppl; 46(2): S43–S59.
61. Breathnach AS. Melanin hyperpigmentation of the skin: melasma, topical treatment with azeleic acid and other therapies. *Cutis* 1996; 57: S36–S45.
62. O'Brien TJ, Dyall-Smith D, Hall AP. Melasma of the arms associated with hormone replacement therapy (letter). *Br J Dermatol* 1999; 141: 592–593.
63. Sialy R, Hassan I, Kaur I, Dash RJ. Melasma in men: a hormonal profile. *J Dermatol* 2000; 27: 64–65.
64. Nguyen QH, Bui TP. Azelaic acid: Pharmacokinetic and pharmacodynamic properties and its therapeutic role in hyperpigmentary disorders and acne. *Int J Dermatol* 1995; 34(2): 75–82.
65. Nordlund JJ. The epidemiology and genetics of vitiligo. *Clin Dermatol* 1997; 15: 875–878.
66. Levin CY, Maibach H. Exogenous ochronosis. An update on clinical features, causative agents and treatment options. *Am J Clin Dermatol* 2001; 2(4):213–217.
67. Goodman RM, Belcher RW. Periorbital hyperpigmentation. *Arch Dermatol* 1969; 100: 169–174.
68. Hacker SM. Common disorders of pigmentation: when are more than cosmetic cover-ups required? *Postgrad Med* 1996; 99: 177–186.
69. Haddock N, Wilkin JK. Periorbital hyperpigmentation. *JAMA* 1981; 246: 835.
70. West TB, Alster TS. Improvement of infraorbital hyperpigmentation following carbon dioxide laser resurfacing. *Dermatol Surg* 1998; 24: 615–616.
71. Kanwar AJ, Dhar S, Kaur S. Treatment of melasma with potent topical corticosteroids. *Dermatology* 1994; 188: 170.
72. Sarkar R, Bhalla M, Kanwar AJ. A comparative study of 20% azelaic acid cream monotherapy versus a sequential therapy in the treatment of melasma in dark-skinned patients. *Dermatology* 2002; 205: 249–254.
73. Arena F, Dixon W, Thomas P, Jimbow K. Glutathione plays a key role in the depigmenting and melanocytotoxic action of N-acetyl-4-S-cysteaminylphenol in black and yellow hair follicles. *J Invest Dermatol* 1995; 104(5):792–797.
74. Jimbow K. N-Acetyl-4-S-Cysteaminylphenol as a new type of depigmenting agent for the melanoderma of patients with melasma. *Arch Dermatol* 1991; 127: 1528–1534.

75. Lowe NJ, Rizk D, Grimes P, Billips M, Pincus S. Azelaic acid 20% cream in the treatment of facial hyperpigmentation in darker-skinned patients. *Clin Ther* 1998; 20(5):945–959.
76. Balina LM, Graupe K. The treatment of melasma 20% azelaic acid versus 4% hydroquinone cream. *Int J Dermatol* 1991; 30(12): 893–895.
77. Sierra-Baldrich E, Tribo MJ, Camarasa JG. Allergic contact dermatitis from kojic acid. *Contact Dermatitis* 1998; 39(2): 86–87.
78. Nakagawa M, Kawai K, Kawai K. Contact allergy to kojic acid in skin care products. *Contact Dermatitis* 1995; 32(9): 9–13.
79. Maeda K, Fukuda M. Arbutin: mechanism of its depigmenting action in human melanocyte culture. *J Pharmacol Exp Ther* 1996; 276(2): 765–769.
80. Yokota T, Nishio H, Kubota Y, Mizoguchi M. The inhibitory effect of glabridin from licorice extracts on melanogenesis and inflammation. *Pigment Cell Res* 1998; 11(6): 355–361.
81. Chan HH, Leung RS, Ying SY, Lai CF, Kono T, Chua JK, Ho WS. A retrospective analysis of complications in the treatment of nevus of Ota with the Q-switched alexandrite and Q-switched ND:YAG lasers. *Dermatol Surg* 2000; 26(11): 1000–1006.
82. Kimbrough-Green CK, Griffiths CE, Finkel LJ, Hamilton TA, Bulengo-Ransby SM, Ellis CN, et al. Topical retinoic acid (tretinoin) for melasma in black patients. A vehicle-controlled clinical trial. *Arch Dermatol* 1994; 130(6): 727–733.
83. Griffiths CE, Finkel LJ, Ditre CM, Hamilton TA, Ellis CN, Voorhees JJ. Topical tretinoin (retinoic acid) improves melasma. A vehicle-controlled, clinical trial. *Br J Dermatol* 1993; 129(4): 415–421.
84. Kligman AM, Willis I. A new formula for depigmenting human skin. *Arch Dermatol* 1975; 111: 40–48.
85. Dogra S, Kanwar AJ, Parsad D. Adapalene in the treatment of melasma: a preliminary report. *J Dermatol* 2002; 29(8): 539–540.
86. Urbanek RW. Tar vitiligo therapy. *J Am Acad Dermatol* 1983; 8: 755.
87. Grimes PE, Morris R, Avaniss-Aghajani, Soriano T, Meraz M, Metzger A. Topical tacrolimus therapy for vitiligo: therapeutic responses and skin messenger RNA expression of proinflammatory cytokines. *J Am Acad Dermatol* 2004; 51: 52–61.
88. Travis LB, Weinberg JM, Silverberg NB. Successful treatment of vitiligo with 0.1% tacrolimus ointment. *Arch Dermatol* 2003; 139: 571–574.
89. Tobin DJ, Peters EMJ, Schallreuter KU. Pigment disorders of the hair and nails. In: Hordinsky MK, Sawaya ME, Scher RK (Eds) *Atlas of Hair and Nails*. Churchill Livingstone, Philadelphia, 2000; 159–160.
90. Brauner GJ. Pigmentation and its disorders in blacks. In: Levine N (Ed) *Pigmentation and Pigmentary Disorders*. CRC Press, Boca Raton, 1993; 439–450.
91. Reintgen DS, McCarty KM Jr, Cox E, Seigler HF. Malignant melanoma in black American and white American populations: comparative review. *JAMA* 1982; 248(15): 1856–1859.
92. Holman CDJ, Armstrong BK. Pigmentary traits, ethnic origin, benign nevi and family history of risk factors for cutaneous malignant melanoma. *J Natl Cancer Inst* 1984; 72: 257–259.
93. Chan HH, Lam LK, Wong DS, Leung RS, Ying SY, Lai CF, Ho WS, Chua JK. Nevus of Ota: a new classification based on the response to laser treatment. *Lasers Surg Med* 2001; 28(3): 267–272.
94. Kilmer SL, Garden JM. Laser treatment of pigmented lesions and tattoos. *Semin Cutan Med Surg* 2000; 19(4): 232–244.
95. Orlow SJ. Congenital disorders of hypopigmentation. *Semin Dermatol* 1995; 14: 27–32.
96. Tassabehji M, Read AP, Newton VE, Patton M, Gruss P, Harris R, Strachan T. Mutations in the PAX4 gene causing Waardenburg's syndrome type 1 and type 2. *Nat Genet* 1993; 3: 26–30.
97. Njoo MD, Nieuweboer-Krobotova L, Westerhof W. Repigmentation of leucodermic defects in piebaldism by dermabrasion and thin split-thickness skin grafting in combination with minigrafting. *Br J Dermatol* 1998; 139(5):829–833.
98. Barsh GS. Genetics of pigmentation: from fancy genes to complex traits. *Trends Genet* 1996; 12: 299–305.
99. Shibahara S. Mutations of the tyrosinase gene in oculocutaneous albinism. *Pigment Cell Res* 1992; 5: 279–283.
100. Castle WE, Allen GM. The hereditary of albinism. *Proc Am Acad Arts Sci* 1903; 38: 603–622.
101. Schnur RE, Selling BT, Holmes SA, Wick PA, Tatsmura YO, Spritz RA. Type I oculocutaneous albinism associated full-length deletion of the tyrosinase gene. *J Invest Dermatol* 1996; 106: 1137–1140.

102. Durham-Pierre D, Gardner JM, Nakatsu Y, King RA, Francke U, Ching A, et al. African origin of an intragenic deletion of the human P gene in tyronisa positive oculocutaneous albinism. *Nat Genet* 1994; 7: 176–179.
103. Schallreuter K, Frenk EU, Wolfe LS, Witkop CJ, Wood JM. Hermansky–Pudlak syndrome in a Swiss population. *Dermatology* 1993; 187: 248–256.
104. Garay SM, Gardella JE, Fazzini EP, Goldring RM. Hermansky-Pudlak syndrome; pulmonary manifestations of ceroid storage disorder. *Am J Med* 1979; 66: 737–747.
105. Norris DA, Tasuya H, Morelli JG. Melanocyte destruction and repopulation in vitiligo. *Pigment Cell Res* 1994; 7: 193–203.
106. Morrelli JG, Kincannon J, Yohn JJ, Zekman T, Weston WL, Norris DA. Leukotriene C, TGF-alpha are stimulators of human melanocyte migration *in vitro*. *J Invest Dermatol* 1992; 98: 290–295.
107. Verallo-Rowell VM, Verallo V, Graupe K, Lopez-Villafuerte L, Garcia-Lopez M. Double-blind comparison of azelaic acid and hydroquinone in the treatment of melasma. *Acta Derm Venereol Suppl (Stockh)* 1989; 143: 58–61.

6 Infectious Diseases of Pigmented Skins: Latinos

Miguel R. Sanchez

INTRODUCTION

Increased poverty, occupational exposures, and travel histories coupled with barriers to health care that include English language illiteracy and high rates of uninsurance contribute to disproportional incidences as well as pronounced severity of bacterial pyodermas, dermatophytosis, arthropod infestations, and sexually transmitted diseases in some Latino communities in the United States. A report by the U.S. Bureau of the Census found poverty rates of 21.7% in U.S.-born Latinos and 28.4% in all Latinos[1] and that 32% of Latinos lack any form of health insurance, the highest number of any major ethnic group.

Another source of potential infections is the influx of Latino immigrants, who have fueled the surge in the Latino population.[2,3] Currently 36% of all Latinos are foreign born. Some of them originate from rural areas endemic for vector-borne and zoonotic diseases that are rarely seen in the United States.

Notably, this spurt in emigration to the United States is coinciding with a significant population migration from rural regions of Latin American countries where there is enhanced risk of exposure to infectious agents that cause tropical infections toward urban and suburban regions.[4] Changes to the local environment, such as deforestation of rainforests, dam building, housing and agriculture in previously uninhabited environments, military expeditions, population displacement, and the popularity of adventure travel, account for the increased number of cases of re-emergent infectious diseases and their expansion to areas outside the traditional geographic boundaries.[5]

Conversely, mobility in the other direction is also promoting propagation of these infections. Peace Corps volunteers, missionaries, ornithologists, biology researchers, soldiers, venturesome vacationers, and laborers inhabit or rove through remote domiciliary or peridomiciliary areas.[6] The hot, humid days and cooler nights in the tropical rainforests of the Amazon and Central America predispose to dermatophytosis, mucocutaneous leishmaniasis, and papular urticaria. On the other hand, the cyclical climate with heavy rainfall followed by periods of aridity, characteristic of the Caribbean islands, the llanos of Venezuela and Colombia, the West Coast of Central America, and the Gran Chaco of South America, provide favorable ecological conditions for fungal and bacterial infections, American trypanosomiasis, filariasis, onchocerciasis, and myiasis.[7,8]

SUPERFICIAL FUNGAL INFECTIONS

Dermatophytosis is one of the more common dermatologic complaints in Latinos living in this country as well as in the tropics[9] (Figure 6.1). There are some interesting observations. Tinea is reportedly less common in Hispanics of African background.[10] Due to the custom of walking barefoot, tinea pedis occurs more often in the rural populations of tropical Latin America than in the urban population.[11] In Latin American countries, pet animals constitute a reservoir for fungus. Keratinophilic fungi were cultured from the haircoats of 67% of cats and 45% of dogs living in the cities of Mexico.[12] The sites of infection vary according to locale and climate. The most prevalent

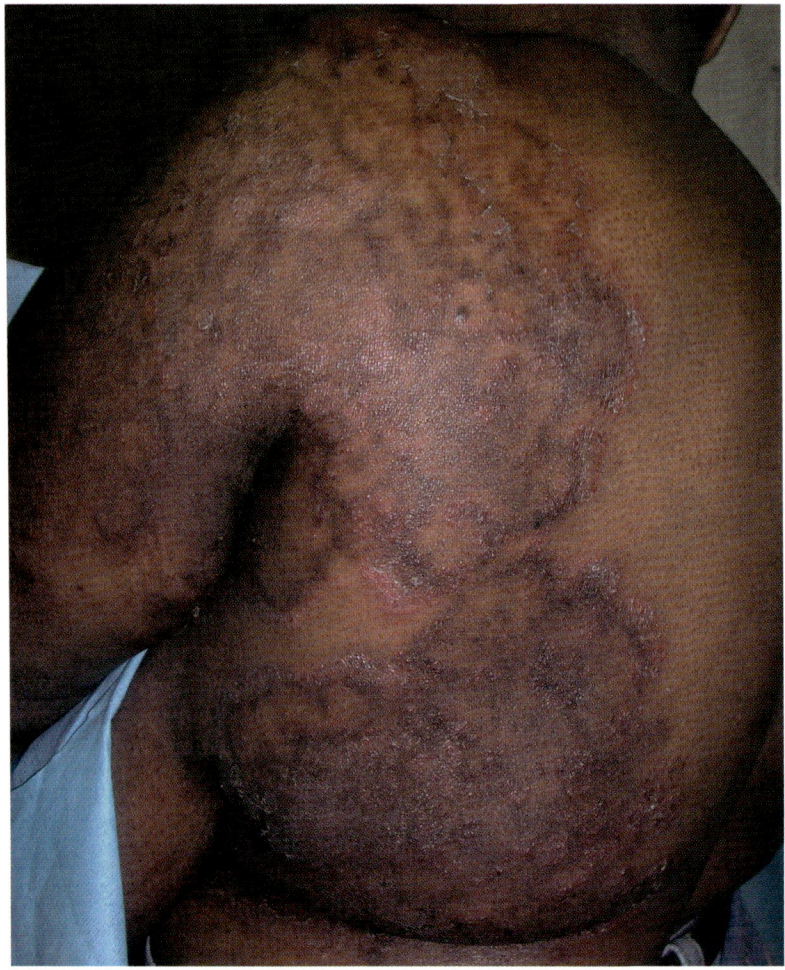

FIGURE 6.1 Extensive tinea corporis caused by trichophyton rubrum and consisting of numerous annular plaques confluent into two adjacent geographic plaques with raised scaly borders.

types of fungal infections in Mexico City are onychomycosis (60%) and tinea pedis (25%), caused predominantly by *Trichophyton (T.) rubrum*.[13] However, in Cuzco, Peru, a high-altitude region with low temperature and dry weather, tinea capitis (13.3%) and onychomycosis (11.1%) were found to be the more common superficial fungal diagnosis, and *Microsporum canis* (52.4%) and *T. mentagrophytes* (35.7%) were cultured more frequently than *T. rubrum* (9.5%).[14] Similar culture results were obtained in a study from Argentina.[15]

There are a number of unusual fungal infections that predominate in the tropics. Tinea imbricata is found in Mexico, Guatemala, and Panama. In the circinate type, the most common of the three varieties, the fungus *Trichophyton concentricum* produces pruritic, achromic patches covered with concentric scaly rings that spread symmetrically and bilaterally over the trunk and extremities but spare intertriginous areas, genitalia, palms, soles, and nails.[16] The concentric pattern is absent in the diffuse type. The exfoliative type is associated with profuse desquamation. Some patients develop a pseudotinea imbricate pattern, usually caused by *T. rubrum* (Figure 6.2).

Tinea nigra caused by *Exophila werneckii* is easily recognized clinically by the presence of one or several brown to black macules that coalesce in a polycyclic pattern in the palm, ventral fingers, interdigital spaces, and, rarely, the soles. Trichosporosis (white piedra) caused by *Trichosporon beigelii* produces soft, gray-white to light brown sleevelike nodules along the hair shafts of

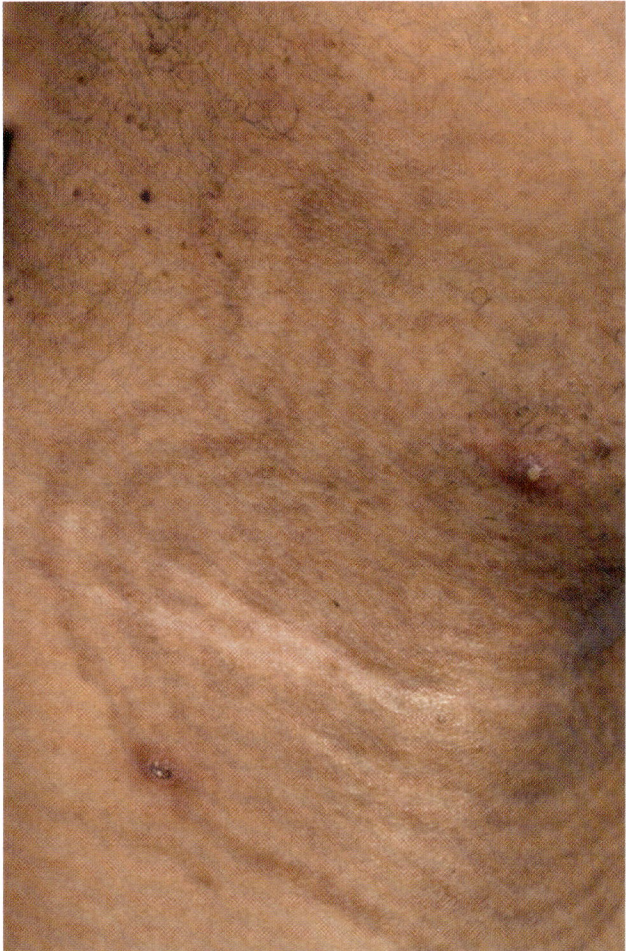

FIGURE 6.2 Concentric patches forming whorling scaly rings characteristic of tinea imbricata.

the axilla, beard, mustache, pubis, and, occasionally, scalp. In contrast, in black piedra, *Piedra hortae* causes brown-black elongated gritty nodules predominantly on the hair shafts of the scalp. The treatment of both infections is therapeutically frustrating and shaving remains the treatment of choice. Oral itraconazole appears to be effective in white piedra and terbinafine in black piedra, but both agents need to be administered for at least 6 weeks.

HUMAN PAPILLOMA VIRUS (HPV)

The prevalence of genital warts has been increasing in the Latino population in the United States. The overall increased incidence in genital HPV infection in the United States as well as many countries in Latin America is the primary reason, but the risk of infection is enhanced by the reluctance of Latino men to use condoms during sexual intercourse and cultural traditions and religious beliefs that preclude women from insisting on such protection. Cases of widespread warts are not uncommon among uninsured immigrants who may be reluctant to access public health clinics (Figure 6.3). Hispanic women are nearly twice (15 vs. 8 cases per 100,000 women) as likely as other women to be diagnosed with cervical cancer at any age.[17] A recent report found high prevalences of HPV type 58 as well as 16 and 18 in Mexican women undergoing colposcopy.[18]

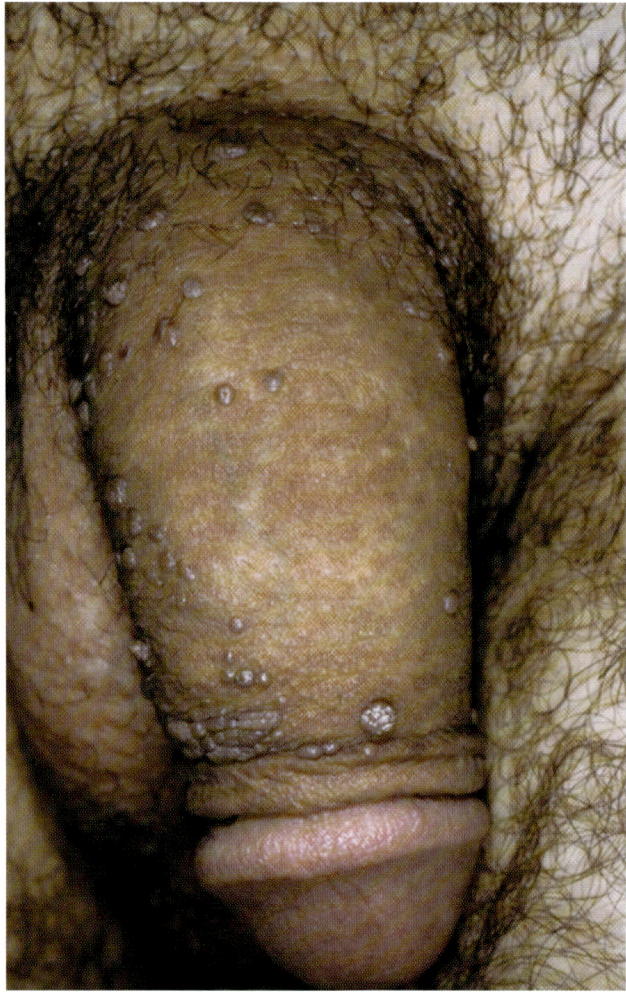

FIGURE 6.3 Condylomata acuminata presenting as multiple hyperkeratotic papules on the penile shaft. Some warts are pigmented due to the darker skin shade.

HEPATITIS

A study conducted by the National Institute on Alcohol Abuse and Alcoholism found that the cirrhosis death rate was 13 per 100,000 persons in Latino men and 19 per 100,000 persons in Latina women, in comparison with 7.4 and 10.5 per 100,000 persons in men and women, respectively, in the overall population. Cirrhosis may result from the effects of alcohol, which some Latinos tend to binge consume, especially on weekends, but also from hepatitis. Although it has been known for some time that the incidence of hepatitis A among Hispanics is more than twice that of non-Hispanics, the recognition that Hispanics are disproportionately represented in the hepatitis C epidemic is more recent. Latinos have more than a 40% greater chance of being infected with the hepatitis C virus than the general population, and reportedly one out of every 50 Hispanics in this country is or has been infected with hepatitis C virus. Although no studies have been conducted, skin manifestations associated with hepatitis C virus infection, such as biliary pruritus, urticaria, lichen planus, acral necrolytic erythema, sialadenitis, leukocytoclastic vasculitis, antiphospholipid syndrome, polyarteritis nodosa, porphyria cutanea tarda, and erythema multiforme, may be more prevalent among Latinos (Figure 6.4).

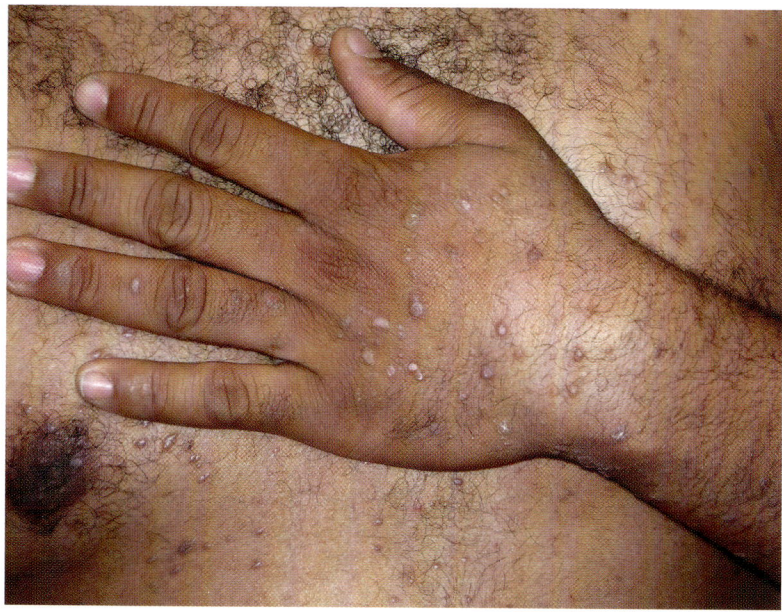

FIGURE 6.4 This eruption, consisting of widespread polygonal, planar, purpuric papules on the trunk and extremities, was the initial presentation of hepatitis C infection in this Dominican man.

SYPHILIS

Syphilis is an infection caused by the spirochete *Trepanema pallidum*, which is transmitted almost exclusively through sexual intercourse. The syphilis rate among Hispanics is about four times that in whites. Ten to ninety days after contact with an infected person, the patient develops one (less commonly, multiple) chancre on the site of treponemal penetration, which is usually the genitals (primary stage). Untreated, the chancre persists for 2–6 weeks and then heals without scarring. Usually 3–12 weeks after the onset of the chancre, the patient develops symptoms of the secondary stage, which consist of a roseolar or papulosquamous eruption in nearly all cases, that characteristically but not necessarily involves the palms and soles. In fact, the distribution may be limited or widespread (Figure 6.5). Fever, lymphadenopathy, pharyngitis, alopecia, myalgias, and fatigue may also be present. Without treatment, the eruption resolves within 12 weeks, and the disease progresses to an asymptomatic stage during which the only abnormal finding is reactive serologic testing. Neurologic damage, aortitis, aortic valve disease, aneurysms, cutaneous gummas, and skeletal abnormalities are the complications that develop in cases that progress to the late stage. Benzathine penicillin continues to be the treatment of choice, with one injection sufficing for the primary, secondary, and early latent (less than 1 year) stages, with three injections each, 1 week apart, needed for latent syphilis of longer duration. Neurosyphilis is treated with at least 18 million units of crystalline penicillin G intravenously daily for 10 to 14 days.

ONCHOCERCIASIS

The filarial nematode *Onchocerca volvulus* infects persons who visit or reside near the habitats of black flies of the genus simulium in endemic regions of southern Mexico, Guatemala, Venezuela, Colombia, and Ecuador.[19,20] The classic lesions are well demarcated, nontender, subcutaneous nodules on the head, face, torso, and, less often, other areas.[20] These encapsulations of female worms and their offspring microfiliariae are most often seen over bony prominences. A hypersensitivity

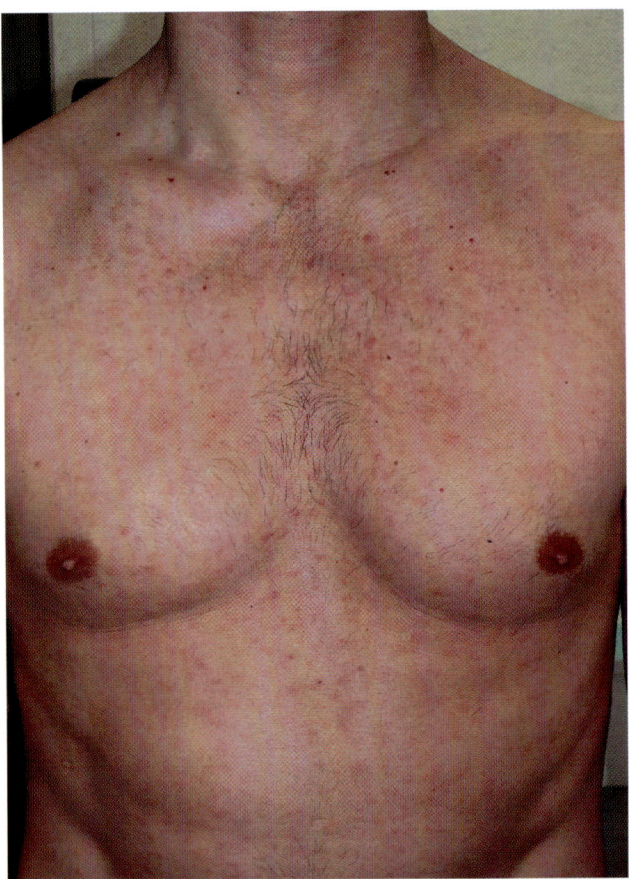

FIGURE 6.5 Bilateral, symmetrically distributed, erythematous patches on the trunk and neck of a man with secondary syphilis.

reaction to dead microfilariae results in itching, followed by lichenification and pattern of depigmentation with follicular hyperpigmentation (leopard skin).[21] Symptoms may not appear for months and even years after departure from endemic areas.[21] Flaps of skin may suspend from enlarged lymph glands, especially in the inguinal region (hanging groin effect). Blindness, usually due to keratitis, is the most dreaded and important long-term complication. The diagnosis is established by finding the adult or microfilarial nematode in suppurative granulation dermal tissue. Diagnostic enzyme-linked immunosorbent assays (ELISA) and polymerase chain reaction (PCR) tests are available.[22] Ivermectin administered in a single dose of 150 μg/kg reduces microfiliariae by 99.5% in 3 months.[23] The dose is repeated at 6–9-month intervals because the drug kills the microfilaria but not the adult worm.

CYSTICERCOSIS

In the United States, this re-emerging infection with the larval stage (*Cysticercus cellulosae*) of the pork tapeworm *Taenia solium* is predominantly seen in Latino immigrants from areas such as Mexico, Central America (especially Guatemala and El Salvador), and South America (Peru and Ecuador). The infection should be considered in natives from these countries with subcutaneous cysts and either decreasing vision, frequent headaches, seizures, focal neurologic findings, or radiculopathy.[24] Cysticercosis is contracted by ingestion of undercooked pork contaminated by feces from individuals who harbor the tapeworm larvae in their gastrointestinal tract.[25] The larvae

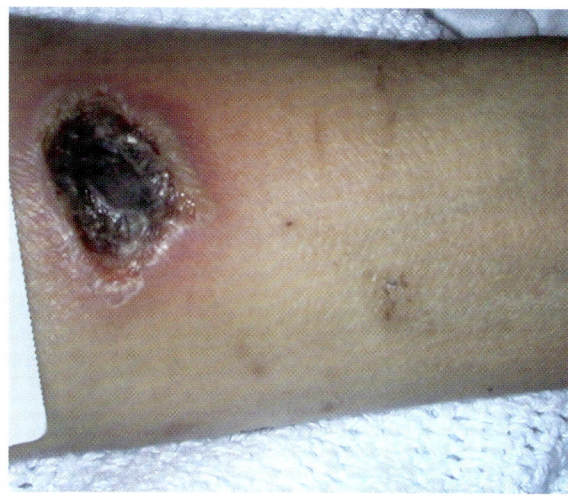

FIGURE 6.6 *Mycobacterium ulcerans* causes well-demarcated ulcers with scalloped, undermined, edematous borders and necrotic base.

penetrate the abdominal wall and migrate to striated muscle, subcutaneous tissue, eyes, brain, liver, or other organs, where they develop into larval cysts (cysticerci). In the skin and muscles, the 1–3-cm firm, rubbery, nontender, deep-seated nodules are often misdiagnosed as pilar cysts[24] (Figure 6.6). Over time, the cysts involve, leaving granulomatous changes and calcification.[24]

The definitive diagnosis consists of demonstrating the larva in histopathologic examination. When biopsy of the cyst is not possible, the diagnosis can be confirmed through a positive enzyme-linked immunoelectrotransfer blot (EITB) with purified *Taenia solium* antigen.[26] This test is not only more sensitive (90% vs. 74%) than enzyme-linked immunosorbent assays (ELISA) but also more specific because components in crude antigens derived from cysticerci do not cross-react with antibodies specific for other helminthic infections, such as echinococcosis and filariasis.[24] Even in patients with intestinal tapeworm infestation, diagnosis with ova and parasite examinations requires multiple stool examinations and is not specific because *T. solium* eggs appear similar to those of the beef tapeworm, which does not cause cysticercosis. Eosinophil counts are not usually elevated.

Treatment consists of complete excision of subcutaneous cysts. The benefits of cysticercoidal therapy in the absence of symptomatic disease are not proven.[25] The recommended treatments of choice are albendazole in a daily oral dose of 15 mg/kg up to a maximum 400 mg twice a day for at least 14 days (8–30 days) or praziquantel 50 mg/kg divided into three daily doses for at least 14 days (8–30 days).[27] Evaluation of symptomatic organs with computed tomography or magnetic resonance imaging scans is needed because cysts cannot be detected radiologically in the absence of calcifications. Previous to initiating treatment with antiparasitic agents, central nervous system (CNS) and eye involvement should be excluded because some patients can develop severe local inflammation that causes permanent eye, brain, or spinal damage. In these cases, prednisone at a daily oral dose of 1 mg/kg should be administered during the initial 4 days of antihelminthic therapy.[27]

MYCOBACTERIUM INFECTION

Cutaneous infection with *Mycobacterium ulcerans* (Buruli ulcer) has become the third most prevalent mycobacterial infection among immunocompetent persons in the world after tuberculosis and leprosy.[28] The infection remains endemic in areas with slow-flowing or stagnant water in Mexico, Peru, and Bolivia.[28] The majority of cases involve children and farmers who reside near swampy areas, river valleys or lakes, and coastal areas of the Amazonian region. The incidence of infection rises following periods of heavy rains and floods. Infection may be acquired from contamination of abrasions or wounds, but aquatic insects may also play a role in transmitting the infection to humans. The initial clinical finding is the sudden appearance in an extremity of one or more firm, 1–2-cm, nontender subcutaneous nodules or larger edematous plaques.[29] *Mycobacterium ulcerans* secretes mycolactone, a lipidic, necrotic, and immunosuppressive toxin[29] that leads to necrosis of the dermis, adipose tissue, and fascia. Rupture of the nodules results in undermined ulcers covered with slough (Figure 6.6).[30] The ulcers may remain small or enlarge to involve an entire arm, leg, or thigh, but pain is never severe. Some patients present only with diffuse, extensive, firm, and occasionally painful nonpitting edema of the infected extremity.[30] The clinical features of the ulcers and poor response to treatment may prompt misdiagnosis of pyoderma gangrenosum.[31]

The clinical diagnosis is substantiated by histological findings, which consist of marked necrosis of the panniculus, with a very sparse inflammatory infiltrate. An acid-fast stain shows bacilli in vast numbers comparable only to lepromatous leprosy. However, the absence of a granulomatous infiltrate excludes *M. leprae* infection.[29]

The bacteria is a nonchromogen that grows slowly over 4–12 weeks at temperatures between 25°C and 37°C, although greater proliferation is observed during growth at temperatures between 30°C and 33°C. Even with optimal conditions, only 55% of cultures are positive.

New PCR techniques allow long-distance transportation of specimens and facilitate confirmation of diagnosis in remote areas. Results of PCR with oligonucleotide-specific capture plate hybridization are at least comparable with culture (45% sensitivity).[32] Better diagnostic techniques will allow earlier diagnosis.[28] The diagnosis of *M. ulcerans* infection should be considered while dealing with a chronic cutaneous ulceration showing necrotizing panniculitis and the presence of a many acid-fast stain bacilli in the necrotic fat. The differential diagnosis includes different types of panniculitis, lupus profundus, α1-antitrypsin deficiency and cryptococcosis, pyoderma gangrenosum, and other forms of ulcers. The treatment of choice is wide surgical resection of the ulcer and skin grafting.[33] Early debridement of all necrotic tissue is essential to prevent spread of the infection. Even without treatment, the ulcers heal spontaneously over months to years but with resulting retractile scars, contractures, deformities, and disability.[33] Osteomyelitis often requires partial amputation of an extremity.[33] Current chemotherapeutic agents have failed to show a consistent rate of response.[28]

Wound infection caused by rapidly growing nontuberculous mycobacteria *M. abscessus*, *M. chelonae*, and *M. fortuitum* following cosmetic surgical procedures such as tissue liposuction, homologous fat tissue injection, and tissue augmentation with silicon or collagen performed in the Dominican Republic, Venezuela, and other Latin American countries have been recently described in a number of reports.[34,35] Infection by these agents has also followed cosmetic procedures such as face-lifts and breast augmentation performed in the United States.[36] Patients develop erythema, nodules, abscesses, and purulent wound drainage within 24 months of the procedures.[35] In most of these cases, the cause was use of gluteraldehyde to sterilize instruments.

Most isolates of *M. abscessus* are susceptible to clarithromycin, amikacin, imipenem, and cefoxitan. Combination chemotherapy with at least two antimicrobial agents to which the isolate is susceptible is recommended because monotherapy has been shown to contribute to the development of resistance.[37] Localized disease typically responds to 6 months of therapy in immunocompetent hosts, and disseminated infections can require more than 6 months of therapy.[38]

CHAGAS DISEASE

Infection with the parasitic flagellate *Trypanosoma cruzi* represents a major public health concern from Mexico to South America as far south as Chile and Argentina.[39] According to estimates, which do not include Mexico or Nicaragua from which adequate statistics are not available, between 16 and 18 million people are infected with Chagas disease and 50,000 die each year.[39] It is the third

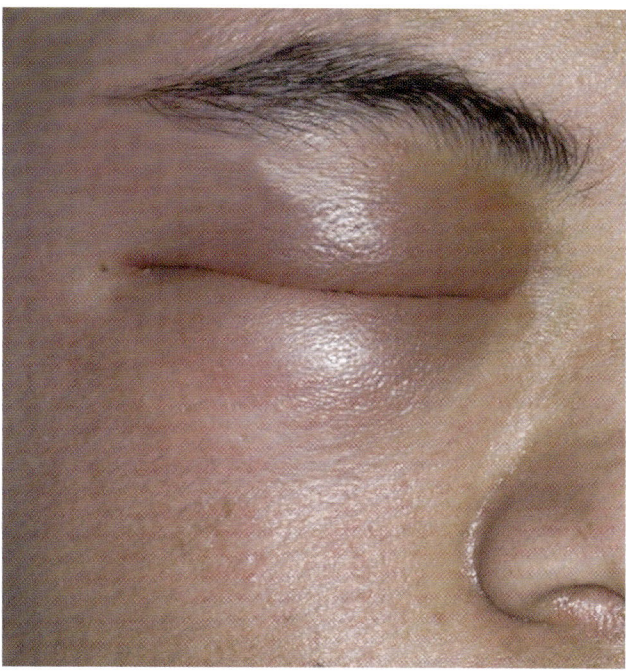

FIGURE 6.7 Unilateral conjunctival edema resulting from a direct bite or from rubbing the feces of a reduviid bug into the eye.

most prevalent parasitic infection in the world, after malaria and schistosomiasis, with approximately 120 million people (25% of the inhabitants of Latin America) at risk of becoming infected.[39] The disease is predominantly found in poor individuals who reside in mud, adobe brick, or palm thatch huts where triatomine bugs (assassin or kissing bugs), known in some countries as vinchucas or barbeiros, inhabit cracks and crevices in the roofs and walls. However, it is being increasingly reported from urban areas and the disease has been traced to some ticks and bedbugs. There are reports of transmission transplacentally and through blood transfusion. The reduviid bug deposits contaminated feces on a person's skin while feeding. The victim inadvertently rubs the feces into mucous membranes, the punctum produced by the insect bite, cuts, excoriations, or abrasions, through which the parasite readily enters the body. The acute disease occurs most frequently in infants and young children. Acute symptoms develop after an incubation period of 7–9 days, but only in 1% of cases, and consist of subcutaneous nodular edema at the portal of entry, the skin (inoculation chagoma), lip, or conjunctiva.[40] In approximately half of the cases, the trypanosomes enter through the conjunctiva, causing unilateral edema of the upper and lower eyelids, chemosis of the conjunctiva, and enlargement of the preauricular lymph nodes, a constellation of findings known as Romaña's sign (Figure 6.7). Erythematous, firm, painful nodules can also develop in distant skin areas through dissemination (hematogenic or metastatic chagomas).[40,41] Myocardial disease probably occurs in all patients but may not be recognized. Other symptoms include fever, fatigue, meningoencephalitis, lymphadenopathy, hepatosplenomegaly, diarrhea, vomiting, anorexia, and a skin eruption (trypanosomide) that can be morbilliform, urticariform, or erythematopolymorphic.[41,42] All symptoms resolve in 4–8 weeks. The reason why recognition of acute disease is important is that after a latent asymptomatic period, 25%–40% of those infected usually progress within 10–25 years to a chronic stage manifested by irreversible symptomatic cardiomyopathy, megaesophagus, or megacolon. Chagas disease can be particularly severe in immunocompromised HIV-infected patients.[40]

Serologic tests such as the Machado–Guerrero complement fixation, hemoagglutination, or ELISA assays become positive 1 month after infection and remain positive indefinitely. PCR assays have also been used to establish diagnosis. Skin biopsy reveals the presence of ovoid or round amastigotes in a dense, mixed-cell infiltrate involving the dermis and hypodermis.[41] Acute disease is diagnosed by thick and thin stained smears, lymph gland biopsy, or blood culture. Treatment with oral administration of either benznidazole in a daily oral dose 5–7 mg/kg (10 mg/kg in children) for at least 60 days or nifurtimox 8 mg/kg (15–20 mg/kg in children) divided into three daily doses for 90–120 days is usually effective in the acute stage and early in the intermediate stage, but the response to antitrypanosome drugs is dismal in the chronic stage.[43]

DENGUE FEVER

Since 1982, epidemics of dengue hemorrhagic fever have been reported from several Latin American countries, including the Dominican Republic, Nicaragua, Panama, Guatemala, Paraguay, Puerto Rico, Costa Rica, Venezuela, Cuba, Mexico, Colombia, Ecuador, and the tropical regions of Bolivia, Paraguay, and Peru.[44] Because of the expansion of the range of its mosquito vector, mainly due to increased temperatures and altered rainfall, dengue fever is again a major health problem in many regions in the north of Argentina after decades of irradication.[45] Epidemic transmission is usually seasonal, with rates increasing during hot, humid months.[46] The disease occurs endemically in both rural and urban areas.[46]

Three to fourteen days following transmission of one of four dengue viruses through the bite of a mosquito of the *Aedes* genus, usually *A. aegypti*, the patient develops an often-mild and self-limited biphasic acute febrile illness with fever, retro-orbital headache, back pain, limb (breakbone) pain, nausea, and vomiting.[47] On the fourth to fifth day, often after the fever subsides, a diffuse morbilliform, occasionally pruritic and desquamative, eruption may appear. In approximately 1% of cases, the patient's condition worsens to dengue hemorrhagic fever with prostration, diaphoresis, restlessness, pallor and circumoral cyanosis, subcutaneous petechiae, and hemorrhage from the nose, gums, venipuncture sites, and the gastrointestinal, genitourinary, and respiratory tracts. Complications include hepatic dysfunction, hypoalbuminemia, hyponatremia, and disseminated intravascular coagulation.[48] The infection may progress to dengue shock syndrome, which is invariably fatal. Thrombocytopenia below 50,000 platelets/mm^3 and prolonged prothrombin times are poor prognostic indicators. The risk of severe infection is highest among immunocompromised persons, children, and persons who have been infected with a second strain of dengue virus.

Dengue hemorrhagic fever is staged according to the severity of clinical findings: Grade I, constitutional symptoms and positive tourniquet test; grade II, spontaneous bleeding of the skin, gums, GI tract; grade III, circulatory failure and agitation; and grade IV, profound shock.[47]

The clinical diagnosis can be confirmed serologically through ELISA detection of acute-phase IgM antibody within 6 or 7 days of onset of illness. Virus-specific nucleic acid sequences can be detected with PCR.

Treatment is nonspecific and consists of supportive care, fluid replacement, red blood cell and platelet transfusions, reducing mortality from approximately 40%–50% to 1%–2%. Anticoagulation with heparin is risky, and high-dose systemic corticosteroids do not improve prognosis.[48] The most effective protection is the use of insect repellents containing *N,N*-diethyl-methyltoluamide (DEET) in a 35% or higher concentration. Live-attenuated vaccines for dengue types 1, 2, and 4 have been developed but are not yet commercially available.

PAEDERUS DERMATITIS

Rove beetles of the species *Paederus* produce the strong vesicant toxin and DNA inhibitor pederin, which circulates in the hemolymph of females.[49] Notably, pederin is not made by beetles but rather by symbiotic bacteria closely related to *Pseudomonas aeuroginosa*.[49] A contender for most powerful animal toxin, pederin is released when the beetle is crushed against the skin. Because the beetles are so small (7–10 mm in length and 0.5–1.0 mm in width), they can be confused with flies, so much so that in Kenya, a similar species of *Paederus* is known as the Nairobi fly. The beetles are attracted to yellow incandescent lights. Within 12–24 h of the beetle's creeping through the skin, the area becomes flushed and patients experience localized symptoms that range from pruritus to intense burning. The lesion resembles a burn from spilled hot liquid. Within hours, pinhead-sized blisters filled with a yellowish fluid, tiny erythematous papules, and, less often, small pustules or bullae erupt and progress to erosions.[50]

The lesions may heal with pigmentation. Through wiping, the toxin may be spread linearly and the lesion may resemble a whiplash mark; in fact, this condition is commonly known as latigazo in Latin America.[51] The more frequently affected body regions are the head (56.6%) and neck (30.9%).[51] Complications include conjunctivitis and genital inflammation from spread of toxin through touching.[51] The differential diagnosis includes contact dermatitis, burns, herpes zoster, bullous impetigo, and phytophotodermatitis.

Since *Paederus* beetles abound in hot, tropical climates, this dermatitis is common in many areas of Central and South America, especially in Paraguay, Ecuador, and Peru. The number of cases soar in years when the weather phenomenon El Niño produces prolonged torrential rainfall and hot climates that lengthen the breeding season and, as a result, increase the population of beetles.[51] Treatment consists of wet to dry compresses, control of symptoms with analgesics or antihistamines, and high-potency corticosteroids, which diminish but do not abolish the reaction.

BARTONELLOSIS (CARRION'S DISEASE)

Infection with the Gram-negative bacillus *Bartonella bacilliforme* is endemic in Andean areas of southern Colombia, Ecuador, and the northern half of Peru, but outbreaks have also been reported from lower areas of the Amazon basin.[52] In Peru, the suspected vector is the nocturnal sandfly *Lutzomya verrucarum* (also implicated in leishmaniasis), but related *Lutzomya* species transmit the disease in other countries. Usually between 16 and 22 days, but sometimes as long as 4 months, after the sandfly bite, the infected person may develop an acute illness called Oroya fever, characterized by high temperatures, headache, musculoskeletal pain, lymphadenopathy, and progressive hemolytic anemia. In some patients the infection results in hepatosplenomegaly, neurologic symptoms, severe hemolysis, and death. Oroya fever is the phase that most often occurs in tourists and migrants who while traveling to endemic areas.[53]

The diagnosis is confirmed by finding the bacillus attached to Giemsa-stained erythrocytes or by culture. During the disease phase or even during the convalescent period, some patients appear to be particularly susceptible to *Salmonella* superinfection and reactivation of toxoplasmosis. The second or eruptive stage of bartonellosis, known as verruga peruana, may emerge 2–8 weeks after resolution of the febrile stage or be the initial manifestation of the disease.

The eruption of discrete, smooth, bright red to purple, vascular, dome-shaped, deep-seated or exophytic, often sessile papules, usually 2–10 mm in width, may be accompanied by mild anemia (Figure 6.8). The number of lesions may vary from one to hundreds and favor the lower and upper extremities and the head over the trunk and abdomen. Even without treatment, the angiomatous lesions may regress spontaneously, usually 3–4 months after their appearance, or they may remain indefinitely. Larger nodules are prone to develop on the knees and elbows. In addition, papules and nodules can develop in mucous membranes, the esophagus, and internal organs. The lesions resemble pyogenic granulomas, proliferative vascular lesions, and Kaposi's sarcoma and are clinically identical to those in bacillary angiomatosis. Notably, pyogenic granulomas may be more common in patients with antibodies to *Bartonella* infection.[54] A recent study of an epidemic of Carrion's disease in Peru found that the attack rates were 13.8% for Oroya fever with 0.7% case-fatality rate and 17.6% for verruga peruana.[55] Histopathologic changes of a nodule show proliferation of endothelial cells and capillaries, a dense histiocytic infiltrate with plasma cells and numerous

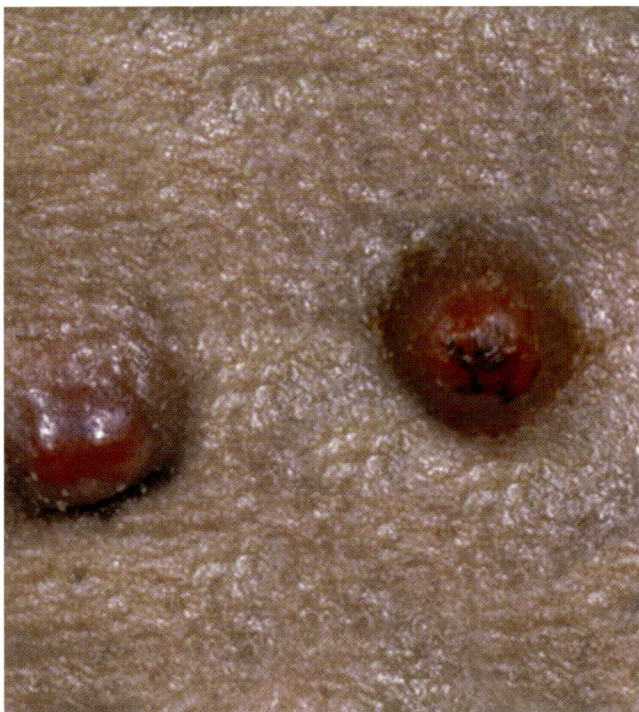

FIGURE 6.8 Exophytic smooth dome-shaped angiomatous nodules characteristic of verruga peruana during the second stage of bartonellosis.

neutrophils that invade the vessels, proliferation of histiocytes and endothelial cells, and proliferation of capillaries.[56]

Treatment with parenteral antibiotics, such as chloramphenicol, is indicated in the acute febrile phase. The bacterium is susceptible to serum concentrations of antibiotics achieved by oral administration of doxycycline, rifampicin, erythromycin, azithromycin, and fluoroquinolone.[57]

CUTANEOUS LARVA MIGRANS

Endemic throughout tropical and subtropical regions in Central and South America as well as the Caribbean and southeastern United States, cutaneous larva migrans is the most common infection acquired by travelers to tropical and subtropical areas of Latin America.[58] In the Western Hemisphere, most cases are attributed to *Ancylostoma braziliense* and *Ancylostoma caninum*, but the disease can be caused by several burrowing hookworms.[58,59] The infection is most commonly acquired while lying down or standing barefoot on moist sand and soil where cats and dogs have passed the hookworm eggs in their feces.[59] The hatched larvae produce proteases that facilitate burrowing through the stratum corneum, hair follicles, and sweat gland orifices and fissures.[59] A stinging sensation may accompany the initial penetration of the larva and within hours an erythematous papule forms at the entrance site. The larva settles in the dermoepidermal junction and begins migration usually 4 days after penetration but occasionally up to weeks longer. It advances from a few millimeters to 5 cm each day, producing an intensely pruritic, erythematous, edematous, serpiginous cord, usually on the feet, hand, arms, and buttocks (Figure 6.9). The tracks average a width of 2–4 mm and can be quite long.[58] Because the location of the larva is 1–2 cm beyond the advancing edge of the lesion, as few as 3% of biopsied skin specimens show the larva.[58] The histopathologic findings depend on the area of the lesion biopsied. Usually there is a spongiotic

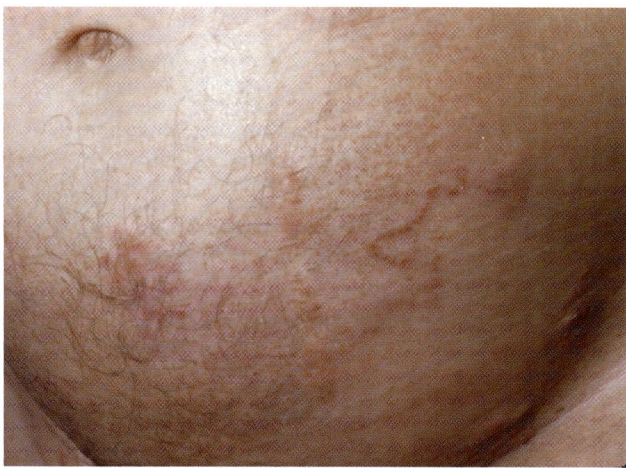

FIGURE 6.9 Elevated erythematous serpiginous tracks in a man with cutaneous larva migrans.

dermatitis with involvement of the follicular infundibula and a dermal infiltrate with eosinophils and neutrophils. If the specimen includes the burrow, round to oval spaces will be present in the lower epidermis. Oral ivermectin, 200 μg/kg as a single dose, or oral albendazole, 400 mg (10–15 mg/kg) daily for 3 days, is highly effective.[60] Daily application of topical 15% thiabendazole cream or thiabendazole suspension (500 mg/5 ml) twice daily for 2 weeks is effective in most cases, but some patients may require treatment with oral thiabendazole 1500 mg twice daily (25 mg/kg per day) for 4 days.[60] The infection is self-limiting, regressing spontaneously in 2–8 weeks[58] but rarely persisting as long as 18 months.[59] The larvae of other nematodes remain in the skin longer. Rarely, larval migration to the gastrointestinal track causes human eosinophilic enterocolitis with abdominal pain, nausea, diarrhea, and anorexia. Ulceration of the terminal ileum or colon is a complication.[61] However, most of these cases never include premonitory skin lesions. Other uncommon complications include erythema multiforme and pulmonary eosinophilia.

CUTANEOUS LARVA CURRENS

Infection with the intestinal roundworm *Strongyloides stercoralis* is common in Latin America. The parasites measure approximately 2–3 mm in length and 30–50 μm in width. The eggs are passed in the feces and hatch into larvae or adult worms that feed on the microflora of fecally enriched soils.[62] The invasive filariform larvae directly penetrates the skin by releasing hydrolytic enzymes, enter dermal vessels, and migrate through blood vessels or lymphatics to the lung, where they are coughed up and swallowed and develop into adult worms in the proximal gut.[62] The worms reproduce internally, with duration of infection up to 65 years recorded. The infection is usually uncomplicated, with mild gastrointestinal symptoms or intermittent pruritus ani except in persons with chronic diseases that lead to immunosuppression, when complications include bowel obstruction, protein-losing enteropathy, respiratory disease, meningitis, and arthritis.[3] Most patients have eosinophilia.

The larvae molt in the perianal region and migrate directly through the skin. The lesions are serpiginous, erythematous, urticarial tracks on the perianal area, buttocks, genitals, groin, and trunk. In contrast to cutaneous larva migrans, the burrow extends rapidly up to 5–10 cm daily, occasionally advancing during observation.[63] The lesions persist for only hours to days, but recurrences are common. Skin biopsy is rarely specific and stool cultures are often negative. Serologic studies are helpful in persons who do not live in endemic areas. Treatment with either albendazole, ivermectin, or thiabendazole is repeated in 1 week.

GNATHOSTOMIASIS

Human infection with the advanced third-stage larvae of *Gnathostoma spinigerum* is emerging as a public health problem in a number of Latin American countries.[64] Increasingly, cases are reported from persons living or visiting western Mexico, Ecuador, coastal Peru, and other countries of South America.[3] The infection is common in China as well as countries in Southeast Asia, especially Thailand and Vietnam.[64] Gnathostomiasis is almost exclusively acquired by eating marinated (ceviche), raw (sushi), or undercooked freshwater fish or shellfish. More rarely, transmission occurs through ingestion of rare chicken and pork. Pickling fish in lemon or lime juice, the standard preparation of the popular dish ceviche, does not destroy the roundworm, which causes this infection.[65] Freshwater fishes that may be infested with gnathostoma larvae include tilapia, catfish, sleepers, and guapotes.[66] Notably, sea bass (corvina) and flounder (lenguado), ocean fishes that visit freshwater estuaries, have been implicated in Peruvian cases.[65] In contrast to other mammals, the larva does not mature into an adult worm in humans. Rather, it migrates through the subcutaneous tissue and internal organs, where it provokes an immune reaction that causes any combination of skin, systemic, ocular, and neurologic disease.

Once ingested, the larva bores through the stomach wall and perigrates through the peritoneal cavity to the liver or to the subcutaneous fat. Nausea and nonspecific abdominal pain are frequent symptoms in the early stage of the disease. Skin lesions appear as early as 3 weeks or even years after ingurgitation of the larva and consist of infiltrated subcutaneous nodules or plaques with surrounding erythema, ranging in size from 3 to 16 cm.[67] In some patients the lesions have been described as ill-defined, erythematous, warm, edematous plaques. The cutaneous lesions may be pruritic, accompanied by burning or stabbing pain, and can be associated with myalgia or arthralgia. The initial lesion is most often present in the abdomen, but lesions may develop in any body area, including the upper and lower extremities, thorax, buttocks, neck, and face (Figure 6.10).[67] As the worm migrates, each skin lesion resolves spontaneously in 1–21 days, but a new lesion develops in the proximity of the previous one in days, or weeks to months, later on distal areas. At first, the

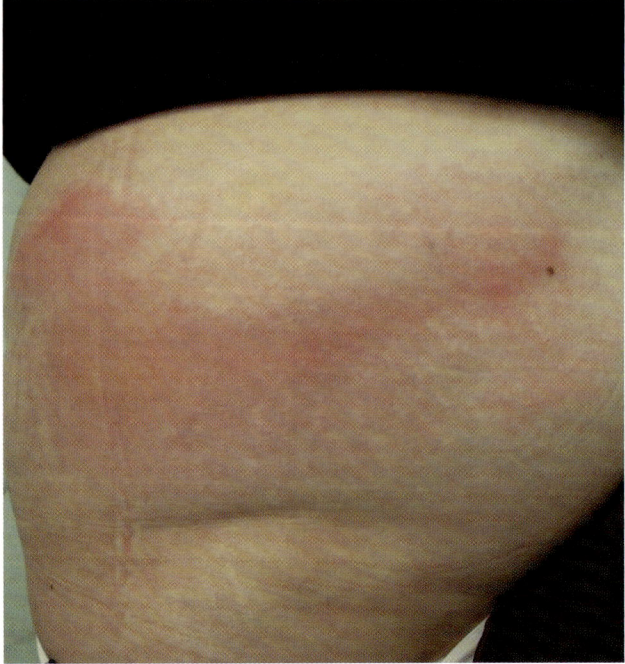

FIGURE 6.10 Indurated edematous urticarial curving plaque in a patient infected with gnathostoma spinigerum.

episodes usually persist for 7–14 days but, over time, they become less frequent and shorter. The migratory episodes may persist for months or years. In some cases, the lesions are superficial, erythematous, serpiginous thin cords that advance at one edge and are caused by migration of the larva through superficial skin. These linear indurations can develop after initiation of antiparasitic therapy.

In one study, the median time from the onset of symptoms to the diagnosis in 16 patients was 12 months.[68] The intermittent nature of the clinical manifestations makes recognition even more challenging. The diagnosis of gnathostomiasis often eludes all but the most experienced health care practitioners. A misdiagnosis of recurrent cellulitis, urticaria, or hypersensitivity reaction to drugs or bites is reinforced by the seeming response to antibiotics, antihistamines, or corticosteroids. Other tropical skin migratory infections, such as sparganosis, cutaneous larva migrans, cutaneous larva currens, *Toxocara* panniculitis, and migrating myiasis, should be considered.[44]

Depending on the organ (lung, gastrointestinal or genitourinary tracts, eye, inner ears) to which the larva migrates, the patient may experience bouts of abdominal pain, cough, hemoptysis, abdominal pain, hematuria, blindness, or decreased hearing. Injury is caused by a combination of direct invasion of the larva, the effect of released enzymatic toxins, and induction of a pernicious immunologic response. CNS invasion is the cause of death in 8%–25% of patients.[69] The most common complication of central nervous system ingress is radiculomyelitis. Subarachnoid hemorrhages, encephalitis, and eosinophilic meningitis are also frequent. One third of those who survive CNS involvement endure long-term sequelae, such as cranial nerve palsies and paralysis of an extremity.[4]

Histologic examination of lesional skin shows the presence of a dense perivascular and interstitial infiltrate with numerous eosinophils in the dermis and subcutaneous fat.[4] Areas of necrosis may be present near the larva; however, the organism is usually not found in the biopsied tissue due to its small size (up to 12.5 by 1.2 mm) and the large diameter of the lesions. In one study of 98 cases, larvae were identified in 26% of cases, whereas in the rest the diagnosis was made on the basis of history, physical findings, and serologic testing.[3] ELISA for IgE antibodies and immunoblots that identify a 24-kDa gnathostoma protein are promising. Although visualization of the constantly migrating larva is rare, a presumptive but reasonably accurate diagnosis can be established by the presence of a migratory eosinophilic panniculitis in biopsied skin from a person who has eaten raw or marinated fish.[70,71] Although the infection typically results in peripheral eosinophilia that may constitute as many as half of the circulating white cells, eosinophil counts may be normal even during the presence of active lesions.

Treatment consists of albendazole 400 mg twice a day for 21 days or ivermectin 200 µg/kg body weight administered as a single dose every 1–2 weeks until resolution of eosinophilia and clinical findings.[71,72] In one study, "cure rates," as defined by reductions in eosinophil counts and ELISA optical density, were achieved in 95.2% of 21 patients treated with ivermectin and 93.8% of 49 patients treated with albendazole.[65] However, these patients were not evaluated over months, and recurrences caused by a re-emerging larva may erupt after apparent cures. In some effectively treated patients, erythematous, nonmigratory inflammatory nodules appear at sites of previous lesions and presumably result from indiscriminant reactivation of T cells following an arthropod bite.

MYIASIS

In Latin America, furuncular myiasis is most often caused in humans as well as other mammals by the "screw-worm" larva of the human botfly *Dermatobia hominis*.[73] In the United States the arthropod-borne infestation is seen in travelers or recently arrived immigrants from warm, humid, lowland forest areas from southern Mexico to Argentina and the Caribbean.[74] Notably, adult female botflies do not directly lay eggs on the host but, rather, attach them to the abdomen of captured blood-sucking arthropods, which then inadvertently deposit them on the host during feeding. The temperature-sensitive eggs hatch on the skin of humans or other warm-blooded mammals into

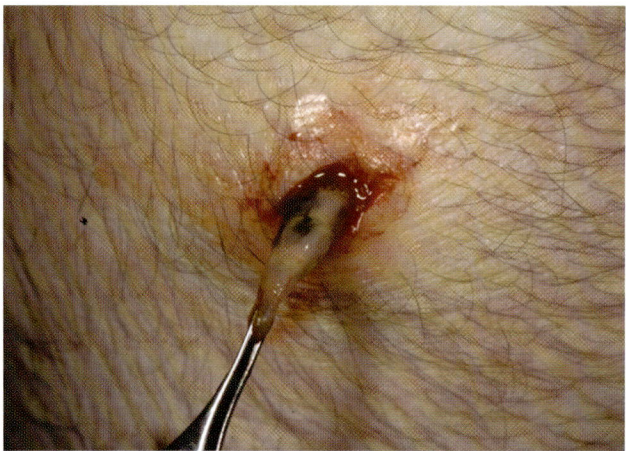

FIGURE 6.11 Botfly being removed from a nodule due to myiasis.

larvae that penetrate the host's skin through the bite wound or along a follicular pore. Within a day, the characteristic lesion, a discrete, pruritic, erythematous papule measuring 2–3 mm in diameter, forms usually on exposed areas such as the scalp, face, and upper or lower extremities.[74] Each lesion contains one or a few larva.[75] The inflamed nodule may become pruritic or tender as it gradually enlarges to a length of 2.0 or more cm. A central punctum develops early from which a serous or serosanguineous exudate drains. From this opening protrude the larval respiratory sinuses in and out of the lesion (Figure 6.11). Unless these tiny white structures are noted, the lesion is often misdiagnosed by inexperienced health providers as a bacterial abscess. Without treatment, the larva matures to a size of up to 2 cm and drops to the soil, where it pupates and molts into an adult fly.[75] Pulling the larva from the tissue is not feasible due to its tapered shape and rows of spines and hooks that grip the tissue cavity. Treatment consists of surgical incision and extraction of the larva under local anesthesia with care not to leave behind a portion of the larva that can result in bacterial infection or granuloma.[59] Suffocation of the larva by occluding the orifice with petrolatum, or other viscous agents, or injection of lidocaine to the base of the nodule, forces the larva to the surface for air, where it can be grasped with forceps.[76]

Unless the lesion becomes secondarily infected by bacteria, an uncommon complication, *D. hominis* myiasis merely results in discomfort. However, myiasis caused by *Cochliomyia hominivorax*, the New World screw worm seen in the United States only rarely in travelers, has been reported to have a mortality of 2.8%, nearly all debilitated individuals.[77] Although infestations are found on tropical and semitropical regions of Central and South America and several Caribbean islands, there is a seasonal spread of the screw worm into the temperate regions of Argentina, Uruguay, and Paraguay.[78] The adult female fly deposits a batch of 10–500 eggs directly onto the edge of any skin wound, or adjacent to mucous membranes such as the nose, oropharynx, conjunctiva, or vulva.[58] The larvae feed on damaged tissue and burrow deeply into adjacent living tissue, including cartilage and bone and potentially brain tissue. A mature larva reaches a length of 15 mm in days. The foul odor of the lesion attracts more botflies to deposit eggs so that there may be hundreds of larvae present. The diagnosis is usually established clinically and confirmed with ultrasound or imaging scans. Irrigation with either chloroform or ether can be attempted, but deep surgical excision is often required.

LEISHMANIASIS

Approximately 75% of leishmaniasis cases in the United States were acquired in Latin America, where this infection is endemic from northern Mexico to northern Argentina, with the exception of Chile and Uruguay.[79] Although leishmaniasis is more common in rural areas, especially those adjacent to wet lands and forests, the infection may also be acquired in the outskirts of some cities abundant with rodents. Unless disturbed, the tiny female *Lutzomyia* sand flies feed between dusk and dawn, transmitting the leishmania protozoa through the bite into macrophages. Characteristically, the latent period varies from 2 to 4 weeks, although it may be longer. New World leishmaniasis presents with three distinct clinical variants, depending on the protozoan species and the immune response. Spontaneously healing lesions are associated with positive antigen-specific T-cell responsiveness. In contrast, diffuse cutaneous, disseminated, and visceral disease develops in persons with impaired T-cell responses, and mucocutaneous disease develops in those with heightened T-cell responsiveness.[80]

Localized cutaneous disease is typically caused by subspecies of the *Leishamnia mexicana complex* (*L. mexicana, L. amazonensis, L. venezuelensis L. gamhamI*, and *L. pifanoi*). Depending on the number of bites, one (occasionally more) small oval or round, erythematous, edematous papule forms at the bite site and eventually ulcerates weeks to months later.[81] Nearly always, the sites are exposed areas, usually the face (especially the ear where the lesion is called chiclero ulcer) and extremities. Patients typically present with a crater surrounded by raised dusky red edges (Figure 6.12). In some patients, the lesions are vegetative and do not ulcerate. Regional adenopathy, satellite lesions, and subcutaneous nodules can be present. Even without treatment, the lesions from the *L. mexicana complex* heal in 1 month to 3 years, leaving depigmented, retracted scars. Associated with anergy and far less responsive to treatment, diffuse cutaneous leishmaniasis is invariably caused *by L. amazonensis, L. pifanoi*, or *L. mexicana* and in the Dominican Republic by an unnamed species.[81] The initial lesion often appears on the face and is followed by diffuse, large, nontender nodules and infiltrated plaques that do not ulcerate on the extremities, buttocks, and other body

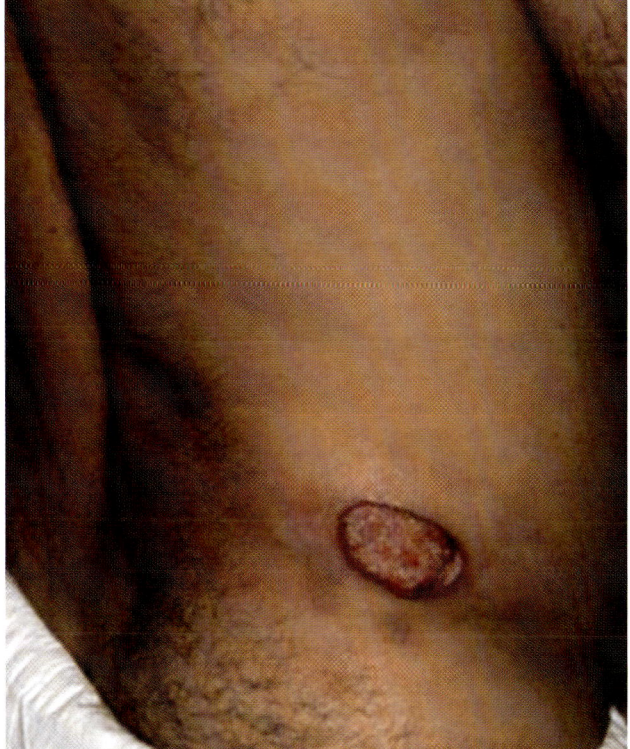

FIGURE 6.12 Slow-growing, sharply demarcated ulcer with indurated margins and granulation tissue at the base caused by *Leishmania braziliensis*.

regions, including the nasal and labial mucosa. The lesions may persist for 20 years. Clinically, the findings resemble lepromatous leprosy. In the mucocutaneous form, typically caused by *L. Viannia braziliensis* complex [*L. (V.) braziliensis, L.(V.) guyanensis, L. (V.) panamensis,* and *L. (V.) peruviana*], the skin lesions are identical to those described earlier but may not heal spontaneously and then only over a longer period of time.[82] However, mucosal lesions then develop on the anterior cartilaginous part of the nasal mucous membranes (tapir's nose) and, without treatment, extend to involve and mutilate the nasal mucosa, oral structures, pharynx, and lips (espundia).[82] The infection progresses to invade the respiratory tract. About 90% of all cases occur in Bolivia, Brazil, and Peru.

Disseminated leishmaniasis is a new and emerging variant of *L. braziliensis* infection. Patients develop a combination of acneiform, ulcerative, papular, and nodular lesions that may range from at least 10 to as many as 300. Lesions have been found in the mucous membranes in 25% of reported cases. In contrast to patients with diffuse cutaneous leishmaniasis, the leishmanin skin test is usually positive. Patients are relatively refractory to therapy with antimony or amphotericin B.

Zoonotic visceral leishmaniasis caused by *Leishmania chagasi*, a long-lasting infectious disease characterized by weight loss, cough, fever, diarrhea, hepatosplenomegaly, and lethargy but no skin signs, has re-emerged in Brazil during the past decade. Patients coinfected with the human immunodeficiency virus and leishmaniasis develop localized skin lesions, diffuse disease, or atypical presentations, depending on the degree of immunosuppression.[80,83]

Cultures from the ulcer edge on Schneider *Drosophila* medium and Novy–MacNeal–Nicolle (NNN) media are unreliable, as organisms are difficult to isolate, especially from older lesions. Monoclonal antibodies or hybridization of tissue touch blots with labeled kinetoplast DNA probes are used for identification of different strains. The Montenegro skin test produces positive results 3 months after the appearance of lesions but does not differentiate between acute and past infection and is no longer available in the United States. Complement fixation tests above 1:8 and immunofluorescent assays above 1:16 are consistent with infection, but a low or absent titer does not exclude infection, especially in the cutaneous form.

Despite insufficient investigational experience, ketoconazole 200 mg daily or itraconazole 400 mg daily are first-line treatments for *L. mexicana* infection.[84] Treatment is recommended for lesions on the face or exposed areas to prevent disfiguring scars and in persons with potentially impaired immunity. Investigational data to support the use of rifampin, dapsone, 15% paromomycin–12% methylbenzethonium chloride ointment, and cryotherapy are also limited.[85,86]

If the organism has not been isolated, the infection should be treated as if it were *L. braziliensis* with sodium stibogluconate (penstostam) or meglumine antimoniate (glucantine) at a dose of 20 mg/kg daily for 20 days.[86] Although this therapy is generally successful, relapses and treatment failures have been reported.[86] In one study from Brazil, the response rates to meglumine antimoniate in cases of localized cutaneous leishmaniasis caused by *Leishmania (Viannia) braziliensis* and *L. (V.) guyanensis* were only 50.8% and 26.3%, respectively.[63] Amphotericin B in liposomes (Ambisome) and pentamidine is reserved for antimony-resistant cases. A new oral investigational drug, miltefosine, appears promising and may revolutionize the treatment of the infection.[86] Steps to avoid sandfly bites include repeated applications of repellents containing DEET to exposed skin and under the edges of clothing and impregnation of clothing with permethrin, as well as protective barriers such as clothing that covers the body and bed nets and window screens with fine mesh netting of 18 or more holes per square inch.

CHROMOMYCOSIS

Infection with several species of dematiaceous (pigmented) fungi (*Fonsecaea pedrosi, Phialophora verrucosa, Cladosporium carrionii, F. compacta, Rhinocladiella aquaspersa, Exophiala jeanselmei, E. spinifera, Ascosubramania melanographoides*), which live as saprophytes in soil and decaying vegetation, is common among Latin American farmers. The vast majority of cases are caused by traumatic inoculation through a splinter of *Fonsecaea pedrosi*.[87] The injury may be so minor as to go unnoticed and may have occurred years before the patient seeks medical advice for the indolent-growing lesion. In one study the average time between the appearance of the disease and medical diagnosis was 14 years.[87] Typically a pink, scaly papule develops at the site of inoculation, usually on the lower extremity.[87,88] The lesion slowly enlarges and evolves into an erythematous psoriasiform or verrucous plaque or nodule, which partially heals with keloid formation (Figure 6.15). Over time, the surface may resemble a cauliflower. In the nodular form, individual, firm, reddish, smooth, moist nodules form and do not coalesce but break down, leaving purulent ulcers with vegetating borders.[88] Satellite lesions form from lymphatic spread or autoinoculation through scratching.

Local complications include frequent recrudescence after therapy, a higher risk of squamous cell carcinoma, and disability from invasion of tendons, muscles, and joints.[87] Rarely, hematogenous dissemination with brain metastasis and an invariably grave prognosis have been reported in immunosuppressed patients.

The clinical diagnosis is confirmed by culture and skin biopsy. The fungus grows within 4 weeks incubated at 30°C in Sabouraud glucose agar and a medium containing cycloheximide, IMA, or BHI agar with 10% sheep blood.[89] Histopathologic examination of infected skin shows pseudoepitheliomatous hyperplasia, acanthosis, and microabscesses in the epidermis as well as acute and chronic granulomatous inflammation, vascular proliferation, and fibrosis. Both dematiaceous hyphae and sclerotic bodies are found in the stratum corneum, but only sclerotic bodies (copper pennies) are found in the areas of dermal inflammation.[89]

Small, localized lesions can be treated with surgical excision, cryotherapy, laser ablation, electrodessication and curettage, or other destructive procedures. In more advanced cases, the best therapeutic strategy seems to be a combination of two drugs chosen according to the results of prior antifungal susceptibility testing.[90] In general, voriconazole, itraconazole, and terbinafine are effective, but the fungi are often resistant to fluconazole. In one study, the best results were obtained with cryosurgery for small lesions and itraconazole combined with cryotherapy for larger lesions. Overall, 31% of cases were cured, 57% improved, and 12% failed treatment.[89] In adults, the dose of itraconazole of 200 mg or more per day for as long as required (or for a period two to three times longer than that required to obtain negative culture results).[89] Itraconazole has also been combined with thiabendazole, amphotericin B, and fluocytosine with varying degrees of success.[90]

HANSEN'S DISEASE

With an aggressive campaign by the World Health Organization to reduce the prevalence of Hansen's disease (HD) below 1 in 10,000 persons in any country, the number of active cases worldwide has been reduced to below 600,000 cases and the disease is a health care problem in only 15 countries, including Brazil and Paraguay.[91] In the United States, out of approximately 110 new cases reported to the national Hansen's Disease program each year, the largest percentage (38%) are Hispanic.[92] It is notable that 27% of all cases were born in the United States. Although most of these patients contracted the disease overseas, some cases without a history of travel abroad are being reported.[92]

Infection with the slow-growing *Mycobacterium leprae* affects predominantly the skin and peripheral nerves. Transmission probably occurs from person to person through respiratory droplets. Infected blood monocytes from broken skin and mucous membranes transport the bacilli to the Schwann cells.[93] The incubation period is approximately 5 years but may be 20 years or longer. Only 1.5% of infected individuals will develop chronic clinically overt infection. Leprosy presents a spectrum disease with two extreme polarities, tuberculoid and lepromatous. Paucibacillary infection is characterized by a Th1-type response with interleukin-2 and interferon-γ production, whereas multibacillary disease has the characteristics of a Th2-type response modulated by interleukins 4 and 10.[93]

Indeterminate HD is frequently the initial form, consisting of one to five small, hypopigmented patches without definite anesthesia or enlarged peripheral nerves. Indeterminate leprosy either resolves spontaneously or progresses towards a tuberculoid or lepromatous form. Polar tuberculoid

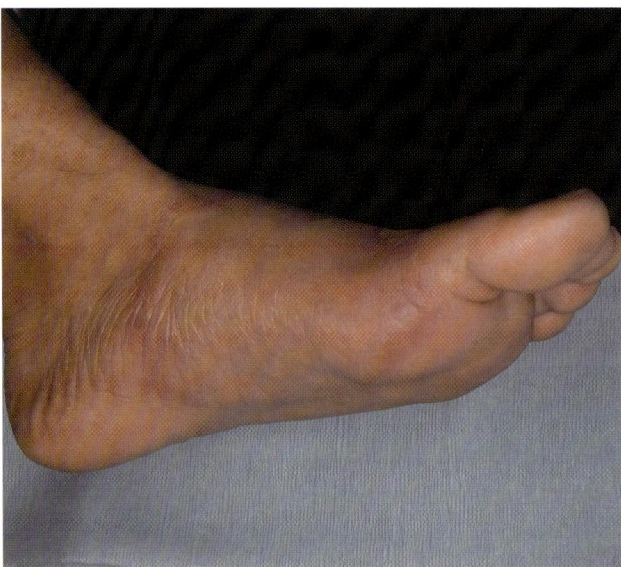

FIGURE 6.13 Single, erythematous annular plaque with dry, anesthetic center and well-defined borders characteristic of borderline tuberculoid leprosy. (i) Can be either one large red patch with well-defined, raised borders or a large hypopigmented asymmetrical spot; (ii) lesions become dry and hairless; (iii) loss of sensation may occur at site of some lesions; (iv) tender, thickened nerves with subsequent loss of function are common; (v) spontaneous resolution may occur in a few years, or it may progress to borderline or, rarely, lepromatous types.

HD presents classically with a single (but occasionally more) sharply outlined, hypopigmented or erythematous, annular, anesthetic, hairless patch or plaque with dry, slightly scaly surface and variable nerve enlargement (Figure 6.13).[93] The most commonly affected nerves are the posterior tibial, followed by the ulnar.[94] In borderline tuberculoid HD there are few to numerous infiltrated, hypoaesthetic to anesthetic plaques with well-defined margins. The skin smear is usually negative but may occasionally show a few mycobacteria.[94] In mid-borderline HD the skin lesions are asymmetrically distributed, erythematous patches and inverted saucerlike, "punched-out" plaques with well-demarcated inner margins but less distinct outer margins.[94] Nerve damage is often prominent.[95] In borderline lepromatous leprosy numerous smooth and shiny papules, plaques and nodules with sloping edges are present. The plaques are commonly annular or serpiginous with ill-defined inner and outer edges (Figure 6.14). In lepromatous leprosy, large areas of the skin are symmetrically affected with numerous papules, plaques, and nodules of varying sizes or complete infiltration of the skin. Testicular atrophy, nasal involvement, and eyebrow alopecia are usually apparent.[76] Sensation loss progresses from the dorsal aspect of the extremities to a glove-and-stocking distribution. The number of bacilli is higher than in borderline lepromatous leprosy.[94] Clinical diagnosis and staging are confirmed by histologic examination of involved skin and slit smears dyed with Fite's Acid Fast stain.[94]

Complications are frequently caused by reactions that occur after or prior to initiation of therapy. Type I reactions are associated with sudden enhancement (upgrading) or reduction (downgrading) of cell-mediated activity, corresponding to progression toward the tuberculoid (reversal reaction) or lepromatous spectrum, respectively.[93] These reactions may occur in all subpolar forms of the disease, although they are more common along the tuberculoid spectrum. The skin lesions become erythematous and edematous. Nerve swelling with associated paresthesias develops.[95] Unless treatment with high-dose systemic corticosteroids is initiated within hours, nerve damage is invariably permanent.

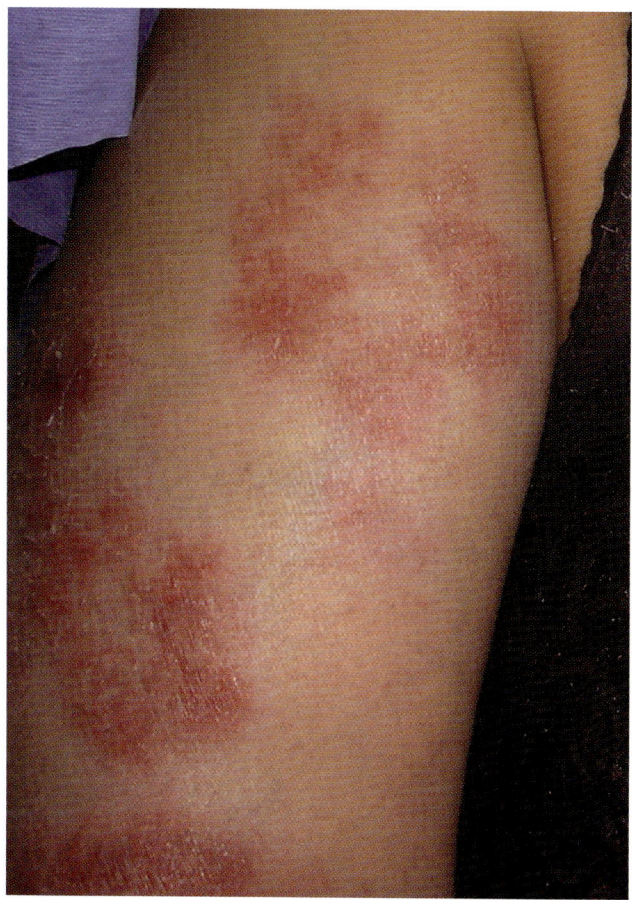

FIGURE 6.14 Erythematous, irregularly shaped, infiltrated plaques with punched-out "inverted saucer" appearance characteristic of borderline lepromatous Hansen's disease.

Erythema nodosum leprosum (Type II reaction) is caused by an immune complex hypersensitivity vasculitis due to an increase in antibody production stimulated by the antigen of killed mycobacteria. The reaction is common in the mid-borderline and borderline lepromatous spectrum. Recurrent attacks of crops of tender, erythematous papules and nodules may be accompanied by fever, orchitis, myositis, osteitis, periostitis, and iridocyclitis (Figure 6.14). The reaction persists for days to months and can be recurrent. Thalidomide is the treatment of choice.

In this country, multidrug regimens involving at least two drugs are recommended.[96] The short-course therapy regimen will be available for evaluations during extended periods of time. For paucibacillary disease, Dapsone 100 mg daily plus rifampin 600 mg daily are prescribed for 1 year. Multibacillary disease is treated with Dapsone 100 mg daily plus rifampin 600 mg daily plus clofazimine 50 mg daily for 2 years.[96] If Dapsone resistance is suspected, the drug is replaced with clofazimine. These regimens are considerably shorter than those previously recommended, and continued clinical assessment is essential to evaluate for relapses and progressive nerve deterioration.[97]

Minocycline, ofloxacin, and clarithromycin have excellent activity against *M. leprae* but are not routinely prescribed. The combination of rifampin, ofloxacin, and minocycline given as a single dose is being used by the World Health Organization for single skin lesions of paucibacillary disease.[98]

RHINOSCLEROMA

This chronic, indolent infection of the nasal tissue by *Klebsiella rhinoscleromatis* characteristically progresses through an exudative, catarrhal stage; a proliferative, granulomatous stage; and a cicatricial stage. Rhinoscleroma is most often reported in persons living within rural, impoverished, sanitation-deprived areas in Mexico, El Salvador, Costa Rica, Colombia, Brazil, Peru, Chile, and Argentina.[99]

The disease begins with a watery nasal discharge that may be accompanied by nasal obstruction and frontal headaches and is often misdiagnosed as viral or allergic rhinitis.[100] The nasal mucosa becomes hyperemic and edematous, covered with edematous tiny bluish-pink papules. The symptoms resolve within months to years, at which time the skin of the nose becomes progressively infiltrated and hardened, and the mucosal papules coalesce to form large, hard, waxy, nonpainful, granulomatous nodules that arise from the floor of the nose and spread to involve both the medial and lateral walls of the nose, leading to nasal obstruction. The lesions spread to involve the nasal tip, alae, and upper lip, resulting in the characteristic "Hebra nose."[100] Complications include ulceration, bleeding, and asphyxiation from complete nasal obstruction.[99] The nodules can extend inward to invade the paranasal sinuses, palate, pharynx, trachea, and, rarely, the brain. Over time, there is partial healing with disfiguring fibrotic scarring, but new granulomatous infiltrations can develop within the scars. Cervical lymphadenopathy may be present.

Histopathologic examination demonstrates a diffuse granulomatous dermal infiltrate with lymphocytes, free-lying plasma cells laden with globulins (Russell bodies), and large, foamy, vacuolated macrophages (Mikulicz cells) in which the phagocytized bacteria can be found. Bacteria inside the foam cells can also be demonstrated in tissue specimens prepared with Warthin–Starry silver, Gram, or Giemsa stains. The diagnosis can further be confirmed through an immunoperoxidase technique and complement fixation and hemagglutination tests.[101]

Treatment consists of surgical debridement and antibiotics to which the organism is susceptible, which have included in various reports ciprofloxacin, streptomycin, tetracycline, and chloramphenicol.[99]

PARACOCCIDIOIDOMYCOSIS (SOUTH AMERICAN BLASTOMYCOSIS)

Caused by *Paracoccidioides braziliensis*, this infection is found in humid forests or lush green mountain areas from northern Mexico to Argentina, with the exception of Chile. Most cases reported are from Brazil, Venezuela, Colombia, and Argentina. Men are affected 15 times more often than women.[102] The primary infection, presumably acquired through airborne inhalation of fungal spores, is usually asymptomatic but the fungus can remain dormant for years or decades within lymph nodes and suddenly reactivate, especially in the presence of immunosuppression.[103] The most typical radiographic pattern is bilateral mixed infiltrates (alveolar and interstitial), mainly located in the middle and lower lobes. Interstitial lesions may have a miliary, nodular, or fibronodular pattern.[104] In contrast to tuberculosis, there is typical absence of hilar adenopathy. However, tuberculosis coexists in up to 10% of patients with paracoccidiomycosis. The majority of cases are diagnosed with the chronic adult form, which is believed to represent reactivation of latent infection and usually presents with painful ulcerated lesions in the mouth, pharynx, nose or larynx, resulting in dysphagia and hoarseness. More than 70% of cases have extrapulmonary disease, which most commonly affects the skin, mucous membranes, or lymph nodes but can also involve the adrenals, abdominal organs, and CNS. The typical lesions are granulomatous papules coalescing into plaques that may ulcerate and small abscesses usually located in the oral–perioral area. Edema, erosions, and ulcers of the lips, as well as granulomatous plaques and ulcers with irregular granulomatous borders on the gingivae and tongue, are common.[105]

The lesions are destructive and heal with fibrotic scars that result in chronic symptoms and organ dysfunction. The appearance may lead to misdiagnosis as squamous cell carcinoma.[106] Patients with mucocutaneous lesions almost always have pulmonary involvement, even in the absence of respiratory symptoms. Bacterial superinfection of ulcerative lesions is more common than that with oral ulcers due to mucocutaneous leishmaniasis.

Under 10% potassium hydroxide smears, the fungus appears as multiple budding yeasts with globose cells between 2 and 30 μm in diameter. The fungus may be cultured from specimens of sputum, purulent exudate, or tissue incubate in Sabouraud dextrose agar at 37°C and grown as cream-colored yeast colonies that assume cerebriform texture. Histopathologic examination shows granulomatous inflammation with focal areas of caseation and pyogenic abscesses.

Detection of the pilot-wheel-shaped yeasts, consisting of spherical cells 10–40 μm in diameter with a thick birefringent cell wall surrounded by several peripheral buds, is facilitated by staining with PAS or silver nitrate. Immunodiffusion assay and complement-fixation tests are positive except in HIV-infected patients, where nearly half of the serologic tests are false negative.[103] In immunocompromised patients skin lesions are more prone to dissemination.[107] Diagnosis through PCR assays appears promising.[108]

The treatments of choice are itraconazole 100–200 mg daily for 6 months or, alternatively, fluconazole 200 mg for 6 months or ketoconazole 200–400 mg daily for 12 months.[104,109] In severe infections, the dose is often doubled. Voriconazole is expected to replace amphotericin B in life-threatening cases.[109]

SPOROTRICHOSIS

Infection by the dimorphic fungus *Sporothrix schenckii* commonly occurs among gardeners, florists, and farmers from Central and South America and the Caribbean.[110] The fungus can be isolated from decaying vegetation, soil, and hay, but cases have also been attributed to contact with animals, especially cats and donkeys.[110,111] In some parts of Peru, the mean annual incidence was recently reported to be 98 cases per 100,000 persons, with children being three times more likely to become infected and to have lesions on the face and neck rather than the extremities.[110]

In immunocompetent persons, the infection usually presents as one of two distinct cutaneous variants.[112] In lymphocutaneous disease (the most common form), painless, firm, erythematous nodules appear, usually 3 weeks to 6 months after infection.[113] As the organism spreads through the lymphatic system, more lesions appear in a linear pattern that is characteristically described as sporotrichoid (Figure 6.15). The nodules subsequently ulcerate and may be covered with copious crusting or become hypertrophic with verrucous changes.[114] The fixed, cutaneous form is more likely to occur in previously infected persons or individuals with strong cell-mediated immunity to *S. schenckii*.[115] The characteristic lesions consist of one or more localized nodular abscesses, ulcers, or hyperkeratotic plaques and more often involve the face, neck, trunk, and legs without lymphatic involvement.[114] In some facial cases the lesions may resemble cystic acne, but the clinical diagnosis that needs to be excluded in early lesions is leishmaniasis. Left untreated, the infection results in disfiguring scars.

Disseminated sporotrichosis is seen in immunocompromised or poorly controlled diabetic patients via hematogenous spread of the fungus from a primary infection site or from a regional lymph node involved in primary infection.[113] The infection may spread to the kidneys, joints, bones, lungs, testes, and CNS.[113] Hyphae with the characteristic bouquet-like conidia can be visualized microscopically after incubation of tissue or pus cultured on Sabouraud or Mycosel media at 25°C. The organism will also grow as a yeast at 35°C.[113] Tissue cultured on Sabouraud's agar yielded hyphae and the characteristic bouquet-like conidia of *S. schenkii* after 2 weeks at 30°C. The organism is often missed in biopsy specimens but when present appears under PAS or silver nitrate

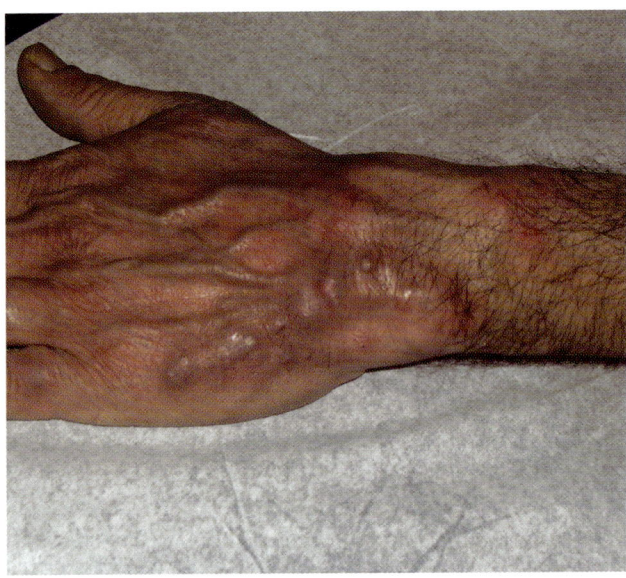

FIGURE 6.15 Inflamed subcutaneous nodules linearly distributed along the lymphatic channels in a characteristic sporotrichoid arrangement.

stains as cigar-shaped structures. Direct fluorescent antibody testing of tissue yields a more rapid diagnosis. The diagnosis can also be confirmed with serum agglutinins, precipitins, and complement-fixing antibodies.[114]

For localized cutaneous disease the treatment of choice is itraconazole at a dose of 200–400 mg daily in two divided doses. Fluconazole (200 mg twice daily), terbinafine (1000 mg daily), ketoconazole (200–400 mg twice daily), and vericonaziole are effective. Due to its low cost, treatment with oral supersaturated potassium iodide solution (1 g/1 cc) at a dose of 300–600 mg three times daily continues to be prescribed.[115] The treatment should be continued for 4 weeks but, unfortunately, adherence is as low as 40% due to the development of gastrointestinal symptoms, especially nausea. Application of external heat is a valuable adjunctive treatment.

Disseminated sporotrichosis can be fatal and requires treatment with itraconazole at higher doses or intravenous amphotericin B at 0.6–1 mg/kg daily for a total dosage of 0.75–3 g or liposomal amphotericin B at a dose of 3 mg/kg daily.[115]

CUTANEOUS *BALAMUTHIA MANDRILLARIS* INFECTION

Infections by species of the free-living soil and water amoebas of the genera acanthamoeba and naegleria cause subacute granulomatous and acute necrotizing meningoencephalitis, respectively. Cutaneous amebiasis caused by these species is associated with disseminated infection in profoundly immunocompromised persons. However, *Balamuthia mandrillaris* has been more recently reported from Peru, Brazil, Mexico, Argentina, and Venezuela, as well as Thailand and Australia, and most of the Latin American cases have had competent immune systems.[112,116,117] *Balamuthia meningoencephalitis* has a prolonged subacute course but is nearly always fatal.[112,116] The CNS findings are preceded by weeks to months by the presence of a single (less often, two or three) erythematous, painless plaque with rubbery to hard edges that measures several centimeters, usually located on the nose but occasionally on the mandible, trunk, or extremities.[118] Because most physicians have no experience with this disease, the infection is clinically misdiagnosed as sarcoid, lupus erythematosus, leishmaniasis, Wegener's granulomatosis, or midline facial granuloma.[118] Although in about 75% of biopsy specimens from lesional tissue, amoebic trophozoites can be detected within the diffuse lymphoplasmocytic infiltrate consisting of histiocytes, ill-defined granulomas and numerous multinucleated giant cells that extends throughout the dermis to the adipose tissue. The definitive diagnosis of *Balamuthia* infection requires culture, specific immunostaining, or immunofluorescent assays.[112]

No treatment has been shown to be effective, but some patients have survived when the diagnosis was established early and treatment was initiated before the development of meningoencephalitis.[119] Albendazole, alone or in combination with itraconazole, or fluconazole for 6–9 months has been effective in a handful of cases.[120] In most cases, there is appearance and progression of CNS disease even while under treatment. Although improvement and disappearance of cutaneous lesions have been reported with intravenous amphotericin B and pentamidine, neither drug prevented the eventual appearance of CNS disease.[120] Success has been reported with an antimicrobial therapeutic regimen that included flucytosine, pentamidine, fluconazole, sulfadiazine, and a macrolide antibiotic (azithromycin or clarithromycin).[121]

CHRONIC INFECTIVE LYMPHOCYTIC PSORIAFORM DERMATITIS

The high prevalence of infection with human T-lymphotrophic virus-1 (HTLV-1) in South American populations is slowly being recognized, with studies from Peru indicating 2%–3% seropositivity among people living in Andean areas of the country and surveys from Brazil, Colombia, and Ecuador finding similarly high rates of infection.[122,123] Among some groups, transmission occurs predominantly through breastfeeding, whereas in others intravenous drug abuse and sexual intercourse are more important means of spread.[123,124]

Infection with HTLV-1 has been associated with the development of acute T-cell leukemia; cutaneous T-cell lymphoma; immunosuppression that leads to hyperkeratotic (Norwegian) scabies; widespread dermatophytosis; opportunistic infection with *Strongyloides stercoralis;* and HTLV-1 associated myelopathy.[125] Another skin disease, chronic infective psoriaform dermatitis, develops at any age but predominantly in young children.[126] The skin findings are clinically and histopathologically similar to those of atopic dermatitis in children and reverse psoriasis or seborrhea in adults. The eruption consists of eczematous plaques with honey-colored crust involving the scalp, periauricular and perinasal areas, axillae, and groin.[126] Other common findings include lymphadenopathy and watery nasal discharge without rhinitis. It is uncertain whether the disease progresses to cutaneous T-cell lymphoma.[127] Adults may have severe xerosis to acquired ichthyosis. Improvement has been reported after administration of antibacterial agents.

LYMPHATIC FILARIASIS

This disease, caused by the nematodes *Wuchereria bancrofti* and *Brugia malayi*, predominantly affects persons living in tropical areas within and adjacent to Brazil, Costa Rica, and the Dominican Republic.[128] The infection is transmitted among humans by mosquitoes of the genera aedes, anopheles, culex, and mansonia during feeding. The larvae mature into mating adults and within 12 months, microfilariae are detectable in the circulation. The infection can persist for 8 years. At least half of all infected persons are clinically asymptomatic, although lymphoscintigraphic and ultrasound studies have demonstrated damage to lymphatics and significant lymphatic dilatation extending several cm beyond the presence of adult filarial worms within lymphatic vessels.[129] Some of these patients have microscopic abnormalities in their urine, such as hematuria or proteinuria. Development of clinical disease is associated with Th2 responses and inflammatory responses that promote lymphatic damage.[130]

Symptoms may appear 5–18 months after a mosquito bite. Acute disease consists of adenolymphangitis with repeated episodes that consist of any combination of lymphedema; fever; inflammation of the inguinal, femoral, or epitrochlear lymph nodes; and skin exfoliation over edematous areas. Lymphatic vessels associated with the spermatic cord provide a preferred location for

W. bancrofti in adult men but not children. Recurrent attacks eventuate in permanent lymphatic damage that produces chronic lymphedema of the legs, arms, scrotum, vulva, and breasts. Progression of lymphedema to elephantiasis is often the result of persistent or repeated bacterial and fungal infections of tissues with compromised lymphatic function.

The most common chronic presentation in patients infected with *W. bancrofti* in men is hydrocoele, which develops after the onset of puberty.[131] Although the hydrocoele may be the only evident clinical sign of infection, in time, patients often develop palpable thickening of the spermatic cord and genital edema. The presence of "dancing" adult worms in the scrotal lymphatics can be shown through ultrasound examination.[132] In women, the breast and retroperitoneal lymphatics are the choice vessels for detection of the parasites. Lymphedema of the extremities, not hydrocoele, is the usual manifestation of brugian filariasis. A dreaded syndrome caused by filarial worms, tropical pulmonary eosinophilia occurs in patients with exuberant immune responses to microfilaria. Signs and symptoms include progressive nocturnal dry cough, wheezing, dyspnea, fever, weight loss, and, occasionally, lymphadenopathy and hepatomegaly. The recommended treatment is diethylcarbamazine (DEC), which in the United States is obtained from the Centers for Disease Control's Parasitic Diseases Drug Service. DEC kills circulating microfilaria and is partially effective against the adult worms and tropical pulmonary eosinophilia. The dose of DEC is 6 mg/kg per day for 12 days in bancroftian filariasis and for 6 days in brugian filariasis, being repeated for 2 days each month for 1 year. Some experts recommend initiating lower doses (approximately 2–3 mg/kg per day) for the first 3 days of treatment in order to decrease the risk of febrile illness due to the massive destruction of nematodes.[133] Ivermectin is very effective in eliminating microfilaremia but has little effect on the adult worms.[134] Albendazole in a single 400-mg dose is macrofilaricidal for *W. bancrofti* if given daily for 2–3 weeks and is an alternative treatment for patients who cannot tolerate DEC.[133]

However, active infection should be documented, as many patients with lymphedema are no longer infected with filarial parasite and would not benefit from antifilarial therapy. In the past, the diagnosis has relied on demonstration of the worm in Giemsa-stained smears of specimens of hydrocoele fluid, urine, or anticoagulated blood diluted in water or formalin (to lyse the red blood cells) obtained between 22:00 and 02:00 (the hours when the worms circulate).[135] The use of polycarbonate filters improved the detection of microfiliariae in body fluids. Although this technique continues to be the diagnostic test of choice for brugian filariasis, it has been replaced by the highly specific and more sensitive ELISA and immunochromatographic ("card test") assays for circulating filarial antigen (CFA) for the diagnosis of *W. bancrofti* infection.[135]

Institution of rigorous hygiene methods and treatment of superinfection with antibiotic and antifungal drugs are essential to prevent worsening of lymphedema. In addition, compression of extremities with bandages and pumps often results in improvement.

Patients who are infected or have live endemic areas of filariasis have higher risks of endomyocardial fibrosis, thrombophlebitis, tenosynovitis, typically monoarticular arthritis, glomerulonephritis, and lateral popliteal nerve palsy.

REFERENCES

1. Money Income in the United States: U.S. Bureau of the Census, U.S. Department of Commerce, 1999.
2. Del Giudice P, Dellamonica J, Durant V, Rahelinrina MP, Grobusch K, Janitschke A, et al. A case of gnathostomiasis in a European traveller returning from Mexico. *Br J Dermatol* 145(3): 487–489, 2001.
3. Rojas-Molina N, Pedraza-Sanchez S, Torres-Bibiano B, Meza-Martinez H, Escobar-Gutierrez A. Gnathostomosis, an emerging foodborne zoonotic disease in Acapulco, Mexico. *Emerg Infect Dis* 5: 264–266, 1999.
4. Bravo F. Emerging infections and the skin. Proceedings of the 49th Montagna Annual Symposium on the Biology of Skin. Snowmass, Colorado, USA. *J Invest Dermatol Symp Proc* 6(3)iv: 167–250, 2001.

5. Brandling-Bennett AE, Pinheiro F. Infectious diseases in Latin America and the Caribbean: are they really emerging and increasing? *Emerg Infect Dis* 2; 1–2; 1996.
6. Institute of Medicine. *Emerging Infections in Latin America. Emerging Infectious Diseases from the Global to the Local Perspective: Workshop Summary.* Washington DC: National Academies Press, pp. 35–51; 2001.
7. Canizares O. In: Parish LC, Millikan LE (Eds) *Global Dermatology: Diagnosis and Management According to Geography, Climate and Culture.* New York: Springer-Verlag; 1994.
8. Epstein PR, Pena OC, Racedo JB. Climate and disease in Colombia. *Lancet* 346: 1243–1244, 1995.
9. Ruiz-Maldonado R, Tamayo Sanchez L, Velazquez E. Epidemiology of skin diseases in 10,000 pediatric patients. *Boletin Medico del Hospital Infantil de Mexico* 34(1): 137–161, 1977.
10. Canizares O. In: Canizares O, Harman RRM (Eds) *Clinical Tropical Dermatology.* Blackwell Publications, 1991.
11. Canizares O. *A Manual of Dermatology for Developing Countries.* 2nd ed. Oxford University Press, 1993.
12. Guzman-Chavez RE, Segundo-Zaragoza C, Cervantes-Olivares RA, Tapia-Perez G. Presence of keratinophilic fungi with special reference to dermatophytes on the haircoat of dogs and cats in Mexico and Nezahualcoyotl cities. *Revista Latinoamericana de Microbiologia* 42(1): 41–44, 2000.
13. Manzano-Gayosso P, Mendez-Tovar LJ, Hernandez-Hernandez F, Lopez-Martinez R. Dermatophytoses in Mexico City. *Mycoses* 37(1–2): 49–52, 1994.
14. Vidotto V, Garcia R, Ponce LM, Valverde M, Bruatto M. Dermatophytoses in Cusco (Peru). *Mycoses* 34(3–4): 183–186, 1991.
15. Mangiaterra ML, Giusiano GE, Alonso JM, Pons de Storni L, Waisman R. Dermatophytosis in the greater Resistencia area, Chaco Province, Argentina. *Revista Argentina de Microbiologia* 30(2): 79–83, 1998.
16. Velasco-Castrejon O, Gonzalez-Ochoa A. Tinea imbricata in the mountains of Puebla, Mexico. *Revista de Investigacion en Salud Publica* 35(2): 109–116, 1976.
17. Kassim S. *Morbid Mortal Wkly Rept* 51(47): 1968–1969, 2002.
18. Gonzalez-Losa Mdel R, Rosado-Lopez I, Valdez-Gonzalez N, Puerto-Solis M. High prevalence of human papillomavirus type 58 in Mexican colposcopy patients. *J Clin Virol* 29(3): 202–205, 2004.
19. Onchocerciasis (river blindness). Report from the eleventh InterAmerican conference on onchocerciasis, Mexico City, Mexico. *Wkly Epidemiol Rec* 26; 77(30): 249–253, 2002.
20. Espinel M. Onchocerciasis: a Latin American perspective. *Ann Trop Med Parasitol* 92 Suppl 1: S157–S160, 1998.
21. Hoerauf A, Buttner DW, Adjei O, Pearlman E. Onchocerciasis. *BMJ* 25; 326(7382): 207–210, 2003.
22. Guevara AG, Vieira JC, Lilley BG, Lopez A, Vieira N, Rumbea J. Entomological evaluation by pool screen polymerase chain reaction of *Onchocerca volvulus* transmission in Ecuador following mass Mectizan. *Am J Trop Med Hyg* 68(2): 222–227, 2003.
23. Gordon J, Boussinesq M, Kamgno J, et al. Effects of standard and high doses of ivermectin on adult worms of *Onchocerca volvulus*: a randomized controlled trial. *Lancet* 360: 203–210, 2002.
24. White AC Jr. Neurocysticercosis: updates on epidemiology, pathogenesis, diagnosis, and management. *Annu Rev Med* 51: 187–206, 2000.
25. White AC Jr. Neurocysticercosis: a major cause of neurological disease worldwide. *Clin Infect Dis* 24(2): 101–113, 1997.
26. Salgado P, Rojas R, Sotelo J. Cysticercosis. Clinical classification based on imaging studies. *Arch Intern Med* 157(17): 1991–1997, 1997.
27. Salinas R, Counsell C, Prasad K. Treating neurocysticercosis medically: a systematic review of randomized, controlled trials. *Trop Med Int Health* 4(11): 713–718, 1999.
28. Evans MR, Thangaraj HS, Wansbrough-Jones MH. Buruli ulcer. *Curr Opin Infect Dis* 13(2): 109–112, 2000.
29. Dega H, Chosidow O, Barete S, Carbonnelle B, Grosset J, Jarlier V. *Mycobacterium ulcerans* infection. *Ann Med Interne (Paris)* 151(5): 339–344, 2000.
30. Palenque E. Skin disease and nontuberculous atypical mycobacteria. *Int J Dermatol* 39(9):659–66, 2000.
31. Van der Werf TS, Stienstra Y, van der Graaf WT. Skin ulcers misdiagnosed as pyoderma gangrenosum. *N Engl J Med* 348(11): 1064–1066, 2003.
32. Portaels F, Aguiar J, Fissette K, et al. Direct detection and identification of *Mycobacterium ulcerans* in clinical specimens by PCR and oligonucleotide-specific capture plate hybridization. *J Clin Microbiol* 35: 1097–1100, 1997.

33. Schierle HP, Lemperle G, Erdmann D. The Buruli type ulcer. *Plast Reconstr Surg* 109(7): 2608, 2002.
34. Anonymous. Rapidly growing mycobacterial infection following liposuction and liposculpture — Caracas, Venezuela, 1996–1998. *MMWR Morbid Mortal Wkly Rep* 47(49): 1065–1067, 1998.
35. Murillo J, Torres J, Bofill L, et al. Skin and wound infection by rapidly growing mycobacteria: an unexpected complication of liposuction and liposculpture. The Venezuelan Collaborative Infectious and Tropical Diseases Study Group. *Arch Dermatol* 136(11): 1347–1352, 2000.
36. Anonymous. *Mycobacterium chelonae* infections associated with face lifts — New Jersey, 2002. *MMWR Morbid Mortal Wkly Rep* 53(9): 192–194, 2003.
37. Wallace RJ, Meier A, Brown BA, et al. Genetic basis for clarithromycin resistance among isolates of *Mycobacterium chelonei* and *Mycobacterium abscessus*. *Antimicrob Agents Chemother* 40(7): 1676–1681, 1996.
38. Villanueva A, Calderon RV, Vargas BA, et al. Report of an outbreak of post-injection abscesses due to *Mycobacterium abscessus*, including management with surgery and clarithromycin therapy and comparison of strains by random amplified DNA polymerase chain reaction. *CID* 24: 1147–1153, 1997.
39. WHO Expert Committee. Control of Chagas disease. World Health Organization Technical Report Series. 905:I-VI, 1–109, 2002.
40. Sartori AM, Sotto MN, Braz LM, et al. Reactivation of Chagas disease manifested by skin lesions in a patient with AIDS. *Trans R Soc Trop Med Hyg* 93(6): 631–632, 1999.
41. La Forgia MP, Pellarano G, de las Mercedes Portaluppi M, et al. Cutaneous manifestation of reactivation of Chagas disease in a renal transplant patient: long-term follow-up. *Arch Dermatol* 139: 104–105, 2003.
42. Gentry LO, Zeluff B, Kielhofner MA. Dermatologic manifestations of infectious diseases in cardiac transplant patients. *Infect Dis Clin North Am* 8: 637–654, 1994.
43. Solari A, Ortiz S, Soto A, Arancibia C, et al. Treatment of Trypanosoma cruzi-infected children with nifurtimox: a 3 year follow-up by PCR. *J Antimicrob Chemother* 48(4): 515–519, 2001.
44. Lange WR, Beall B, Denney SC. Dengue fever: a resurgent risk for the international traveler. *Am Fam Physician* 45: 1161–1168, 1992.
45. Seijo A, Cernigoi B, Deodato B. Dengue imported from Paraguay to Buenos Aires. Clinical and epidemiological report of 38 cases. *Medicina (Buenos Aires)* 61: 137–41, 2001.
46. Dengue and Dengue Haemorrhagic fever in the Americas: Guidelines for Prevention and Control; 1997.
47. WHO. *Dengue Haemorrhagic Fever: Diagnosis, Treatment, Control*. Geneva: World Health Organization; 1986.
48. Cunningham R, Milton K. Dengue haemorrhagic fever. *BMJ* 302: 1083–1084, 1991.
49. Piel J. A polyketide synthase-peptide synthetase gene cluster from an uncultured bacterial symbiont of Paederus beetles. *Proc Natl Acad Sci USA* 99(22): 14002–14007, 2002.
50. Veraldi S, Suss L. Dermatitis caused by *Paederus fuscipes* Curt. *Int J Dermatol* 33(4): 277–278, 1994.
51. Alva-Davalos V, Laguna-Torres VA, Huaman A, Olivos R, Chavez M, Garcia C, Mendoza N. Epidemic dermatitis by *Paederus irritans* in Piura, Peru at 1999, related to El Nino phenomenon. *Revista Da Sociedade Brasileira de Medicina Tropical* 35(1): 23–28, 2002.
52. Maguiña C, Gotuzzo E. Bartonellosis new and old. Emerging and re-emerging diseases in Latin America. *Infect Dis Clin North Am* 14: 1–22, 2000.
53. Alexander B. A review of bartonellosis in Ecuador and Colombia. [Historical Article]. *Am J Trop Med Hyg* 52(4): 354–359, 1995.
54. Lee J, Lynde C. Pyogenic granuloma: pyogenic again? Association between pyogenic granuloma and bartonella. *J Cutan Med Surg* 5(6): 467–470, 2001.
55. Kosek M, Lavarello R, Gilman RH, et al. Natural history of infection with *Bartonella bacilliformis* in a nonendemic population. *J Infect Dis* 182(3): 865–872, 2000.
56. Bhutto AM, Nonaka S, Hashiguchi Y, Gomez EA. Histopathological and electron microscopical features of skin lesions in a patient with bartonellosis (verruga peruana). *J Dermatol* 21(3): 178–184, 1994.
57. Sobraquès M, Maurin M, Birtles RJ, Raoult D. *In vitro* susceptibilities of four *Bartonella bacilliformis* strains to 30 antibiotic compounds. *Antimicrob Agents Chemother* 43(8): 2090–2092, 1999.
58. Kain KC. Skin lesions in returned travelers. *Med Clin North Am* 83(4): 1077–1102, 1999.

59. Jelinek T, Maiwald H, Nothdurft HD, Loscher T. Cutaneous larva migrans in travelers: synopsis of histories, symptoms, and treatment of 98 patients. *Clin Infect Dis* 19: 1062–1066, 1994.
60. Bouchaud O, Houze S, Schiemann R, Durand R, Ralaimazava P, Ruggeri C, Coulaud JP. Cutaneous larva migrans in travelers: a prospective study, with assessment of therapy with ivermectin. *Clin Infect Dis* 31(2): 493–498, 2000.
61. Sherman SC. Radford N. Severe infestation of cutaneous larva migrans. *J Emerg Med* 26(3): 347–349, 2004.
62. Ly MN, Bethel SL, Usmani AS, Lambert DR. Cutaneous *Strongyloides stercoralis* infection: an unusual presentation. *J Am Acad Dermatol* 49(2 Suppl Case Reports): S157–S160, 2003.
63. Smith JD, Goette DK, Odom RB. Larva currens. Cutaneous strongyloidiasis. *Arch Dermatol* 112: 1161–1163, 1976.
64. Menard A, Dos Santos G, Dekumyoy P, Ranque S, Delmont J, Danis M, et al. Imported cutaneous gnathostomiasis: report of five cases. *Trans R Soc Trop Med Hyg* 97(2): 200–202, 2003.
65. Chappuis F, Farinelli T, Loutan L. Ivermectin treatment of a traveler who returned from Peru with cutaneous gnathostomiasis. *Clin Infect Dis* 33: E17–E19, 2001.
66. Camacho SP, Willms K, Ramos MZ, del Carmen de la Cruz Otero M, Nawa Y, Akahane H. Morphology of *Gnathostoma* spp. isolated from natural hosts in Sinaloa, Mexico. *Diaz Parasitol Res* 88(7): 639–645, 2002.
67. Rusnak J, Lucey D. Clinical gnathostomiasis: case report and review of the English language literature. *Clin Infect Dis* 16: 33–50, 1993.
68. Moore DA, McCroddan J, Chiodini PL. Gnathostomiasis: an emerging imported disease. *Emerg Infect Dis* 9: 647–650, 2003.
69. Costa H, Bravo F, Valdez L, et al. Paniculitis migratoria eosinofílica en el Perú (Gnathostomiasis humana). *Folia Dermatológica Peruana* 12: 21–35, 2001.
70. Ligon BL. Gnathomiasis. A review of a previously localized zoonosis now crossing numerous geographic boundaries. *Sem Ped Inf Dis* 16(2), 137, 2005.
71. Kraivichian P, Kulkumthorn M, Yingyourd P, Akarabovorn P, Paireepai CC. Albendazole for the treatment of human gnathostomiasis. *Trans R Soc Trop Med Hyg* 86: 418–421, 1992.
72. Nontasut P, Bussaratid V, Chullawichit S, Charoensook N, Visetsuk K. Comparison of ivermectin and albendazole treatment for gnathostomiasis. *Southeast Asian J Trop Med Publ Health* 31: 374–377, 2000.
73. Powers N, Yorgensen M. Myiasis in humans: an overview and a report of two cases in the Republic of Panama. *Mil Med* 61(8): 495–497, 1996.
74. Lucchina L, Wilson M, Drake L. Dermatology and the recently returned traveler: infectious diseases with dermatologic manifestations. *Int J Dermatol* 36(3): 167–181, 1997.
75. Jelinek T, Nothdurft H, Rieder N, Loescher T. Cutaneous myiasis: review of 13 cases of travelers returning from tropical countries. *Int J Dermatol* 39(9): 689–694, 2000.
76. Brewer T, Wilson M, Gonzalez E, et al. Bacon therapy and furuncular myiasis. *JAMA* 270: 2087–2088, 1993.
77. Seppänen M, Virolainen-Julkunen A, Kakko I, Vilkamaa P, Meri S. Myiasis during adventure sports race. *CDC Emerg Infect Dis* 10(1): 1, 2004.
78. Noutsis C, Millikan L. Myiasis. *Dematol Clin* 12(4): 729–736, 1994.
79. Desjeux P. The increase in risk factors for leishmaniasis worldwide. *Trans R Soc TropMed Hyg* 95(3): 239–243, 2001.
80. Choi CM, Lerner EA. Leishmaniasis: recognition and management with a focus on the immunocompromised patient. *Am J Clin Dermatol* 3(2): 91–101, 2002.
81. Andrade-Narvaez FJ, Vargas-Gonzalez A, Canto-Lara SB, Damian-Centeno AG. Clinical picture of cutaneous leishmaniases due to Leishmania (Leishmania) mexicana in the Yucatan Peninsula, Mexico. *Memorias do Instituto Oswaldo Cruz* 96(2): 163–167, 2001.
82. Romero GA, Guerra MV, Paes MG, Macedo VO. Comparison of cutaneous leishmaniasis due to *Leishmania (Viannia) braziliensis* and *L. (V.) guyanensis* in Brazil: therapeutic response to meglumine antimoniate. *Am J Trop Med Hyg* 65(5): 456–465, 2001.
83. Daudén E, Peñas PF, Rios L, Jimenez M, Fraga J, Alvar J, García-Diez A. Leishmaniasis presenting as a dermatomyositis-like eruption in AIDS. *J Am Acad Dermatol* 35: 316–319, 1996.

84. Amato VS, Padilha AR, Nicodemo AC, et al. Use of itraconazole in the treatment of mucocutaneous leishmaniasis: a pilot study. *Int J Infect Dis* 4(3): 153–157, 2000.
85. Weigel MM, Armijos RX. The traditional and conventional medical treatment of cutaneous leishmaniasis in rural Ecuador. *Pan Am J Publ Health* 10(6): 395–404, 2001.
86. Croft SL, Yardley V. Chemotherapy of leishmaniasis. *Curr Pharm Des* 8(4): 319–342, 2002.
87. Minotto R, Bernardi CD, Mallmann LF, et al. Chromoblastomycosis: a review of 100 cases in the state of Rio Grande do Sul, Brazil. *J Am Acad Dermatol* 44: 585–592, 2001.
88. Silva JP, de Souza W, Rozental S. Chromoblastomycosis: a retrospective study of 325 cases on Amazonic Region (Brazil). *Mycopathologia* 143(3): 171–175, 1998–1999.
89. Bonifaz A, Carrasco-Gerard E, Saul A. Chromoblastomycosis: clinical and mycologic experience of 51 cases. *Mycoses* 44(1–2): 1–7, 2001.
90. Poirriez J, Breuillard F, Francois N, et al. A case of chromomycosis treated by a combination of cryotherapy, shaving, oral 5-fluorocytosine, and oral amphotericin B. *Am J Trop Med Hyg* 63(1–2): 61–63, 2000.
91. Anonymous. Elimination of leprosy in the Americas. *Epidemiol Bull* 21: 5–6, 2000.
92. Levis WR, Vides EA, Cabrera A. Leprosy in the Eastern United States. *JAMA* 283(8): 1004–1005, 2000.
93. Jacobson RR, Krahenbuhl JL. Leprosy. *Lancet* 353(9153): 655–660, 1999.
94. Ramos-e-Silva M, Rebello PF. Leprosy. Recognition and treatment. *Am J Clin Dermatol* 2(4): 203–211, 2001.
95. Haimanot RT, Melaku Z. Leprosy. *Curr Opin Neurol* 13(3): 317–322, 2000.
96. Solomon S, Kurian N, Ramadas P, Rao PS. Incidence of nerve damage in leprosy patients treated with MDT. *Int J Leprosy Other Mycobacterial Dis* 66(4): 451–456, 1998.
97. Rodriguez G, Pinto R, Laverde C, Sarmiento M, Riveros A, Valderrama J, Ordonez N. Relapses after multibacillary leprosy treatment. *Biomedica* 24(2): 133–139, 2004.
98. Grosset JH. Newer drugs in leprosy. *Int J Leprosy Other Mycobact Dis* 69(2 Suppl): S14–S18, 2001.
99. Andraca R, Edson RS, Kern EB. Rhinoscleroma: a growing concern in the United States? Mayo Clinic experience. *Clin Proc* 68(12): 1151–1157, 1993.
100. Fernandez-Vozmediano JM, Armario Hita JC, Gonzalez Cabrerizo A. Rhinoscleroma in three siblings. *Pediatr Dermatol* 21(2): 134–138, 2004.
101. Tapia Collantes A. Dermatology in the tropics. *Revista Medica de Panama* 20(3): 65–71, 1995.
102. Miyaji M, Kamei K. Imported mycoses: an update. *J Infect Chemother* 9(2): 107–113, 2003.
103. Benard G, Duarte AJ. Paracoccidiodiomycosis: a model for evaluation of the effects of human immunodeficiency virus infection on the natural history of endemic tropical diseases. *Clin Infect Dis* 31: 1032–1039, 2000.
104. Trent JT, Kirsner RS. Identifying and treating mycotic skin infections. *Adv Skin Wound Care* 16(3): 122–129, 2003.
105. Godoy H. Reichart PA. Oral manifestations of paracoccidioidomycosis. Report of 21 cases from Argentina. *Mycoses* 46(9–10):412–7, 2003
106. Meneses-Garcia A, Mosqueda-Taylor A, Morales-de la Luz R, Rivera LM. Paracoccidioidomycosis: report of 2 cases mimicking squamous cell carcinoma. *Oral Surg Oral Med Oral Pathol Oral Radiol Endodontics* 94(5): 609–613, 2002.
107. Bakos L, Kronfeld M, Hampe S, Castro I, Zampese M. Disseminated paracoccidioidomycosis with skin lesions in a patient with acquired immunodeficiency syndrome. *J Am Acad Dermatol* 20(1): 854–855, 1989.
108. Gomes GM, Cisalpino PS, Taborda CP, de Camargo ZP. PCR for diagnosis of paracoccidiodomycosis. *J Clin Microbiol* 38: 3478–3480, 2000.
109. Shikanai-Yasuda MA, Benard G, Higaki Y, et al. Randomized trial with itraconazole, ketoconazole and sulfadiazine in paracoccidiodomycosis. *Med Mycol* 40(4): 411–417, 2002.
110. Lyon GM, Zurita S, Casquero J, et al. Sporotrichosis in Peru Investigation Team. Population-based surveillance and a case-control study of risk factors for endemic lymphocutaneous sporotrichosis in Peru. *Clin Infect Dis* 36(1): 34–39, 2003.
111. Schubach TM, Schubach A, Okamoto T, et al. Evaluation of an epidemic of sporotrichosis in cats: 347 cases (1998–2001). *J Am Vet Med Assoc* 224(10): 1623–1629, 2004.

112. Bravo F, Sanchez MR. New and re-emerging cutaneous infectious diseases in Latin America and other geographic areas. *Dermatol Clin* 21(4): 655–668, 2003.
113. Queiroz-Telles F, McGinnis MR, Salkin I, Graybill JR. Subcutaneous mycoses. *Infect Dis Clin North Am* 17(1):59–85, 2003.
114. De Araujo T, Marques AC, Kerdel F. Sporotrichosis. *Int J Dermatol* 40(12): 737–742, 2001.
115. Bustamante B, Campos PE. Endemic sporotrichosis. *Curr Opin Infect Dis* 14(2): 145–149, 2001.
116. Riestra-Castaneda JM, Riestra-Castaneda R, Gonzalez-Garrido AA, et al. Granulomatous amebic encephalitis due to Balamuthia mandrillaris (Leptomyxiidae): report of four cases from Mexico. *Am J Trop Med Hyg* 56(6): 603–607, 1997.
117. Taratuto AL, Monges J, Acefe JC, et al. Leptomyxid amoeba encephalitis: report of the first case in Argentina. *Trans R Soc Trop Med Hyg* 85(1): 77, 1991.
118. Pritzker AS, Kim BK, Agrawal D, et al. Fatal granulomatous amebic encephalitis caused by *Balamuthia mandrillaris* presenting as a skin lesion. *J Am Acad Dermatol* 50(2 Suppl): S38–S41, 2004.
119. Recavarren-Arce S, Velarde C, Gotuzzo E, Cabrera J. Amoeba angeitic lesions of the central nervous system in Balamuthia mandrilaris amoebiasis. *Hum Pathol* 30(3): 269–273, 1999.
120. Schuster FL, Visvesvara GS. Opportunistic amoebae: challenges in prophylaxis and treatment. *Drug Resist Update* 7(1): 41–51, 2004.
121. Deetz TR, Sawyer MH, Billman G, Schuster FL, Visvesvara GS. Successful treatment of Balamuthia amoebic encephalitis: presentation of 2 cases. *Clin Infect Dis* 37(10): 1304–1312, 2003.
122. Gotuzzo E, Arango C, de Queiroz-Campos A, Isturiz RE. Human T-cell lymphotropic virus-I in Latin America. *Infect Dis Clin North Am* 14(1): 211–239, 2000.
123. Sanchez-Palacios C, Gotuzzo E, Vandamme AM, Maldonado Y. Seroprevalence and risk factors for human T-cell lymphotropic virus (HTLV-I) infection among ethnically and geographically diverse Peruvian women. *Int J Infect Dis* 7(2): 132–137, 2003.
124. Trujillo L, Munoz D, Gotuzzo E, et al. Sexual practices and prevalence of HIV, HTLV-I/II, and Treponema pallidum among clandestine female sex workers in Lima, Peru. *Sex Transm Dis* 26(2): 115–118, 1999.
125. Goncalves DU, Guedes AC, Proietti AB, et al. Interdisciplinary HTLV-1/2 Research Group. Dermatologic lesions in asymptomatic blood donors seropositive for human T cell lymphotropic virus type-1. *Am J Trop Med Hyg* 68(5): 562–565, 2003.
126. La Grenade L, Manns A, Fletcher V, et al. Clinical, pathologic, and immunologic features of human T-lymphotrophic virus type I-associated infective dermatitis in children. *Arch Dermatol* 134(4): 439–444, 1998.
127. Hanchard B, LaGrenade L, Carberry C, et al. Childhood infective dermatitis evolving into adult T-cell leukaemia after 17 years. *Lancet* 338(8782–8783): 1593–1594, 1991.
128. Laurence BR. The global dispersal of bancroftian filariasis. *Parasitol Today* 5(8): 260–264, 1989.
129. Melrose WD. Lymphatic filariasis: new insights into an old disease. *Int J Parasitol* 32(8): 947–960, 2002.
130. Lammie PJ, Cuenco KT, Punkosdy GA. The pathogenesis of filarial lymphedema: is it the worm or is it the host? *Ann N Y Acad Sci* 979: 131–142, 2002.
131. Richens J. Genital manifestations of tropical diseases. *Sex Transm Infect* 80(1): 12–7, 2004.
132. de Cassio Saito O, de Barros N, Chammas MC, Oliveira IR, Cerri GG. Ultrasound of tropical and infectious diseases that affect the scrotum. *Ultrasound Q* 20(1): 12–8, 2004.
133. Melrose WD. Chemotherapy for lymphatic filariasis: progress but not perfection. *Expert Rev Anti Infect Ther* 1(4): 571–577, 2003.
134. Hoerauf A, Adjei O, Buttner DW. Antibiotics for the treatment of onchocerciasis and other filarial infections. *Curr Opin Invest Drugs* 3(4): 533–537, 2002.
135. Walther M, Muller R. Diagnosis of human filariases (except onchocerciasis). *Adv Parasitol* 53: 149–193, 2003.

7 Cutaneous Manifestations of Systemic Disease in Pigmented Skins

Yamini V. Saripalli and Sharon Bridgeman-Shah

INTRODUCTION

Human skin has many functions and its condition/appearance often gives clues to systemic disease that may or may not be otherwise clinically evident. For this reason, it is of benefit to discuss the role of the skin as it relates to internal disease. Features of skin involvement in systemic disease may include primary lesions such as papules, plaques, nodules, vesicles or bullae, or may be secondary such as pruritus, redness, hyperkeratosis, or hyperpigmentation.

Because the skin is the largest organ of the body and an organ of homeostasis, it is not surprising that systemic conditions can somehow manifest as cutaneous changes. As such, a high index of suspicion for internal disease and a thorough dermatologic examination are key when evaluating a patient with new or peculiar skin changes. Even when a presenting symptom may seem unrelated to the skin, all organ systems, including the skin, should receive a thorough physical examination. Simple clues may aid in early recognition and treatment of systemic disease in addition to lab work recommendations when systemic symptoms are not present.

SARCOIDOSIS

Sarcoidosis is a multisystem disease that features noncaseating, epithelioid granulomas as its hallmark.[1] The etiology of sarcoidosis is unknown but current hypotheses revolve around immunologic, genetic, infectious, or environmental causes.[2,3] The disease is more common in the African-American population and has an incidence of 64/100,000 vs. only 14/100,000 in Caucasians.[3,4] In addition to its high prevalence in the African-American population, these individuals are found to have more severe cutaneous disease than other ethnic groups.[5]

Although cutaneous involvement is present in 20%–35% of cases, sarcoidosis can involve almost any organ, including the lymphatic, ophthalmologic, pulmonary, cutaneous, hematologic, cardiac, neurological, and gastrointestinal systems.[1,3,4] A Taiwanese study found that more than 50% of their study subjects who presented with cutaneous sarcoidosis had systemic involvement.[1] Other cases have reported Chinese patients presenting with cutaneous sarcoidosis and having coexisting pulmonary or hepatic sarcoidosis.[6,7]

Histologically, sarcoidosis consists of noncaseating granulomas composed of lymphocytes and monocytic phagocytes.[2] In African-American and Asian populations, large-vessel vasculitis is a more common complication than the small vessel vasculitides seen in Caucasian races.[8]

Clinically, cutaneous sarcoidosis may mimic other entities. As such, skin biopsy may be of tremendous benefit if there is any doubt as to the etiology of otherwise-common skin conditions. It is also helpful for patients with known systemic sarcoidosis or with new, unremitting, cutaneous lesions of any kind.

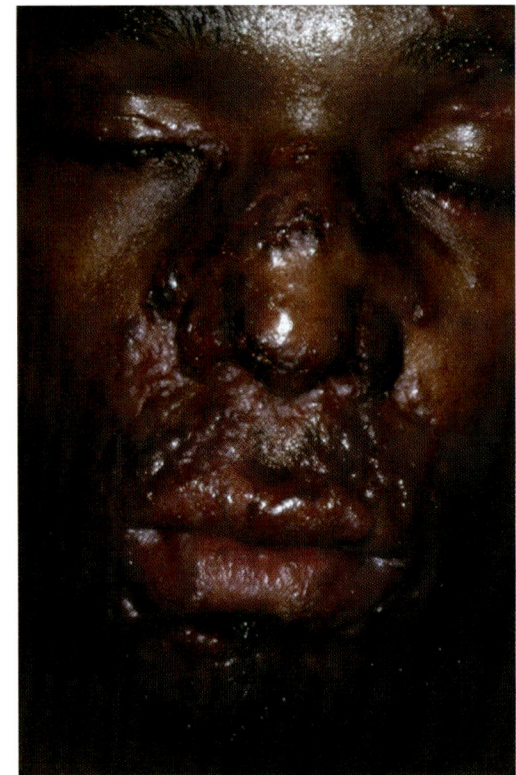

FIGURE 7.1 An African-American male with disfiguring sarcoidosis affecting the upper lip and nasolabial folds. (Courtesy of Rebat M. Halder, M.D.)

The clinical presentation of cutaneous sarcoidosis is extremely varied. Histologically, sarcoidosis has been identified in some lesions of cicatricial alopecia, xanthelasma, and annular lichen planus and also in ichythiotic, verrucous, lichenoid, clubbing, ulcerative, hypopigmented patches, and plaques and scars.[2,5,9] Characteristic erythema nodosum skin lesions consisting of tender nodules on the anterior pretibial area are less prevalent in African-Americans.[10,11] More common in these individuals are waxy, papular lesions that are usually on the face but that can also be on the upper back and extremities.[2,11,12]

In pigmented skins, some variants of sarcoidosis can be disfiguring, in contrast to other skin types (Figures 7.1–7.4). Lupus pernio is a variant of sarcoidosis consisting of chronic, indurated, shiny papules and plaques on the face specifically on the nose, lips, cheeks, and ears (Figure 7.5).[2,5,10] Lupus pernio occurring on the nasal alar rim is associated with systemic involvement.[2,3] This form of disease is prevalent in black South African individuals[4] as well as in African-Americans with sarcoidosis. There are also case reports of African-American and African persons in which sarcoidosis presented solely as isolated lesions on the scrotum and penis,[13] leonine facies consisting of nodules and plaques,[14] and dactylitis.[4] The cicatricial alopecia variant of sarcoidosis has been found to be more prevalent in African-American females and is often associated with systemic involvement.[7] A recent retrospective study of 147 patients with sarcoidosis found seven cases of ulcerative sarcoidosis in which all patients were African-American.[15] More than 50% of these patients were female and the lesions usually occurred in the pretibial region.[15] The authors also note that lupus pernio with nasal involvement can coincide with ulcerative sarcoidosis. This combination suggests that individuals with lupus pernio may have a more disfiguring outcome.

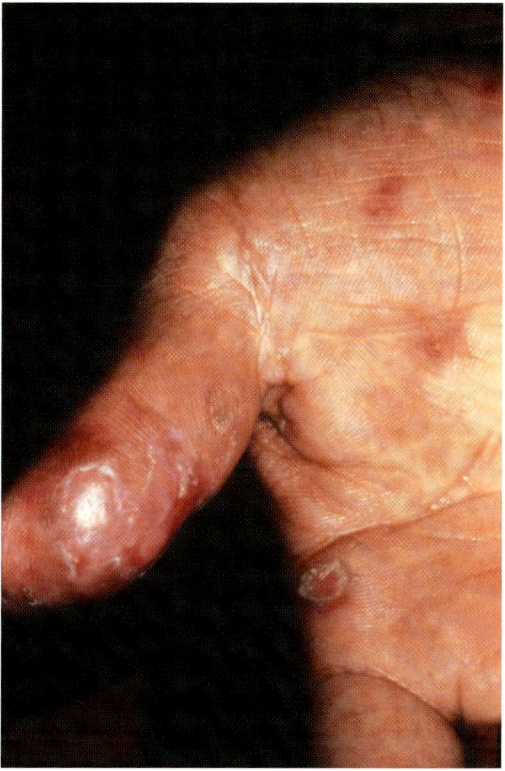

FIGURE 7.2 A patient with ulcerative sarcoidosis on the first digit of the right hand. (Reproduced from Halder RM. *Dermatol Clin* 2003; 21: 679–687. With permission from Elsevier.)

The minimum baseline workup for a patient who presents with cutaneous sarcoidosis includes liver function tests (LFTs), renal function tests, complete blood count (CBC), erythrocyte sedimentation rate (ESR), and calcium and angiotensin-converting enzyme (ACE) levels.[3] Treatment varies, depending on the presence or absence of systemic involvement and the severity of the disease. The mainstay of treatment consists of topical or intralesional steroids for cutaneous lesions and oral glucocorticoids for severe, extensive lesions.[2] Several immunosuppressants/modulators and antimalarials such as plaquenil,[16] methotrexate,[17] thalidomide,[5,18] azathioprine,[12,19,20] cyclophosphamide,[12,19,20] chlorambucil,[12,19,20] cyclosporine,[12,19,20] and allopurinol[21] have been used in refractory cases of cutaneous sarcoidosis. In addition, pulse dye laser has been used with some success in lupus pernio.[22]

Because of its prevalence, severity, and variability in pigmented skins, physicians should be aware of both the presentation and treatment options of sarcoidosis in these populations.

AUTOIMMUNE DISEASE

SCLERODERMA

Scleroderma is an autoimmune disease defined as a hardening of the skin that makes it immobile.[11] There are two variants of the disease: systemic and limited (Figure 7.6). The systemic form has an increased incidence in African-Americans and is associated with a worse prognosis.[23] Some current evidence also shows an increased occurrence of the diffuse variant in Hispanic patients.[24] In addition, ninety percent of scleroderma patients have a positive antinuclear antibody.[25] Individuals with limited

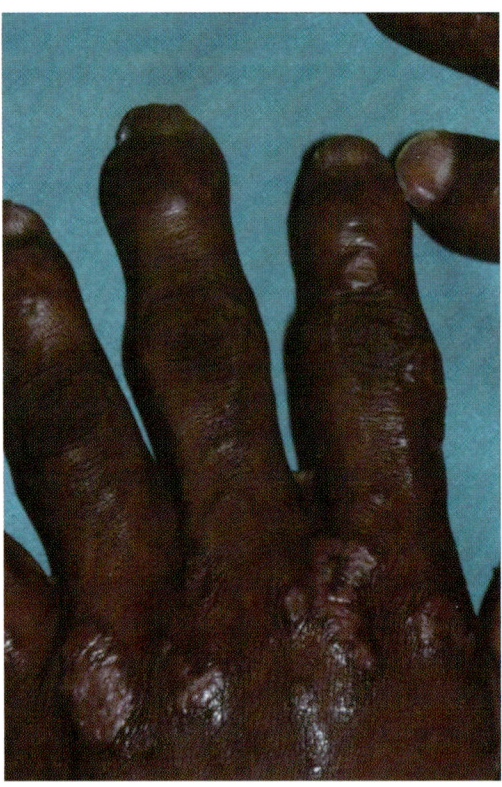

FIGURE 7.3 Plaque-type lesions of sarcoidosis and associated disfigurement on the left hand of an African-American individual. (Courtesy of Rebat M. Halder, M.D.)

disease may have anticentromere antibodies (seen in the CREST [calcinosis, Raynaud's phenomenon, esophageal dysphagia, and telangiectasias] syndrome),[23,26] but those with diffuse disease can have anti Scl 70 (antitopoisomerase I) antibodies, which can be associated with a poor outcome.[27] An antinucleolar pattern is most specific for scleroderma.[26] In the diffuse disease variant, patients may also have anti RNA polymerase I and III antibodies in the absence of anti Scl 70 antibodies which has also been found more commonly in African-American individuals.[24,28] It is interesting to note that when compared to Caucasian populations, African-Americans have a higher incidence of anti Scl 70 (37% vs. 17%) and a lower incidence of anticentromere antibody (4% vs. 36%).[27] This evidence suggests that African-Americans are more prone to a worse prognosis than other ethnic populations.[27] Other factors associated with a poor prognosis include male sex and proteinuria.[29]

Histology of affected skin in scleroderma reveals abundant collagen in both the dermis and subcutaneous tissue.[23] Clinically, some characteristic features of the disease include Raynaud's phenomenon and facial induration.[23] It is the facial disfigurement that usually most worries patients.[30] A study of 78 Indian patients found skin thickening as the most common presenting symptom of scleroderma, and 100% of their patients had cutaneous involvement.[31] The affected skin area can either be hypo- or hyperpigmented, but in darker skin types (i.e., African-Americans and South Asians) there can be a characteristic "salt and pepper" appearance of perifollicular hyperpigmentation (Figure 7.7) occurring on the forearms, trunk and hands.[11,23] Other common physical findings include telangiectasias of the lips and palms, calcinosis cutis near joints, and cutaneous ulcers.[23] Cutaneous ulcers can be very difficult to treat and are more common in African-American and Hispanic individuals.[23,24] Some patients will have internal organ involvement such as diastolic cardiac dysfunction, renal failure, lead pipe esophagus, and restrictive pulmonary disease.[23,31]

Cutaneous Manifestations of Systemic Disease in Pigmented Skins 151

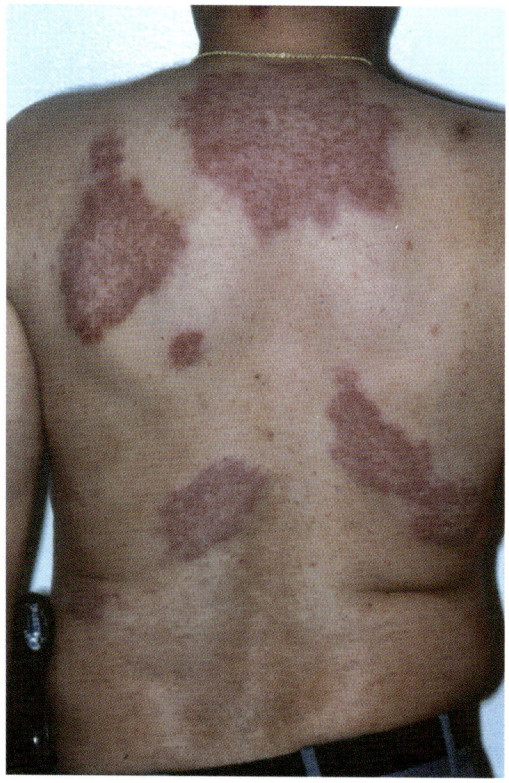

FIGURE 7.4 Erythematous plaques with hyperpigmented borders on the back of a patient with sarcoidosis.

Treatment of scleroderma can be very difficult. Physical therapy, massage, warmth, as well as avoiding cold and smoking should be key treatment elements in all patients.[11,23] Calcium channel blockers are useful in treating Raynaud's phenomenon, and intravenous prostaglandins have been used with some success in refractory cases.[32] Because of the proximity to the underlying bone, debridement of ulcers is usually not recommended, and occlusive dressings or skin equivalents should be used instead.[23] Cutaneous sclerosis can be very resistant to treatment.[23] There are current trials using penicillamine because it interrupts the cross-linking of collagen.[33] The growth factor relaxin has been used with some success and has been shown to increase collagenase activity as well as decrease skin scores.[34] In addition some patients show response to phototherapy using UVA wavelengths.

Scleroderma is associated with a severe morbidity in both the limited and diffuse forms. It is important to recognize the clinical presentations in pigmented races such as African-Americans and Hispanics because of their tendency to have more severe, diffuse disease and characteristic skin findings.

LUPUS ERYTHEMATOSUS

Systemic lupus erythematosus (SLE) is associated with skin findings approximately 70%–90% of the time.[34,35] Cutaneous lupus erythematosus (CLE) can be divided into three different types, including chronic CLE (CCLE), subacute CLE (SCLE), and acute CLE (ACLE).[35,36] There are several theories on the pathogenesis of LE. Genetic influences seem to play the greatest role in predisposing individuals to developing LE.[37] The gene for developing LE is located on the long arm of chromosome 1.[38] More specifically, ACLE is associated with HLA DR2 and HLA DR3,[39] and SCLE is associated with HLA B8, DR3, DRW52, DQ1, and DQ2.[40] Environment also affects

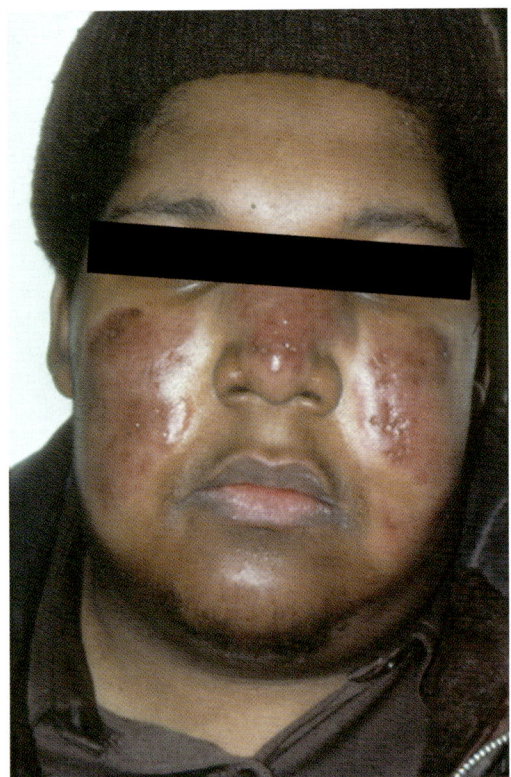

FIGURE 7.5 Lupus pernio affecting the nasal bridge and cheeks of an African American male with sarcoidosis. (Reproduced from Halder RM. *Dermatol Clin* 2003; 21: 679–687. With permission from Elsevier.)

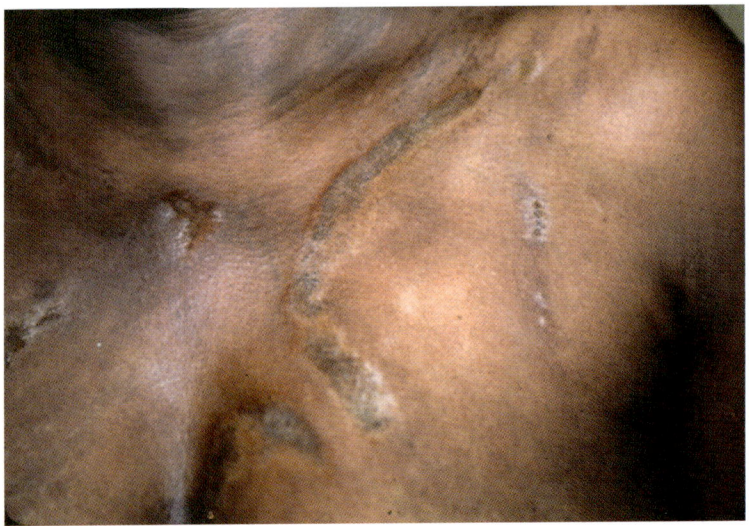

FIGURE 7.6 Morphea, a localized variant of scleroderma, affecting the chest of an African-American female.

the development of LE. More than 60% of patients with CLE develop an exacerbation upon exposure to UVA and UVB light rays.[41] This photosensitivity is thought to develop from keratinocyte-induced apoptosis.[36] Photosensitivity is associated with the existence of anti Ro/SSA and anti La/SSB

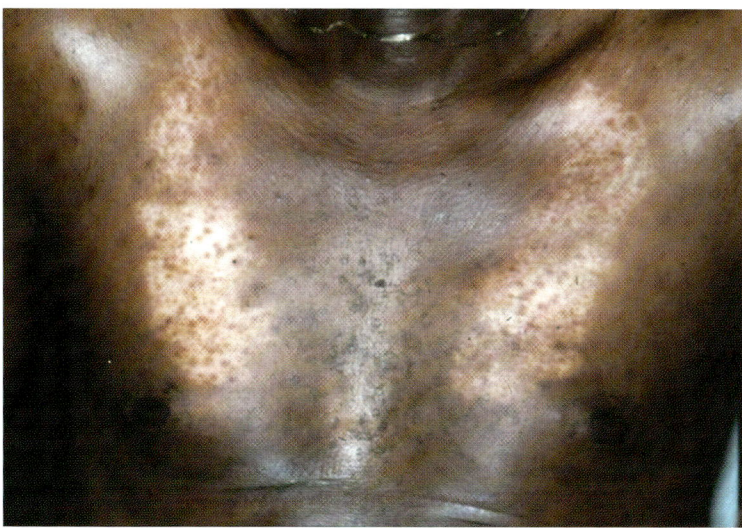

FIGURE 7.7 Characteristic "salt and pepper" perifollicular hyperpigmentation associated with scleroderma in an African-American male. (Reproduced from Halder RM. *Dermatol Clin* 2003; 21: 679–687. With permission from Elsevier.)

antibodies.[41,42] Cellular immune mechanisms are also implicated in the pathogenesis of LE. Most CLE lesions are positive for cell markers CD28, CDB7-1, and CDB7-2,[43] but the most prominent cell marker in DLE is CD45RA.[44] Interleukin-2 (IL-2) and interferon-gamma can be found in DLE lesions.[45] Other immune mechanisms in the etiology of LE include antibody formation. The antinuclear antibody (ANA) is positive in 95% of patients with SLE.[46] Although both anti-double-stranded DNA (DSDNA) and anti-Smith antibody can be present in SLE, the latter is more specific for the disease.[47] SCLE is associated with anti Ro/SSA antibody, but DLE and lupus panniculitis lesions do not have any specific associated antibodies.[47,48]

SLE is more common in females than males and has a four times greater incidence in African-American women.[48,49] African-American patients affected by SLE have an earlier onset of disease and a higher incidence of nephritis, pneumonitis, and discoid LE (DLE).[50] As such, this racial group has a higher mortality from SLE than other ethnic groups.[51,52] Similar findings were found in Hispanic groups, along with a greater occurrence of cardiac and renal complications than Caucasian individuals.[53,54]

Clinically, SLE is diagnosed based on the American Rheumatologic Association (ARA) criteria, which can be one of the following as a result of LE: DLE lesion, malar erythema (Figure 7.8), serositis, nonerosive arthritis, photosensitivity, nephropathy, CNS disorder, hematologic disorder, oral ulcers, positive ANA, or an immunologic disorder.[42] Systemic manifestations of SLE include arthralgias and thrombosis and involve the renal, cardiac, pulmonary, and CNS systems.[11] This systemic involvement is more common in African-Americans.[11] Specifically, blacks have a higher incidence of discoid lesions as well as renal, pulmonary, and immunologic (decreased complement) involvement.[55] CLE classically appears as a butterfly malar rash but can also present as bullous, vascular, mucous membrane, or ulcerative lesions.[11] Microscopically, these lesions have upper dermal edema lymphohistiocytic and fibrinoid infiltrates as well as vasodilatation with RBC extravasation.[48]

There are many variants of CCLE, including DLE, hypertrophic DLE, and lupus panniculitis.[36] Patients with more generalized lesions have a tendency toward a more severe disease course than those with lesions above the neck.[35] DLE lesions are sharply demarcated erythematous or hyperkeratotic plaques or papules with adherent scale in the follicular orifices.[11,56,57] The underside of these lesions has a characteristic "carpet tack" sign.[11] Most lesions are commonly found on the face and scalp, but in blacks another common site for lesions is the conchal bowl of the ear.[11] The

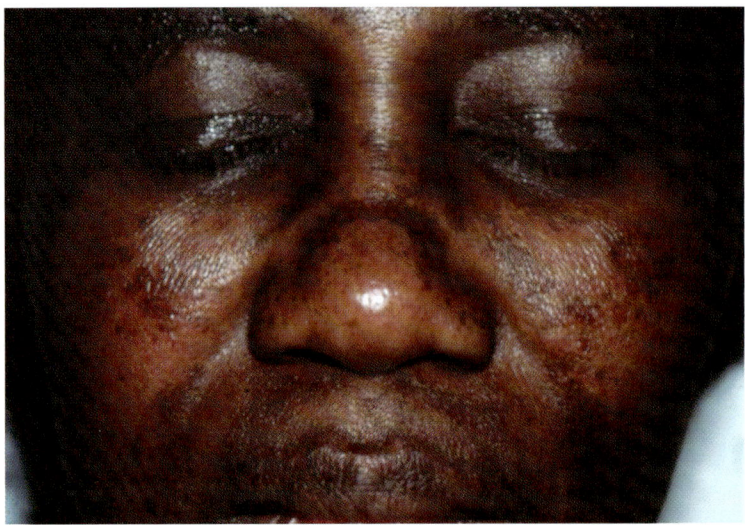

FIGURE 7.8 Hyperpigmented patches occurring in a malar distribution in a patient with cutaneous lupus erythematosus.

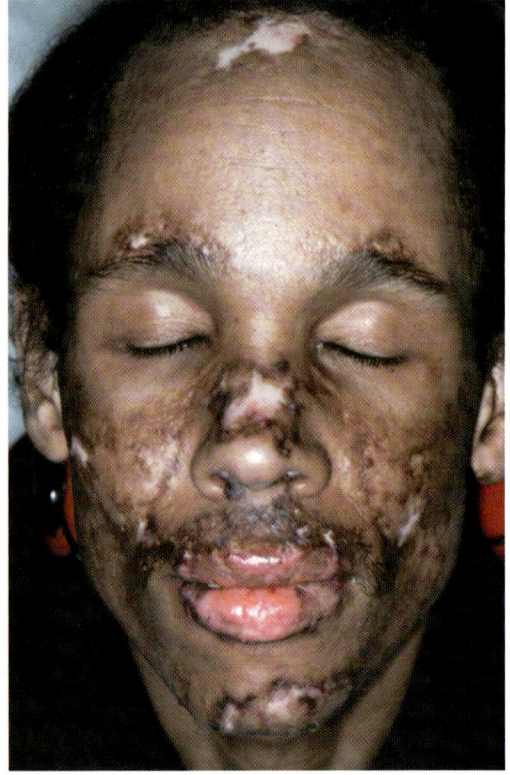

FIGURE 7.9 Disfiguring discoid lupus erythematosus with perilesional hyperpigmentation on the face of an African-American male.

lesions in DLE can be very disfiguring secondary to the large amount of inflammation that extends deep into the dermis (Figures 7.9 and 7.10).[57] In addition, DLE lesions tend to leave dyspigmentation with hypopigmented to depigmented central patches surrounded by hyperpigmented peripheries.[11,48]

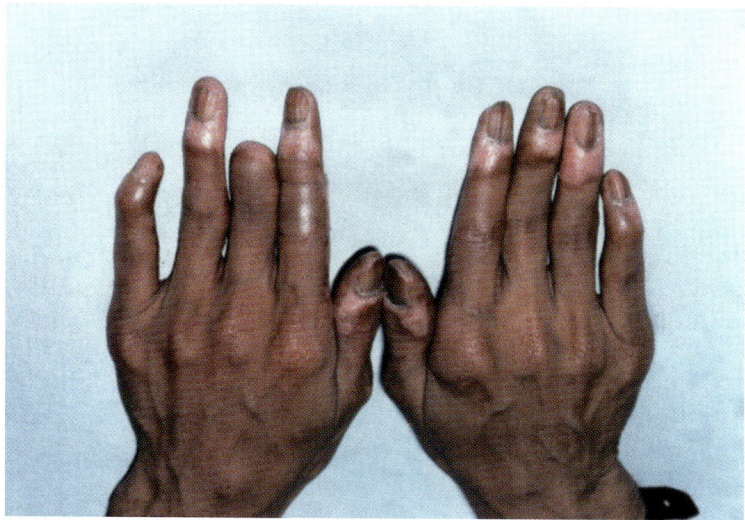

FIGURE 7.10 Discoid lupus erythematosus affecting the distal phalanges and causing digit destruction.

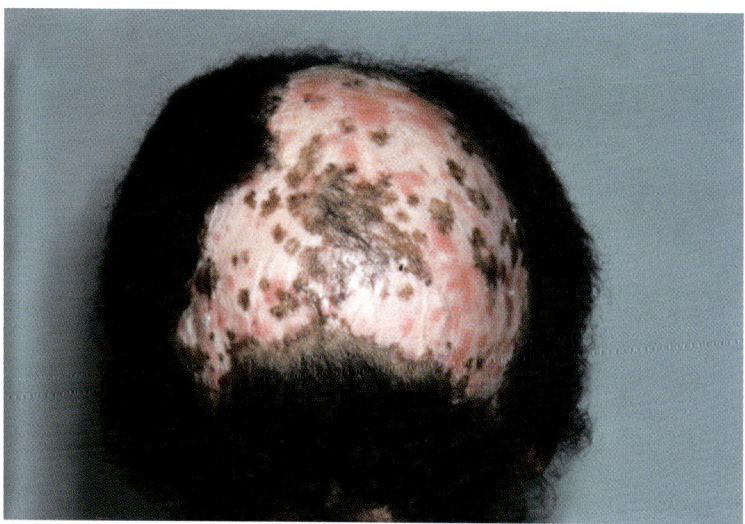

FIGURE 7.11 Scarring alopecia and hyperpigmentation in the same individual in Figure 7.9 from discoid lupus erythematosus.

The scalp lesions of DLE can cause scarring alopecia whereas the alopecia, associated with SLE is nonscarring (Figures 7.11 and 7.12).[48] Lupus panniculitis has an increased occurrence in association with DLE lesions.[58] Lupus panniculitis consists of severe inflammation in the deep dermis and subcutaneous fat that causes disfiguring indurated plaque or nodular lesions associated with severe pain, scarring, erythema, and ulceration.[48,58,59] Histological findings include paraseptal and lobular inflammation extending deep into the dermis.[60] One study found that Asians typically have a higher prevalence of disease and a younger age of disease onset when compared to Caucasian populations.[60]

SCLE is the most photosensitive subset of CLE.[48] Clinically these lesions occur in a photodistributed area and are nonscarring.[36] SCLE usually spares the midface and involves the arms and

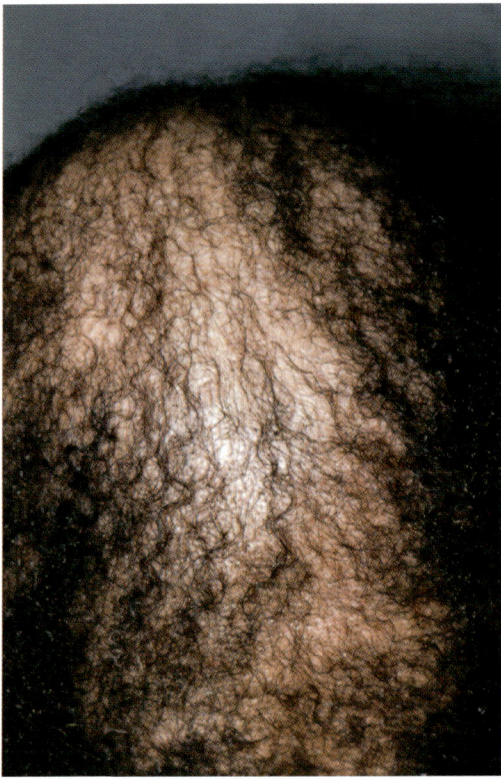

FIGURE 7.12 Nonscarring alopecia in an African-American female with systemic lupus erythematosus.

neck.[61] Lesions can appear psoriasiform, papulosquamous, eczematous, or annular and can be isolated or involve systemic disease.[36]

SCLE has a high progression rate to SLE and is associated with anti-Ro antibody.[36,62] ACLE has a 100% chance of progression to SLE, especially lupus nephritis. In addition, ACLE is associated with anti-DS-DNA and usually has an abrupt presentation in correlation with a systemic illness.[63,64] Localized lesions typically show a butterfly malar rash, and more generalized lesions consist of a generalized lupus dermatitis.[36] Patients may also have a thinning hair line, nail fold telangiectasias, and cuticle abnormalities.

The goal of treatment is not only to prevent disease evolution but also to improve appearance. Treatment for CLE consists of a two-pronged approach. Patient education about daily sunscreen use, sun avoidance, and protective clothing is extremely important.[11,36,48] In addition, there are several medications that are currently being used. Topical and intralesional steroids are the mainstay of treatment for cutaneous disease.[11] DLE lesions may require a high-potency steroid, even if located on the face.[48] Severe cases may require systemic steroids, antimalarials, or immunosuppressive drugs.[11] Antimalarials such as hydrochloroquine can be used, but it is imperative that patients have ophthalmologic exams every 6 months because of the risk of retinopathy with the use of this class of drugs.[65] Other side effects from antimalarial drugs include blue-gray hyperpigmentation, bleaching of hair, gastrointestinal upset, myopathy, cardiomyopathy, and lowering of the seizure threshold.[65–67] Patients should be advised about smoking cessation because smoking has been shown to decrease antimalarial drug efficacy.[68] Other medications used with some success in refractory CLE include azathioprine (especially for SCLE and acral DLE),[69,70] methotrexate,[71–74] cyclophosphamide,[36] cytarabine,[75] cyclosporine,[76] mycophenolate mofetil (MMF),[77] and dapsone (especially for DLE, and bullous or vascular CLE).[69,78] Clofazimine[79] and retinoids[65,67,80,81] have been useful in DLE lesions as well. Thalidomide has also been used with some success in refractory

CLE cases, but patients should be monitored for peripheral neuropathy.[82,83] There are currently no surgical options because new lesions may occur at the manipulation site.[69] However, pulse dye laser has been used in CLE vascular lesions and SCLE lesions with some success.[84] The risks of this treatment, however, include the development of CLE itself, pigmentary changes, or hyperpigmentation.[36]

DERMATOMYOSITIS

Dermatomyositis (DM) is an autoimmune disease that primarily affects the skin and skeletal muscle, causing severe limb girdle weakness.[85] DM is twice as common in women and blacks as in men and whites.[86] However, in nonwhite ethnic groups, DM is more common in men.[87] The disease has a bimodal age distribution and is manifest typically by a symmetrical proximal extensor inflammatory myopathy.[88] There are several theories regarding the etiology of this disorder. One theory is that it may be caused by a polymorphism of the gene-encoding tumor necrosis factor (TNF)-alpha 308 A.[85] Presence of this polymorphism is linked to increased disease chronicity, calcinosis, and increased TNF-alpha levels.[89] Another possible etiology for DM may be drug-induced disease, with offending agents including atorvastatin, pravastatin, simvastatin,[90,91] alfuzosin,[92] noinsteroidal anti-inflammatory drugs (NSAIDs), D-penicillamine,[87] and phenytoin.[93] Viral etiologies of DM may include both parvovirus B19 and Epstein–Barr virus (EBV).[94]

There are several autoantibodies that may be found in DM patients. Approximately 40%–60% of patients with dermatomyositis have a positive antinuclear antibody.[87] Myositis-specific antibodies include MI-2, SRP, PM/Scl, and Ro/SS-A, as well as the antisynthetase antibody group consisting of anti Jo-1, PL-7, PL-12, and OJ.[95] Ro-S2, RO-60, and U1RNA autoantibodies are also associated with DM.[95] Because fewer than 20% of patients will be positive for these antibodies, routine testing is not recommended.[95] Other novel autoantibodies associated with DM include MJ[95] and PMS1.[96] Additional serum markers of DM disease activity and inflammation include VWF Ag, CD19+ B cells, VCAM-1, and E-selectin.[87] Both VCAM and E-selectin are released from inflamed muscular and cutaneous tissue.[97] Patients who have antisynthetase antibodies may also develop the antisynthetase syndrome consisting of arthritis, Raynaud's phenomenon, and interstitial lung disease.[89] This syndrome is linked with a more severe and chronic course in juvenile DM.[89]

DM may be classified into two basic types: amyopathic DM and classic DM. Amyopathic DM has the associated skin findings of DM but patients lack any muscle findings or elevation in muscle enzymes for 6 months or longer.[87] Amyopathic DM is found more commonly in Asians.[87] In classic DM, patients have both the characteristic DM skin findings and evidence of muscle inflammation.[87] Major criteria for diagnosing DM have been proposed and three characteristic skin findings include the heliotrope rash, Gottron's papules, and Gottron's sign. The heliotrope rash consists of a periorbital, scaly, macular erythema, often violaceous in color.[98] Gottron's papules are violaceous papules or plaques on the dorsum of the interphalangeal and metacarpophalangeal joints.[87] Gottron's sign includes similar skin changes on the knuckles, elbows, medial malleoli, or knees.[87] Violaceous patches involving the lateral thighs and hips are known as Holster's sign.[87] Any of the above mentioned lesions can have scale, hyperkeratosis, pigment changes, and telangiectasias.[87] Clinical signs of DM feature the characteristic poikiloderma that may consist of hyperpigmentation, telangiectasias, epidermal atrophy, follicular hyperkeratosis, ulcerations, and subepidermal bullous changes on the extensor surfaces and/or the periorbital areas.[86,87] Patients may also develop mucinous papules or plaques on the palmar creases.[99,100] Pityriasis rubra pilaris appearing as a perifollicular keratosis, usually on the upper extremities and gingival telangiectasias (in juvenile DM patients), may occur as well.[101–103] Histologically, epidermal basement degeneration, vacuolization of the basal layer, and lymphocyte and mucin infiltration of the dermis are present.[86]

Internally, patients may develop a symmetric myopathy involving the proximal muscles (biceps and triceps), and they may also acquire a nonerosive arthritis.[86] Patients often develop fibromyalgia during the course of their disease,[87,104] and magnetic resonance imaging may show functional metabolic changes in the involved muscle groups.[87] Calcinosis, which is usually caused by a vasculitis/vasculopathy associated with DM, occurs in 25% of juvenile DM cases.[86,87] Patients with juvenile DM have a 40%–50% lifetime risk of developing calcinosis.[86] Approximately 15%–30% of patients with DM develop pulmonary disease that is usually manifest as a diffuse interstitial fibrosis.[86] Pulmonary disease has been found to occur more often in Japanese patients with DM.[87] DM may also cause cardiac conduction and rhythm abnormalities.[105] In 25% of adult DM cases, there may be an association with underlying malignancy.[86] The cutaneous manifestations of DM usually precede the malignancy findings.[86,87] Increased age, creatinine kinase, and severity of skin disease are associated with an increased risk for malignancy.[106] It has been noted that systemic manifestations of DM have a negative correlation with malignancy.[106] Some studies have found an increased incidence of nasopharyngeal cancer in Asian patients.[86,107,108] Although they are not specific or sensitive, sequential tumor marker levels such as CEA, CA-125, CA-15, MUC1, and TPS can be used to monitor for the development of malignancy.[87,109]

Topical steroids and sunscreens are the mainstay of treatment for DM skin lesions.[86] Systemic corticosteroids with a taper of several months to years are used in severe disease.[86] Other medications that have been used as an adjunct and in refractory disease include antimalarials (such as aminoquinolone),[86] etanercept,[110,111] cyclosporine, chlorambucil, cyclophosphamide,[86] dapsone,[112] intravenous immunoglobulin,[113] methotrexate,[114] cyclosporine,[115] fludarabine,[116] and MMF.[98] Diltiazem and aluminum hydroxide have been used in treating calcinosis with limited success.[117–119]

DM is an autoimmune disease that has a more severe course in African-Americans. In addition, Asians affected by the disease are at increased risk for nasopharyngeal cancer. Physicians should be aware of these consequences so that they can initiate early and aggressive treatment.

HEMATOLOGIC DISEASE

HERMANSKY–PUDLAK SYNDROME (SEE ALSO CHAPTERS 5 AND 18)

A specific entity termed Hermansky–Pudlak syndrome explicitly affects the Puerto Rican population. This disease affects 1 in 1800 people in Northwest Puerto Rico, and it is the most frequent genetic illness in the territory.[120] Individuals affected by this disease are found to be homozygous for a 16-base-pair repetition on exon 15 of the HPS1 gene.[121] This gene has been isolated to chromosome 10q23.[121]

The clinical syndrome consists of oculocutaneous albinism that can lead to blindness, platelet dysfunction, and progressive systemic disease.[120] Patients have blue to brown eye color and can develop photophobia and strabismus.[120] Cutaneously, patients have a creamy white, lightly pigmented skin and freckling.[120] Because of their decreased pigmentation, patients have an increased likelihood of developing solar damage as well as squamous cell and basal cell carcinomas.[121]

Patients can also present with acanthosis nigricans in the neck and axilla.[121] Other systemic complications include pulmonary fibrosis, inflammatory bowel disease, and renal disease. Because of their low platelet count and tendency to bleed, up to 13% of individuals die from bleeding events.[121] There is no specific treatment for this syndrome. Dermatologically, patients should have regular skin exams to evaluate for skin cancers.

ENDOCRINE DISEASE — DIABETES MELLITUS

Diabetes has a high prevalence in several ethnic groups. South Asian Indians have approximately a four times greater incidence of diabetes mellitus than Caucasian populations of European descent.[122] In addition, African-American, Native American, and Hispanic ethnic groups have about a two times greater incidence of diabetes mellitus compared to non-Hispanic white ethnic groups.[123,124] According to the latest estimates, by the year 2025, approximately half of diabetic patients worldwide will be of Asian or Pacific Island origin.[125] It is important to note these racial groups with a high incidence of diabetes because about 30% of diabetic patients will develop cutaneous manifestations of their disease at some point in their lifetime.[126]

WAXY SKIN

Waxy skin is a disease entity seen in approximately 2% of diabetic patients.[127] Most diabetics usually have an increase in skin thickness and elasticity and decreased skin extensibility,[127,128] and there are several theories as to the cause of this. One primary theory states that there is an abnormal increase in collagen metabolism or synthesis[129] caused by insulin-like growth factor.[130] Other theories include hypoxia secondary to angiopathy resulting in greater fibroblast synthesis[130,131] and abnormal nonenzymatic glycosylation of collagen.[132] The increased glycosylation causes the collagen fibers to be resistant to enzymatic removal.[128] Clinically, waxy skin appears as thick, shiny skin and in non-insulin-dependent diabetes mellitus (NIDDM) can be associated with the diabetic hand syndrome, consisting of decreased joint mobility, waxy skin, sclerodactyly, and stiffened joints.[128] Prevalence of this syndrome ranges from 8% to 50%.[133] Waxy skin can also appear as pebbled papules on the finger extensors or the periungual area.[134] Histology shows increased dermal and connective tissue thickness and decreased glands surrounding the hair follicles.[129] Tight glucose control has been shown to decrease skin thickness.[127] Other treatments include topical and intralesional steroids, intralesional insulin, PUVA, methotrexate, prostaglandin E1, and pentoxifylline.[131,135,136]

DERMOPATHY

Diabetic dermopathy (i.e., shin spots, pigmented pretibial papules) is the most common cutaneous sign of diabetes mellitus.[137–139] Although they are not pathognomonic for diabetes or related to blood glucose levels, these lesions can often precede the diagnosis of diabetes mellitus and have an greater prevalence with increased age and disease duration.[140,141] Diabetic dermopathy eventually develops in approximately 70% of diabetic patients.[35,128,142] The etiology of these lesions is unknown, but one study induced these lesions with thermal (both heat and cold) injury.[143–146] Another theory attributes diabetes-related vasculopathy as a possible cause for diabetic dermopathy. Clinically these lesions appear as bilateral, asymmetrical, erythematous, well-circumscribed papules or plaques on the extensor surface of the legs, forearms, and lateral malleoli.[128,147–149,150] These lesions eventually regress to hyperpigmented, brown, atrophic, scaly macules.[128] Histological examination of these lesions reveals a thin, atrophic epidermis with thickened vessels in the papillary dermis and a mild perivascular lymphohistiocytic infiltrate often containing hemosiderin accumulation.[128,151,152] There is no effective treatment for these skin lesions, and they usually remain clinically asymptomatic.[153,154] However, because diabetic dermopathy is often associated with internal complications of diabetes such as retinopathy, nephropathy, and neuropathy, both internal screening and aggressive blood glucose control are key to prevent further problems.[128,137]

ACANTHOSIS NIGRICANS

Acanthosis nigricans (AN) is a condition that is most commonly seen in diabetes and insulin resistance.[128,155,156] A direct association has been observed between the degree of AN and the amount of fasting plasma insulin concentration.[157] AN usually precedes the diagnosis of diabetes mellitus, and the cause of this condition seems to be related to insulin-like growth factor (ILGF) present on keratinocytes as well as dermal fibroblast proliferation.[158] AN is very common in obese patients, and several studies have found an increased incidence in African-American and Hispanic individuals up to two times greater than Caucasians.[148,157] Clinically, AN presents as velvety, verrucous plaques most severe on the neck but also involving flexural areas such as the axillae, areolae, submammary areas, hands, groin, and umbilicus (see Figure 7.13).[143,144,148,159] Histologically, AN shows papillomatosis, hyperkeratosis, and acanthosis in the epidermis.[159,160] The epidermis appears dark secondary to excessive keratin deposits.[159] AN presenting on the palms or soles has been specifically

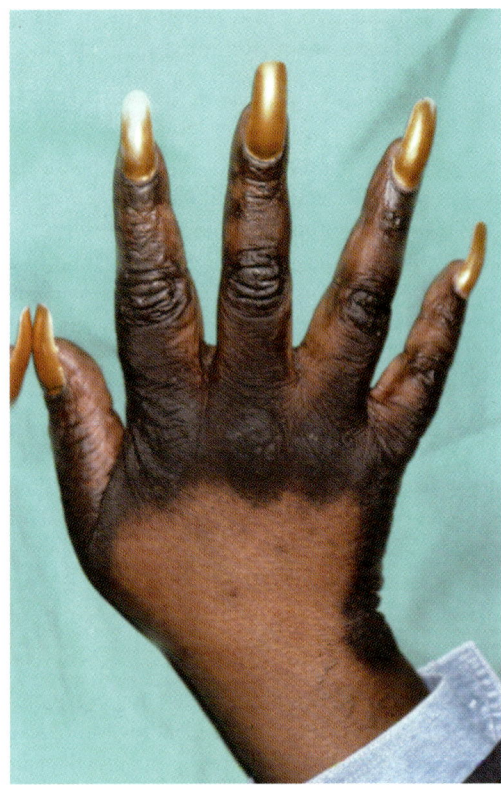

FIGURE 7.13 Acanthosis nigricans on the right hand of a patient. (Courtesy of Rebat M. Halder, M.D.)

associated with both gastrointestinal and genitourinary malignancies.[144] AN has also been associated with systemic conditions such as polycystic ovary disease and lipodystrophy as well as medication administration including nicotinic acid and corticosteroids.[138,149] Both retinoic acid and salicylic acid have had some success in cosmetic treatment of these lesions,[138] most likely secondary to their keratolytic properties. Other effective treatments include weight loss and dietary fish oil.[159,160] It is most important, however, to find the underlying cause of AN because of its possible association with malignancy.[143]

DIABETIC FOOT ULCERS

Approximately 70% of lower limb amputations in the United States may be attributed to diabetic foot ulcers (DFU) (Figure 7.14).[128] Etiologies include peripheral neuropathy in 60%–70% of cases and peripheral vascular disease in 15%–20% of patients.[128] Treatment of these lesions varies, depending on the severity of disease. If adequate blood supply is present, even in the face of impaired sensation, debrided DFUs can heal in a few weeks.[161] It is important as dermatologists to know that skin grafts or growth factors cannot solely be substituted for necessary treatments such as revascularization, debridement, or weight-bearing avoidance.[162,163] The main treatment for these lesions is to prevent their occurrence through appropriate foot care, inspection, and footwear to avoid pressure leading to callus formation.[164–166]

NECROBIOSIS LIPOIDICA DIABETICORUM

Necrobiosis lipoidica diabeticorum (NLD) affects approximately 0.3%–1.6% of diabetic patients, and it is three times more common in women.[167,168] Some study populations have estimated approximately 65% of their diabetic patients to be affected by NLD,[167–169] and type I diabetic

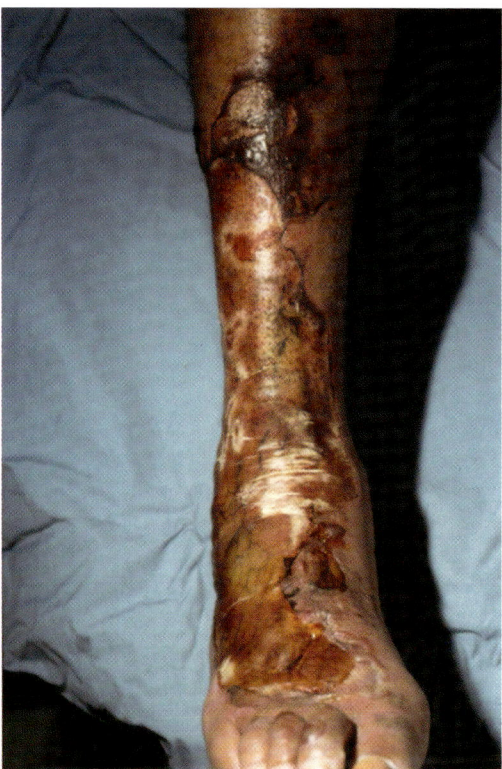

FIGURE 7.14 Diabetic ulcer causing epidermal loss and necrosis on the right lower extremity of a patient.

patients develop NLD almost two decades earlier than type II diabetic patients.[170] About 90% of patients with NLD eventually develop diabetes mellitus, have a baseline abnormal glucose tolerance, or have parents with diabetes mellitus.[156] Theories about the etiology of NLD include microangiopathy, decreased neutrophil margination, peripheral vascular disease, nonenzymatic glycosylation, delayed hypersensitivity, obliterative endarteritis, and anticollagen antibody immune mediated vasculitis.[168,170] NLD is clinically characterized by single or multiple, pretibial, yellowish brown, telangiectatic, atrophic plaques that are surrounded by raised violaceous borders.[128,168,170] These lesions have a tendency to ulcerate spontaneously or from trauma.[150] Patients tend to have a decreased sensation in the affected areas but can develop symptoms such as pruritus and dysesthesia.[168] Histology of these lesions shows diffuse granulomatous dermatitis with a loss of elastic tissue, a thickened basement membrane, and endothelial cell swelling.[128,168] There has been no proven efficacious treatment for NLD, and blood glucose levels do not affect skin disease outcome.[168] Both topical and intralesional steroids have been used at the lesional borders with some success.[168] In an effort to decrease platelet aggregation and thromboxane A2 production or increase fibrinolysis, several medications, including stanozol, inositol niacinate, nicofuarnose, ticlodipine, and pentoxifylline, have been used anecdotally.[168] Other subjective treatment reports include niacinamide,[171] topical retinoids,[172] cyclosporine,[173,174] granulocyte-monocyte colony stimulating factor (GM-CSF), bovine collagen,[175,] PUVA,[176,177] and MMF.[178]

DIABETIC BULLAE

About 0.5% of diabetic patients develop diabetic bullae (DB). DB consist of tense, sudden-appearing, painless, noninflamed bulla on the lower legs, dorsum of the feet, and occasionally on the forearms and hands.[128,144] Although the cause of DB is unknown, hypotheses include immunologic mechanisms; abnormalities in calcium, magnesium, or carbohydrate metabolism; or peripheral vascular disease.[138,179–183] Histological examination of nonhemorrhagic DB reveals an intraepidermal split without acantholysis,[184,185] and hemorrhagic lesions show a subepidermal split.[186] These lesions are not usually treated because they tend to resolve in approximately 1 month, though they may recur.[187]

HEPATIC DISEASE

LICHEN PLANUS

Lichen planus (LP) is a chronic inflammatory disease of the skin and mucous membranes that primarily affects females in the age range 30–60 years.[188,189] LP can often affect the gingival and buccal mucosa in 75% of LP cases, and this variant in particular is associated with liver disease and diabetes as well as the development of oral cancer.[188] There is a 2–13.5 greater incidence of hepatitis C in patients with LP when compared with controls.[190] The strongest association of LP with hepatitis C has been found in Japanese and Mediterranean races.[189] Thirty percent of patients with LP have variant subsets of LP including LP pigmentosus (LPP).[191] LPP clinically appears as pigmented macules, and a possible cause for this variant has been attributed to paraphenylenediamine.[191] LPP was once thought to predominantly affect individuals from the Indian subcontinent; however, this has not been proven to date.[192] Clinically, LP presents as pruritic, polygonal, flat-topped, violaceous papules with fine white lines in areas of trauma on the flexor surfaces of the extremities as well as on the penis.[189–193] Histology of LP lesions shows an acanthotic, hyperkeratotic, sawtooth epidermis and hypergranulosis with a lymphocytic infiltrate in the dermis.[189]

There are several types of LP. Oral LP shows a reticular, lacy pattern of white raised lines known as Wickham's striae usually on the tongue and gingival and labial mucosa.[194] Oral LP is closely linked with hepatitis C virus.[190,195,196] Actinic LP (i.e., LP subtropicus, LP tropicus) has been noted around the world; however, a large number of cases have been reported from the Mediterranean region.[189] Actinic LP presents as ruddy, brown, hyperpigmented plaques involving the forehead, face, dorsal side of the arms, hands, and neck. Acute LP (i.e., eruptive LP, exanthematous LP) is a widely disseminated, sudden-onset variant that affects the trunk, dorsal side of the feet, and the anterior wrists.[189] This resolves spontaneously in 3–6 months but can leave residual hyperpigmentation.[189] Annular LP presents with papular lesions that have central sparing and spread peripherally.[189] Large plaques with central depression and atrophy as well as hyperpigmentation are characteristic of atrophic LP, whereas ulcerative LP presents as painful ulcers on the palms and soles.[189] These ulcerations pose a risk for developing into squamous cell carcinoma, as do the lesions of hypertrophic LP.[189] Hypertrophic LP (i.e., LP verrucosus) displays thick, hyperkeratotic plaques typically on the dorsal foot, and these lesions can last for many years.[189] Lichen planopilaris consists of keratotic plugs surrounded by a violaceous rim on the scalp and other hair-bearing areas and can cause a scarring alopecia. Nail LP has classic findings of lateral nail thinning, longitudinal ridging, and fissuring.[189] Other variants of LP include the bullous, pemphigoides, and linear types.

With respect to hepatitis C and LP, some theories state that the hepatitis C virus replicates inside lymphocytes and then presents on the skin.[156] The association with hepatitis C and LP is more common in the mucosal and generalized LP variants.[192] Moreover, this connection between oral LP and hepatitis C virus has been linked to HLA DR6.[189,195] In Chinese and Japanese individuals, oral LP has been associated with HLA DR9.[189] Contact allergens from gold, mercury, copper, and other metals may also be involved in the etiology of LP.[189]

Patients with oral and cutaneous LP can have spontaneous remission of their disease. Hepatitis C and associated oral LP treated with interferon (IFN) have shown equivocal results.[197–199] Treatment of LP consists of topical or intralesional steroids, systemic corticosteroids, retinoids, and PUVA.[189] Resistant cases have successfully been treated with cyclosporine and griseofulvin.[193,200,201]

PRURITUS IN HEPATIC DISEASE

In order of decreasing incidence, Southeast Asian and Pacific, African, and Mediterranean populations have the highest rates of hepatitis C and associated liver disease. Because of the high incidence of hepatic disease in Asian populations,[202] it is important to know about the pathophysiology and management of hepatitis-related symptoms such as pruritus when treating these patients. Any type of hepatic disease and associated complications can present with pruritus, and this symptom can affect up to 25% of patients with jaundice.[203,204] Many diseases that cause cholestasis, including primary biliary cirrhosis (PBC), primary sclerosing cholangitis (PSC), obstructive choledocholithiasis, hepatitis C, and malignancy, may be associated with pruritus.[205–208] Drug-induced cholestasis can be caused by drugs such as the phenothiazines, estrogens, and tolbutamide.[206,209] Although the etiology of pruritus in liver dysfunction is unknown, there are several theories regarding its pathogenesis. Because of the liver's inability to clear toxins or because of increased toxin production, endogenous opioid or other toxin buildup may cause pruritus.[203,207,210–212] A long-standing theory attributes bile acid buildup as a possible cause of hepatic pruritus.[213] Although this theory has yet to be proven, bile salts may indirectly increase pruritus by amplifying the amount of pruritic metabolites in the body.[213–215] Pruritus of hepatic origin often involves the palms and soles, and because of persistent scratching individuals may develop prurigo nodularis.[156]

Liver transplant results in complete and immediate resolution of pruritus.[213,216] Other symptomatic treatments that can provide mild relief include topical emollients with menthol or camphor, anesthetics, steroids, and oral antihistamines.[205,217–219] General treatment of pruritus includes avoiding heat and keeping the skin cool.[204] Cholestyramine has been shown to decrease pruritus and is thought to decrease pruritogenic factors by binding to bile acid resins in the gastrointestinal tract.[205,220] Through a similar mechanism, opioid antagonists such as naloxone and naltrexone are also effective by decreasing the amount of endogenous opioids in the body.[221–223] Codeine offers similar results without the withdrawal side effects[224] and ondansetron also works by modulating serotonin.[225–227] Doxepin is an antidepressant that helps alleviate pruritus through its antihistamine properties.[228–229] UVB light treatment twice weekly has been found to be very useful in the treatment of pruritus.[230,231] Extracorporeal plasmapheresis provides transient relief of pruritus through plasma perfusion with charcoal beads.[232] Medications such as rifampin and phenobarbital are also thought be effective through their induction of the hepatic microsomal enzyme system that theoretically reduces the amount of toxic metabolites in the body.[233–236]

CRYOGLOBULINEMIA AND HEPATITIS C

Although hepatitis C can cause a leukocytoclastic vasculitis or polyarteritis nodosa, cryoglobulinemia is one of the primary cutaneous manifestations of hepatitis C infection.[22] The disease is thought to manifest secondary to viral antigen deposition and immune complexes such as rheumatoid factor or complement, in the skin that precipitate at cold temperatures.[237–239] Type II cryoglobulinemia is caused by polyclonal IgG and monoclonal IgM, and type III cryoglobulinemia is caused by polyclonal IgM and IgG deposition.[239] Cryoglobulinemia can present on the skin with palpable purpura, livedo reticularis, urticarial plaques, cold-induced urticaria, and Raynaud's phenomenon.[240] Systemically the disease can present with signs of arthralgias and fatigue.[240] When a patient presents with cryoglobulinemia, the initial laboratory work should consist of an enzyme-linked immunosorbent assay antibody test for hepatitis C virus. If this is positive, a follow-up hepatitis C polymerase chain reaction should be ordered, as this is a more specific test than the prior.[237,238] Patients who are positive for both tests should be referred to a hepatologist for possible IFN and ribavarin treatment.[156,212,237,241] Treatment of cryoglobulinemia includes addressing the underlying disease as well as administering systemic corticosteroids and immunosuppressants.[242]

RENAL DISEASE

GENERAL

Almost all patients with chronic renal failure (CRF) will develop associated skin changes.[243] The most common cutaneous finding in CRF patients is pruritus and xerosis secondary to decreased sebum production.[240,243] The cutaneous manifestations of renal disease are extremely important in ethnic populations because end-stage renal disease (ESRD) is more common in African-American individuals.[243] Moreover, African-American patients with renal disease more often develop ESRD. It is interesting to also note that both African-American and Hispanic individuals experience the side effects of renal disease/renal transplant medications more frequently than other ethnic groups.[243] For example, a study of 30 children with ESRD found that African-American and Hispanic patients on cyclosporine develop both hypertrichosis and gingival hypertrophy more often than other ethnic groups.[243] This study also found that secondary to darker pigmentation, these individuals had a greater tendency toward cosmetically disfiguring skin changes.[243]

CRF patients also have a tendency to develop anemia of chronic disease and bleeding tendencies due to platelet dysfunction.[240] Individuals with ESRD may also develop a yellowish hue because of the increased urochromes and carotene deposition in the skin.[240] Metabolic abnormalities in calcium and phosphate metabolism secondary to parathyroid dysfunction may cause calcinosis cutis, which presents as nodules or plaques on the joints and fingers.[240] These nodules clear when the metabolic disturbance resolves.[240] A more serious complication of parathyroid dysfunction is calciphylaxis. Calciphylaxis is associated with high mortality and consists of painful, symmetric, purpuric plaques that may be located on the abdomen, hands, fingers, and buttocks.[240] Again, treatment involves medically and, in emergencies, surgically, treating the parathyroid dysfunction.[240]

KYRLE'S DISEASE

Kyrle's disease is a hereditary genodermatosis caused by a problem in protein glycosylation that results in defective dermal–epidermal differentiation.[244,245] Although Kyrle's disease is usually associated with renal failure, it can also be linked to hepatic disease and type II diabetes.[244,246] The disease seems to be more prevalent in African-American individuals, and one study noted that all the patients with Kyrle's disease and renal failure were African-American.[247] The onset of disease is usually between 30 and 50 years, and the etiology involves an inciting event disrupting epidermal cell replication, thereby causing keratin plug production.[143] Clinically, the disorder presents as 1–4-mm hyperkeratotic, plugged, follicular papules on the tibial and extensor areas of the lower extremities.[145,244–246] Histological examination of these lesions reveals a lymphohistiocytic infiltration of the dermis with an atrophic epidermis filled with keratin plugs.[145,244] A variant of Kyrle's disease, called acquired perforating disorder (APD), has a similar pathogenesis involving keratin plug formation.[240] APD affects 10% of ESRD patients on hemodialysis (HD)[240] and is more common in African-American individuals as well as ESRD patients with type 2 diabetes (Figure 7.15).[240] Treatment of both of these disease entities is not particularly effective.[240] Topical and intralesional steroids have had mild success, and UVB light treatment may help decrease the pruritus associated with these lesions.[248]

PRURITUS IN RENAL DISEASE

Because of the high incidence of ESRD in the above-mentioned ethnic populations, physicians should know how to treat the pruritus that often accompanies ESRD. Pruritus, both generalized and local, can be related to systemic disease,[208,213,263] and pruritus secondary to renal disease can affect up to 90% of patients on HD.[248–250] Patients on HD are affected more often and more severely than individuals using peritoneal dialysis (PD). Several theories exist about the etiology of renal pruritus. These include the accumulation of nondialyzable substances, malfunction of the parathyroid

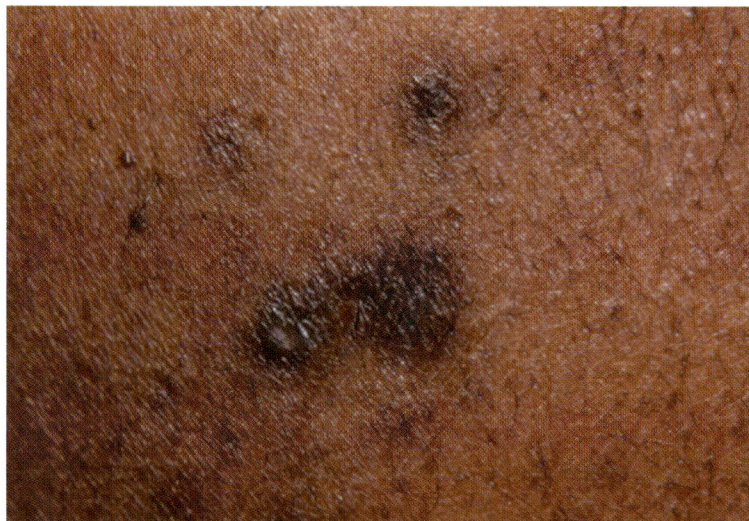

FIGURE 7.15 Hyperkeratotic, hyperpigmented papules characteristic of Kyrle's disease. (Courtesy of Rebat M. Halder, M.D.)

gland, neuropathy, opioid accumulation, xerosis, mast cell proliferation, increased vitamin production, and impaired hidrosis mechanisms.[208,251–259] Some theories are not well supported because for example, lack of therapeutic efficacy of antihistamines somewhat disproves the mast cell proliferation theory. The pruritus in renal disease can be constant or intermittent, but pruritus secondary to renal disease is often more severe than pruritus from other causes.[260] The height of symptoms have been noted when individuals have missed two dialysis sessions and are lowest one day after HD.[261,262] Pruritus in both hepatic and renal disease is worsened by heat, sweat, and xerosis.[248] Xerosis is one of the prominent skin findings in patients with renal failure, and on clinical examination, excoriations in various stages are often present.[240]

Treatment of renal pruritus has some overlap with treatment of hepatic pruritus. Again, topical emollients such as those mentioned prior offer little if any relief to patients.[240,250,263] Anesthetic agents may cause a mild decrease in pain and pruritus of any cause.[264] Capsaicin is another topical agent that has been helpful in alleviating pruritic symptoms by modulating substance P levels.[265–267] Both azelastin, an antiallergy medication and ondansetron, a 5HT-3 blocker, effectively treat pruritus through histamine and serotonin modulation.[268] Similar to the treatment of hepatic pruritus, UVB exposure as well as UVA and combination light exposure has been shown to cause a significant improvement in pruritic symptoms up to 90% in some studies.[240,269] These are administered 2–5 times per week or until a minimal erythema dose is achieved.[204] Oral activated charcoal (up to 5 months after treatment), and thalidomide have also been shown to be useful in pruritus treatment.[204,208,254,270] Epogen administration has also had some efficacy in relieving renal pruritus,[269] but studies with naltrexone and renal pruritus have produced equivocal results.[252,272] Altering dialysate concentrations of divalent ions such as calcium and magnesium has also been shown to improve pruritus symptoms.[257,273] A successful nontraditional treatment modality is transelectrical nerve stimulation by centrally inhibiting pruritus.[274–276]

SYSTEMIC MEDICATION REACTIONS

Almost any systemic medication can induce a skin eruption. However, there are several common offenders in a typical drug eruption which include drugs containing the sulfa moiety, quinolone, and penicillin classes of antibiotics (see Figures 7.16–7.19).[277] There are several proposed mechanisms for these reactions, including IgE antibody formation, keratinocyte apoptosis, and reactive

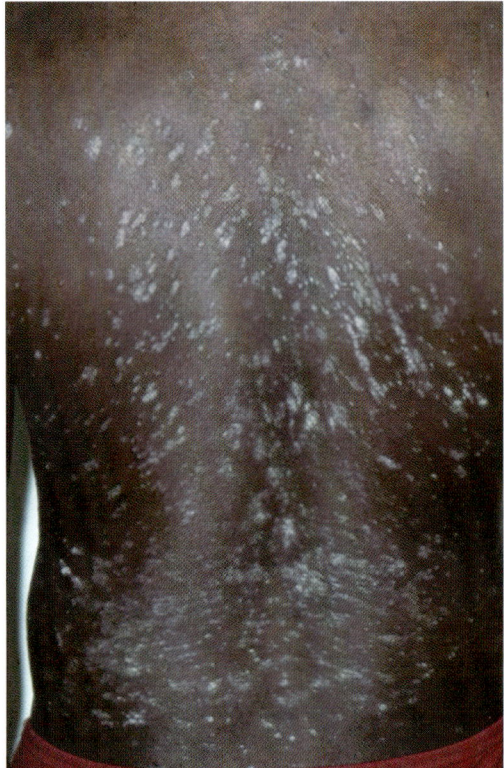

FIGURE 7.16 Cutaneous drug eruption on the back secondary to plaquenil.

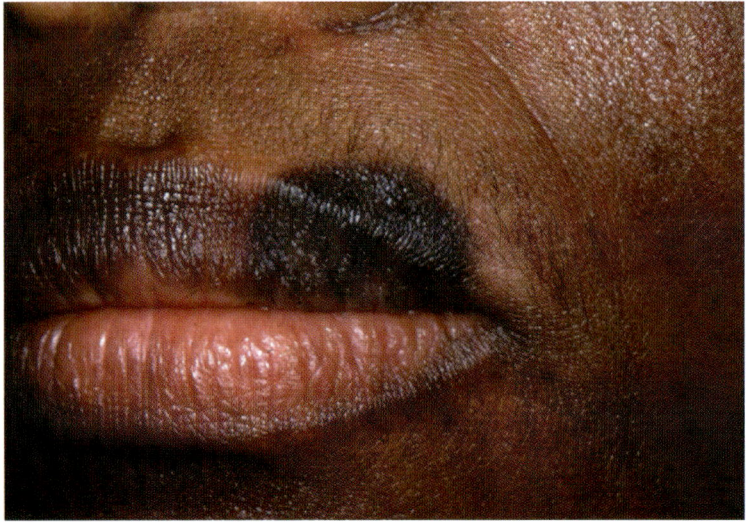

FIGURE 7.17 Fixed drug eruption secondary to minocycline on the upper lip.

intermediates from the liver causing a rash and fever.[277] The mainstay of treatment for these reactions is avoiding the offending agent; however, if an antibiotic is necessary for life-saving measures, then a patient can usually be desensitized to the agent.[277]

Cutaneous Manifestations of Systemic Disease in Pigmented Skins

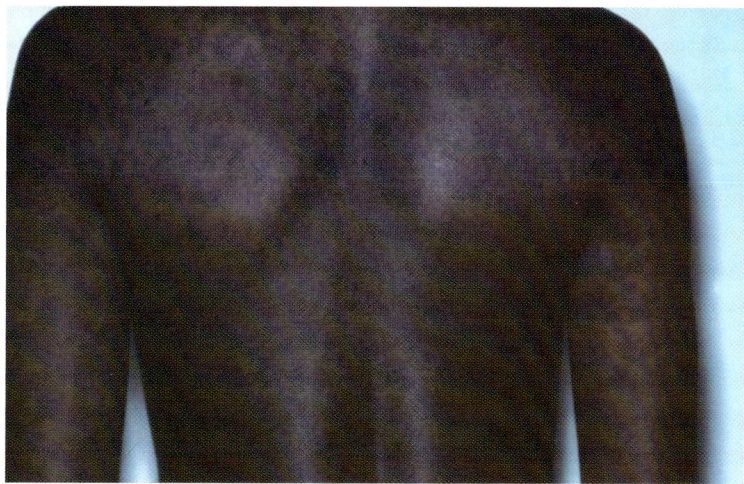

FIGURE 7.18 Morbiliform eruption secondary to cephalosporin antibiotics on the back of an African-American female. (Courtesy of Rebat M. Halder, M.D.)

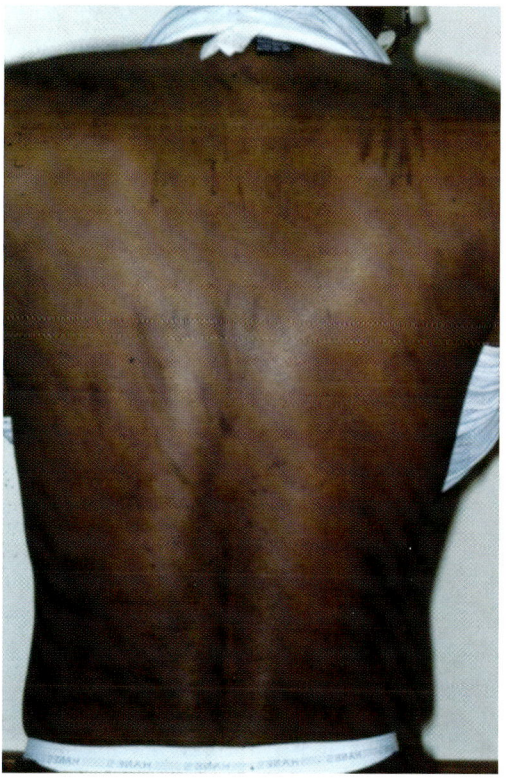

FIGURE 7.19 Flagellate hyperpigmentation on the back of a patient secondary to bleomycin use. (Courtesy of Rebat M. Halder, M.D.)

Some drugs can cause a drug eruption and systemic symptoms resembling systemic lupus erythematosus (SLE). Several of these medications are cardiovascular agents, including the beta-blocker antihypertensives, the arterial vasodilator hydralazine, and alpha-2 agonists as well as drugs that induce the hepatic CYP 450 system such as phenytoin and isoniazid.[278–281] The cardiovascular medications mentioned are particularly important in African-Americans and South Asian Indians because of the high incidence of hypertension and associated coronary artery disease (CAD) that occur in these populations. African-Americans have a 50% greater mortality rate from CAD compared to all other ethnic groups in the United States.[282] South Asian Indians have a 40% greater incidence of CAD when compared with white populations of European descent.[283] African-Americans have the highest incidence of hypertension worldwide that tends to occur earlier in life when compared to other populations.[282] Because this ethnic group also has high prevalence of stage 3 hypertension, African-Americans often require many medications to control their hypertension.[282] Several of these medications can cause cutaneous eruptions.

Atenolol is a beta-receptor-blocking antihypertensive used in the treatment of acute myocardial infarction and angina.[284] This drug can cause a psoriasiform eruption, skin necrosis, or vasculitis. There have also been reports of SLE and its cutaneous findings with a positive antinuclear antibody occurring in a patient several months after initiation of atenolol therapy.[284]

Hydralazine has been a well-known cause of drug-induced SLE in which patients may have both antinuclear and antihistone antibodies.[285] Hydralazine-induced skin eruptions may also present as an eczematous or urticarial picture and may sometimes be associated with Sweet's syndrome.[285,286] This drug, along with phenytoin and isoniazid, shows a homogeneous ANA pattern on skin biopsy.

Yohimbine, originally from the yohimbine tree found in West Africa, is an alkaloid alpha-2 agonist used as an aphrodisiac.[287] There has been a report of an allergic dermatitis in an African-American male occurring 3 days after initiation of this drug.[287] During this same time period, the patient also developed renal failure, Raynaud's phenomenon, eosinophilia, and a positive antinuclear (ANA) antibody.[287] All of these symptoms improved upon cessation of yohimbine.[287] Methyldopa, another central-acting alpha agonist, has also been reported to cause an SLE picture that can be accompanied by an eczematous or lichenoid eruption on the hands and feet.[286]

Other cardiovascular drugs can induce photosensitivity. These include (but are not limited to) the thiazide diuretics and the antiarrhythmic amiodarone.[279,291,292] This photosensitivity can last for several years after the medication has been stopped.[284] Thiazides have also been associated with eczema and erythema multiforme, and patients can sometimes have detectable anti-SSA and anti-Ro antibodies. Amiodarone is an antiarrhythmic used for SVT and other arrhythmias. Up to 75% of patients on this drug develop a dose-dependent photosensitivity within 4 months of being on the drug.[289] Once the drug is stopped, it can take up to a year for the photosensitivity to resolve.[289] In a study of 103 patients on amiodarone at a minimal cumulative dose of about 40 g, individuals were found to have photosensitivity appearing within 30 min to 2 h of sun exposure that usually faded in approximately 1–2 days. This study also noted a decrease in the minimal erythema dose as well as the development of a characteristic slate-gray hyperpigmentation. Some theories regarding the etiology of this hyperpigmentation include drug-induced melanin accumulation, buildup of the drug itself, drug-induced pigment synthesis, or iron deposit from drug-induced endothelial destruction.[290] Another hypothesis is that amiodarone binds to phospholipids in the cell that prevent lysosomal destruction of the drug and, therefore, cause the medication to accumulate.[291–293] These pigment deposits can occur in the cornea as well. It is interesting to note that, histologically, the perivascular dermal inflammation of lymphocytes and histiocytes is present in both normal and pigmented (secondary to medication) skin.[291] However, the amount of pigment in each cell has been noted to be greater in hyperpigmented skin. Astute judgment is imperative in obtaining a medication history from a patient with naturally deeply pigmented skin because the gray-blue hue may not be easy to detect.

Allopurinol is a xanthine oxidase inhibitor used in the treatment of gout. It is of greater interest in African-American males because they are twice as likely to have gout than Caucasian males[295] in a toxic epidermal necrolysis (TEN) picture. The hypersensitivity syndrome caused by allopurinol, as well as sulfa and anticonvulsant medications, is characterized by fever, lymphadenopathy, nephritis, eosinophilia, and mucous membrane involvement and can have up to an 8% mortality.[295]

One study noted that this allergic hypersensitivity is more common in men with renal failure,[294] most likely secondary to decreased excretion of the drug. This is of particular interest in African-Americans because ESRD is more common in these individuals than in Caucasian populations (see section on hepatic disease in this chapter). Allopurinol, as well as antimalarials, sulfa, oxicams, pyrazolone, anticonvulsants, and NSAIDs, may also cause life-threatening drug reactions such as Stevens–Johnson (S-J) syndrome and TEN.[297] S-J syndrome consists of erythematous macules and epidermal necrosis, and many consider this condition to be a more limited form of TEN. Some have used body surface area as a means to differentiate S-J syndrome and TEN.[297] This method defines S-J syndrome as involving less than 10% of the epidermis, TEN as involving greater than or equal to 30% of the epidermis, and anything in between as an S-J syndrome/TEN overlap. TEN is characterized by necrosis of the entire epidermis and inflammation of the dermis. Clinically, these lesions classically occur on the face, neck, and trunk and often heal over 3–6 weeks with scars that, when involving the face, can cause blindness.[297,298] These patients typically require an intensive care unit and are treated similarly to burn patients secondary to their large amount of water loss.[297]

Treatment modalities for drug-induced skin eruptions remain essentially the same for all races. These include withdrawal of the offending agent, topical and systemic (for severe disease) steroids,[284,288] supportive care, and treatment of any systemic involvement.

Where treatment varies is in the management of postinflammatory changes that are usually more profound in the pigmented races. Sunlight avoidance is key with respect to the photosensitizing agents, and there has also been some anecdotal evidence that initial PUVA treatment with concomitant systemic steroid treatment can be useful.[288]

Because of the high incidence of SLE in African-Americans[49] and the less noticeable visible erythema and pigment changes in darker skin types, it is important to be aware of the drugs that can induce an SLE syndrome as well as those that induce pigmentation changes and photosensitivity. When seeing a patient on allopurinol, a drug that may be more commonly used in the African-American population, it is important to keep in mind the wide range of reactions that may occur.

CONCLUSION

Many systemic diseases manifest themselves in the skin. As dermatologists, it is important to recognize the various types and severity of disease presentation as well as different treatment options, depending on the particular affected ethnic group.

REFERENCES

1. Chao SC, Yan JJ, Lee JY. Cutaneous sarcoidosis among Taiwanese. *J Formos Med Assoc* 2000; 99(4): 317–323.
2. Katta R. Cutaneous sarcoidosis: a dermatologic masquerader. *Am Fam Phys* 2002; 65: 1581–1584.
3. English JC, Patel PJ, Greer KE. Sarcoidosis. *J Am Acad Dermatol* 2001; 44: 725–743.
4. Jacyk WK. Cutaneous sarcoidosis in black South Africans. *Int J Dermatol* 1999; 38(11): 841–845.
5. Lee JB, Kolbenzer PS. Disfiguring cutaneous manifestation of sarcoidosis treated with thalidomide: a case report. *J Am Acad Dermatol* 1998; 39: 835–838.
6. Lee JY, Mak CP, Kao HF. Extrathoracic sarcoidosis in a Chinese man presenting with multiple, large plaques and tumors. *J Formos Med Assoc* 1992; 91(12): 1200–1204.
7. Katta R, Nelson B, Chen D, Roenigk H. Sarcoidosis of the scalp: a case series and review of the literature. *J Am Acad Dermatol* 2000; 690–692.
8. Fernandes SR, Singsen BH, Hoffman GS. Sarcoidosis and systemic vasculitis. *Semin Arthritis Rheum* 2000; 30(1): 33–46.
9. Jacyk WK. Sarcoidosis in the West African. A report of eight Nigerian patients with cutaneous lesions. *Trop Geogr Med* 1984; 36(3): 231–236.

10. Minus HR, Grimes PE. Cutaneous manifestations of sarcoidosis in blacks. *Cutis* 1983; 32(4): 361–363, 372.
11. Halder RM. Cutaneous diseases in the black races. *Dermatol Clin* 2003; 21: 679–687.
12. Baughman PR. Sarcoidosis. In: Weatherall DJ, Ledingham JGG, Warrell DA (Eds) *Oxford Textbook of Medicine*, 3rd ed. Oxford: Oxford University Press, 1995; 2831.
13. Wei H, Friedman KA, Rudikoff D. Multiple indurated papules on penis and scrotum. *J Cutan Med Surg* 2000; 4(4): 202–204.
14. Kendrick CG, Brown RA, Reina R, Ford BP, Reed RJ, Nesbitt LT Jr. Cutaneous sarcoidosis presenting as leonine facies. *Int J Dermatol* 1999; 38(11): 841–845.
15. Yoo SS, Mimouni D, Nikolskaia OV, Kouba DJ, Sauder DN, Nousari CH. Clinicopathologic features of ulcerative-atrophic sarcoidosis. *Int J Dermatol* 2004; 43: 108–112.
16. Zic JA, Horowitz DH, Arzubiaga C, King LE. Treatment of cutaneous sarcoidosis with chloroquine. Review of the literature. *Arch Dermatol* 1991; 127: 1034–1040.
17. Webster GF, Razsi LK, Sanchez M, Shupack JL. Weekly low-dose methotrexate therapy for cutaneous sarcoidosis. *J Am Acad Dermatol* 1991; 24: 451–454.
18. Rousseau L, Beylot-Barry M, Doutre MS, Beylot C. Cutaneous sarcoidosis successfully treated with low doses of thalidomide. *Arch Dermatol* 1998; 134: 1045–1046.
19. Anonymous. Statement on sarcoidosis: joint statement of the American Thoracic Society (ATS), the European Respiratory Society (ERS), and the World Association of Sarcoidosis and Other Granulomatous Disorders (WASOG) adopted by the ATS board of directors and by the ERS executive committee, February 1999. *Am J Resp Crit Care Med* 1999; 160: 736–755.
20. Baughman RP, Lower EE. Steroid-sparing alternative treatments for sarcoidosis. *Clin Chest Med* 1997; 18: 853–864.
21. Pfau A, Stolz W, Karrer S, Szeimies RM, Landthaler M. Allopurinol in treatment of cutaneous sarcoidosis. *Hautarzt* 1998; 49: 216–218.
22. Jackson JM. Hepatitis C and the skin. *Dermatol Clin* 2002; 20(3): 449–458.
23. Falanga V. Scleroderma (systemic sclerosis). In: Bolognia JL, Jorizzo JL, Rapini RP (Eds) *Dermatology*, 1st ed. New York: Mosby, 2003; pp. 625–631.
24. Reveille JD, Fischbach M, McNearney T, Friedman AW, Aguilar MB, Lisse J, et al.; GENISOS Study Group. Systemic sclerosis in 3 US ethnic groups: a comparison of clinical, sociodemographic, serologic, and immunogenetic determinants. *Semin Arthritis Rheum* 2001; 30(5): 332–346.
25. Odom RB, James WG, Berger TG. Dermal and subcutaneous tumors. In: *Andrew's Diseases of the Skin: Clinical Dermatology*, 9th ed. Philadelphia: Saunders, 2000; 775.
26. Steen VD, Powell DL, Medsger RA Jr. Clinical correlations and prognosis based on serum auto antibodies in patients with systemic sclerosis. *Arthritis Rheum* 1988; 31: 196–201.
27. Reveille JD, Durban E, Goldstein R, Moreda R, Arnett FC. Racial differences in the frequencies of scleroderma-related autoantibodies. *Arthritis Rheum* 1992; 35(2): 216–218.
28. Medsger TA Jr. Systemic sclerosis. In: Koopman WH (Ed) *Arthritis and Allied Conditions*. Baltimore: Williams and Wilkins, 1997; pp. 1433–1455.
29. Altman RD, Medsger RA Jr, Bloch RA, Michel BA. Prediction of survival in systemic sclerosis (scleroderma). *Arthritis Rheum* 1991; 34: 403–413.
30. Paquette D, Falanga V. The psychosocial dimensions of scleroderma: a survey. *Arthritis Rheum* 2000; 43: 1522.
31. Krishnamurthy V, Porkodi R, Ramakrishnan S, Rajendran CP, Madhavan R, Achuthan K, et al. Progressive systemic sclerosis in south India. *J Assoc Physicians India* 1991; 39(3): 254–257.
32. Wigley FM, Wise RA, Seibold JR, McCloskey DA, Kujala G, Medsger TA Jr, et al. Intravenous iloprost infusion in patients with Raynaud phenomenon secondary to systemic sclerosis. A multicenter, placebo-controlled, double-blind study. *Ann Intern Med* 1994;120(3): 199–206.
33. Stone JH, Wigley FM. Management of systemic sclerosis: the art and science. *Semin Cutan Med Surg* 1998; 17: 55–64.
34. Seibold JR, Korn JH, Simms R, Clements PJ, Moreland LW, Mayes MD, et al. Recombinant human relaxin in the treatment of scleroderma. A randomized, double-blind, placebo-controlled trial. *Ann Intern Med* 2000;132(11): 871–879.
35. Tebbe B, Orfanos CE. Epidemiology and socioeconomic impact of skin disease in lupus erythematosus. *Lupus* 1997; 6: 96–104.

36. Patel P, Werth V. Cutaneous lupus erythematosus: a review. *Dermatol Clin* 2002; 20: 373–385.
37. Drake CG, Kotzin BL. Genetic and immunological mechanisms in the pathogenesis of systemic lupus erythematosus. *Curr Opin Immunol* 1992; 4: 733–40.
38. Michel M, Johanet C, Meyer O, et al. Familial lupus erythematosus: clinical and immunologic features of 125 multiplex families. *Medicine (Baltimore)* 2001; 80: 153–158.
39. McCauliffe DP. Cutaneous lupus erythematosus. *Semin Cutan Med Surg* 2001; 20: 14–26.
40. Werth VP, Dutz JP, Sontheimer RD. Pathogenetic mechanisms and treatment of cutaneous lupus erythematosus. *Curr Opin Rheumatol* 1997; 9: 400–409.
41. Hansan T, Nyberg F, Stephansson E, et al. Photosensitivity in lupus erythematosus, UV photoprovocation results compared with history of photosensitivity and clinical findings. *Br J Dermatol* 1997; 136: 699–705.
42. Ioannides D, Golden B, Buyon J, et al. Expression of SS-A/Ro and SS-/La antigens in skin biopsy specimens of patients with photosensitive forms of lupus erythematosus. *Arch Dermatol* 2000; 136: 340–346.
43. Denfeld RW, Kind P, Sonteheimer RD, et al. *In situ* expression of B7 and CD28 receptor families in skin lesions of patients with lupus erythematosus. *Arthritis Rheum* 1997; 40: 814–821.
44. Hasan T, Stephannson E, Ranki A. Distribution of naïve and memory T-cells in photoprovoked and spontaneous skin lesion soft discoid lupus erythematosus and polymorphous light eruption. *Acta Derm Venereol* 1999; 79: 437–442.
45. Toro JR, Finlay D, Dou X, et al. Detection of type 1 cytokines in discoid lupus erythematosus. *Arch Dermatol* 2000; 136: 1497–1501.
46. Odom RB, James WG, Berger TG. Connective tissue diseases. In: *Andrew's Diseases of the Skin: Clinical Dermatology*, 9th ed. Philadelphia: Saunders, 2000; 172–204.
47. Egner W. The use of laboratory tests in the diagnosis of SLE. *J Clin Pathol* 2000; 53: 424–432.
48. Lela A. Lupus erythematosus. In: Bolognia JL, Jorizzo JL, Rapini RP (Eds) *Dermatology*, 1st ed. New York: Mosby, 2003; pp. 600–613.
49. Hochberg MC. The epidemiology of systemic lupus erythematosus. In: Wallace DJ, Hahn BH (Eds) *Dubois' Lupus Erythematosus*, 4th ed. Philadelphia: Lea and Febiger, 1993; 49–57.
50. Hochberg MC, Boyd RE, Ahearn JM, et al. Systemic lupus erythematosus: a review of clinico-laboratory features and immunogenetic markers in 150 patients with emphasis on demographic subsets. *Medicine* 1985; 64: 285–295.
51. McCarty DJ, Manzi S, Medsger TA Jr, et al. Incidence of systemic lupus erythematosus. Race and gender differences. *Arthritis Rheum* 1995; 38: 1260–1270.
52. Petri M. The effect of race on incidence and clinical course in systemic lupus erythematosus: the Hopkins Lupus Cohort. *J Am Med Womens Assoc* 1998; 53: 9–12.
53. Alarcon GS, Roseman I, Bartolucci AA, et al. Systemic lupus erythematosus in three ethnic groups: II. Features predictive of disease activity early in its course. LUMINA Study Group. Lupus in minority populations, nature versus nurture. *Arthritis Rheum* 1998; 41: 1173–1180.
54. Reveille JD, Moulds JM, Ahn C, et al. Systemic lupus erythematosus in three ethnic groups: I. The effects of HLA class II, C4, and CR1 alleles, socioeconomic factors, and ethnicity at disease onset. LUMINA study group. Lupus in minority populations, nature versus nurture. *Arthritis Rheum* 1998; 41: 1161–1172.
55. White G. Common diseases in the darker-skinned adult. In: Johnson B, Ronald G, White G (Eds) *Ethnic Skin: Medical and Surgical*. St. Louis: Mosby, 1998; pp. 43–120.
56. Crowson AN, Magro C. The cutaneous pathology of lupus erythematosus: a review. *J Cutan Pathol* 2001; 28: 1–23.
57. de Berker D, Dissaneyeka M, Burge S. The sequelae of chronic cutaneous lupus erythematosus. *Lupus* 1992; 1: 181–186.
58. Marten PB, Moder KG, Ahmed I. Lupus panniculitis: clinical perspectives from a case series. *J Rheumatol* 1999; 26: 68–72.
59. Ng PPL, Tan SH, Tan T. Lupus erythematosus panniculitis: a clinopathologic study. *Int J Dermatol* 2002; 41: 488–490.
60. Watanabe T, Tsuchdida T. Lupus erythematosus profundus: a cutaneous marker for a distinct clinical subset? *Br J Dermatol* 1996; 134: 123–125.
61. Sontheimer RD. Subacute cutaneous lupus erythematosus. *Clin Dermatol* 1985; 3: 58–68.

62. Sontheimer RD, Provost TT. In: Sontheimer RD, Provost TT (Eds) *Cutaneous Manifestations of Rheumatic Disease*. Baltimore: Williams and Wilkins, 1996; 1–71.
63. Yung A, Oakley A. Bullous systemic lupus erythematosus. *Australas J Dermatol* 2000; 41: 234–237.
64. Gilliam JN, Sontheimer RD. Distinctive cutaneous subsets in the spectrum of lupus erythematosus. *J Am Acad Dermatol* 1981; 4: 471–475.
65. Werth V. Current treatment of cutaneous lupus erythematosus. *Dermatol Online J* 2001; 7. http://dermatology.org/cdlib
66. McCauliffe DP. Cutaneous lupus erythematosus. *Semin Cutan Med Surg* 2001; 20: 14–26.
67. Callen J. Therapy for cutaneous lupus. *Dermatologic Ther* 2001; 14: 61–69.
68. Dalziel K, Going G, Cartwright PH, et al. Treatment of chronic discoid lupus erythematosus with an oral gold compound (auranofin). *Br J Dermatol* 1986; 115: 211–216.
69. Callen JP. Management of skin disease in lupus. *Bull Rheum Dis* 1997; 6: 145–157.
70. Ashinoff R, Werth VP, Franks AG Jr. Resistant discoid lupus erythematosus of palms and soles; successful treatment with azathioprine. *J Am Acad Dermatol* 1998; 19: 961–965.
71. Boehm IM, Boehm GA, Bauer R. Management of cutaneous lupus erythematosus with low-dose methotrexate: indication for modulation of inflammatory mechanisms. *Rheumatol Int* 1998; 18: 59–62.
72. Bohm L, Uerlich M, Bauer R. Rapid improvement of subacute cutaneous lupus erythematosus with low-dose methotrexate. *Dermatology* 1997; 194: 307–308.
73. Bottomley WW, Goodfield MJ. Methotrexate for the treatment of discoid lupus erythematosus. *Br J Dermatol* 1995; 133: 655–656.
74. Goldstein E, Carey W. Discoid lupus erythematosus: successful treatment with oral methotrexate. *Arch Dermatol* 1994; 130: 938–939.
75. Yung RL, Richardson BC. Cytarabine therapy for refractory cutaneous lupus. *Arthritis Rheum* 1995; 38: 1341–1343.
76. Saeki Y, Ohshima S, Kurimoto I, et al. Maintaining remission of lupus erythematosus profundus (LEP) with cyclosporin A. *Lupus* 2000; 9: 390–392.
77. Pashinian N, Wallace DJ, Klinenberg JR. Mycophenolate mofetil for systemic lupus erythematosus. *Arthritis Rheum* 1998; 41:S110.
78. Lindskov R, Reymann F. Dapsone in the treatment of cutaneous lupus erythematosus. *Dermatologica* 1986; 172: 214–217.
79. Krivanek JF, Paver WK. Further study of the use of clofazimine in discoid lupus erythematosus. *Australas J Dermatol* 1980; 21: 169.
80. Reid C. Drug treatment of cutaneous lupus. *Am J Clin Dermatol* 2000; 1: 375–379.
81. Ruzicka T, Meurer M, Braun-Falco O. Treatment of cutaneous lupus erythematosus with etreinate. *Acta Derm Venereol* 1985; 65: 324–329.
82. Kyriakas KP, Konotchrisopolous CJ, Panteleos DN. Experience with low-dose thalidomide in chronic discoid lupus erythematosus. *Int J Dermatol* 2000; 39: 218–222.
83. Ordi-Ros J, Cortes F, Cucurull E, et al. Thalidomide in the treatment of cutaneous lupus refractory to conventional therapy. *J Rhematol* 2000; 27: 1429–1433.
84. Raulin C, Schmidt C, Hellwig S. Cutaneous lupus erythematosus — treatment with a pulse dye laser. *Br J Dermatol* 1999; 141: 1046–1050.
85. Santmyire-Rosenberger B, Dugan EM. Skin involvement in dermatomyositis. *Curr Opin Rheumatol* 2003; 15(6): 714–722.
86. Jorizzo JL. Dermatomyositis. In: Bolognia JL, Jorizzo JL, Rapini RP (Eds) *Dermatology*, 1st ed. New York: Mosby, 2003; 625–631.
87. Sontheimer RD. Dermatomyositis: an overview of recent progress with emphasis on dermatologic aspects. *Dermatol Clin* 2002; 20: 387–408.
88. Ichikawa E, Furuta J, Kawachi Y, et al. Hereditary complement (C9) deficiency associated with dermatomyositis. *Br J Dermatol* 2001; 144: 1080–1083.
89. Pachman LM, Liotta-Savis MR, Hong DK, et al. TnF alpha 308 A allele in juvenile dermatomyositis: association with increased production of tumor necrosis factor alpha, disease duration and pathologic calcifications. *Arthritis Rheum* 2000; 43: 1080–1083.
90. Hill C, Zeitz C, Kirkham B. Dermatomyositis with lung involvement in a patient treated with simvastatin. *Aust N Z J Med* 1995; 25: 745–746.

91. Khattak FH, Morris IM, Branford WA. Simvastatin associated dermatomyositis (letter; comment). *Br J Rheumatol* 1994; 33: 199.
92. Vela-Casassempre P, Borras-Blasco J, Navaroo-Ruiz A. Alfuzosin associated dermatomyositis. *Br J Rheumatol* 1998; 37: 1135–1136.
93. Dimackie MM, Vriesendorp FJ, Heck KA. Phenytoin-induced dermatomyositis: case report and literature review. *J Child Neurol* 1998; 13: 577–580.
94. Yamashita K, Hosokawa M, Hirohashi S, et al. Epstein-Barr virus associated gastric cancer in a patient with dermatomyositis. *Intern Med* 2001; 40: 96–99.
95. Targoff IN. Update on myositis specific and myositis associated autoantibodies. *Curr Opin Rheumatol* 200; 12: 475–481.
96. Rosen A, Casciola-Rosen L. Clearing the way to mechanisms of autoimmunity. *Nat Med* 2001; 7: 664–665.
97. Kubo M, Ihn H, Yamne K, et al. Increased serum levels of soluble vascular ell adhesion molecule-1 and soluble E-selectin in patients with polymyositis/dermatomyositis. *Rheumatology (Oxford)* 2000; 143: 392–398.
98. Gelber AC, Nousari HC, Wigley FM. Mycophenolate mofetil in the treatment of severe skin manifestations of dermatomyositis: a series of 4 cases. *J Rheumatol* 2000; 27: 1542–1545.
99. Euwer RL, Sontheimer RD. Dermatomyositis, In: Sontheimer RD, Provost TT (Eds) *Cutaneous Manifestations of Rheumatic Disease*. Baltimore: Williams and Wilkins, 1996; 73–114.
100. Del Pozo J, Almagro M, Martinez W, et al. Dermatomyositis and mucinosis. *Int J Dermatol* 2001; 40: 120–124.
101. Lupton JR, Figueroa P, Berberian BJ, et al. An unusual presentation of dermatomyositis: the type Wong variant revisited. *J Am Acad Dermatol* 2000; 43: 908–912.
102. Wong KO. Dermatomyositis: a clinical investigation of 23 cases in Hong Kong. *Br J Dermatol* 1969; 81: 544–547.
103. Ghali FE, Stein LD, Fine JD, et al. Gingival telangiectases: an underappreciated physical sign of juvenile dermatomyositis. *Arch Dermatol* 1999; 135: 1370–1374.
104. Plamondon S, Dent PB. Juvenile amyopathic dermatomyositis: results of a case finding descriptive survey. *J Rheumatol* 2000; 27: 2031–2034.
105. Askari AD, Huettner TL. Cardiac abnormalities in polymyositis/dermatomyositis. *Semin Arthritis Rheum* 1982; 12: 208–219.
106. Chen YJ, Wu Cy, Shen JL. Predicting factors of malignancy in dermatomyositis and polymyositis: a case-control study. *Br J Dermatol* 2001; 144: 825–831.
107. Airio A, Pukkala E, Isomaki H. Elevated cancer incidence in patients with dermatomyositis: a population based study. *J Rheumatol* 1995; 22: 1300–1303.
108. Sigurgeirsson B. Skin disease and malignancy: an epidemiological study. *Acta Derm Venereol Suppl (Stockh)* 199; 178: 1–110.
109. O'Gradaigh D, Merry P. Tumor markers in dermatomyositis: useful or useless? (letter). *Br J Rheumatol* 1998; 37: 914.
110. One member's story. Enbrel use restored his strength. In: Curry TR (Ed) *The Outlook for the Inflammatory Myopathies*. Myositis Association of America, 2000.
111. Saadeh CK. Etanercept effective in polymyositis, dermatomyositis refractory to conventional therapy. In: Curry TR (Ed) *The Outlook for the Inflammatory Myopathies*. Myositis Association of America, 2001.
112. Cohen JB. Cutaneous involvement of dermatomyositis can respond to Dapsone therapy. *Int J Dermatol* 2002; 41(3): 182–184.
113. Dalakas MC. Controlled studies with high-dose intravenous immunoglobulin in the treatment of dermatomyositis, inclusion body myositis and polymyositis. *Neurology* 1998; 51 (suppl 5): S37–S45.
114. Al-Mayouf S, Al Mazyed A, Bahabri S. Efficacy of early treatment of severe juvenile dermatomyositis with intravenous methylprednisolone and methotrexate. *Clin Rheumatol* 2000; 19: 138–141.
115. Nawata Y, Kurasawa K, Takabayashi K, et al. Corticosteroid resistant interstitial pneumonitis in dermatomyositis/polymyositis: prediction and treatment with cyclosporine. *J Rheumatol* 1999; 26: 1527–1533.
116. Adams EM, Pucino F, Yarboro C, et al. A pilot study: use of fludarabine for refractory dermatomyositis and polymyositis and examination of endpoint measures. *J Rheumatol* 1999; 26: 352–360.

117. Ichiki Y, Akiyama T, Shimozawa N, et al. An extremely severe case of cutaneous calcinosis with juvenile dermatomyositis and successful treatment with diltiazem. *Br J Dermatol* 2001; 144: 894–897.
118. Oliveri MB, Palermo R, Matualen C, et al. Regression of calcinosis during diltiazem treatment in juvenile dermatomyositis. *J Rheumatol* 1996; 23: 2152–2155.
119. Vinen CS, Patel S, Buckner FE. Regression of calcinosis associated with adult dermatomyositis following diltiazem therapy. *Rheumatology (Oxford)* 2000; 39: 333–334.
120. Sanchez MR. Cutaneous diseases in Latinos. *Dermatol Clin* 2003; 21: 689–697.
121. Toro J, Turner M, Gahl WA. Dermatologic manifestations of Hermansky–Pudlak syndrome in patients with and without a 16-base pair duplication in the HPS1 gene. *Arch Dermatol* 1999; 135: 774–780.
122. McKeigue PM, Shah B, Marmot MG. Relation of central obesity, and insulin resistance with high diabetes prevalence and cardiovascular risk in South Asians. *Lancet* 1991;337: 382–386.
123. How many Hispanic Americans have diabetes? http://diabetes.niddk.nih.gov/dm/pubs/hispanicamerican/#c. Accessed on October 12, 2004.
124. How many African Americans have diabetes? http://diabetes.niddk.nih.gov/dm/pubs/africanamerican/#2. Accessed on October 12, 2004.
125. Why is diabetes more common in Asians and Pacific Islanders? http://www.joslin.harvard.edu/api/why_common.shtml. Accessed on October 12, 2004.
126. Perez MI, Kohn SR. Cutaneous manifestations of diabetes mellitus. *J Am Acad Dermatol* 1994; 30: 519–531.
127. Nikkels-Tassoudji N, Henry F, Letawe C, Pierard-Franchimont C, Lefebvre P, Pierard GE. Mechanical properties of the diabetic waxy skin. *Dermatology* 1996; 192(1): 19–22.
128. Ferringer T, Miller OF. Cutaneous manifestations of diabetes mellitus. *Dermatol Clin* 2002; 20: 483–492.
129. Knowles HB. Joint contractures, waxy skin, and control of diabetes. *N Engl J Med* 1981; 305: 217–218.
130. Wilson BE, Newmark JJ. Severe scleroderma diabeticorum and insulin resistance. *J Am Board Fam Pract* 1995; 8: 55–57.
131. Ikeda Y, Suehiro T, Abe T, et al. Severe diabetic scleroderma with extensions to the extremities and effective treatment using prostaglandin E1. *Intern Med* 1998; 37: 861–864.
132. Buckingham BA, Uitto J, Snadborg C, Keen T, Kaufman F, Landing B. Scleroderma like syndrome and the non-enzymatic glycosylation of collagen in children with poorly controlled insulin dependent diabetes (IDDM). *Pediatr Res* 1982; 15 (a part 2): 626.
133. Brik R, Berant M, Vardi P. The scleroderma-like syndrome of insulin-dependent diabetes mellitus. *Diabetes Metab Rev* 1991; 7: 120–128.
134. Libecco JF. Finger pebbles and diabetes: a case with broad involvement of the dorsal fingers and hands. *Arch Dermatol* 2001; 137: 510–511.
135. Lieberman LS, Rosenbloom AL, Riley WJ, et al. Reduced skin thickness with pump administration of insulin. *N Engl J Med* 1980; 303: 940–941.
136. Seyger MMB, van den Hoogen FHJ, de Mare S, et al. A patient with severe scleroderma diabeticorum, partially responding to low-dose methotrexate. *Dermatology* 1999; 198: 177–179.
137. Shemer A, Bergman R, Linn S, Kantor Y, Friedman-Birnbaum R. Diabetic dermopathy and internal complications in diabetes mellitus. *Int J Dermatol* 1998; 37(2): 113–5.
138. Sibbald RG, Landolt SJ, Toth D. Skin and diabetes. *Endocrinol Metab Clin North Am* 1996; 25: 463–472.
139. Yosipovitch G, Hodak E, Vardi P, et al. The prevalence of cutaneous manifestations in IDDM patients and their association with diabetes risk factors and microvascular complications. *Diabetes Care* 1998; 21: 506–509.
140. Melin H. An atrophic circumscribed skin lesion in the lower extremities of diabetics. *Acta Med Scand* 1964; 176 (Suppl 423): 9–75.
141. Danowski TS, Sabeh G, Sarver ME, et al. Shin spots and diabetes mellitus. *Am J Med Sci* 1966; 251: 570–575.
142. Huntely AC. The cutaneous manifestations of diabetes mellitus. *J Am Acad Dermatol* 1982; 7: 427–455.
143. Stulberg DL, Clark N, Tovey D. Common hyperpigmentation disorders in adults: Part II. Melanoma, seborrheic keratoses, acanthosis nigricans, melasma, diabetic dermopathy, tinea versicolor and postinflammatory hyperpigmentation. *Am Fam Phys* 2003; 68: 1963–1968.

144. Callen JP. Dermatologic signs of systemic diseases. In: Bolognia JL, Jorizzo JL, Rapini RP (Eds) *Dermatology*, 1st ed. New York: Mosby, 2003; 711–726.
145. Cunningham SR, Walsh M, Matthews R, Fulton R, Burrows D. Kyrle's disease. *Am Acad Dermatol* 1987; 16(1 Pt 1): 117–123.
146. Melin H. An atrophic circumscribed skin lesion in the lower extremities of diabetics. *Acta Med Scand* 1964; 176 (suppl 423): 9–75.
147. Stuart CA, Pate CJ, Peters EJ. Prevalence of acanthosis nigricans in an unselected population. *Am J Med* 1989; 87: 269–272.
148. Acanthosis nigricans. In: Rook A, Wilkinson DSD, Ebling FJG (Eds) *Textbook of Dermatology*. Oxford: Blackwell Scientific, 1979; 1307–1310.
149. Flier JS. Metabolic importance of acanthosis nigricans. *Arch Dermatol* 1985; 121: 193–194.
150. Feingold KR, Elias PM. Endocrine skin interactions. *J Am Acad Dermatol* 1987; 17: 921–940.
151. Jelinker JE. *The Skin in Diabetes*. Philadelphia: Lea and Febiger, 1986; 58–72.
152. Lever WF, Schaumburg-Lever G. *Histopathology of the Skin*. Philadelphia: Lippincott, 1990; 302–308.
153. Haroon TS. Diabetes and skin — a review. *Scott Med J* 1974; 19: 257–267.
154. Stawiski MA, Voorhees JJ. Cutaneous signs of diabetes mellitus. *Cutis* 1976; 18: 415–421.
155. Flier JS, Eastman RC, Minaker KL, Matteson D, Rowe JW. Acanthosis nigricans in obese women with hyperandrogenism and characterization of an insulin-resistant state distinct from the type A and type B syndromes. *Diabetes* 1985; 34: 101–107.
156. Paron NG, Lambert PW. Cutaneous manifestations of diabetes mellitus. *Prim Care* 2000; 27: 371–383.
157. Stuart CA, Gilkison CR, Keenan BS, Nagamani M. Hyperinsulinemia and acanthosis nigricans in African Americans. *J Natl Med Assoc* 1997; 89(8): 523–7.
158. Cruz PD. Excess insulin binding to insulin-like growth factor receptors: proposed mechanism of acanthosis nigricans. *J Invest Dermatol* 1992; 98: 82s-85s.
159. Stuart CA, Gilkison CR, Smith MM, et al. Acanthosis nigricans as a risk factor for non-insulin dependent diabetes mellitus. *Clin Pediatr* 1998; 37: 73–80.
160. Sheretz EF. Improved acanthosis nigricans with lipodystrophic diabetes during dietary fish oil supplementation. *Arch Dermatol* 1988; 124: 1094–1096.
161. Steed DL, Donohoe D, Webster MX, et al. Effect of extensive debridement and treatment on the healing of diabetic foot ulcers. Diabetic Ulcer Study Group. *J Am Coll Surg* 1996; 183: 61–64.
162. Sorensen JC. Living skin equivalents and their application in wound healing. *Clin Podiatr Med Surg* 1998; 15: 129–137.
163. Grayson ML, Biggons GW, Balogh K, et al. Probing bone in infected pedal ulcers. *JAMA* 1995; 273: 721–723.
164. Cavanaugh PR, Ulbrech JS, Capputo GM. Biomechanical aspects of diabetic foot disease: etiology, treatment and prevention. *Diabet Med* 1996; 3: s17-s22.
165. Crane M, Branch P. The healed diabetic foot. *Clin Podiatr Med Surg* 1998; 15: 155–174.
166. Soulier SM. The use of running shoes in the prevention of plantar diabetic ulcers. *J Am Podiatr Med Assoc* 1986; 76: 395–400.
167. Muller SA, Winkkelmann RK. Necrobiosis lipoidica diabeticorum. A clinical and pathological investigation of 171 cases. *Arch Dermatol* 1966; 93: 272–281.
168. Howard A, White CR. Necrobiosis lipoidica. Chapter non infectious granulomas. In: Bolognia JL, Jorizzo JL, Rapini RP (Eds) *Dermatology*, 1st ed. New York: Mosby, 2003; 1463–1465.
169. Marinella MA. Necrobiosis lipoidica diabeticorum. *Lancet* 2002; 360: 1143.
170. Jelinek JE. Cutaneous manifestations of diabetes mellitus. *Int J Dermatol* 1994; 33: 605–617.
171. Lowitt MH, Dover JS. Necrobiosis lipoidica. *J Am Acad Dermatol* 1991; 25: 735–748.
172. Heymann WR. Necrobiosis lipoidica treated with topical tretinoin. *Cutis* 1996; 58: 53–54.
173. Smith K. Ulcerating necrobiosis lipoidica resolving in response to cyclosporine-A. *Dermatol Online J* 1997; 3: 2.
174. Darvay A, Acland KM, Russell-Jones R. Persistent ulcerated necrobiosis lipoidica responding to treatment with cyclosporine. *Br J Dermatol* 1999; 141: 725–727.
175. Spencer EA, Nahass GT. Topically applied bovine collagen in the treatment of ulcerative necrobiosis lipoidica diabeticorum. *Arch Dermatol* 1997; 133: 817–818.
176. Patel GK, Harding KG, Mills CM. Severe disabling Koebnerizing ulcerated necrobiosis lipoidica successfully managed with topical PUVA. *Br J Dermatol* 2000; 143: 668–669.

177. McKenna DB, Cooper EJ, Tidman MJ. Topical psoralen plus ultraviolet: a treatment for necrobiosis lipoidica. *Br J Dermatol* 2000; 143: 1333–1335.
178. Reinhard G, Lohmann F, Uerlich M, et al. Successful treatment of ulcerated necrobiosis lipoidica with mycophenolate mofetil. *Acta Derm Venereol* 2000; 80: 312–313.
179. Goodfield MJD, Millard LG. The skin diabetes mellitus. *Diabetologia* 198; 31: 567–575.
180. Lipsky BA, Baker PD, Ahroni JH. Diabetic bullae: 12 cases of purportedly rare cutaneous disorder. *Int J Dermatol* 2000; 39: 196–200.
181. Derighetti M, Hohl D, Karyenbuhl BH, et al. Bullosis diabeticorum in a newly discovered type 2 diabetes mellitus. *Dermatology* 2000; 200: 366–367.
182. Basarab T, Munn SE, McGrath J, et al. Bullosis diabeticorum: a case report and literature review. *Clin Exp Dermatol* 1995; 20: 218–220.
183. Patterson JW. Skin changes in diabetes mellitus: a review. *Mil Med* 1983; 148: 135–140.
184. Allen GE, Hadden DR. Bullous lesions of the skin diabetes. *Br J Dermatol* 1970; 82: 216–220.
185. Cantwell AR, Martz W. Idiopathic bullae in diabetics: bullosis diabeticorum. *Arch Dermatol* 1967; 96: 42–44.
186. Kurwa A, Roberts P, Whitehead R. Concurrence of bullous and atrophic skin lesions in diabetes mellitus. *Arch Dermatol* 1971; 103: 670–675.
187. Rocca FF, Pereyra E. Phlyctenar lesions in the feet of diabetic patients. *Diabetes* 1963; 12: 220–222.
188. Lozada-Nur F, Miranda C. Oral lichen planus: epidemiology, clinical characteristics, and associated diseases. *Semin Cutan Med Surg* 1997; 16(4): 273–7.
189. Shiohara T, Kano Y. Lichen planus and lichenoid dermatoses. In: Bolognia JL, Jorizzo JL, Rapini RP (Eds) *Dermatology*, 1st ed. New York: Mosby, 2003; 175–184.
190. Conklin RJ, Blasberg B. Oral lichen planus. *Dermatol Clin* 1987; 5(4): 663–673.
191. Bhutani LK. Ashy dermatosis or lichen planus pigmentosus: what is in a name? *Arch Dermatol* 1986; 122: 133.
192. Samman PD. Lichen planus an lichenoid eruptions. In: Rook A, Wilkinson DS, Ebling FJG (Eds) *Textbook of Dermatology*. London: Blackwell Scientific, 1979; 2: 1483–1502.
193. Boyd AS, Neldner KH. Lichen planus. *J Am Acad Dermatol* 1991; 25(4): 593–619.
194. Mignogna MD, Lo Muzio L, Lo Russo L, Fedele S, Ruoppo E, Bucci E. Oral lichen planus: different clinical features in HCV-positive and HCV-negative patients. *Int J Dermatol* 2000; 39(2): 134–139.
195. Carrozzo M, Francia Di Celle P, Gandolfo S, Carbone M, Conrotto D, Fasano ME, et al. Increased frequency of HLA-DR6 allele in Italian patients with hepatitis C virus-associated oral lichen planus. *Br J Dermatol* 2001; 144(4): 803–808.
196. Nagao Y, Kameyama T, Sata M. Hepatitis C virus RNA detection in oral lichen planus tissue (letter). *Am J Gastroenterol* 1998; 93: 850.
197. Beaird LM, Kahloon N, Franco J, Fairly JA. Incidence of hepatitis C in lichen planus. *J Am Acad Dermatol* 2001; 44: 311–312.
198. Jubert C, Pawlotsky JM, Pouget F, et al. Lichen planus and hepatitis C virus related chronic active hepatitis. *Arch Dermatol* 1994; 130: 73–76.
199. Moshe L, Arber N, Bben-Amitai D, et al. Successful interferon treatment for lichen planus associated with chronic active hepatitis due to hepatitis C virus infection. *Acta Derm Venereol* 1997; 77: 171–172.
200. Ho VC, Gupta AK, Ellis CN, Nickoloff BJ, Voorhees JJ. Treatment of severe lichen planus with cyclosporine. *J Am Acad Dermatol* 1990; 22(1): 64–68.
201. Pigatto PD, Chiapino G, Birgardi A, et al. Cyclosporine A for the treatment of severe lichen planus. *Br J Dermatol* 1990; 122: 121–123.
202. Lok ASF. Hepatitis B and C in Asians. http://www.fcmsdocs.org/Conference/9th/9hepatitisbandcinasians.html. Accessed on October 12, 2004.
203. Bergasa NV. Pruritus in chronic liver disease: mechanisms and treatment. *Curr Gastroenterol Rep* 2004; 6(1): 10–16.
204. Etter L, Meyers SA. Pruritus in systemic disease: mechanisms and management. *Dermatol Clin* 2002; 20: 459–472.
205. Garden J, Ostrow J, Roenigk H. Pruritus in hepatic cholestasis: pathogenesis and therapy. *Arch Dermatol* 1985; 121: 1415–1420.
206. Gilchrest B. Pruritus: pathogenesis, therapy, and significance in systemic disease states. *Arch Intern Med* 1982; 142: 101–105.

207. Fisher D, Wright T. Pruritus as a symptom of hepatitis C. *J Am Acad Dermatol* 1994; 30: 629–632.
208. Berhnhard JD. *Itch: Mechanisms and Management of Pruritus*. New York: McGraw-Hill, 1994.
209. Krajnik M, Zylicz Z. Pruritus in advanced internal diseases: pathogenesis and treatment. *Netherlands J Med* 2001; 58: 27–40.
210. Bonacini M. Pruritus in patients with chronic human immunodeficiency virus, hepatitis B and C virus infections. *Dig Liver Dis* 2000; 32: 621–625.
211. Carson CW, Conn DL, Czaja AJ, et al. Frequency and significance of antibodies to hepatitis C virus in polyarteritis nodosa. *J Rheumatol* 1993; 20: 304–309.
212. Edwards L. The interferons. *Dermatol Clin* 2001; 19: 139–146.
213. Weisshaar E, Kucenik MJ, Fleischer AB, Bernhard JD. Pruritus and dysesthesia. In: Bolognia JL, Jorizzo JL, Rapini RP (Eds) *Dermatology*, 1st ed. New York: Mosby, 2003; 102–109.
214. Freedman M, Holzbach R, Ferguson D. Pruritus in cholestasis: no direct causative role for bile acid retention. *Am J Med* 1981; 70: 1011–1016.
215. Ghent C, Bloomer J, Klatskin G. Elevations in skin tissue levels of bile acids in human cholestasis: relation to serum levels and to pruritus. *Gastroenterology* 1977; 73: 1125–1130.
216. Bergasa NV, Mehlman JK, Jones EA. Pruritus and fatigue in primary biliary cirrhosis. *Baillieres Best Pract Res Clin Gasteoenterol* 2000; 14: 643–655.
217. Fleischer A, Michales J. Pruritus in cancer patients. *J Geriatr Dermatol* 1995; 3: 172–181.
218. Bromm B, Scharein E, Darsow U, et al. Effects of menthol and cold on histamine-induced itch and skin reactions in man. *Neurosci Lett* 1995; 187: 157–160.
219. Yosipovitch G, Szolar C, Hui X, et al. Effect of topically applied menthol on thermal, pain and itch sensations and biophysical properties of the skin. *Arch Dermatol Res* 1996; 288: 245–248.
220. Carey J, Williams G. Relief of the pruritus of jaundice with a bile acid sequestering resin. *JAMA* 1961; 176: 432–435.
221. Bergasa N, Alling D, Talbot T, et al. Effects of naloxone infusions in patients with the pruritus of cholestasis. *Ann Intern Med* 1995; 123: 161–167.
222. Bergasa N, Alling D, Talbot T, et al. A controlled trial of naloxone infusions for the pruritus of chronic cholestasis. *Gastroenterology* 1992; 102: 544–549.
223. Wolfhagen F, Sternieri E, Hop W, et al. Oral naltrexone treatment for cholestatic pruritus: a double-blind placebo controlled study. *Gastroenterology* 1997; 113: 1264–1269.
224. Zylicz Z, Krajnik M. Codeine for pruritus in primary biliary cirrhosis. *Lancet* 1999; 353: 813.
225. Raderer M, Muller C, Scheithauer W. Ondansetron for pruritus due to cholestasis. *N Engl J Med* 1994; 330: 1540.
226. Schworer H, Hartmann H, Ramadori G. Relief of cholestatic pruritus by a novel class of drugs: 5-hydroxytryptamine type 3 (5-HT3) receptor antagonists: effectiveness of ondansetron. *Pain* 1995; 61: 33–37.
227. Schworer H, Ramadori G. Improvement of cholestatic pruritus by ondansetron. *Lancet* 1993; 341: 1277.
228. Kantor G. Pruritus. In: Sams W, Lynch P (Eds) *Principles and Practice of Dermatology*. New York: Churchill Livingstone, 1996; 881–885.
229. Childs N. CNS-related itch is hard to treat. *Skin Allerg News* 1999; 30: 16.
230. Cerio R, Murphy G, Sladen G, et al. A combination of phototherapy and cholestyramine for the relief of pruritus in primary biliary cirrhosis. *Br J Dermatol* 1987; 116: 265–267.
231. Hanid M, Levi A. Phototherapy for pruritus in primary biliary cirrhosis. *Lancet* 1980; 2: 530.
232. Datta D, Sherlock S. Treatment of pruritus of cholestasis by plasma perfusion through USP-charcoal-coated glass beads. *Lancet* 1980; 2: 53–55.
233. Bachs L, Elena M, Pares A, et al. Comparison of rifampin with phenobarbitone for treatment of pruritus in biliary cirrhosis. *Lancet* 1989; 1: 574–576.
234. Cynamon H, Andres J, Iafrate R. Rifampin relieves pruritus in children with cholestatic liver disease. *Gastroenterology* 1990; 98: 1013–1016.
235. Ghent C, Carruthers S. Treatment of pruritus in primary biliary cirrhosis with rifampin: results of double blind, crossover, randomized trial. *Gastroenterology* 1988; 94: 488–493.
236. Stiehl A, Thaler M, Admirand W. The effects of phenobarbital on bile salts and bilirubin in patients with intrahepatic and extrahepatic cholestasis. *N Engl J Med* 1972; 286: 858–861.

237. Agnello V, Abel G. Localization of hepatitis C virus in cutaneous vasculitic lesions in patients with type II cryoglobulinemia. *Arthritis Rheum* 1997; 40: 2007–2015.
238. Sansonno D, Cornacciulo V, Iacobelli AR, et al. Localization of hepatitis C virus antigens in liver and skin tissues of chronic hepatitis C virus-infected patients with mixed cryoglobulinemia. *Hepatology* 1995; 21: 305–312.
239. Jackson JM. Hepatitis C and the skin. *Dermatol Clin* 2002; 20: 449–458.
240. Knable AL. Cutaneous nephrology. *Dermatol Clin* 2002; 20: 513–521.
241. National Institutes of Health. Management of hepatitis C. NIH consensus statement online 1997; 15: 1–41.
242. Davis M, Su W. Cryoglobulinemia: recent findings in cutaneous and extracutaneous manifestations. *Int J Dermatol* 1996; 35: 240–248.
243. Silverberg NB, Singh A, Laude TA. Cutaneous manifestations of chronic renal failure in children of color. *Pediatr Dermatol* 2001; 18: 199–204.
244. Golusin Z, Poljacki M, Matovic L, Tasic S, Vuckovic N. Kyrle's disease. *Med Pregl* 2002; 55(1–2): 47–50.
245. Detmar M, Ruszczak Z, Imcke E, Stadler R, Orfanos CE. Kyrle disease in juvenile diabetes mellitus and chronic renal failure. *Hautkr* 1990; 65(1): 53–61.
246. Salomon RJ, Baden TJ, Gammon WR. Kyrle's disease and hepatic insufficiency. *Arch Dermatol* 1986; 122: 18–19.
247. Hood AF, Hardegen GL, Zarate AR, et al. Kyrle's disease in patients with chronic renal failure. *Arch Dermatol* 1982; 118: 85–88.
248. Robinson-Bostom L, DiGiovanna J. Cutaneous manifestations of end-stage renal disease. *J Am Acad Dermatol* 2000; 43: 975–986.
249. Kato A, Hameda M, Masuyama T, et al. Pruritus and hydration state of stratum corneum in hemodialysis patients. *Am J Nephrol* 2000; 20: 437–442.
250. Murphy M, Carmichael A. Renal itch. *Clin Exp Dermatol* 2000; 25: 103–106.
251. Mettang T, Fischer FP, Dollenbacher U, Kuhlman U. Uremic pruritus is not related to beta-endorphin serum levels in hemodialysis patients. *Nephrol Dial Transplant* 1998; 13: 231–232.
252. Peer G, Kvitiy S, Agami O, et al. Randomized crossover trial of naltrexone in uremic patients. *Lancet* 1996; 348: 1552–1554.
253. Szepietowski J, Scwartz R. Uremic pruritus. *Int J Dermatol* 1998; 37: 247–253.
254. Berne B, Vahlquist A, Fischer T, et al. UV treatment of uremic pruritus reduces the vitamin A content of the skin. *Eur J Clin Invest* 1984; 14: 203–206.
255. De Kroes S, Smeenk G. Serum vitamin A levels and pruritus in patients on hemodialysis. *Dermatologica* 1983; 166: 199–202.
256. Fantini F, Baraldi A, Sevignanni C, et al. Cutaneous innervation in chronic renal failure patients. *Acta Derm Venereol* 192; 72: 102–105.
257. Graf H, Kovarik J, Summvoll H, et al. Disappearance of uremic pruritus after lowering dialysate magnesium concentration. *BMJ* 1979; 3: 1478–1479.
258. Massry S, Popovtzer M, Coburn J, et al. Intractable pruritus as a manifestation of secondary hyperparathyroidism in uremia: disappearance of itching after subtotal parthryoidectomy. *N Engl J Med* 1968; 279: 697–700.
259. Tan J, Haberman H, Codlman A. Identifying effective treatments for uremic pruritus. *J Am Acad Dermatol* 1991; 25: 811–818.
260. Zucker I, Yosipovitch G, David M, Gafter U, Boner G. Prevalence and characterization of uremic pruritus in patients undergoing hemodialysis: uremic pruritus is still a major problem for patients with end-stage renal disease. *J Am Acad Dermatol* 2003; 49(5): 842–846.
261. Stahle-Backdahl M. Uremic pruritus. Clinical and experimental studies. *Acta Derm Venereol Suppl (Stockh)* 1989; 145: 1–38.
262. Yosipovitch G, Zucker I, Boner G, et al. A questionnaire for the assessment of pruritus: validation in uremic patients. *Acta Derm Venereol* 2001; 81: 108–111.
263. Botero F. Pruritus as a manifestation of systemic disorders. *Cutis* 1978; 21; 873–880.
264. Weisshaar E, Heyer G, Forster G, et al. Antipruritic effect of antihistaminic and local anesthetic topical agents after iontophoretic histamine stimulation. *Hautzart* 1996; 47: 355–360.

265. Breneman D, Cardone J, Blumsack R, et al. Topical capsaicin for treatment of hemodialysis-related pruritus. *J Am Acad Dermatol* 1992; 26: 91–94.
266. Cho Y, Liu H, Huang T, et al. Uremic pruritus: roles of parathyroid hormone and substance P. *J Am Acad Dermatol* 1997; 36: 538–543.
267. Bernstein J. Capsaicin in dermatologic disease. *Semin Dermatol* 1988; 7: 304–309.
268. Balaskas E, Bamihas G, Karamouzis M, et al. Histamine and serotonin in uremic pruritus: effect of ondansetron in CAPD pruritic patients. *Nephron* 1998; 78: 395–402.
269. Gilchrest B, Rowe J, Brown R, et al. Relief of uremic pruritus with ultraviolet phototherapy. *N Engl J Med* 1977; 297: 136–138.
270. Silva SRB, Viana PCF, Lugon NV, et al. Thalidomide for the treatment of uremic pruritus: a crossover randomized double-blind trial. *Nephron* 1994; 67: 270–273.
271. De Marchi S, Cecchin E, Villalta D, et al. Relief of pruritus and decreases in plasma histamine concentrations during erythropoietin therapy in patients with uremia. *N Engl J Med* 1992; 326: 969–974.
272. Pauli-Magnus C, Klumpp S, Alscher DM, et al. Naltrexone does not relieve uremic pruritus: results of a randomized, double blind, placebo controlled cross over study. *J Am Soc Nephrol* 2000; 11: 514–519.
273. Brown M, George C, Dunstan C, et al. Prurigo nodularis and aluminum overload in maintenance hemodialysis. *Lancet* 1992; 340: 48.
274. Duo L. Electrical needle therapy of uremic pruritus. *Nephron* 1987; 47: 179–183.
275. Monk B. Transcutaneous electronic nerve stimulation in the treatment of generalized pruritus. *Clin Exp Dermatol* 1993; 18: 67–68.
276. Tang W, Chan L, Lo K, et al. Evaluation on the antipruritic role of transcutaneous electrical nerve stimulation in the treatment of pruritic dermatoses. *Dermatology* 1999; 199: 237–241.
277. Shepherd GM. Hypersensitivity reactions to drugs: evaluation and management. *Mt Sinai J Med* 2003; 70(2): 113–125.
278. Stevens MB. Drug-induced lupus. *Hosp Pract* 1992; 27: 27–36.
279. Brown CW, Deng JS. Thiazide diuretics induce cutaneous lupus-like adverse reaction. *J Toxicol Clin Toxicol* 1995; 33: 729–733.
280. Fritzler MJ, Rubin RL. Drug-induced lupus. In: Wallace DJ, Hahn BH, Quismorio FP Jr, et al (Eds) *Dubois Lupus Erythematosus*, 4th ed. Philadelphia: Lea and Febiger, 1993; 442–453.
281. Zamber RW, Starkebaum G, Rubin RL, et al. Drug induced systemic lupus erythematosus due to ophthalmic timolol. *J Rheumatol* 1992; 19: 977–979.
282. Hypertension in racial and ethnic minorities. http:///www.blackhealthcare.com/BHC/Hypertension/Epidemiology.asp. Accessed on October 12, 2004.
283. Balarajan R. Ethnic differences in mortality from ischemic heart disease and cerebrovascular disease in England and Wales. *BMJ* 1991; 302: 560–564.
284. McGuiness M, Frye RA, Deng JS. Atenolol-induced lupus erythematosus. *J Am Acad Dermatol* 27; 298–299.
285. Ramsey-Goldman R, Franz T, Solano FX, Medsger TA Jr. Hydralazine induced lupus and Sweet's syndrome. Report and review of the literature. *Rheumatology* 1990; 17(5): 682–684.
286. Thestrup-Pedersen K. Adverse reactions in the skin from anti-hypertensive drugs. *Dan Med Bull* 1987; 34 Suppl 1: 3–5.
287. Sandler B, Aronson P. Yohimbine-induced cutaneous drug eruption, progressive renal failure and lupus-like syndrome. *Urology* 1993; 41: 343–345.
288. Robinson HN, Morison WL, Hood AF. Thiazide diuretic therapy and chronic photosensitivity. *Arch Dermatol* 1985; 121: 522–524.
289. Rappersberger K, Honigsmann H, Ortel B, Tanew A, Konrad K, Wolff K. Photosensitivity and hyperpigmentation in amiodarone-treated patients: incidence, time course, and recovery. *J Invest Dermatol* 1989; 93: 201–209.
290. Dereure O. Drug-induced skin pigmentation. Epidemiology, diagnosis and treatment. *Am J Clin Dermatol* 2001; 2(4): 253–262.
291. Riva E, Marchi S, Pesenli M, Bizzi A, Cini M, Veneroni E, et al. Amiodarone induced phospholipidosis. Biochemical, morphological, and functional changes in the lungs of rats chronically treated with amiodarone. *Biochem Pharmacol* 1987; 36: 3209–3214.

292. Shaik NA, Downar E, Butany J. Amiodarone — an inhibitor of phospholipase activity: a comparative study on the inhibitory effects of amiodarone, chloroquine, chlorpromazine. *Mol Cell Biochem* 1987; 76: 163–172.
293. Hostetler KY, Giordano JR, Jellison EJ. *In vitro* inhibition of lysosomal phospholipase A1 of rat lung by amiodarone and desethyl-amiodarone. *Biochim Biophys Acta* 1988; 959: 316–321.
294. What are the risk factors for gout? http://www.umm.edu/patiented/article/what_risk_factors _gout000093_5.htm. Accessed on September 9, 2004.
295. Nedorost ST, Stevens SR. Diagnosis and treatment of allergic skin disorders in the elderly. *Drugs Aging* 2001; 18: 827–835.
296. Arellano F, Sacristan JA. Allopurinol hypersensitivity syndrome: a review. *Ann Pharmacother* 1993; 27: 337–343.
297. Bastuji-Garin S, Rzany B, Stern RS, Shear NH, Naldi L, Roujeau JC. Clinical classification of cases of toxic epidermal necrolysis, Stevens-Johnson syndrome, and erythema multiforme. *Arch Dermatol* 1993; 129: 92–96.
298. Fritsch PO, Sidoroff A. Drug-induced Stevens-Johnson syndrome/toxic epidermal necrolysis. *Am J Clin Dermatol* 2000; 1: 349–360.

8 Skin Cancer in Pigmented Skins

Rebat M. Halder and Collette J. Ara

INTRODUCTION

When one thinks of skin cancer, the patient prototype is that of a fair-haired, fair-eyed individual of European decent. Skin cancer does occur in people of color, although the relative risk remains low. Because of increased pigmentation and melanosomal dispersion of the skin, people of color have added protection against the ultraviolet rays of the sun. The average natural sun protective factor (SPF) of black skin is approximately 13.1,[1] making sun-induced skin cancers less prevalent. Increased skin cancer rates can be attributed to childhood sun exposure, increased outdoor recreational activities (even during the winter, e.g., skiing), and destruction of the ozone layer. There is now a trend toward increased skin cancer rates in most ethnic groups. People of color have higher morbidity and mortality rates for several types of skin cancer as compared to white counterparts. This is probably secondary to late presentation and treatment. Certain types of skin cancer are more prevalent in whites as compared to other groups.

Blacks have an incidence of malignant melanoma 5 to 18 times less than whites, whereas Hispanics have a higher incidence than blacks. Hispanics have an incidence 3.5 to 4.5 times less than whites, according to one study.[2] Melanoma in non-sun-exposed skin, especially in palmar, plantar, and subungual areas, is most commonly seen in Asians, Native Americans, African and North American blacks. The acral lentiginous form of melanoma was once thought to be more commonly found in blacks than whites, but in more recent studies there was no significant difference found.[3]

AFRICAN-AMERICANS, AFRO-CARIBBEANS, AND AFRICANS

The most deadly skin cancer found in African-Americans is melanoma, specifically the acral lentiginous type. It has been commonly misdiagnosed and treated as a plantar wart, tinea nigra palmaris, or even, in some cases talon noir. According to a retrospective study at Tulane University School of Medicine from 1958 to 1990 in which 82 black patients with acral lentiginous melanoma were followed and treated by the surgical service,[4] there was a trend toward decreased survival observed in black males with this type of cancer. There was a strong relationship between decreased survival and increased Clark's level. The overall incidence of malignant melanoma in the black population is lower than that of whites, and this also include acral lentiginous melanoma, although this is the most common type seen in blacks (Figure 8.1).

Cancer incidence tabulation from western Washington state and metropolitan Atlanta between 1974 and 1984 found that plantar melanoma was 1.7 million per year for blacks and 2.0 million per year for whites. These data argue that in North America there is little difference between blacks and whites for this type of malignancy and that the perceived difference is due to the decreased incidence of melanoma on nonpalmar and nonplantar surfaces in blacks. The literature states that it is not less likely that acral lentiginous melanoma arises in a precursor nevus or dysplastic nevus, however there have been such cases in the literature. There are also other types of melanoma found in African-Americans, including nodular and superficial spreading types. However, acral lentiginous

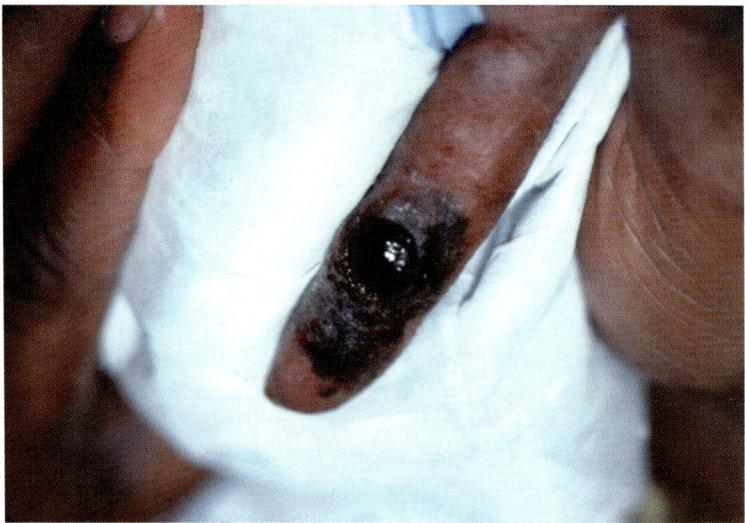

FIGURE 8.1 Nodular acral lentiginous melanoma in an African-American man. (Reproduced from Halder RM. *Dermatol Clin* 2003; 21: 725–732. With permission from Elsevier.)

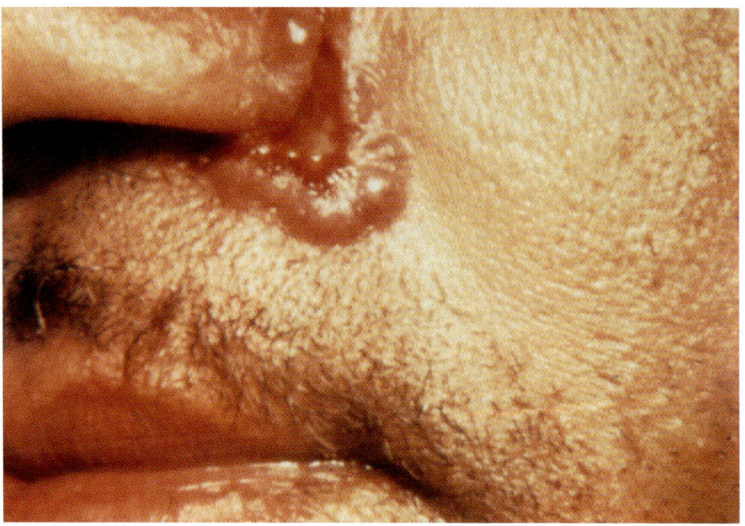

FIGURE 8.2 Basal cell carcinoma in a fair-skinned African-American man. (Reproduced from Halder RM. *Dermatol Clin* 2003; 21: 725–732. With permission from Elsevier.)

melanoma has a poor prognosis because of its deep invasion at time of presentation, with a 5-year survival rate of less than 50%.[3] There has been one reported case of a Spitz's nevus described in an 11-year-old African-American girl, which, as in any patient population, is a difficult lesion, both clinically and histologically.[5]

There are many studies in the literature that have reported that, for incidence of nonmelanoma skin cancer in blacks, squamous cell carcinoma is more prevalent than basal cell carcinoma (BCC). As in white patients, exposure to ultraviolet light is the major etiological factor in BCC. However, darker skin pigmentation protects against the adverse effects of UVB irradiation, which is thought to be the cause of skin cancer development.[1,6] The darker the pigmentation, the more protection is afforded. BCC in blacks occurs more commonly in those with fair skin (Figure 8.2). A history of previous radiation exposure or therapy, trauma, arsenic ingestion, nevus sebaceous, immunosuppression, basal

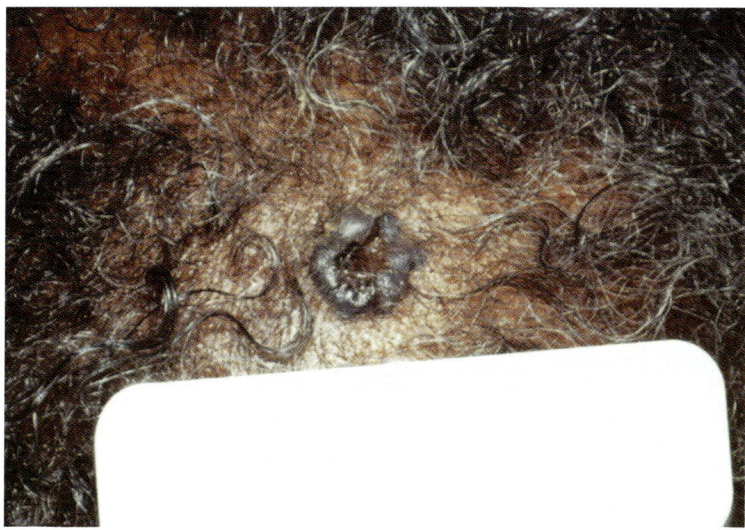

FIGURE 8.3 Pigmented basal cell carcinoma of the scalp in an African-American woman.

cell nevus syndrome, and long-term ulceration, especially in those with connective tissue disease, can predispose to developing BCC.[1] BCC in black patients may evolve from other causes. The literature shows that the BCCs found in blacks are more prevalent in women than in men and less common on the nose and trunk.[7] Presentation tends to be with older individuals, usually 50 years of age and above, but the prevalence of BCC in non-sun-exposed skin is equal between blacks and whites.[6]

There have been reports of different types of BCCs found in blacks that include a diverse presentation from superficial basal cell to perianal basal cell carcinoma to patients with multiple tumors.[8] Usually the BCC is of the pigmented type and may be diagnosed clinically as seborrheic keratosis or melanoma (Figure 8.3). The histopathology of many of these lesions has shown a positive correlation between the maximum depth of tumor invasion and the maximum diameter of the lesion. There have been BCCs that have arisen in scars and then have developed metastasis in black patients.[1] Morpheaform BCCs are an uncommon histological subtype found in African-American patients, but there has been a case in which an African-American female patient underwent Mohs micrographic surgery as the primary therapy for this tumor.[9] In another rare case, a report of an African-American male with dark complexion had a giant BCC infiltrating almost the entire scalp.[10] This patient also had widespread metastatic bone marrow involvement that produced a myelophthisic anemia. There was a case of a 70-year-old black man with a BCC that arose from a gunshot wound in his shoulder and metastasized to axillary lymph nodes.[11] The development of skin cancers in areas treated with x-ray for benign lesions is rare, but such cases have been reported in the literature. One was a case of a black male who developed two BCCs in the hair-covered scalp 3 decades after he had undergone epilation of the scalp by x-ray for treatment of tinea capitis.[12]

As previously stated, squamous cell carcinoma (SCC) is the most common skin cancer in African-Americans, with the majority found in non-sun-exposed areas. Contrary to the white population where SCC is primarily found in sun-exposed areas, the higher morbidity of SCC in black patients is due not to delayed diagnosis and treatment but also to the fact that SCC in non-sun-exposed areas are usually more biologically aggressive.[1]

In one study of African patients, the peak incidence for SCC of the skin was in the 40s age range, and the most commonly affected site was the lower limb, followed by the head and neck. The genital area was the third most commonly affected site. The scalp and the lip were more commonly affected in females than in males. Chronic trauma, chronic ulcers, scars, and albinism were the main predisposing risk factors for the lower limb and the scalp[13] (Figure 8.4). Ultraviolet

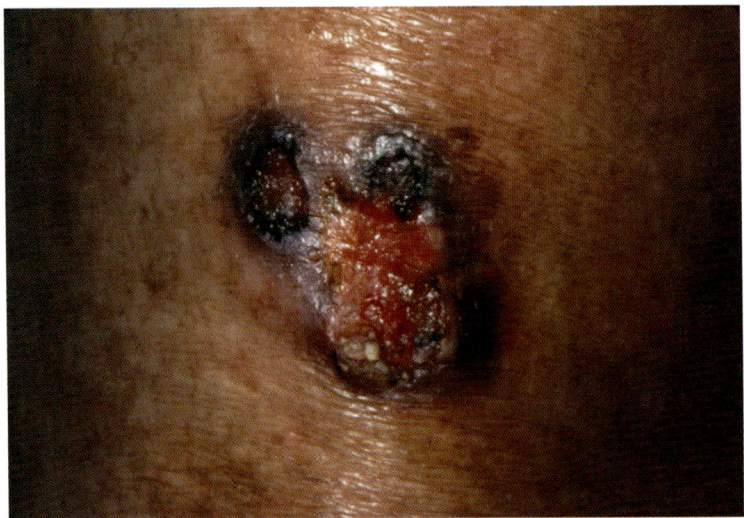

FIGURE 8.4 Squamous cell carcinoma in a chronic ulcer in an African-American woman.

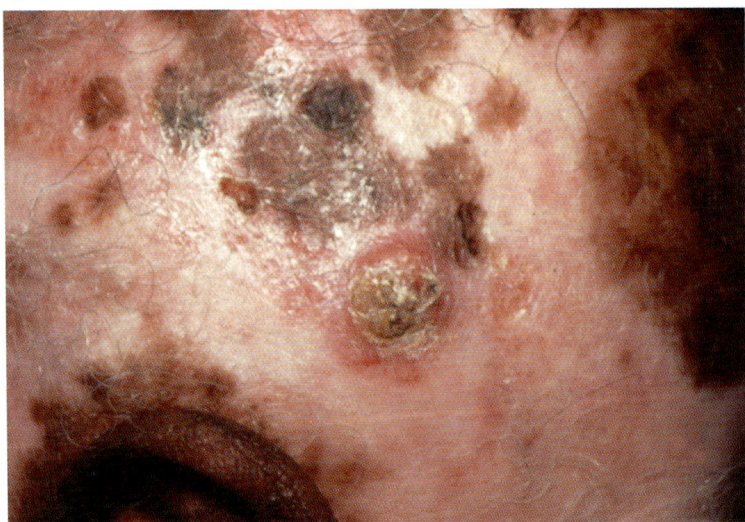

FIGURE 8.5 Squamous cell carcinoma in lesions of chronic discoid lupus erythematosus in an African-American woman. (Reproduced from Halder RM. *Dermatol Clin* 2003; 21: 725–732. With permission from Elsevier.)

radiation was the main predisposing risk factor for the head and neck. Smegma of the uncircumcised penis was thought to be a risk factor for most cases of SCC that developed on the penis.[13] Histologically, most cases of SCC on the penis were found to be SCC *in situ*.[14]

There have been many case reports cited in the literature in which SCC was noted to occur in scars of chronic discoid lupus erythematosus (DLE) in black patients (Figure 8.5). In a review it was found that there was an increased tendency of the cancer to metastasize in patients with DLE.[15] It was postulated that sun exposure of the hypopigmented lesions may have been one of the causative factors.

Bowen's disease in blacks clinically presents as nonspecific scaling, hyperkeratotic, pigmented lesions, some of which have been misdiagnosed as malignant melanoma. Bowen's disease will rarely show pigmentation outside the groin area in whites, but in blacks the nongenital lesions usually show pigmentation[1] (Figure 8.6). It affects black women twice as frequently as black men

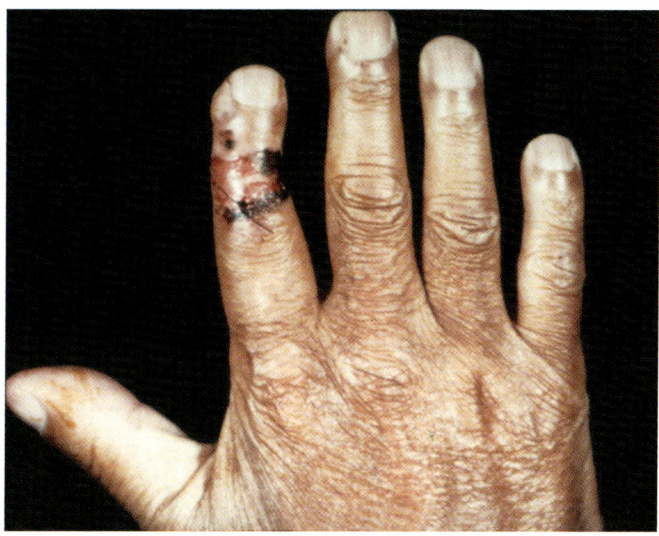

FIGURE 8.6 Pigmented Bowen's disease of the first finger in an African-American man.

and most commonly in non-sun-exposed skin.[16] Invasive disease did occur in five of 19 patients, and three died subsequently.[17] In a study done between 1942 and 1982, there was a series of 19 patients that had Bowen's disease, and lesions on non-sun-exposed skin occurred three times more commonly than on sun-exposed skin. The most common locations were the lower extremities.[17] When Bowen's disease occurs in blacks, it tends to present in an atypical fashion. There has been a report in the literature of a verrucous form of Bowen's disease occurring in a black patient.[18]

Dermatofibrosarcoma protuberans (DFSP) has a pigmented variant that is rare and accounts for 1%–5% of dermatofibrosarcomas. The pigmented variant is a multinodular spindled cell neoplasm of the dermis or subcutaneous tissue that occurs predominantly in blacks. It occurs primarily on the trunk and less frequently on upper and lower extremities and the head and neck. It may clinically resemble a keloid, so that those keloid-like lesions in blacks not occurring secondary to trauma or that demonstrate rapid growth necessitate biopsy[7] (Figure 8.7). Histologically, it is

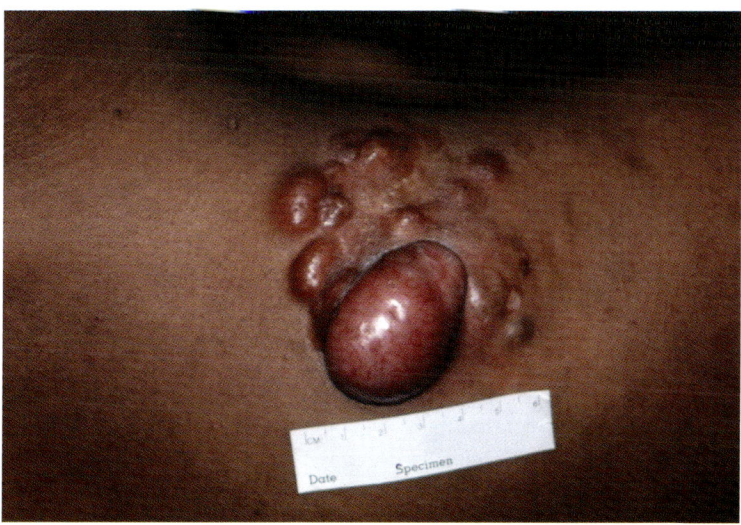

FIGURE 8.7 Dermatofibrosarcoma protuberans on the shoulder of an African-American man. (Courtesy of Beverly A. Johnson, M.D.)

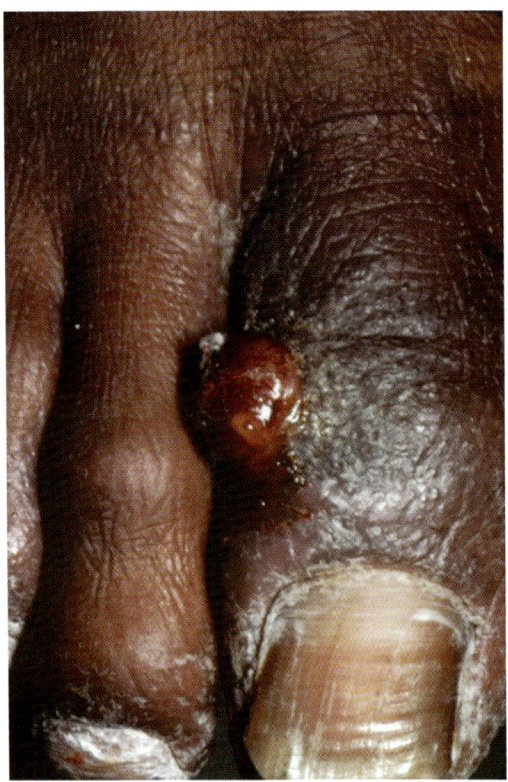

FIGURE 8.8 Kaposi's sarcoma appearing pyogenic granuloma-like on the foot of an African-American man with AIDS.

distinguished from the normal variant of DFSP by containing a small population of melanin-containing dendritic cells. These lesions have been considered variants of neurofibroma but are S-100 protein negative. They have a high local recurrence rate but distant metastasis has been noted. Surgical excision with close follow-up is indicated.

Kaposi's sarcoma, a malignant neoplastic process manifests as vascular tumors. It now occurs most commonly in immunocompromised patients with AIDS (Figures 8.8 and 8.9). The incidence of these tumors occurs in higher in proportion blacks compared to other races, and both blacks and men suffer relatively greater morbidity. Black patients with both AIDS and Kaposi's sarcoma tend to have more rapid disease progression.[16] There is a relative rarity of cutaneous cancers among African blacks but the predominance of Kaposi's sarcoma may be explained by the high prevalence of human immunodeficiency virus in Africa.[19]

Mycosis fungoides, a subset of cutaneous T-cell lymphoma, classically presented as erythematous and/or hyperpigmented patches and tumors in African-Americans, Afro-Caribbeans, and Africans (Figure 8.10). A newly recognized variant of mycosis fungoides, presenting as nonscaling hypopigmented patches in patients of African, Afro-Caribbean, African-American, Hispanic, and Asian descent, has recently been noted.[20] The latency period for diagnosis is usually about 6 years, and the mean age of diagnosis is about 34 years, which is an earlier onset than the nonhypopigmented variant. It tends to respond well to treatment with long remissions, with a tendency for relapse, which usually responds to another course of therapy. The lesions may clinically resemble tinea versicolor, generalized pityriasis alba, postinflammatory hypopigmentation, hypopigmented sarcoidosis, and vitiligo (Figures 8.11 and 8.12). The skin involvement is more central than acral and pruritus is commonly reported. Histopathological changes and cell marker studies show a relative loss of the CD7 antigen.[21]

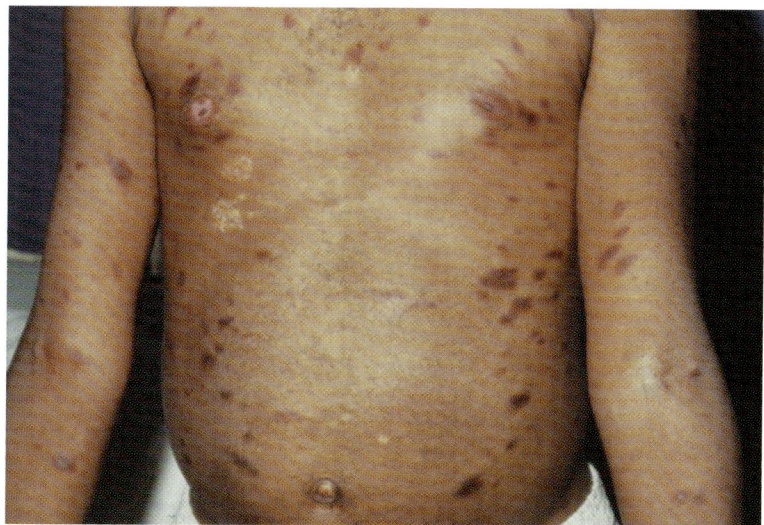

FIGURE 8.9 Generalized Kaposi's sarcoma in an African-American man with AIDS. (Courtesy of Beverly A. Johnson, M.D.)

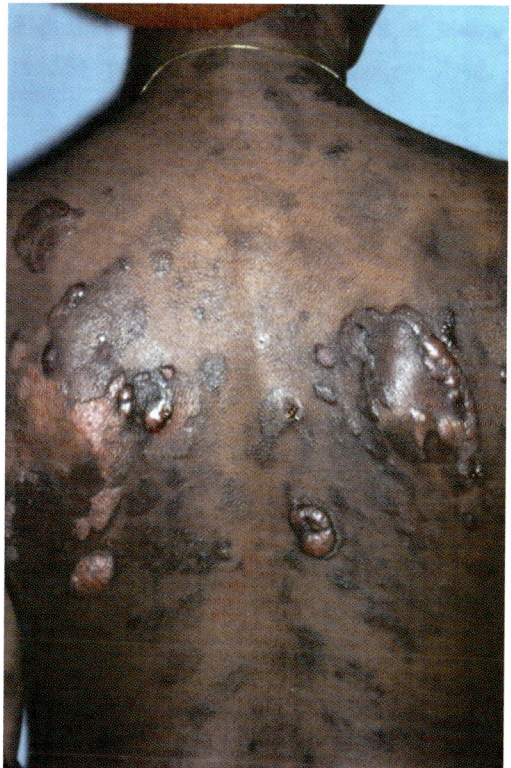

FIGURE 8.10 Tumor stage mycosis fungoides in an African woman.

There are atypical variants of skin cancer lesions that are reported to occur in black patients. Microcystic adnexal carcinoma is a relatively uncommon adnexal neoplasm that can display aggressive local invasion.[22] The central face is the most commonly affected area, and tumors have a benign appearance.[22] Granular cell tumors are uncommon tumors that are thought to be of Schwann cell

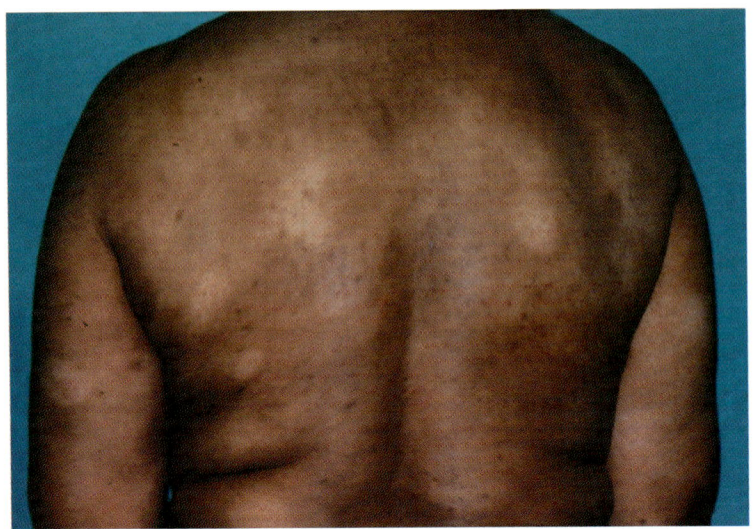

FIGURE 8.11 Hypopigmented mycosis fungoides in an African-American man.

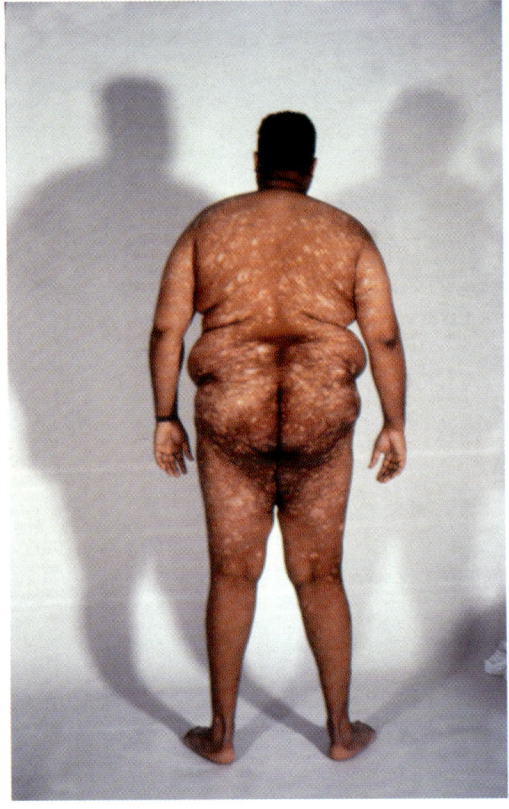

FIGURE 8.12 Generalized lesions of hypopigmented mycosis fungoides in an African-American man.

origin.[23] They clinically present as reddish-brown to flesh-colored papules, usually with a smooth surface and are occasionally pruritic or tender. They are usually benign tumors, but malignant variants have been reported, with blacks female being affected several times more often than whites.[23]

Merkel cell carcinoma has an annual age-adjusted incidence per 100,000 of 0.2 for whites and 0.01 for blacks. There is an increased incidence with sun exposure, with the face being the most common site.[24]

In mixed-race populations of South Africa that are composed of native African and Asian (predominantly East Indian) ancestry, the type and anatomical distribution of skin cancers reflect the disease pattern of black populations, but the overall 5-year survival rate was similar to that seen in white populations.[25]

HISPANICS

Malignant melanoma is the most prevalent form of skin cancer in Hispanics. One study postulated that Hispanic patients present with advanced disease because they do not consider themselves to be at risk for development of skin cancer, and they have a decreased tendency to burn.[26] Skin cancer awareness is usually directed toward white, non-Hispanic populations, with less emphasis on self-examination of the skin, sun protection and sun avoidance in Hispanics. In a descriptive analysis performed at Jackson Memorial Hospital in Miami, a total of 54 cases of melanoma in Hispanics was reviewed. Most of the lesions occurred on the trunk, arm, shoulder, leg, and hip. Interestingly, in this study Hispanic patients did better overall than the non-Hispanics in treatment outcome and survival.[27]

There was a comparison of incidence of melanoma in Hispanic vs. non-Hispanic Caucasian populations and in blacks done in a study between 1973 and 1981. The incidence among whites was 8.0 per 100,000, ten times that of U.S. blacks. The incidence among Hispanic patients from Puerto Rico and New Mexico was 1.6 to 3.7 times that of blacks. The anatomical distribution among New Mexico whites and New Mexico Hispanics were similar, even for both genders. The most common anatomical distribution of melanoma for Puerto Rican Hispanics was the leg, similar to that of U.S. blacks.[28] Another study noted that nearly half the tumors were located on the extremities, most notably on the feet, as seen in blacks and Japanese[29] (Figure 8.13). The most commonly recognized clinicohistologic type was superficial spreading melanoma, followed by acral lentiginous, nodular, and lentigo maligna melanoma.[29]

There was a report that cited three Hispanic patients with oculodermal melanocytosis and uveal melanoma who underwent enucleation.[30] Melanocanthoma is a rare lesion composed of the simultaneous benign proliferation of the keratinocyte and the melanocyte.[31] There are distinct clinical differences between mucosal and skin lesions. The skin lesions occur almost exclusively in older white patients. This is in contrast to the mucosal lesions that occur almost exclusively in black patients, and is associated with a history of traumatic irritation. The mucosal lesions usually develop rapidly after trauma, so some have thought it to be a reactive phenomenon rather than a true neoplasia.[31]

Pigmented basal cell carcinoma is a common neoplasm found in Hispanic patients. Because basal cell epitheliomas and carcinomas tend to be pigmented in Hispanics, they many times have been diagnosed clinically as melanoma[32,33] (Figure 8.14). A study that compared pigmented basal cell carcinoma in Hispanics to whites found the incidence to be twice as frequent in Hispanics.[32] A skin cancer registry in New Mexico between 1964 and 1992 found an average of 2.2 lesions per person in Hispanics, of which BCC was 6.6 times more common than SCC.[34] The incidence of nonmelanoma skin cancers increased with age, and rates were higher for non-Hispanic males than females, although Hispanics in general had much lower rates than non-Hispanic whites, with no sex difference.[34] When BCC does occur in Hispanics, it presents with multiple or subsequent lesions as compared to SCC, which usually has only one primary site. The subsequent lesions of BCC were diagnosed within 1 year of the first presenting lesion, and new lesions continued to present for more than 10 years.[34]

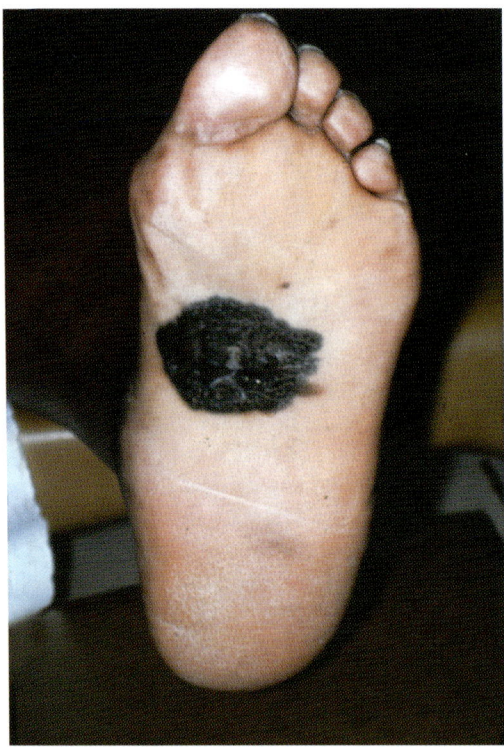

FIGURE 8.13 Melanoma on the sole of the foot in a Hispanic man.

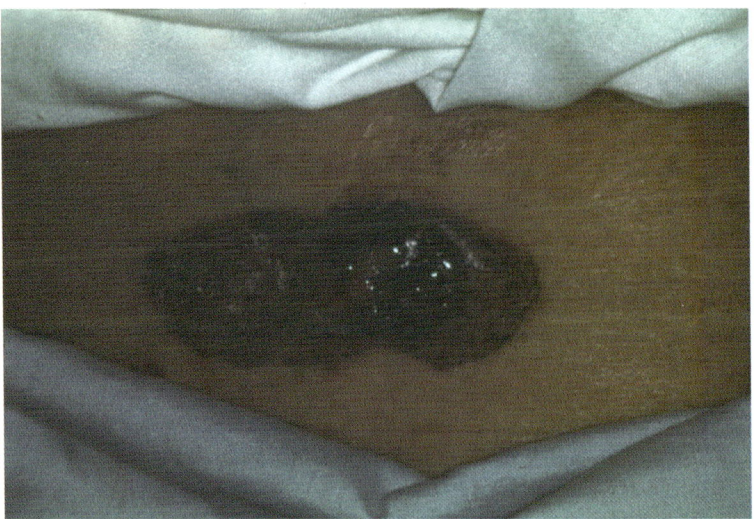

FIGURE 8.14 Pigmented basal cell carcinoma on the abdomen of a Hispanic woman.

A study done in native Puerto Ricans with nonmelanoma skin cancer to measure DNA repair found that these patients had a lower DNA repair capacity from ultraviolet light. The authors concluded that UV radiation is a risk factor for nonmelanoma skin cancer in native Puerto Ricans.[35]

As with other patients of skin of color, mycosis fungoides usually presents with either erythematous or hypopigmented patches; however, Hispanic patients usually compare with white patient populations with respect to morbidity and mortality (Figure 8.15). A study from New Mexico found

Skin Cancer in Pigmented Skins

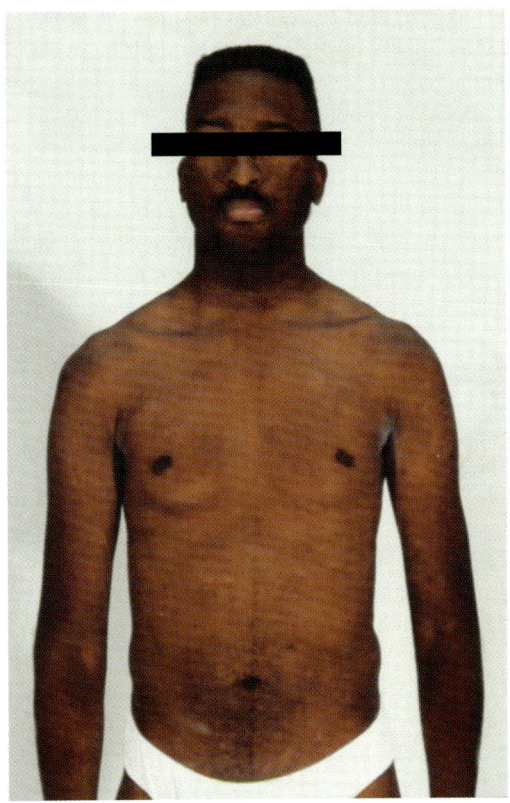

FIGURE 8.15 Generalized lesions of hypopigmented mycosis fungoides in a dark-skinned Puerto Rican man.

that the incidence of leukemias, mycosis fungoides, and lymphomas was comparable among the three dominant ethnic groups: Native Americans, Hispanics, and non-Hispanic white patients.[34]

ASIANS

A study was done in Kasai City in 1992 to characterize the prevalence and incidence of skin cancer in Japanese patients. A high prevalence rate of actinic keratosis was noted most likely secondary to UVB radiation exposure. Sunscreen application did decrease incidence after proper patient education.[36]

In Asians, the plantar surface is the most common site for cutaneous melanoma, and the most common type of melanoma arising in this region is the acral lentiginous type. There have been other types noted, as described in a rare case of superficial spreading melanoma arising in a longstanding melanocytic nevus on the sole of a Korean patient.[37] A study in Taiwan described the incidence rates of different types of melanoma found in the Taiwanese patient populations. Acral lentiginous melanoma was the most common type (54%), followed by nodular melanoma (about 30%), superficial spreading melanoma, and lentigo maligna melanoma.[38] During the study certain patterns were noted. The overall survival of melanoma revealed that age of onset greater than 55 years, male gender, ulceration of tumor, and tumor thickness were contributory factors toward poorer prognosis.[38] They concluded that histologic subtypes other than acral lentiginous melanoma with advanced stages (III and IV) had a poorer prognosis.[38]

Another study indicates that in Japan, sun-exposed SCC may be relatively less involved with p53 mutation and that non-sun-exposed SCC acquires more genetic alterations than sun-exposed SCC.[39] Melanomas found in many Japanese patients had tetraploid mutations not caused by p53 mutations or deletion. This suggests that there is no positive relationship between tetraploidy and poorer prognosis. The mutational loss of the p53 gene might be a marker of aggressive forms of malignant forms of melanoma.[40]

In a study of the non-Caucasian population of Hawaii, which is composed primarily of ethnic Japanese and Chinese, the incidence of malignant melanoma was not substantially different from that of the remainder of the United States.[41] In that study melanoma, although unusual, was not rare. Although lesions on the palms and soles were more common, as were subungual melanomas, primary tumors on other skin sites accounted for the majority of patients in the non-Caucasian population of Hawaii. The substantial difference in primary tumor thickness suggested that the poorer outcomes for non-Caucasian patients with cutaneous melanoma may be explained, at least in part, by a delay in diagnosis.[41]

Little is known of the incidence of Spitz nevus on palmar surfaces. The Japanese literature noted the incidence to be about 2% with the mean age of 17.8 years, and all four of the cases were women.[42] On clinical examination, these were black macules or small elevated nodules extending from 3.5 to 8.0 mm in size. The backs of the hands and insteps have almost the same incidence as that of the palms and sole; however, it is still a rare tumor on the palms and soles.[42] A rare case of leptomeningeal melanomatosis that was associated with multiple cutaneous pigmented nevi was reported in an Asian.[43]

Nevus of Ota is a congenital pigmentary disorder usually involving the parts of the face supplied by the first and second branches of the trigeminal nerve. Ipsilateral ocular melanosis is usually associated in about two thirds of the cases, and its occurrence is highest among Asians. Malignant transformation of nevus of Ota has been found in the literature, mostly in the Caucasian population. There have been only four cases of melanomas associated with nevus of Ota with ocular melanosis that have been described.[44] One of the cases involved a man who had this melanoma without ocular melanosis, but the location of the tumor to the orbital apex and its extension to the sphenocavernous area were responsible for ipsilateral loss of vision without proptosis.[44] This finding has not been previously found in any case of nevus of Ota without ocular melanosis.

There have been multiple reports in the Japanese literature of patients with hyperkeratotic papular porokeratosis palmaris et plantaris disseminata who developed multiple squamous cell carcinomas on the lesional sites of the palms and soles.[45] There was a family history of hyperkeratotic papules found in most cases. There were nine squamous cell carcinomas that developed in a Japanese woman with linear porokeratosis, arranged linearly with the tumor arising on the left side of the body. This would represent a type 2 segmental manifestation of disseminated superficial porokeratosis that showed a systemized pattern of involvement and pronounced susceptibility to developing into a malignancy.[46]

Basal cell carcinomas and Bowen's disease are predominantly pigmented in Asians. Because of their pigmented clinical appearance, many of these lesions have been diagnosed and treated as malignant melanoma.[47]

Nonmelanoma skin cancer is uncommon but not rare among the Chinese population of Hong Kong. The incidence of basal cell carcinoma among this population in 1990 and 1999 was 0.32 and 0.92 per 100,000, respectively, whereas that of squamous cell carcinoma was 0.16 and 0.34 per 100,000, respectively.[47] Pigmented basal cell carcinoma was the most common type of nonmelanoma skin cancer, about 60%, in Chinese patients during this study, in contrast to rodent ulceration in Caucasians.[47] Multiple skin cancers, recurrences, and subsets of new skin cancers were less frequently seen in the Chinese group than in the Caucasian group.

A study conducted to examine time trends and ethnic differences among Asians in Singapore found that from 1968 to 1977 the incidence of basal cell carcinoma increased 3% annually, melanoma remained constant, and squamous cell carcinoma decreased 0.9% annually.[48] Basal cell carcinoma age-standardized incidence rates were highest among Chinese, then Malays and last, Indians. A similar pattern was noted for squamous cell carcinoma and melanoma. The incidence rates of skin cancer increased in Singapore during the period 1968–1997, with fairer-skinned Chinese having a higher incidence.

Merkel cell carcinoma is a rare neoplasm in Asians, but there have been case reports that have shown its association with other skin cancers, such as Bowen's disease. There was a case of an 85-year-old Japanese woman who developed hyponatremia after excision of the tumor from her left cheek, which was considered to be an incidental finding most likely caused by postoperative stress and indapamide.[49] The histopathology showed characteristics of both Merkel cell carcinoma and Bowen's disease.

As with other patients of skin of color, the hypopigmented form of mycosis fungoides is prevalent in Asians and is characterized by early onset and good response to therapy but with high recurrence rates.[50]

NATIVE AMERICANS

All forms of skin cancer are uncommon among Native Americans. As with other skins of color, the subtype of malignant melanoma presenting predominantly with predilection for palms, soles, and subungual locations is most common.[51] Because of late detection, advanced disease states are commonly found at the time of initial presentation in Native Americans.

As with Hispanic patients, the incidence of nonmelanoma skin cancers among Native American New Mexico residents was that BCC was higher than SCC, but was much less prevalent when compared with New Mexico whites.[34] Basal cell carcinomas in Native Americans tend to be pigmented.

PUBLIC HEALTH ISSUES FOR SKIN CANCER IN PIGMENTED SKINS

There is a need for patients of skin of color to be educated toward a better understanding of factors that improve sun protection practices which will lead to a decrease in prevalence of skin cancer. Use of sunscreen and protective clothing and shade-seeking, especially during the peak sun hours from 10 a.m. to 2 p.m., should be emphasized. There have been studies done to estimate the risk of skin cancer in blacks as a function of average annual surface levels of UVB radiation.[52]

Sun exposure is an increasing etiologic factor for patients of skin of color, but little is known of their sun-protection behavior. About 6% of African-Americans have reported to be extremely sensitive to the sun and experience severe sunburn, and 9% reported mild burning, according to one study.[53] Fifty-three percent of subjects (47% men and 57% women) reported that they were likely to wear protective clothing, seek shade, or use sunscreen lotion.[53] Educational background, history of sun burning, and age association contributed to better sun protection with sunscreen lotions.[53] More education about sun protection and early detection by routine skin examinations would help to reduce the morbidity and mortality of skin cancer in people of color.

Acral lentiginous melanoma is the prevalent form of melanoma in people of color, with a poor prognosis secondary to late diagnosis and, therefore, treatment. Squamous cell carcinoma is the prevalent form of nonmelanoma skin cancer in people of color. The pigmented form of basal cell cancer is found more commonly. Although most physicians do not immediately associate skin cancer with people of color, it does formidably exist. The approach to skin self-examination (SSE) and skin cancer prevention does differ among racial groups. Caucasians and Hispanics are more likely than African-Americans to report having used a sunscreen.[54] Caucasians perform SSE more frequently than Hispanics. African-Americans performed SSE as frequently as Hispanics,[54] but follow-up in African-Americans by a dermatologist was less prevalent.

In general, little is known about awareness of skin cancer, risk perception, and performance of SSE by people with skin that rarely burns.[55] In a study by Pipitone et al., these factors were studied in a Hispanic vs. non-Hispanic white population.[55] Hispanic individuals reported decreased skin sensitivity and tendency to burn. They believed that they were at average or below-average risk for skin cancer. None reported ever being taught SSE. Fifteen percent of Hispanics had performed SSE within the last year, compared with 32% of non-Hispanics. The authors conclude that people without sun sensitivity did not perceive themselves as being at risk, did not learn the warning signs of skin cancer, and did not perform SSE. Awareness of melanoma and nonmelanoma skin cancer and perception of risk among patients of skin of color is less than that among Caucasians, which may contribute to presentation of care at an advanced stage.[55]

Indeed, the incidence rates for both melanoma and nonmelanoma skin cancer will continue to rise in patients of skin of color due to factors such as the decreased ozone layer and more participation in recreational activities (golf, tennis, water and snow skiing, sunbathing) that have been previously practiced primarily by Caucasians. These factors will play a more important part in the pathogenesis of skin cancer in pigmented skins. They are an addition to factors that have been discussed in this chapter that predispose certain racial and ethnic groups to developing certain skin cancers. SSE is becoming very important for people with pigmented skins and should be taught to all patients, regardless of skin color. This awareness is an essential public health education issue.

REFERENCES

1. Johnson BL, Moy R, White GM. *Ethnic Skin: Medical and Surgical.* Toronto: Mosby, 1998.
2. Kalter DC, Goldberg LH, Rosen T. Darkly pigmented lesions in dark-skinned patients. *J Dermatol Surg Oncol* 1984; 10(11): 876–881.
3. Stevens NG, Liff JM, Weiss NS. Plantar melanoma: is the incidence of melanoma of the sole of foot really higher in blacks than whites? *Int J Cancer* 1990; 45(4): 691–693.
4. Sutherland CM, Mather FJ, Muchmore JH, Carter RD, Reed RJ. Acral lentiginous melanoma. *Am J Surg* 1993; 166(1): 64–67.
5. Bovenmyer DA. Spitz's nevus in a black child. *Cutis* 1981; 28(2): 186–188.
6. Chorum L, Norris JE, Gupta M. Basal cell carcinoma in blacks: a report of 15 cases. *Ann Plast Surg* 1994; 33(1): 90–95.
7. Abreo F, Sanusi ID. Basal cell carcinoma in North American blacks. Clinical and histopathologic study of 26 patients. *J Am Acad Dermatol* 1992; 27(5 Pt 1): 787–788.
8. Kaidbey KH, Agin PP, Sayre RM, Kligman AM. Photoprotection by melanin — a comparison of black and Caucasian skin. *J Am Acad Dermatol* 1979; 1(3): 249–260.
9. Lesher JL Jr, d'Aubermont PC, Brown VM. Morpheaform basal cell carcinoma in a young black woman. *J Dermatol Surg Oncol* 1988; 14(2): 200–203.
10. Schwartz RA, De Jager RL, Janniger CK, Lambert WC. Giant basal cell carcinoma with metastases and myelophthisic anemia. *J Surg Oncol* 1986; 33(4): 223–226.
11. Lambert WC, Kasznica J, Chung HR, Moore D. Metastasizing basal cell carcinoma developing in a gunshot wound in a black man. *J Surg Oncol* 1984; 27(2): 97–105.
12. Walther RR, Grossman ME, Troy JL. Basal-cell carcinomas on the scalp of a black patient many years after epilation by x-rays. *J Dermatol Surg Oncol* 1981; 7(7): 570–571.
13. Amir H, Mbonde MP, Kitinya JN. Cutaneous squamous cell carcinoma in Tanzania. *Cent Afr J Med* 1992; 38(11): 439–443.
14. Hubbell CR, Rabin VR, Mora RG. Cancer of the skin in blacks. V. A review of 175 black patients squamous cell carcinoma of the penis. *J Am Acad Dermatol* 1988; 18(2 Pt 1): 292–298.
15. Caruso WR, Stewart ML, Nanda VK, Quismorio FP Jr. Squamous cell carcinoma of the skin in black patients with discoid lupus erythematosus. *J Rheumatol* 1987; 14(1): 156–159.
16. Halder RM, Bang KM. Skin cancer in blacks in the United States. *Dermatol Clin* 1988; 6(3): 397–405.
17. Mora RG, Perniciaro C, Lee B. Cancer of the skin in blacks. III. A review of nineteen black patients with Bowen's disease. *J Am Acad Dermatol* 1984; 11(4 Pt 1): 557–562.
18. Schamroth JM, Weiss RM, Grieve TP. Verrucous Bowen's disease in a black patient. A case report. *S Afr Med J* 1987; 71(8): 527–528.

19. Barro-Traore F, Traore A, Konate I, et. al. Epidemiological features of tumors of the skin and mucosal membranes in the department of dermatology at the Yalgado Ouedraogo National Hospital, Quagadougou, Burkina Faso. *Sante* 2003; 13: 101–104.
20. Stone ML, Styles AR, Cockerell CJ, Pandya AG. Hypopigmented mycosis fungoides: a report of 7 cases and review of the literature. *Cutis* 2001; 67(2): 133–138.
21. Whitmore SE, Simmon-O'Brien E, Rotter FS. Hypopigmented mycosis fungoides. *Arch Dermatol* 1994; 130(4): 476–480.
22. Peterson CM, Ratz JL, Sangueza OP. Microcystic adenexal carcinoma: first reported case in an African-American man. *J Am Acad Dermatol* 2001; 45(2): 283–285.
23. Peters JS, Crowe MA. Granular cell tumor of the toe. *Cutis* 1998; 62(3): 147–148.
24. Miller RW, Rabkin CS. Merkel cell carcinoma and melanoma: etiological similarities and differences. *Cancer Epidermiol Biomarkers Prev* 1999; 8(2): 153–158.
25. Swan MC, Thidson DA. Malignant melanoma in South Africans of mixed ancestry: a retospective analysis. *Melanoma Res* 2003; 13: 415–419.
26. Pipitone M, Robinson JK, Camara C, Chittineni B, Fisher SG. Skin cancer awareness in suburban employees: a Hispanic perspective. *J Am Acad Dermatol* 2002; 47(1): 118–123.
27. Feun LG, Raub WA Jr, Duncan RC. Melanoma in a southeastern Hispanic population. *Cancer Detect Prev* 1994; 18(2): 145–152.
28. Bergfelt L, Newell GR, Sider JG, Kripke ML. Incidence and anatomic distribution of cutaneous melanoma among United States Hispanics. *J Surg Oncol* 1989; 40(4): 222–226.
29. Vazquez-Botet M, Latoni D, Sanchez JL. Malignant melanoma in Puerto Rico. *Bol Assoc Med PE* 1990; 82(10): 454–457.
30. Infante de German-Ribon R, Singh AD, Arevalo JF. Choroidal melanoma with oculodermal melanocytosis in Hispanic patients. *Am J Ophthalmol* 1999; 128(2): 251–253.
31. Goode RK, Crawford BE, Callihan MD, Neville BW. Oral melanoacanthoma. Review of the literature and report of cases. *Oral Surg Oral Med Oral Pathol* 1983; 56(6): 622–628.
32. Bigler C, Feldman J, Hall E, Padilla RD. Pigmented basal cell carcinoma in Hispanics. *J Am Acad Dermatol* 1996; 34(5 Pt 1): 751–752.
33. White EA, Rabinovitz HS, Greene RS, Olivero M, Kopf A. Pigmented basal carcinoma in a burn scar. *Cutis* 2003; 71: 404–406.
34. Hoy WE. Nonmelanoma skin carcinoma in Albuquerque, New Mexico: experience of a major health care provider. *Cancer* 1996; 77(12): 2489–2495.
35. Matta JL, Villa JL, Ramos JM, Sanchez J, Chompre G, Ruiz A, Grossman L. DNA repair and nonmelanoma skin cancer in Puerto Rican populations. *J Am Acad Dermatol* 2003; 49: 433–439.
36. Araki K, Nagano T, Ueda M, Kwahio F, Watanabe S, Yamaguchi N, Ichihashi M. Incidence of skin cancers and precancerous lesions in Japanese, risk factors and prevention. *J Epidemiol* 1999; 9(6 Suppl): S14–S21.
37. Cho K, Han KH, Minn KW. Superficial spreading melanoma arising in a longstanding melanocytic nevus on the sole. *J Dermatol* 1998; 25(5): 337–340.
38. Chen YJ, Wu CY, Chen JT, Shen JL, Chen CC, Wang HC. Clinicopathologic analysis of malignant melanoma in Taiwan. *J Am Acad Dermatol* 1999; 41(6): 945–949.
39. Hayashi M, Tamura G, Kato N, Ansai S, Kondo S, Motoyama T. Genetic analysis of cutaneous squamous cell carcinomas arising from different areas. *Pathol Int* 2003; 53: 602–607.
40. Satoh S, Hashimoto-Tamaoki T, Furuyama J, Mihara K, Namba M. High frequency of tetraploidy detected in malignant melanoma in Japanese patients by fluorescence *in situ* hybridization. *Int J Oncol* 2000; 17(4): 707–715.
41. Johnson, DS, Yamane S, Morita S, Yonehara C, Wong JH. Malignant melanoma in non-Caucasians: experience from Hawaii. *Surg Clin North Am* 2003; 83: 275–282.
42. Banba K, Fujioka A, Takasu H, Ishibashi A, Ohta M. Spitz nevus on the palmar surface. *J Dermatol* 2000; 27(5): 333–336.
43. Oka H, Kameya T, Hata T, Kawano N, Fujii K, Yada K. Leptomeningeal melanomatosis with multiple cutaneous pigmented nevi: tumor cell proliferation and malignant transformation in an autopsy case. *J Neurooncol* 1999; 44(1): 41–45.
44. Reichert S, Berrod JP, Rozot P, Schmutz JL. Melanoma developed on nevus of Ota without ocular melanoma. Apropos of an anatomo-clinical case. *J Fr Ophtalmol* 1996; 19(5): 389–394.

45. Seishima M, Izumi T, Oyama Z, Maeda M. Squamous cell carcinoma arising from lesions of porokeratosis palmaris et plantaris disseminata. *Eur J Dermatol* 2000; 10(6): 478–480.
46. Murata Y, Kumano K, Takai T. Type 2 segmental manifestation of disseminated superficial porokeratosis showing a systematized pattern of involvement among pronounced cancer proneness. *Eur J Dermatol* 2001; 11(3): 191–194.
47. Cheng SY, Luk NM, Chong LY. Special features of non-melanoma skin cancer in Hong Kong Chinese patients: 10-year retrospective study. *Hong Kong Med J* 2001; 7(1): 22–28.
48. Koh D, Wang H, Lee J, Chia KS, Lee HP, Goh CL. Basal cell carcinoma, squamous cell carcinoma and melanoma of the skin: analysis of the Singapore Cancer Registry data 1968–1997. *Br J Dermatol* 2003; 148: 1161–1166.
49. Anzai S, Sato T, Takayasu S, Asada Y, Terashi H, Takasaki S. Postoperative hyponatremia in a patient with ACTH-producing Merkel cell carcinoma. *J Dermatol* 2000; 27(6): 397–400.
50. Akaraphanth R, Douglass MC, Lim HW. Hypopigmented mycosis fungoides: treatment and a 6(1/2)-year follow-up of 9 patients. *J Am Acad Dermatol* 2000; 42(1 Pt 1): 33–39.
51. Black WC, Wiggin C. Melanoma among southwestern American Indians. *Cancer* 1985; 55(12): 2899–2902.
52. Pennello G, Devesa S, Gail M. Association of surface ultraviolet B radiation levels with melanoma and nonmelanoma skin cancer in United States blacks. *Cancer Epidemiol Biomarkers Prev* 2000; 9(3): 291–297.
53. Hall HI, Rogers JD. Sun protection behaviors among African-Americans. *Ethn Dis* 1999; 9(1): 126–131.
54. Friedman LC, Bruce S, Weinberg AD, Cooper HP, Yen AH, Hill M. Early detection of skin cancer: racial/ethnic differences in behaviors and attitudes. *J Cancer Educ* 1994; 9(2): 105–110.
55. Pipitone M, Robinson JK, Canara C, Chittineni B, Fisher SG. Skin awareness in suburban employees: a Hispanic perspective. *J Am Acad Dermatol* 2002; 47: 118–123.

9 Intrinsic Skin Aging in Pigmented Races

Monte O. Harris

INTRODUCTION

Never before have so many people lived for so long. Life expectancy has nearly doubled over the last century, with individuals expecting and almost demanding to be productive well into their eighth decade. At the onset of the 21st century, there is an unprecedented quest for wellness in conjunction with maintaining youthful vigor and appearance.

Our faces serve as a primary interface with society and, for better or worse, herald the visible stigmata of growing old. Changes in the face attributed to aging reflect a complex interplay between the nature and position of skin, subcutaneous soft tissues, and the bony facial skeleton. Individuals exhibit signs of facial aging at variable rates; however, the overall progression is believed to be consistent for all individuals. Interactions between intrinsic and extrinsic factors ultimately determine the timing of clinical changes seen in the aging face. Intrinsic factors are uncontrollable, largely determined by heredity and genetics, whereas extrinsic factors relate to environmental exposure, health, and lifestyle. Facial structure and skin pigment as determined by racial background are considered intrinsic. Extrinsic factors tend to be more controllable, influenced by individual habits such as sun exposure, cigarette smoking, diet, and exercise.

People with skin of color constitute a heterogeneous group of races whose skin is of darker pigmentation when compared with individuals of Northern European descent. These pigmented populations include individuals of African, Asian, Latino, Arabic, Mediterranean, and Indian descent. Because of frequent migrations of ethnic groups throughout the continents, racially mixed populations are increasingly commonplace. Individuals with skin of color are by far the fastest-growing segment of the American population. Currently, one third of the U.S. population is non-Caucasian, and predictions indicate that more than 50% of the population will be non-Caucasian by the year 2050.

GENERAL CONSIDERATIONS

The overwhelming majority of literature pertaining to the aging face has traditionally featured the Caucasian patient. Likewise, conventional facial rejuvenation procedures have been fashioned from a Northern European aging face reference point. Currently, there are a number of unanswered questions with regard to the progression of aging in darker-skinned individuals. Is the process of facial aging the same for people with skin of color when compared to the Caucasian model? Second, if changes occur, at what point in the overall facial aging process do they arise? Last, is there a morphological basis for the differences, if they exist? Although much is understood regarding the intrinsic photoprotective role of skin color, there is a paucity of literature discussing the relationship between facial morphology in darker-pigmented people and the aging face. It has been commonly accepted that individuals with skin of color exhibit less severe facial aging when compared to their lighter-complexioned counterparts. This concept is unchallenged if facial aging is addressed from the singular perspective of cutaneous photodamage. When taking into account features of aging such as fat atrophy and gravitational soft tissue redistribution, people with skin of color have a tendency toward premature aging in some areas and delayed aging in others (Figure 9.1).

ANTHROPOLOGIC CONSIDERATIONS AND FACIAL CHARACTERISTICS

People with skin of color show a marked diversity of facial shapes. Frequently, there is gross evidence of mixed ethnic heritage, with facial structure blended from each of the racial components (Figure 9.2). The literature defines most facial differences among ethnic groups, based upon anthropologic studies of young adults. Apart from skin color and hair, the most defining characteristics of pigmented people lie in the morphology of the eyes, nose, and lips. Anthropologic studies have elucidated variations in facial structure for individuals with skin of color, particularly those of Asian, Latino, and African descent, when compared with Caucasian standards.[1–5] These observations serve as the foundation for understanding the impact of facial morphology on the progression of facial aging.

ASIAN MORPHOLOGY

Asian is an inclusive term describing individuals from a wide variety of ethnically similar groups including Chinese, Korean, Japanese, Thai, Malaysian, Filipino, and Polynesian. The Asian face is characterized by increased bizygomatic distance and relative deficiency of the maxilla, creating a flat image with protruding zygomas and a shallow midface.[2] Le et al. reported that horizontal anthropologic measurements were significantly greater in the faces of Asians when compared with those of their Caucasian counterparts.[2] The dominant characteristics of the Asian face are a wider intercanthal distance in relation to a shorter palpebral fissure, a much wider soft nose within wide facial contours, a smaller mouth width, and a lower face smaller than the forehead height.[2] Wide prominent mandibular angles are often noted, which accentuates a square facial shape.

LATINO MORPHOLOGY

The modern-day Latino population is one of mixed heritage with ethnic contributions from the indigenous Americas, Europe, and Africa. Despite multiethnic lineage, common features of the Latino face include an increased bizygomatic distance, bimaxillary protrusion, and higher convexity angle compared with the Caucasian, giving the face a broad appearance with a somewhat rounded profile.[6] Caribbean Latino anthropometric indexes tend to reflect African-American values as a result of racial admixture introduced by the trans-Atlantic slave trade.[4] South American Latinos show greater similarity to Caucasian norms.[4] Central American indexes typically fall somewhere in between.[4] Swlerenga et al. evaluated cephalometric differences between adult Mexican-American, African-American, and white patients.[7] The overall skeletal trend of Mexican-Americans was a longer maxillary and mandibular length than African-American or Caucasian men and a flatter mandibular plane.[7] Mexican-American women, similar to African-American women, are slightly more maxillary protrusive than Caucasian women.[7] The incidence of microgenia is higher than in the Caucasian population.

AFRICAN-AMERICAN MORPHOLOGY

African-Americans are individuals of remote African ancestry who were born in North America. The ethnic origins of the African-American population are linked to the trans-Atlantic slave trade of the 17th and 18th centuries. Facial features of modern-day African-Americans commonly reflect a multicultural ancestry resulting from generations of racial admixture in the United States.

Significant differences exist between average Caucasian and African-American facial features.[3] When compared with Caucasians, the average African-American profile shows bimaxillary protrusion,

Intrinsic Skin Aging in Pigmented Races 199

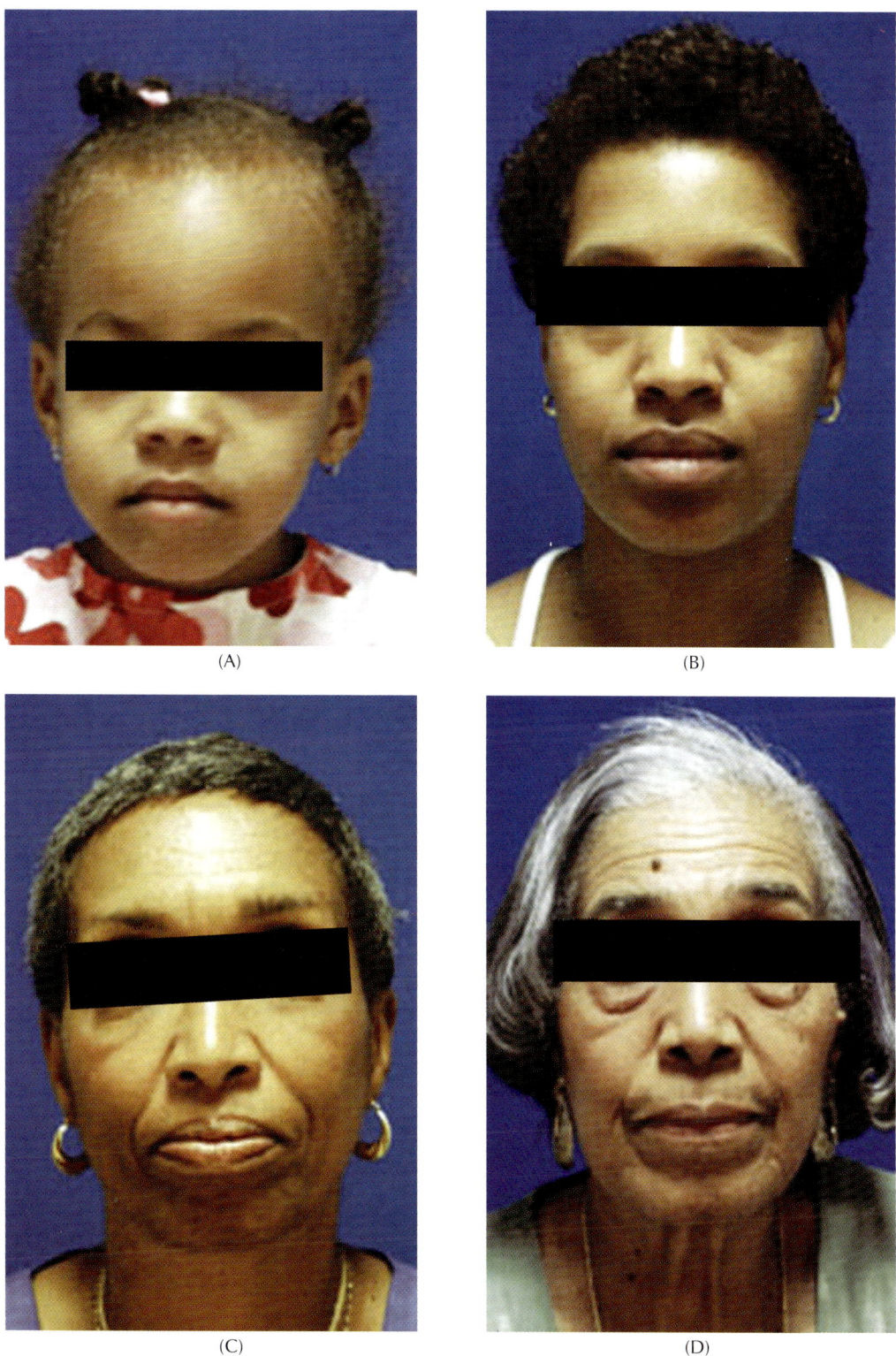

FIGURE 9.1 Progression of facial aging in African-American family across four generations, ages 2, 34, 56, and 80 (A–D, respectively). Note the pronounced nature of eye and midface aging in contrast to a relatively preserved jaw line with the absence of jowling (C,D).

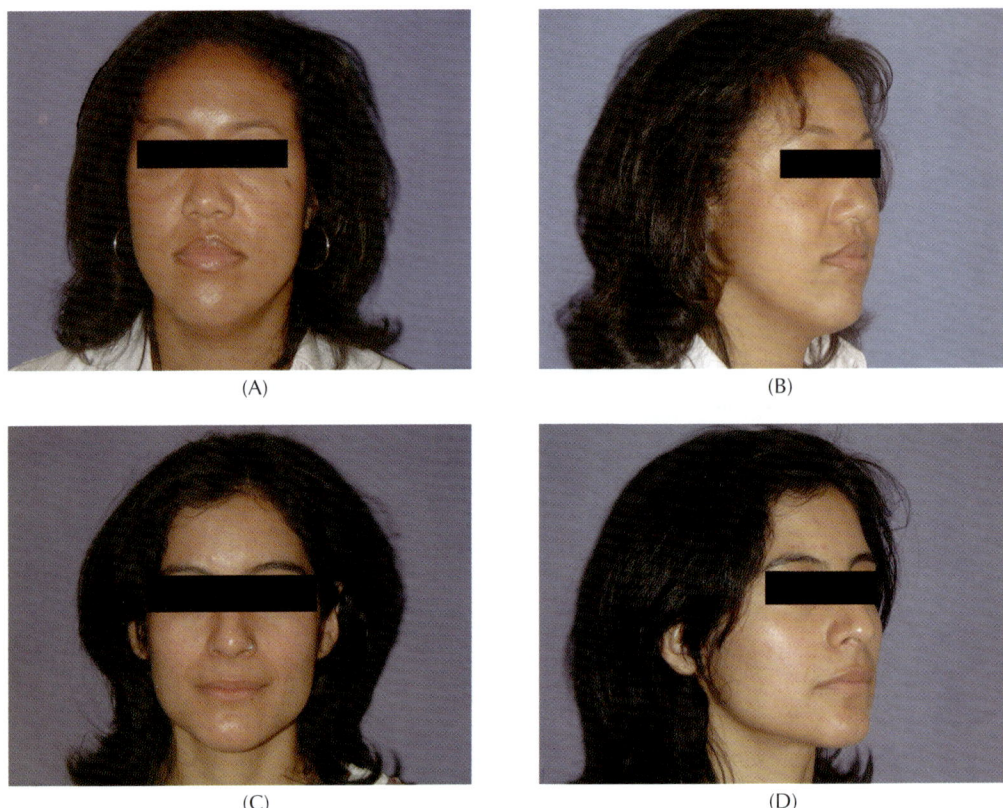

FIGURE 9.2 Individuals of mixed ethnic heritage with facial features blended from each racial component. (A,B) Forty-two-year-old female with African and Asian ethnic origins. (C,D) Twenty-eight-year-old female with Latino and Native American ethnic origins.

increased facial convexity, decreased nasal and osseous chin projection, wide nasal base, and increased soft tissue thickness of the midface, lips, and chin.[8] In 1984, Migliori and Gladstone determined the normal range of globe protrusion for white and black adults.[9] Hertel exophthalometry demonstrated that black adult globes were 2 mm more prominent than white adult globes.[9] In general, African-Americans tend to have more proptotic eyes when compared to whites. African-Americans have fuller, more procumbent lips than Caucasians.[9,10] Upper and lower lip projection is also significantly greater than Caucasians. African-American profiles are more protrusive than the Caucasian profiles due to underlying hard tissue. Sutter and Turley noted a proportionately higher percentage of midface height at 20% in African-Americans when compared with Caucasian samples.[8] Caucasians had the greatest upper and lower soft tissue face height, whereas the African-American had the greatest middle face height. This vertical maxillary excess may also be associated with underprojection of the chin.

MORPHOLOGICAL FACIAL AGING

The modern concept of facial aging features a synergistic relationship between photodamage, fat atrophy, gravitational soft tissue redistribution, and bone remodeling. The general progression of facial aging has been well described in the literature.[11–13]

In the current aging face model, the onset of morphological aging is commonly observed in the upper face during the thirties and gradually progresses to the lower face and neck over the next

Intrinsic Skin Aging in Pigmented Races

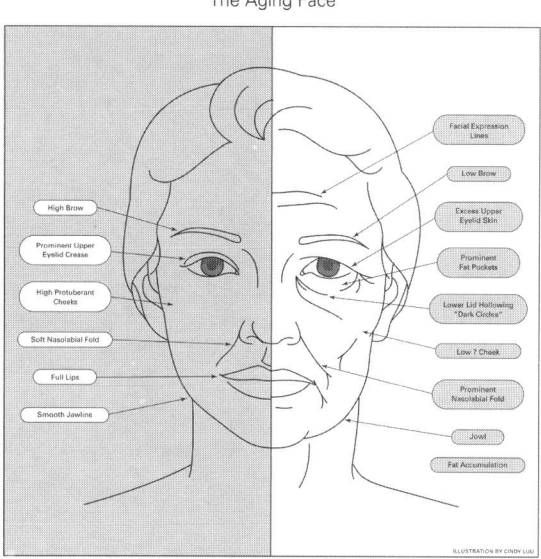

FIGURE 9.3 Morphological signs of facial aging.

several decades (Figure 9.3). Early signs of facial aging can be visualized in the periorbital region. Excess skin of the upper eyelids frequently appears as a result of brow ptosis and upper eyelid skin laxity in the late thirties. Descent of the lateral portion of the eyebrow may produce a relative excess of upper eyelid skin, causing "hooding" during the same period. Weakening of the inferior orbital septum and prolapse of the underlying intraorbital fat produce the characteristic "bags" under the eyes. Lower eyelid fat prolapse may occur as early as the second decade in individuals with a familial predisposition; however, this typically becomes noticeable in individuals by their mid-forties. Photodamage further accentuates the aging changes in the periorbital region with the development of periocular and brow rhytides.

The midface is bounded by the malar eminence and anterior border of the masseter laterally, the inferior orbital rim superiorly, and the nasolabial fold medially. Conceptually, the lower eyelid/orbital rim junction may be viewed as the roof of the midface. As a result, lower eyelid signs of aging usually occur with midface aging during the thirties. In the midface, malar soft tissue abutting the inferior orbital rim descends accumulating as fullness along the nasolabial fold. Malar soft tissue atrophy and ptosis result in periorbital hollowing and tear trough deformity in the fourth decade.

Gravitational soft tissue redistribution, particularly in the lower face, has been considered to be a hallmark of the aging face.[11–13] The lower face soft tissues are supported in a youthful anatomic position by a series of retaining ligaments within the superficial musculo-aponeurotic system (SMAS).[14] First described in 1974, the SMAS represents a discrete fascial layer that envelops the face and forms the basis for resuspending sagging facial tissues.[15] In youth, the SMAS fascia envelope maintains tension on the muscles of the face and offsets to a large degree soft tissue sagging. Beginning in the late thirties, gradual ptosis of the SMAS and skin elastosis sets the stage for jowl formation. Accumulation of submandibular fat and sagging of the submandibular gland may also play a role in interrupting the smooth contour of a youthful jaw line. Changes in the neck are intimately related to changes in the lower face because the SMAS is anatomically continuous with the platysma muscle. In the forties, sag of the SMAS-platysma unit along with submandibular fat redistribution gradually blunts the junction between jaw and neck. Cervicomental laxity in conjunction with excess submental fat deposits may create a "double chin" appearance in individuals regardless of age. In the fifties, diastasis and hypertrophy of the anterior edge of the platysma muscle may produce vertical banding in the cervicomental area. From the sixth to eighth decade, facial aging is further exaggerated by progressive soft tissue atrophy and bony remodeling of the maxilla and mandible, creating a relative excess of sagging skin.

ETHNIC CONSIDERATIONS — FACIAL AGING

Current opinion suggests that individuals with skin of color exhibit less severe facial aging when compared with whites. Much of this acknowledgment is based upon the fact that individuals with darker-pigmented skin are less susceptible to sun-induced photodamage.[16] Likewise, preservation of dermal elasticity due to the photoprotective effect of melanin offsets, to some degree, facial sagging that accompanies advanced age. Although it is beyond the scope of this chapter to individually discuss each race constituting the diverse group of people with skin of color, certain key distinctions in aging for people with skin of color should be appreciated when compared with Caucasian counterparts.

Although the current aging face model establishes a point of reference, it does not address the impact of racial variation in facial structure on the overall progression of aging. By understanding how anthropologic facial features impact morphological aging, common themes related to the progression of facial aging can be applied across ethnic groups. There is currently a lack of published data specifically evaluating the dynamic relationship between facial morphology and aging in people with skin of color. The majority of our perceptions regarding morphologic facial aging among people with skin of color have arisen simply from observations by plastic surgeons.

UPPER FACE

Brow ptosis in African-Americans seems to occur to a lesser degree and a decade later in life than in Caucasians.[17] Whereas descent of the brow becomes noticeable in the Caucasian patient in the third decade, it is typically not a significant feature of African-American aging until much later. For individuals of Latino descent, brows tend to be implanted at a lower level with respect to the supraorbital rim.[6] Accordingly, a tendency toward sagging brow facial soft tissues at an earlier age has been noted in Latinos.[6] In the Asian, small changes in brow position can be quite apparent. With absence of a supratarsal fold in the Asian eye, descent of thick juxtabrow tissues in the lateral orbit may create a prematurely tired appearance. In African-Americans, prolapse of the lacrimal gland commonly masquerades as lateral upper eyelid fullness.[18]

Significant variations exist in position of the supratarsal fold or upper eyelid crease among individuals with skin of color. Presence of a well-defined supratarsal fold gives the impression of a larger palpebral fissure and, thus, a more youthful "bright-eyed" appearance. The position of the supratarsal fold is determined largely by the point of fusion of the orbital septum to the levator aponeurosis. In African-Americans, the upper eyelid crease typically sits approximately 6 to 8 mm above the lid margin, in contrast to individuals of Northern European descent, whose upper lid crease rests 8 to 10 mm above the lid margin.[19] In Asians, a low point of fusion between the orbital septum and levator aponeurosis typically results in absence of a supratarsal crease, allowing orbital fat to extend close to the level of the upper lid margin. As skin laxity progresses with age, the combination of a perceived smaller palpebral fissure and upper eyelid fullness may lead to more pronounced stigmata of aging in the Asian eye.

As aging progresses, proptosis in individuals of African and Hispanic descent is commonly accompanied by rounding of the lateral canthus and scleral show. In individuals of Asian descent, lower eyelid malposition with aging may be less severe because additional support to the lower lid is provided by an overlying hypertrophic obicularis oculi.

MIDFACE

Early aging is evident in individuals of African, Asian, and Hispanic descent in the midface region. The classic signs of midface aging include tear trough deformity, infraorbital hollowing, malar fat

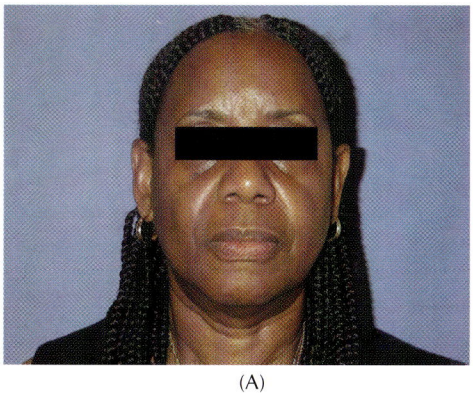 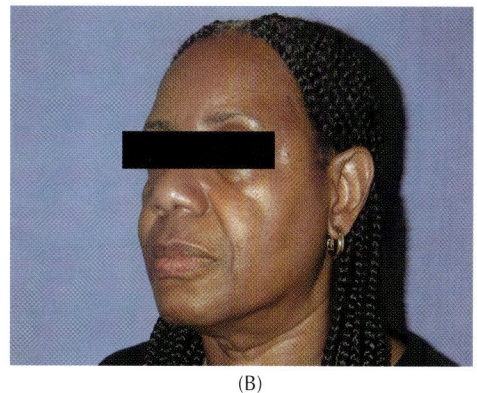

(A) (B)

FIGURE 9.4 (A,B) Sixty-five-year-old African-American woman exhibiting clinical signs of midface aging. Note the downward migration of the malar fat pad leading to infraorbital hollowing and deepening of the nasolabial fold.

ptosis, nasojugal groove prominence, and deepening of the nasolabial fold (Figure 9.4). In individuals with skin of color, predisposition to midface aging is likely a consequence of three factors: the relationship of eyes to the infraorbital rim, basic midface skeletal morphology, and skin thickness.

Globe position relative to the inferior orbital rim becomes interesting when considered in the context of the aging face. Pessa and colleagues discovered that the globe–orbital rim relationships change with age.[20] In the youthful face, the cheek mass lies anterior to the cornea. This has been called a positive vector and is associated with youth. In the aging face, the cheek mass tends to lie posterior to the cornea, forming a negative vector relationship. These vector relationships have significance when analyzing facial aging in people with skin of color. As a result of a tendency toward proptosis, it is also more likely for individuals of African, Hispanic, and Asian descent to develop a negative vector relationship sooner and exhibit features consistent with midface aging.

With midface aging, the malar fat pad descends from its location overlying the inferior orbital rim and accumulates along the nasolabial fold.[21] Consequently, there is a loss of soft tissue cushioning along the inferior orbital rim and zygomatic eminence, creating a hollowing appearance. Hypoplasia of the orbital rim and maxilla may accentuate this process.[22] As previously noted, bimaxillary protrusion in the presence of infraorbital hypoplasia is a common morphological theme for individuals of African, Asian, and Hispanic descent.[2,8] In this population, a thicker dermis with denser subcutaneous tissue may add additional weight to a hypoplastic infraorbital bony scaffold. In patients with orbital rim hypoplasia and thick skin, midface aging changes may occur much earlier and are usually more pronounced. Infraorbital hollowing is quite noticeable in individuals of African descent at an early age as malar fat atrophies and descends with time. In the aging Asian face, the zygomatic bone protrudes more and becomes more angulated with inferior migration of the skin and the subcutaneous tissues from the malar area. Particularly in the early stages of aging, this is often indicated by excessive hollowness in the malar region, which creates a more elderly appearance.[23] In Latinos, malar soft tissues ptosis is common along with early appearance of frowning of the oral commisure.[6]

LOWER FACE

Individuals of African descent demonstrate lower face aging evidenced by jowling in a delayed fashion. In some cases, excess localized submental fatty deposits may be present due to bony chin underprojection despite having a smoothly contoured jaw line. In contrast, Asians may have a tendency to jowl formation as a result of fat accumulation in the buccal space. It has been suggested that ptosis of the buccal fat during the aging process contributes to early jowl formation in Asians following standard facelifting procedures.[24] Fat accumulation in the neck, producing the "double chin," is less common in Asians under age 40 than in younger Caucasians, but it becomes more common after age 40 in association with increasingly redundancy of the cervical skin.[23]

REJUVENATION PROCEDURES

There is a growing interest in cosmetic therapy among people of color. Once a secret weapon for the privileged, cosmetic surgery is now attracting a diverse multicultural patient base with less invasive procedures to enhance appearance. Facial plastic surgery performed on Latinos, Asians, and African-Americans has increased dramatically in recent years. According to the American Academy of Facial Plastic and Reconstructive Surgery (AAFPRS), procedures performed on Hispanics have tripled (up 200%), on African-Americans have more than quadrupled (up 323%), and on Asian Americans have increased 340%.

In darker-pigmented populations, despite improved dermal elasticity, morphological changes of aging tend to predominate in the upper and midface regions. Lower face aging is typically not as pronounced as in the Caucasian population, with the exception of submental fat accumulation. Diffuse morphological facial aging is rare before the sixth decade. Individuals with darker-pigmented skin also have a significantly higher risk of scar formation and postinflammatory hyperpigmentation. Consequently, it is important to customize surgical rejuvenation measures to specifically address the localized stigmata of aging in a minimally invasive manner.

Surgical rejuvenation of the upper face in individuals with skin of color is best achieved by endoscopic brow lifting and blepharoplasty. Endoscopic techniques for lifting the brow are well tolerated in individuals with skin of color because of smaller incisions and less risk of scarring. Blepharoplasty is a minimally invasive procedure involving removal of excess eyelid skin and sculpting of prolapsed fat. Excision of redundant skin and fat helps to reduce the signs of aging in the upper and lower eyelids. Blepharoplasty can be performed safely on people with skin of color without significant risk of adverse scarring. Because of the thinness of the eyelid skin, the possibility of keloid or hypertrophic scarring is almost nonexistent. Upper-lid blepharoplasty in individuals of African and Hispanic descent does not vary significantly from the standard procedure for Caucasians (Figure 9.5). Typically, upper-lid blepharoplasty in individuals of African descent will require more aggressive lipocontouring, sculpting of the brow fat pocket, and repositioning of a prolapsed lacrimal gland. Because of variation in upper lid anatomy for Asians, upper-lid blepharoplasty requires special attention for management of the upper eyelid crease. Creation of a uniform upper eyelid crease-fold complex and orbital fat contouring are frequent requests for the Asian patient.

Special consideration is necessary when performing lower-eyelid surgery in individuals with skin of color. The morphological combination of proptosis and infraorbital hypoplasia places individuals with skin of color at higher risk for lower-lid malposition following blepharoplasty. The transconjunctival approach is recommended as a means of minimizing the chance of lower-lid retraction and eliminating the risk of adverse scarring from a transcutaneous incision.[18] At times, a secondary lower-lid pinch excision of skin is undertaken to remove excess skin following removal of protruding lower-lid fat pads. Lower-lid tightening procedures may also be necessary to stabilize the lid and prevent a downward pull after surgery.

Reversal of midface aging can be addressed by volume replacement and repositioning of ptotic malar fat. Autologous fat transplantation has been championed by many as an effective means to restore volume loss in the midface. Contemporary fat infiltration techniques stress the importance of multilayer microdroplet infiltration using blunt cannulas.[25,26] Facial fat transfer is particularly useful for improving infraorbital hollowing and camouflaging infraorbital rim exposure by malar fat ptosis (Figures 9.6 and 9.7). The outer thighs, buttocks, and abdomen are common donor sites.

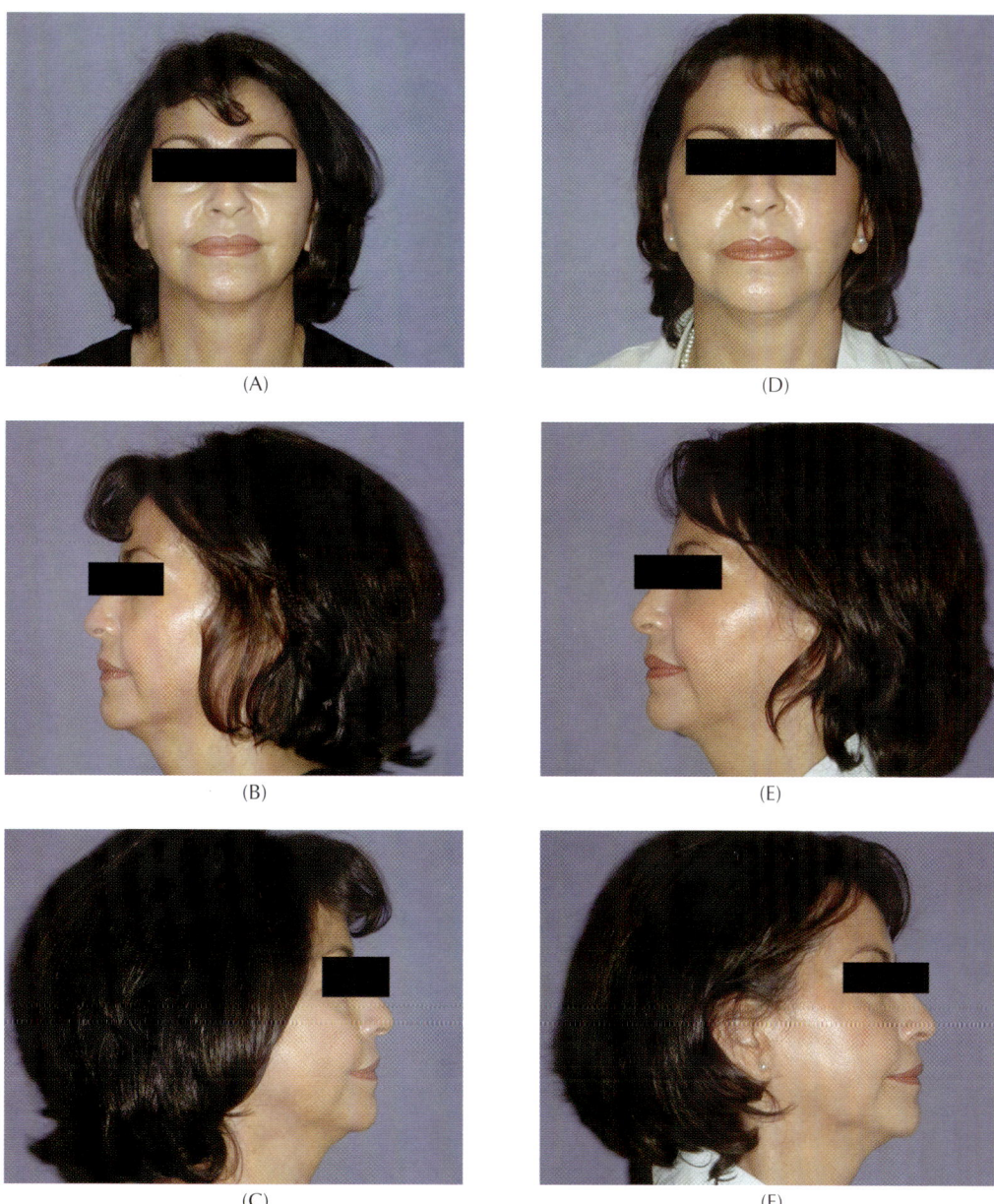

FIGURE 9.5 (A–C) Preoperative upper blepharoplasty in patient of Latino descent. (D–F) Three-month postoperative view following upper-lid blepharoplasty.

Repositioning of a ptotic malar fat pad by a percutaneous suture technique has gained recent popularity.[27,28] The procedure is a simplified method of malar fat pad elevation to rejuvenate the midface. The percutaneous cheek lift repositions the malar fat pad through a small incision just posterior to the temporal hairline. Gore-Tex bolsters affixed to a nonabsorbable suture are then placed percutaneously to elevate the malar fat pad. These rejuvenation techniques may manifest in time as ideal procedures for addressing midface aging in a minimally invasive manner for individuals with skin of color (Figure 9.8).

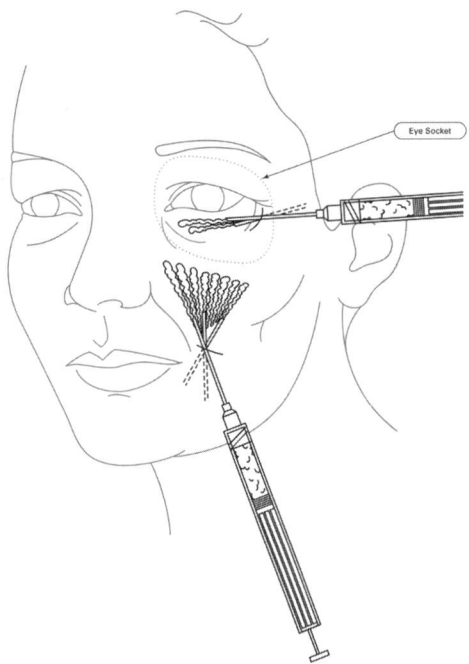

FIGURE 9.6 Facial fat transfer.

Submandibular liposuction may be a favorable alternative to the facelift in individuals with skin of color. The frequent combination of isolated submandibular fat accumulation without excessive jowling in the presence of thicker skin with preserved elastic integrity makes suction lipectomy a favorable cosmetic procedure. Where the Caucasian patient often requires a facelift to diminish the loose skin created by submandibular liposuction, the individual with skin of color, with thicker skin and preserved elastic integrity, frequently does not. The risk of hypertrophic scarring associated with the facelift incision in pigmented skin is also avoided.

CONCLUSION

The modern concept of facial aging features a synergistic relationship between photodamage, fat atrophy, gravitational soft tissue redistribution, and bone remodeling. Over recent years, the number of individuals with skin of color seeking means to offset visible signs of aging has grown exponentially. With an underlying appreciation for the interplay between facial structure and morphological aging, common themes across darker-pigmented populations emerge. Despite the photoprotective effect of melanin, facial aging is quite evident in individuals with skin of color, particularly around the eyes and cheeks. Lower-face aging is not as pronounced as in the Caucasian population. As a result, similar principles for facial rejuvenation may be applied across populations with skin of color. Contemporary approaches to facial rejuvenation feature minimally invasive operations to combat localized stigmata of aging. With a "less is more" focus, facial cosmetic surgery now offers safe and effective options for the patient with skin of color to restore a more youthful appearance.

Intrinsic Skin Aging in Pigmented Races

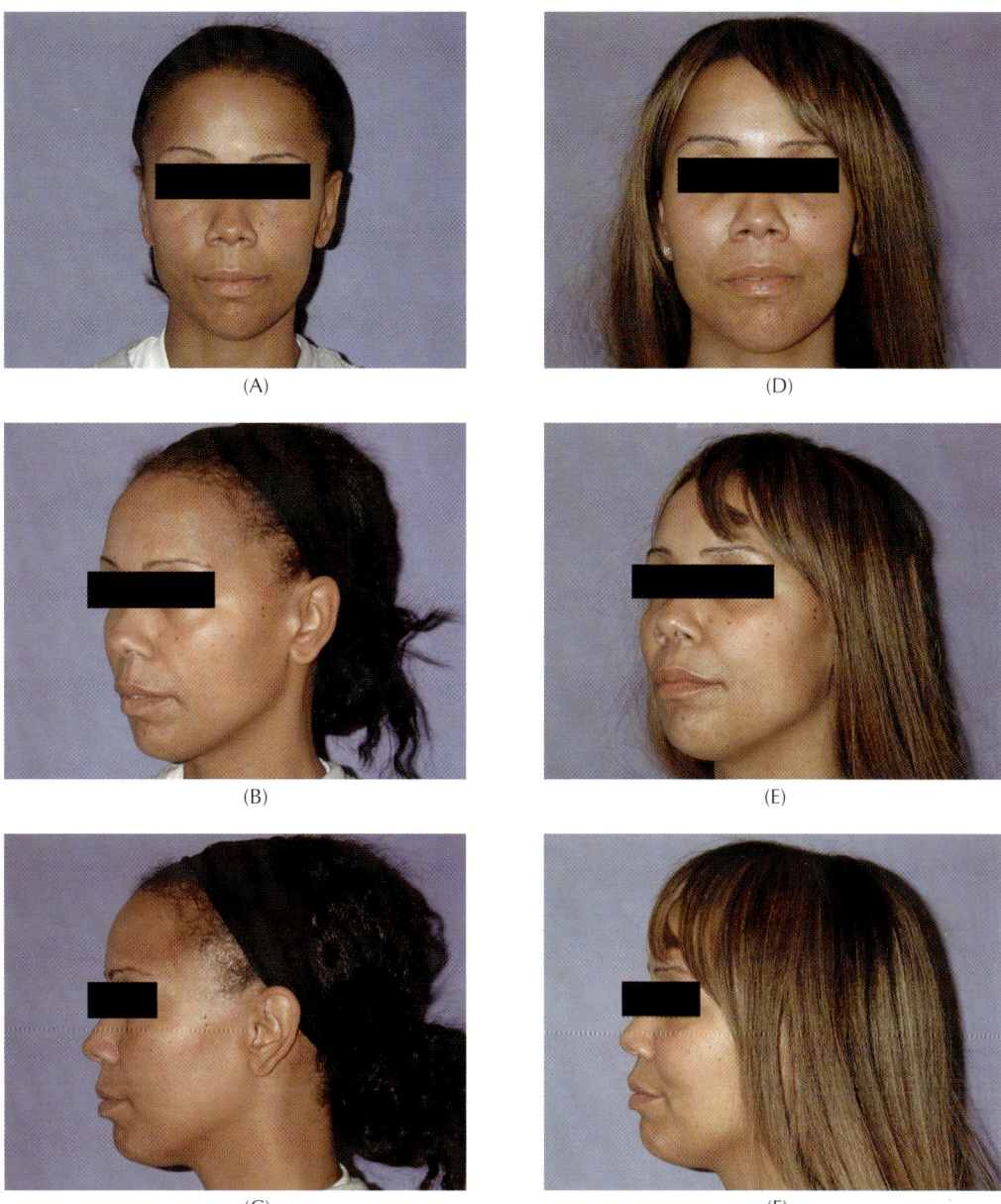

FIGURE 9.7 (A–C) Preoperative view of 38-year-old female with midface soft tissue loss of volume. (D–F) Three-month postoperative view following midface facial fat transfer. Note the rounded, more youthful contours of cheeks following fat transfer.

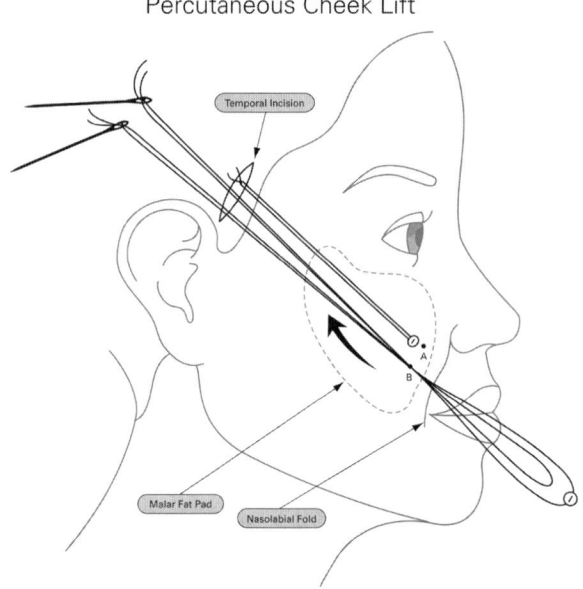
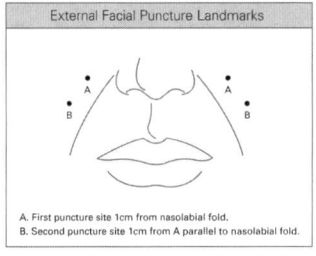
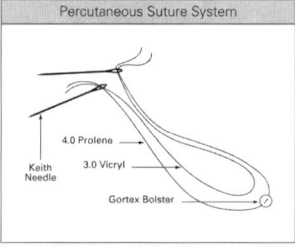

FIGURE 9.8 Percutaneous midface lift.

REFERENCES

1. Farkas LG, Forrest CR, Litsas L. Revision of neoclassical facial canons in young adult Afro-Americans. *Aesth Plast Surg* 2000; 24: 179–184.
2. Le TT, Farkas LG, Ngim RC, Levin LS, Forrest CR. Proportionality in Asian and North American Caucasian faces using neoclassical facial canons as criteria. *Aesth Plast Surg* 2002; 26: 64–69.
3. Porter JP, Olson KL. Anthropometric facial analysis of the African-American female. *Arch Facial Plast Surg* 2001; 3: 191–197.
4. Milgrim LM, Lawson W, Cohen AF. Anthropometric analysis of the female Latino nose: revised aesthetic concepts and their surgical implications. *Arch Otolaryngol Head Neck Surg* 1996; 122: 1079–1086.
5. Porter JP, Lee JI. Facial analysis: maintaining ethnic balance. *Facial Plast Surg Clin North Am* 2002; 10: 343–349.
6. Ramirez OM. Facial surgery in the Hispano-American patient. In: Matory WE (Ed) *Ethnic Considerations in Facial Aesthetic Surgery*. Philadephia: Lippincott-Raven, 1998; 307–320.
7. Swlerenga D, Oesterle LJ, Messersmith ML. Cephalometric values for adult Mexican-Americans. *Am J Orthod Dentofac Orthop* 1994; 106: 146–155.
8. Sutter RE, Turley PK. Soft tissue evaluation of contemporary Caucasian and African-American female facial profiles. *Angle Orthod* 1998; 68(6): 487–496.

9. Migliori ME, Gladstone GJ. Determination of the normal range of exopthalmometric values for black and white adults. *Am J Ophthalmol* 1984; 98: 438–442.
10. Baretto RL, Mathog RH. Orbital measurement in black and white populations. *Laryngoscope* 1999; 109: 1051–1054.
11. Gonzales-Ulloa M, Flores ES. Senility of the face — basic study to understand its causes and effects. *Plast Reconstr Surg* 1965; 36: 239–246.
12. Ellis DA, Ward DK. The aging face. *J Otolaryngol* 1986; 15: 217–223.
13. Fedok FG. The aging face. *Facial Plast Surg* 1996; 12: 107–115.
14. Stuzin JM, Baker TJ, Gordon HL. The relationship of the superficial and deep facial fascias: relevance to rhytidectomy and aging. *Plast Reconstr Surg* 1992; 89: 441–449.
15. Mitz V, Peyronie M. The superficial musculoaponeurotic system (SMAS) in the parotid and cheek area. *Plast Reconstr Surg* 1976; 58: 80.
16. Kaidbey KH, Agin PP, Sayre RM, Kligman AM. Photoprotection by melanin — a comparison of black and Caucasian skin. *J Am Acad Dermatol* 1979; 1: 249–260.
17. Matory WE. Aging in people of color. In: Matory WE (Ed) *Ethnic Considerations in Facial Aesthetic Surgery*. Philadephia: Lippincott-Raven, 1998; 151–170.
18. Bosniak SL, Zilkha MC. *Cosmetic Blepharoplasty and Facial Rejuvenation*. New York: Lippincott-Raven, 1999.
19. Matory WE. Definitions of beauty in the ethnic patient. In: Matory WE (Ed) *Ethnic Considerations in Facial Aesthetic Surgery*. Philadephia: Lippincott-Raven, 1998; 61–83.
20. Pessa JE, Desvigne LD, Lambros VS, Nimerick J, Sugunan B, Zadoo VP. Changes in ocular globe-to-orbital rim position with age: implications for aesthetic blepharoplasty of the lower eyelids. *Aesthetic Plast Surg* 1999; 23: 337–342.
21. Hester TR, Codner MA, McCord CD, Nahai F. Transorbital lower-lid and midface rejuvenation. *Op Tech Plast Reconstr Surg* 1998; 5: 163–185.
22. Flowers RS. Tear trough implants for correction of tear trough deformity. *Clin Plast Surg* 1993; 20: 403–415.
23. Shirakable Y. The Oriental aging face: an evaluation of a decade of experience with the triangular SMAS flap technique. *Aesth Plast Surg* 1988; 12: 25–32.
24. McCurdy JA Jr. *Cosmetic Surgery of the Aging Asian Face*. New York: Thieme Medical, 1990.
25. Coleman SR. Facial recontouring with lipostructure. *Clin Plast Surg* 1997; 24: 347–367.
26. Donofrio LM. Structural autologous lipoaugmentation: a pan-facial technique. *Dermatol Surg* 2000; 26: 1129–1134.
27. Keller GS, Namazie A, Blackwell K, Rawnsley J, Khan S. Elevation of the malar fat pad with a percutaneous technique. *Arch Facial Plast Surg* 2002; 4: 20–25.
28. Sasaki GH, Cohen AT. Meloplication of the malar fat pads by percutaneous cable-suture technique for midface rejuvenation: outcome study (392 cases, 6 years' experience). *Plast Reconstr Surg* 2002; 110: 635–654.

10 Photoaging in Pigmented Skins

Rebat M. Halder and Georgianna M. Richards

INTRODUCTION

People of skin of color constitute the majority of the world's population. These include Asians who can be subdivided into East Asians (Chinese, Japanese, Koreans), Southeast Asians (Indonesians, Malaysians, Singaporeans, Thais, Cambodians, Vietnamese), and South Asians (Bangladeshis, Indians, Pakistanis, Sri Lankans). Those from East Asia tend to be lighter in skin color, although Koreans are more brown skinned than Chinese or Japanese. Southeast Asians are brown in skin color. East Asians and Southeast Asians are of Mongoloid ethnic background. South Asians are of Caucasian ethnic background but have brown to dark brown skin.[1]

Hispanics are another large group that constitute individuals of skin of color. There are European Hispanics who are of Caucasian ethnic origin and are lighter in skin color. However, a large number of Hispanics worldwide are brown skinned. Some Hispanics can be of mixed ancestry, having Caucasian and Native Indian heritage. There are also some Hispanics with black heritage. The geographic areas for brown-skinned Hispanics include North America, Mexico, Central and South America, and the Caribbean.[1]

Blacks are also a large group of people of skin of color. For the purposes of discussion in this chapter, the term black includes those from the African continent, African-Americans, and Afro-Caribbeans. Thus, the term skin of color includes an extremely heterogeneous group of peoples. Patients of skin of color can be anywhere within Fitzpatrick's skin phototype 3–6. With this wide range of skin colors, patients of skin of color vary considerably in their response to sunlight, sun exposure, and, ultimately, photodamage and photoaging.[1]

In general, all races are susceptible to photoaging.[2] However, it is clear that those who fall within Fitzpatrick's skin phototype 4–6 are less susceptible. This is most likely due to the photoprotective role of melanin.[3,4] It has been shown that the mean protective factor (PF) for UVB black epidermis is 13.4, as compared to 3.4 for white epidermis.[5] The mean UVB transmission by black epidermis was found to be 5.7%, compared with 29.4% for white epidermis. For UVA, the mean PF of black epidermis is 5.7, which is significantly higher than that of white epidermis, 1.8.[5] Thus, the mean UVA transmission by black epidermis was 17.5%, compared with 55.5% for white epidermis, so that about three to four times more UVA reaches the upper dermis of whites than that of blacks. The main site of UV filtration in white skin is the stratum corneum, whereas in black skin it is the malpighian layers.[5] The malpighian layers of black skin remove twice as much UVB radiation as the stratum corneum.[5] For UVA, possibly even greater removal of radiation occurs in black malpighian layers.[5] Other factors besides melanin may be responsible for natural photoprotection. However, any major differences in the thickness or composition of the epidermal layers in the two racial groups have not been demonstrated[5,6] so that these observed differences in transmission of UVB and UVA are likely to be due mainly to melanin.[5] Although these studies were performed on black skin, the data can probably be extrapolated to most persons of Fitzpatrick's skin types 4–6.

PHOTOAGING IN EAST AND SOUTHEAST ASIANS

The largest number of studies conducted to date on photoaging in patients of skin of color have been in East and Southeast Asians (Chinese, Japanese, Koreans, Malaysians, Singaporeans, Thais).[2,7–11] In these regions of the world, photoaging is common because of the proximity to the equator.[2]

The clinical features of photoaging in East and Southeast Asians are primarily discrete pigmentary changes. These include actinic lentigines — flat, pigmented, seborrheic keratoses — and mottled hyperpigmentation (Figure 10.1). Solar-induced facial melasma is more common in this group than in whites and should be considered a form of actinic dyspigmentation in this instance.[2] In Asian cultures, the standard of beauty is flawless facial skin, uniform in color and texture;[2,7,8] thus, the pigmentary changes of photoaging become significant cosmetic problems. In a study of 61 Thai subjects, of whom 80% were women, Kotrajaras and Kligman found unexpected histological findings of photodamage. Most of the subjects were Fitzpatrick's type 4. However, Thailand is in a tropical zone with approximately 12 h of continuous sunshine almost year round. The population makes little effort to protect the skin from excessive sun exposure; thus, the clinical signs of photoaging appear in Thais by the age of 40.[8] Skin biopsies were taken from the cheek over the lateral zygomatic process, avoiding lesional skin such as lentigos or keratoses. There was an extraordinary degree of dermal photodamage, which was found in practically all of the subjects over the age of 50. Even subjects in their thirties showed a surprising degree of actinic damage. The epidermis of those subjects over the age of 50 showed atrophy, atypia, and dysplasia.[8] There was poor polarity and disorderly differentiation. The quantity of melanin in the keratinocytes was high. Basilar keratinocytes had dense clusters of highly melanized melanosomes. Subepidermal melanophages were found in most subjects in this study. They were often numerous, large, packed with pigment, and sometimes scattered throughout the reticular dermis. This pigment dumping is a characteristic feature of darkly pigmented races after various chemical and physical traumas.[8] Dermal changes were severe. There was marked elastosis presenting as twisted fibers, in various

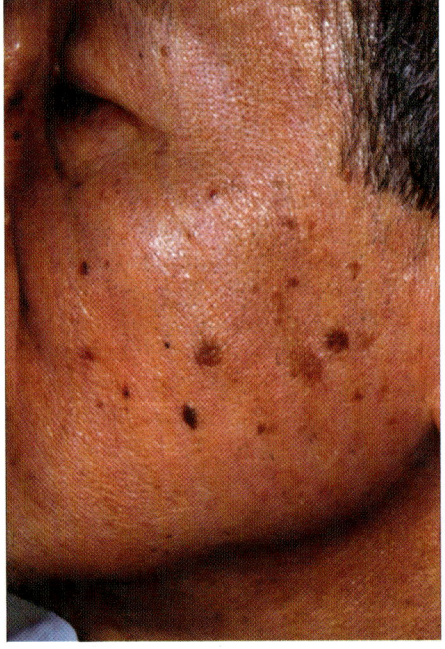

FIGURE 10.1 Photoaging shown as pigmented lesions in an Asian male. (Reproduced from Halder RM. *Dermatol Clin* 2003; 21: 725–732. With permission from Elsevier.)

stages of amorphous degeneration. This finding in older Thai individuals was almost equivalent to that of end-stage photodamaged Caucasian skin, with the amorphous degeneration and twisted fibers described.[8] Elastotic tissue almost completely replaced the collagen network. A later study by Griffiths et al. that consisted of 45 photoaged Asian patients (23 Chinese, 22 Japanese) indicated that wrinkling was not a prominent feature of photoaging in Asian skin.[2] Histologic diagnoses of photoaging in this patient group included seborrheic keratoses, benign keratoses (seborrheic keratosis without horn-cyst formation), actinic lentigo, and solar elastosis.

The largest study to date of Asian patients with photoaging was done by Goh and included more than 1500 patients of skin type 3 or 4 of Singaporean, Indonesian, or Malaysian background, aged 30–50 years.[7] Singaporeans were of Chinese ancestry. The main features of photoaging included hyperpigmentation, tactile roughness, and also coarse and fine wrinkling (Figure 10.2).

A more recent study by Chung et al., however, indicates that wrinkling may be a major feature of photoaging in Asians.[10] In this study that was limited to only Koreans aged 30–92 years (236 men and 171 women), seborrheic keratosis was the major pigmentary lesion associated with photoaging in men, whereas in women it was hyperpigmented macules. The number of hyperpigmented macules and seborrheic keratoses increased with each decade of age ($p < 0.05$). In those 60 years and older, seborrheic keratosis was more common in men than in women ($p < 0.001$). In those 50 years and older, hyperpigmented macules were found more frequently in women than in men ($p < 0.01$).

The most striking feature of this study was the finding of moderate to severe wrinkling associated with photodamage that becomes apparent at about age 50 years in Koreans. Women tended to have more severe wrinkling, and the risk of developing wrinkling was higher in women (prevalence odds ratio, 3.7). This was also the first study to demonstrate a relationship between cigarette smoking and wrinkling in Asians, which has previously been demonstrated in Caucasian subjects.[12–15] In this present study by Chung et al.,[10] cigarette smoking was present in 194 subjects ranging from 0 to 0.9 pack-years and in 213 subjects ranging from 1 to 120 pack-years. After controlling for age, sex, and sun exposure, an association between cigarette smoking and wrinkling

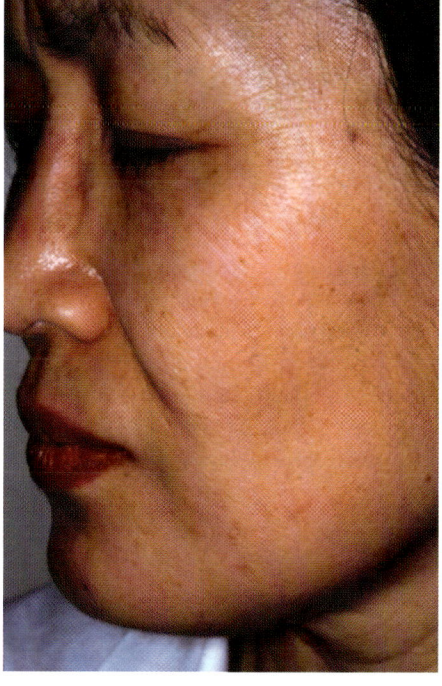

FIGURE 10.2 Photoaging as fine wrinkling and minimal pigmented lesions in an Asian female.

showed a significant trend with increasing pack-years. There was also an association between exposure to the sun and development of wrinkling. Sun exposure of more than 5 h per day was associated with a 48-fold increased risk for wrinkling, compared with 1–2 hours per day. A combined effect of sun exposure and cigarette smoking in Koreans was also seen. Sun exposure of more than 5 h per day and a smoking history of more than 30 pack-years were associated with a 4.2-fold increased risk of wrinkling, compared with a 2.2-fold increase for nonsmokers with 1–2 h of daily sun exposure. In another recent study by Chung et al. that was also limited to Koreans, 21 subjects (12 men, 9 women), with three subjects for each decade of life from the third to ninth, were evaluated to quantify the effects of photoaging on cutaneous vascularization over time[11]. Previous studies on photoaged skin have focused for the most part on end-stage dermal vascular changes. Punch biopsies were taken from chronically sun-exposed skin (crow's feet area of the face). Immunostaining was done with a specific antibody for the CD 31 antigen (platelet endothelial cell adhesion molecule (PECAM-1)) and was examined through computer-assisted morphometric analysis. Chung et al found that photoaged skin showed significantly reduced numbers of dermal vessels, in particular in the sub-epidermal areas that had extensive matrix damage. There was an inverse relationship of vessel numbers and age of the subject in photodamaged skin. The conclusion was that in Korean skin, chronic photodamage results in a gradual decrease in the number and size of dermal vessels over decades of sun exposure, most likely due to degenerative changes of the dermal extracellular matrix. This is an interesting study, as it was done in Koreans of skin type 5 only. A similar study has never been conducted in Caucasians.

Another recent study on photoaging in Asians was conducted by Kwon et al.[16] A total of 303 Korean brown-skinned males aged 40–70 years were examined for seborrheic keratoses, one of the signs of photoaging in Asians. The mean overall prevalence of seborrheic keratoses was 88.1%. A considerable increase in the prevalence of seborrheic keratoses was shown from 78.9% at 40 years to 93.9% at 50 years and 98.7% in those over 60 years. They were considerably more frequent on sun-exposed areas, with the majority of lesions concentrated on the face and the dorsae of the hands. The size of each lesion also became significantly larger by decade. The estimated area covered by seborrheic keratosis per percentage body surface area on sun-exposed areas was 5.7, 11.2, and 18.3 times greater than partially exposed areas at ages 40, 50, and 60 years, respectively.[16] More than 6 h per day of lifetime cumulative sunlight exposure were found to have a 2.28 times higher risk of seborrheic keratoses than fewer than 3 h of daily sun exposure. Seborrheic keratoses are common in Korean males aged 40–70 years, with both aging and cumulative sunlight exposure being independent contributory factors.[16]

PHOTOAGING IN BLACKS

Photoaging occurs in blacks but is presently uncommon. Although unusual, it is more often seen in African-Americans than in African or Afro-Caribbeans. This may be because African-Americans are often a heterogeneous mixture of African, Caucasian, and Native American ancestry. Published studies on photoaging in blacks have been limited to African-Americans. Thus, this section will focus on photoaging in the African-American population. In an earlier portion of this chapter, data were presented on the efficient filtering capacity of black skin for UVA and UVB as compared to white skin. This is due mainly to increased melanin in black skin.

In African-Americans, photoaging appears primarily in lighter-complexioned individuals and may not be apparent until the late fifth or sixth decades of life.[17] Clinically the features of photoaging in African-Americans are fine wrinkling and mottled pigmentation (Figures 10.3 and 10.4).

In a study by Montagna and Carlisle of 19 black and 19 white females who had lived in Tucson, Arizona, for two or more years, there were few histological findings of photoaging in blacks. Biopsy specimens were taken from the malar eminences of the subjects. Histological findings showed that in white sun-exposed skin, the stratum lucidum is usually distorted. Black sun-exposed skin, on the other hand, rarely showed any evidence of alteration in the stratum lucidum.[18] In addition, the

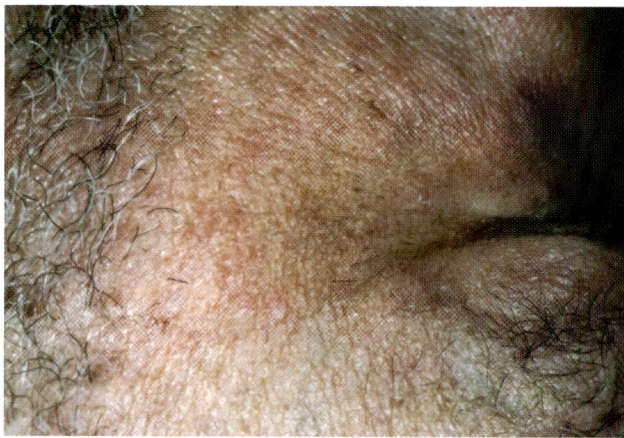

FIGURE 10.3 Photoaging appearing as fine wrinkling and mottled pigmentation in a fair-skinned African-American male.

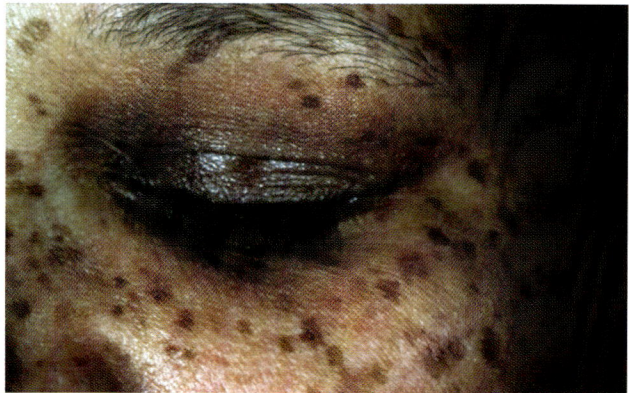

FIGURE 10.4 Photoaging appearing as multiple pigmented lesions in a fair-skinned African-American female. (Reproduced from Halder RM. *Dermatol Clin* 2003; 21: 725–732. With permission from Elsevier.)

stratum lucidum remained compact and unaltered in black sun-exposed skin regardless of age, whereas in white sun-exposed skin it was swollen and distinctly cellular.

Oxytalan fibers were still found in the papillary dermis of sun-exposed skin of 50-year-old black subjects, but these fibers were usually lacking in sun-exposed skin of white persons of the same age. Oxytalan fibers were found in the facial skin of white subjects only in their twenties and early thirties, but they seemed to disappear in the sun-exposed skin of persons aged 40 years and older. No solar elastosis was seen in specimens of black sun-exposed skin. Older black subjects appeared to have an increase in the number and thickness of elastic fibers that separated the collagenous fiber layer in the reticular dermis. Single-stranded elastic fibers in younger subjects resembled braids in older (50 years) subjects. Elastic fibers in the sun-exposed skin of a 45-year-old light-skinned black female resembled those in white sun-exposed skin in both distribution and amount.[18]

The facial skin of black women in the study had elastic fibers that stained differently from those of white skin with the hematoxylin and Lee stain. Photodamaged white skin showed only elastic fibers in the papillary and reticular dermis stained pink, and the wide ribbonlike fibers in the intermediate dermis stained blue.[19] All dermal elastic fibers in black sun-exposed skin stained pink, similar to the sun-protected skin of white individuals. In a light-skinned 45-year-old black woman, the elastic fibers stained similarly to those in white skin.[18]

The majority of the white women aged between 45 and 50 years had wrinkles present beside the lateral canthi of the eyes and at the corners of the mouth, whereas none of the black women showed any obvious wrinkles. Long-term sun exposure to black skin resulted in only minor changes compared with the profound alterations present in sun-exposed white skin. The presence of a greater number of melanosomes and their distribution in black skin likely protect the epidermis from photodamage.[18]

One key factor in the dermal photodamage of white skin is the presence of elastotic material.[19] Elastotic tissue, once it is formed, is constantly resorbed and replaced with other elastotic tissue and large collagenous fiber bundles. This results in shrinkage and reduction of the dermal volume. This process occurs less precipitously in the facial skin of young and middle-aged black women.[18]

The presence of abundant fiber fragments in black skin could be due to degradation products in addition to newly synthesized fibers. The fiber fragments, hypertrophied multinucleated fibroblasts, and macrophages are numerous in black skin. These histological characteristics represent active biosynthesis degradation and turnover and may be responsible for the clean appearance of black dermis as compared to the damaged dermis of sun-exposed white skin.

PHOTOAGING IN HISPANICS

There are no studies in the literature that specifically address photoaging in Hispanics. Sanchez found, however, that photoaging was the third most common dermatologic diagnosis in 1000 Hispanic patients treated in a dermatology private practice, accounting for 16.8% of visits.[20]

Photoaging in European and fair-skinned Hispanics most likely occurs with the same frequency and degree as in Caucasians, so that the clinical manifestation is primarily wrinkling rather than pigmentary alterations. Wrinkling appears at the same age that it would appear in Caucasians. Darker-skinned Hispanics who are type 4 and 5 and live in hot tropical climates such as Mexico, Central and South America will have clinical manifestations of photoaging that are similar to those of South Asians and African-Americans. These manifestations include fine wrinkling and mottled pigmentation occurring in the late fourth through sixth decades of life. However, with many years of occupational sun exposure, there are some darker-skinned Hispanics who have marked deep wrinkling. No histological studies could be located in the literature that specifically address photoaging in Hispanics.

SUMMARY OF PHOTOAGING IN PIGMENTED SKINS

At the present time, photoaging in skin of color has variable presentations. Asians and fair-skinned Hispanics have wrinkling as one of the clinical manifestations that were not previously described as being common in these populations. Wrinkling is not as common a manifestation of photoaging in blacks, South Asians, or darker-skinned Hispanics. In general, melanin still gives protection against photodamage in patients of color. Within most pigmented racial groups, the lighter-colored individuals have evidence of photodamaged skin. Pigmentary manifestations of photoaging are common in skin of color, including seborrheic keratosis, actinic lentigines, mottled hyperpigmentation, and solar-induced facial melasma.

A significant component of photoaging in patients of skin of color may be related to the fact that they live in sunny, hot, tropical areas. It has been previously accepted that increased skin melanin affords protection against photoaging. However, because photoaging now appears to be a global problem as shown by both clinical and histological studies, it may be that there are other factors that contribute to the degree of photodamage observed in patients of skin of color. It has been shown that many patients of skin of color do not protect themselves with sunscreen when exposed to the sun.[21–23] Many times this is by choice, as patients of skin of color do not often believe or understand that they need protection when involved in either occupational or recreational sun exposure. Studies have shown that sunscreen use is less prevalent in African-Americans and Hispanic populations than in Caucasians.[21,22] Hispanics, however, use sunscreen more frequently than African-Americans.

Patients of skin of color worldwide now engage in recreational activities that involve sun exposure. Previously these activities were engaged in primarily by Caucasians and include water and snow skiing, playing tennis, golfing, and sunbathing on the beach. With access to these activities, many patients of skin of color still do not observe sun protection and may be exposed to the sun for prolonged periods of time.[23] There will certainly be an increase in photodamaged patients of skin of color if public education concerning sun exposure in this segment of the population is not addressed well.

The reasons why patients of color are prone to photoaging are not completely known. Even though the efficient UV filtering capacity of pigmented skin was described earlier in the chapter, it may be that high UV exposure overwhelms the filtering capacity of melanin in hot, sunny climates.[8] Many patients of skin of color live in sunny and hot areas of the world. The question is whether infrared radiation also contributes to photodamage. There is evidence that chronic exposure to natural or artificial heat sources can lead to histological changes that resemble those induced by ultraviolet radiation, including elastosis and carcinoma.[24] Also, infrared radiation can potentiate the photodamaging effects of ultraviolet radiation that have been demonstrated in animals.[25]

THERAPY OF PHOTOAGING OF PIGMENTED SKINS

Because the manifestation of photoaging in pigmented skins consists primarily of dyspigmentation such as actinic lentigines, mottled hyperpigmentation, and solar-induced melasma, topical therapy is useful.

Retinoids

Topical Tretinoin

Topical tretinoin has the effect of partially reversing signs of photodamage on facial skin. In a 1986 study in which this was first reported,[26] the clinical signs such as fine wrinkling, blotchiness, and altered surface texture improved after 6 months of treatment. Structural corrections of the features associated with photodamaged skin were also noted histologically. In a study of 61 volunteers with a mean age of 63 years, 80% of whom were women, topical tretinoin was used in a 0.05% cream applied nightly on the forehead and spread over the entire face. Thirty-five patients were treated for 6 months and 26 for 1 year, and they were scored for changes in fine wrinkles and hyperpigmentation at bimonthly visits. There was only slight improvement in the majority of subjects after 6 months. Seventy-one percent showed moderate improvement, with 19% showing marked improvement after 1 year of treatment. For fine wrinkles, moderate to marked improvement was shown in almost 90% of subjects, with 60% showing improvement after 6 months. Hyperpigmentation improved in 65% of the patients after 12 months.[8]

Marked improvement of photodamaged skin was also seen in a group of patients of skin type 3 or 4 aged 30–50 years. They presented with wrinkling and uneven pigmentary patches and improved markedly after 3 months of treatment with topical tretinoin, with even further improvement when treatment was continued for up to 12 months.[7] Tretinoin 0.05% cream was applied after cleansing at night, and in the morning, tretinoin 0.1% was applied. The tretinoin cream was reduced to 0.25% if adverse events occurred and increased to 0.1% if side effects were tolerable at both morning and night applications. The skin was cleansed by scrubbing each night and morning prior to tretinoin cream application, using an abrasive containing 25% aluminum oxide and 75% aqueous calamine cream initially. A scrubbing agent containing 50% aluminum oxide and 50% aqueous calamine was used twice a day after a month. The soap contained lactoserum and lactic acid.[7]

In a 40-week study of Chinese and Japanese patients with photoaging, both groups had comparable improvement in global response to 0.1% tretinoin. The study demonstrated that hyperpigmented lesions, which are predominant in the Chinese and Japanese facial skin, lighten with topical tretinoin therapy, as noted in Caucasian skin.[27] Chinese and Japanese primarily have hyperpigmented lesions and only a small degree of wrinkling in response to photoaging when compared with Caucasians. The presence of wrinkling in this study, therefore, was insufficient to be evaluated.[27] Some of the effects of photoaging in blacks, such as hyperpigmentation, have been effectively treated with tretinoin. A study lasting 40 weeks using topical tretinoin therapy on black skin showed increases in the degree of compaction of the stratum corneum; increases in the thickness of epidermis, granular cell layer, mitotic figures, and spongiosis; with a decrease in the epidermal melanin content.[28]

Systemic Retinoid Therapy

Oral isotretinoin has been used as a treatment for cutaneous photoaging in Hispanic patients. The study was done in El Salvador.[29] Treatment was given as an adjunct to cosmetic surgery and assessment made on the basis of improvement in discoloration, wrinkles, oiliness, thickness, size of follicular pores, and general skin improvement; significant improvement was noted when compared with surgery alone. Skin tone and elasticity improved, with minimal adverse events. This study is mentioned but the use of isotretinoin is not advocated by the authors of this chapter for use in treating photoaging.

BLEACHING AGENTS

The dyschromias associated with photoaging in pigmented skins may be effectively treated with topical hydroquinone-containing products. The treatment requires twice-daily application directly to the involved area for 3 months.[30] Other bleaching agents that can be used include kojic acid, arbutin, and azelaic acid (see Chapter 5). Triple-combination therapy using hydroquinone, tretinoin, and topical corticosteroid is also effective for pigmentary manifestations of photoaging if used once daily in pigmented skins.[31]

CHEMICAL PEELS

Chemical peeling agents used to resurface the skin of people of color improve the textural and pigmentary skin changes that are associated with photoaging (see Chapter 11).

MICRODERMABRASION

Microdermabrasion is used for resurfacing the skin and has been well tolerated in darker skin types. Good results in improving fine wrinkles, skin texture, and pigmentary abnormalities have been shown in a study by Rubin and Greenbaum, in which normalization of the stratum corneum increased collagen deposition in the papillary dermis, and epidermal thickening was observed[32] (see Chapter 11).

PHOTOREJUVENATION

Full-face photorejuvenation for Asian patients using intense pulsed light with integrated contact cooling has been found to be safe, effective, and associated with fewer post-treatment complications than other, more invasive treatments.[33] In a study of 73 patients, at least five full-face treatments were given at 3–4-week intervals. Evaluations of improvement were done by the patients and treating physician 1 month after the third and fifth treatments. Improvement was evaluated in pigmentation, telangiectasia, fine wrinkles, skin texture, and overall improvement. Histological changes were also evaluated.[33] Results showed improvement in pigmentation, telangiectasia and fine wrinkle reduction, and smoother skin texture. Subjective ratings by the patients and physicians after the fifth treatment showed greater than 60% improvement in more than 80% of the patients. Histologically, there was strong staining of Types I and II collagen.

Conventional modalities of treatment have been used to meet the needs of Japanese patients with photoaged skin. These therapies, including collagen injections, rhytidectomies, and laser treatments, have been done based on the patients' symptoms. Pigmented lesions, telangiectasia, deteriorating smoothness of skin texture, and fine and coarse wrinkles are some of the features that are increasingly being treated.[34]

In the United States and Europe, more ablative methods of dermabrasion, laser resurfacing, and phenol peeling have been used. Laser resurfacing using pulsed CO_2 laser and Er:YAG to improve various symptoms of photoaging has become increasingly popular in recent years[35] and may be applicable to some Hispanic and Asian populations (including East and South Asians).

In another study of 97 Japanese patients between the ages of 22 and 70 years with photoaged skin, treatment using intense pulsed light was given three to six times at 2–3-week intervals. The parameters used for treatment through the cutoff filter of 550 or 570 nm were total fluence of 28–32 J/cm^2 with a double pulse mode of 2.5–4.0/4.0–5.0 ms and a delay time of 20.0/40.0 ms between pulses.[34] After evaluation and rating by physicians and patients at the end of treatment, good or excellent was given to more than 90% for pigmentation, to more than 83% for telangiectasia, and to more than 65% for skin texture.[34] Photorejuvenation was found to be safe and effective in Asian skin of types IV or V. The procedure has been more beneficial in this skin type, which has a tendency to develop pigmentation and other complications through other skin rejuvenation procedures (see also Chapter 14).

REFERENCES

1. Halder RM, Richards GM. Photoaging in patients of skin of color. In: Rigel DS, Weiss RA, Lim HW, Dover JS (Eds) *Photoaging*. New York: Marcel Dekker, 2004; 55–63.
2. Griffiths CE, Goldfarb MT, Finkel LJ, Roulia V, Bonawitz M, Hamilton TA, Ellis CN, Voorhees JJ. Topical tretinoin treatment of hyperpigmented lesions associated with photoaging in Chinese and Japanese patients: a vehicle-controlled trial. *J Am Acad Dermatol* 1994; 30: 76–84.
3. Pathak MA, Fitzpatrick TB. The role of natural photoprotective agents in human skin. In: Fitzpatrick TB, Pathak MA, Harber LC, Seiji M, Kukita A (Eds) *Sunlight and Man*. Tokyo: University of Tokyo Press, 1974; 725–750.
4. Kligman AM. Solar elastosis in relation to pigmentation. In: Fitzpatrick TB, Pathak MA, Harber LC, Seiji M, Kukita A (Eds) *Sunlight and Man*. Tokyo: University of Tokyo Press, 1974; 157–163.
5. Kaidbey KH, Agin PP, Sayre RM, Kligman AM. Photoprotection by melanin — a comparison of black and Caucasian skin. *J Am Acad Dermatol* 1979; 1: 249–260.
6. Weigand DA, Haygood C, Gaylor JR. Cell layers and density of negro and Caucasian stratum corneum. *J Invest Dermatol* 1974; 62: 563–568.
7. Goh SH. The treatment of visible signs of senescence: the Asian experience. *Br J Dermatol* 1990; 122(Suppl 35): 105–109.
8. Kotrajaras R, Kligman AM. The effect of topical tretinoin on photodamaged facial skin: the Thai experience. *Br J Dermatol* 1993; 129: 302–309.
9. Griffiths CE. Assessment of topical retinoids for the treatment of Far-East Asian skin. *J Am Acad Dermatol* 1998; 39(2): S104–S107.
10. Chung JH, Lee SH, Youn CS, Park BJ, Kim KH, Park KC, Cho KH, Eun HC. Cutaneous photodamage in Koreans. *Arch Dermatol* 2001; 137:1043–1051.
11. Chung JH, Yano K, Lee MK, Youn CS, Seo JY, Kim KH, Cho KH, Eun HC, Detmar M. Differential effects of photoaging vs. intrinsic aging on the vascularization of human skin. *Arch Dermatol* 2002; 138:1437–1442.
12. Daniell HW. A study in the epidemiology of "crow's feet." *Ann Intern Med* 1971; 75: 873–880.

13. Kadunce DP, Burr R, Gress R, Kanner R, Lyon JL, Zone JJ. Cigarette smoking: risk factor for premature facial wrinkling. *Ann Intern Med* 1991; 114: 840–844.
14. Ernster VL, Grady D, Miike R, Black D, Selby J, Kerlikowske K. Facial wrinkling in men and women, by smoking status. *Am J Public Health* 1995; 85: 78–82.
15. Smith JB, Fenske NA. Cutaneous manifestations and consequences of smoking. *J Am Acad Dermatol* 1966; 34: 717–732.
16. Kwon OS, Hwang EJ, Bae JH, Park HE, Lee JC, Youn JI, Chung JH. Seborrheic keratosis in the Korean males: causative role of sunlight. *Photodermatol Photoimmunol Photomed* 2003; 19: 73–80.
17. Halder RM. The role of retinoids in the management of cutaneous conditions in blacks. *J Am Acad Dermatol* 1998; 39(2 Pt 3): S98–S103.
18. Montagna W, Carlisle K. The architecture of black and white facial skin. *J Am Acad Dermatol* 1991; 24: 929–937.
19. Montagna W, Kirchner S, Carlisle K. Histology of sun-damaged human skin. *J Am Acad Dermatol* 1989; 21: 907–918.
20. Sanchez MR. Cutaneous disease in Latinos. *Dermatol Clin* 2003; 21: 689–697.
21. Hall HI, Jones SE, Saraiya M. Prevalence and correlates of sunscreen use among US high school students. *J Sch Health* 2001; 71(9): 453–457.
22. Friedman LC, Bruce S, Weinberg AD, Cooper HP, Yen AH, Hill M. Early detection of skin cancer: Racial/ethnic differences in behaviors and attitudes. *J Cancer Educ* 1994; 9: 105–110.
23. Halder RM, Bridgeman-Shah S. Skin cancer in African Americans. *Cancer* 1995; 75(2 Suppl): 667–673.
24. Kligman LH. Intensification of ultraviolet-induced dermal damage by infra-red radiation. *Arch Dermatol* 1982; 272: 229–238.
25. Kligman AM. Aging, light and heat. In: *Psoralens in Cosmetics and Dermatology. Proceedings of the International Symposium (SIR)*. Paris: Pergamon Press, 1981; 57–64.
26. Kligman AM, Grove GL, Hirose R, Leyden JJ. Topical tretinoin for photoaged skin. *J Am Acad Dermatol* 1986; 15: 836–859.
27. Griffiths CEM, Goldfarb MT, Finkel LJ, Roulia V, Bonawitz M, Hamilton TA, Ellis CN, Voorhees JJ. Topical tretinoin (retinoic acid) treatment of hyperpigmented lesions associated with photoaging in Chinese and Japanese patients: a vehicle-controlled trial. *J Am Acad Dermatol* 1994; 30: 76–84.
28. Bulengo-Ransby SM, Griffiths CEM, Kimbrough-Green CK, Finkel LJ, Hamilton TA, Ellis CN, Voorhess CN. Topical tretinoin (retinoic acid) therapy for hyperpigmented lesions caused by inflammation of the skin in black patients. *N Engl J Med* 1993; 328: 1438–1443.
29. Hernandez-Perez E, Khawaja HA, Alvarez TYM. Oral isotretinoin as part of the treatment of cutaneous aging. *Dermatol Surg* 2000; 26: 649–652.
30. Taylor SC. Treatment of photoaging in African American and Hispanic patients. In: Rigel DS, Weiss RA, Lim HW, Dover JS (Eds) *Photoaging*. New York: Marcel Dekker, 2004; 365–377.
31. Galderma Laboratories. Data on file.
32. Rubin MG, Greenbaum SS. Histologic effects of aluminum oxide microdermabrasion on facial skin. *J Aesth Dermatol Cosmet Surg* 1999; 1: 14.
33. Negishi K, Wakamatsu S, Kushikata N, Tezuka Y, Kotani Y, Shiba K. Full-face photorejuvenation of photodamaged skin by intense pulsed light integrated contact cooling: initial experiences in Asian patients. *Lasers Surg Med* 2002; 30(4): 298–305.
34. Negishi K, Tezuka Y, Kushikata N, Wakamatusu S. Photorejuvenation for Asian skin by intense pulsed light. *Dermatol Surg* 2001; 27(7): 627–631.
35. Goldberg DJ, Cutler KB. The use of the erbium: YAG laser for the treatment of class III rhytids. *Dermatol Surg* 1999; 25: 713–715.

11 Pharmacological Agents for Pigmented Skins

Pearl E. Grimes

INTRODUCTION

With the introduction of numerous new pharmacologic agents for dermatological use over the past several decades, clinicians have more tools in their armamentarium than ever before. Simultaneously, the demographic of the patients seen in dermatology practices has also undergone a major paradigm shift. Patients with pigmented skin are the most rapidly growing segment of the population, and this trend is expected to continue well into the next century. Although many treatments for dermatologic conditions may not vary with level of pigmentation, physiological differences in skin of color may make certain therapies imprudent or even harmful. A thorough understanding of the subtleties involved in treating skin of color with a wide variety of pharmacologic agents is critical for a successful modern dermatologic practice.

This chapter will provide an overview of the most important pharmacologic agents used in dermatology today and give special emphasis to the application of these therapies in patients with skin of color.

RETINOIDS

Retinoids (i.e., tretinoin, tazarotene, and adapalene) mediate cellular responses primarily through activation of nuclear retinoid receptors.[1] There are two types of nuclear retinoic acid receptors: the retinoic acid receptors (RARs) and the retinoid X receptors. Each type of receptor contains three receptor subtypes: alpha, beta, and gamma.[1,2] Among the commonly prescribed retinoids, tretinoin activates the RARs alpha, beta, and gamma directly and the retinoid X receptors indirectly (through conversion of tretinoin to 9-cis-retinoic acid).[1,3] Conversely, tazarotenic acid, the metabolite of tazarotene, selectively binds to RARs beta and gamma and is unable to directly or indirectly activate retinoid X receptors.[2] This difference in receptor activity may explain the varying efficacy of the different retinoids in the treatment of dermatologic conditions.

Topical retinoids are useful for the treatment of a variety of cutaneous disorders, including acne, psoriasis, photodamage, melasma, and enlarged pores. However, use of the products can be associated with retinoid dermatitis and may lead to postinflammatory hyperpigmentation. This problem tends to be common in darker racial/ethnic groups.[4]

TRETINOIN

Multiple studies document the efficacy and safety of tretinoin for treatment of acne vulgaris, photodamage, postinflammatory hyperpigmentation, and melasma. Since its introduction 3 decades ago, tretinoin has been a leading treatment for acne vulgaris and numerous clinical trials confirm its efficacy.[5,6] However, several recent clinical trials suggest that the newer retinoids, such as tazarotene and adapalene, are at least as effective in reducing clinical signs of acne and are better tolerated than tretinoin.[5,6] In a randomized clinical trial of 143 patients with mild to moderate facial acne, it was reported that tazarotene 0.1% gel was more effective than tretinoin 0.025% gel in reducing the open comedone count, the total noninflammatory lesion count, and the total inflammatory lesion count.[6] Peeling, erythema, dryness, burning, and itching associated with tazarotene never exceeded trace levels.

In the treatment of photodamage, topical application of tretinoin, a Vitamin A derivative naturally found in the body, has been shown to improve fine wrinkles, mottled hyperpigmentation, and roughness.[7] Histologically, the improvement in the appearance of photoaged skin is associated with the ability of tretinoin to compact the stratum corneum, thicken the epidermis, and reduce melanin content.[8,9] In addition, tretinoin has been found to induce collagen synthesis while inhibiting some of the metalloproteinases responsible for dermal collagen degradation.[8,10] Several recent clinical trials have reported that topical application of tretinoin provides a statistically significant improvement in fine wrinkling, coarse wrinkling, and yellowing..[11] Further, a histological study by Bhawan and associates found that topically applied tretinoin significantly increased epidermal thickness, increased granular layer thickness, decreased melanin content, and improved stratum corneum compaction.[12] Interestingly, it has been suggested that tretinoin may also reduce signs of aging in non-sun-exposed skin. In a study by Kligman and associates, patients aged 68–79 years were asked to apply 0.025% tretinoin cream to the inner aspect of one thigh and to apply a placebo cream to the other, one daily for 9 months.[7] At the end of the evaluation period, skin treated with tretinoin displayed a marked increase in visible epidermal thickness and resulted in a more undulating dermoepidermal junction with prominent rete ridges. Dermal changes noted included increases in glycosaminoglycan deposition, elastic fibers, and new blood vessel formation. The authors concluded that the magnitude of tretinoin-induced change in aged protected skin may be even greater than that in photodamaged skin.

Topical tretinoin has also been found to improve melasma. In a double-blind, vehicle-controlled trial, 38 women applied topical 0.1% tretinoin cream or vehicle to the face once daily for 40 weeks.[13] At the end of the treatment, 68% of the tretinoin-treated patients were clinically rated as improved or much improved, compared with only 5% in the vehicle group. Colorimetry demonstrated a 0.9-unit lightening of tretinoin-treated skin, compared with a 0.3-unit darkening with vehicle. Histologically, epidermal pigment was reduced 36% following tretinoin treatment, compared with a 50% increase following treatment with the vehicle cream. Moderate side effects, including erythema and desquamation, occurred in 88% of tretinoin patients, compared with 29% of vehicle patients. Tretinoin has also been shown to improve the appearance of actinic lentigines.[7,9,14,15]

The use of tretinoin in skin of color has also been evaluated. In an evaluation of the efficacy of tretinoin in the treatment of hyperpigmented lesions associated with photoaging in Asian (Chinese and Japanese) patients, 45 photoaged Asian patients were randomized to treatment with tretinoin or vehicle for 40 weeks.[16] At the end of the treatment period, hyperpigmented lesions of the face and hands were lighter or much lighter in 90% of the tretinoin group, compared with 33% of the vehicle group. Moreover, colorimetry demonstrated significant lightening of the lesions after tretinoin treatment compared with vehicle. The authors concluded that tretinoin cream significantly lightens the hyperpigmentation of photoaging in Asian patients. Conversely, others reported that a combination of 0.1% tretinoin and 0.1% hydrocortisone for 6 months actually worsened pigmentation in Japanese women with melasma. Further, more than 25% of the patients dropped out due to irritation.[17]

In a study of topical tretinoin for the treatment of hyperpigmented lesions caused by inflammation of the skin in black patients, 54 patients were randomized to 40 weeks of treatment with 0.1% tretinoin cream or vehicle.[18] After 40 weeks of treatment, the facial hyperpigmented lesions of the tretinoin-treated patients were significantly lighter than those of the vehicle-treated patients. Colorimetry demonstrated a 40% lightening of the lesions in the tretinoin group, compared with an 18% lightening in the vehicle group. Tretinoin also lightened normal skin in this patient population. The authors concluded that topical application of tretinoin significantly lightens post-inflammatory hyperpigmentation in black patients.

TAZAROTENE

Tazarotene is a newly introduced synthetic retinoid that mediates cell differentiation and proliferation.[19] Tazarotene, a prodrug of tazarotenic acid, has been proven effective for the treatment of psoriasis (both as a monotherapy and in combination with various other treatments including UVB phototherapy and topical corticosteroids)[2,20] and acne vulgaris[21,22] and as a topical treatment for photodamage.[1]

In the treatment of psoriasis, tazarotene normalizes keratinocyte differentiation, reverses keratinocyte hyperproliferation, and has been shown to have better anti-inflammatory effects than any of the other currently available topical retinoids.[21] When used alone or as combination therapy, tazarotene has been shown to effectively ameliorate the clinical symptoms of psoriasis.[19,20,23] However, it is most commonly used in combination with a topical corticosteroid or phototherapy.[21] In a large study by Tanghetti, 1393 patients with mild to moderate stable plaque psoriasis applied tazarotene 0.05% or 0.1% gel once daily for up to 12 weeks, either as monotherapy or in combination with other topical psoriasis therapies.[23] The adjunctive use of an emollient and/or a corticosteroid enhanced the efficacy of tazarotene treatment and increased the percentage of patients who were satisfied with their treatment. Adjunctive steroid use also enhanced tolerability, and the authors concluded that the optimal treatment regimen was combination therapy with tazarotene and a corticosteroid.

In the treatment of acne vulgaris, tazarotene has greater comedolytic activity than the other available topical retinoids.[21] Tazarotene ameliorates acne by normalizing hyperkeratinization and by exerting significant anti-inflammatory effects. The inhibition of leukocytic activity, release of proinflammatory cytokines and other mediators, and expression of transcription factors and toll receptors involved in immunomodulation has been demonstrated in *in vitro* and *in vivo* evaluations, suggesting a multiple mechanism of action for tazarotene. The efficacy of tazarotene for the treatment of acne vulgaris have been well documented, even when compared to the other commercially available retinoid preparations. In a recent study, there was a 78% incidence of treatment success (defined as at least 50% global improvement) with the application of tazarotene, compared with only 52% of patients who were randomized to adapalene.[22] Moreover, tazarotene provided significantly greater reductions in overall disease severity, noninflammatory lesion count, and inflammatory lesion count. Similarly, an evaluation of tazarotene and tretinoin 0.1% gel for the treatment of acne vulgaris determined that tazarotene therapy was superior to tretinoin therapy.[24] The efficacy of tazarotene for the treatment of inflammatory lesions may be further enhanced when used in combination with erythromycin and benzoyl peroxide.[25] The efficacy of tazarotene for treatment of postinflammatory hyperpigmentation and acne has been assessed in darker racial ethnic groups. Fifty-six patients completed the 18-week double-blind study. Tazarotene cream was applied once daily. When compared to vehicle, tazarotene produced a significantly greater reduction in acne lesions as well as improvement in postinflammatory hyperpigmentation. The drug was well tolerated in darker-skinned patients.[26]

Several recent clinical trials have demonstrated that tazarotene is effective for the treatment of photodamaged skin. In a 1-year evaluation, 563 patients with facial photodamage applied 0.1% tazarotene cream to one half of their faces and vehicle cream to the other half in a double-masked fashion for 24 weeks.[27] Patients then continued treatment with tazarotene for an additional 28 weeks. At week 24, compared with the vehicle cream, tazarotene treatment was associated with a significantly greater occurrence of treatment success (defined as at least 50% global improvement) and at least a one-grade improvement in fine wrinkling, pore size, mottled hyperpigmentation, lentignes, elastosis, irregular depigmentation, roughness, and the overall assessment of photodamage. Moreover, Kang et al. also found tazarotene improved mottled pigmentation and fine wrinkles and that these improvements were comparable to those seen with tretinoin cream.[1]

Tazarotene has been widely reported to be safe and well tolerated. The most commonly reported adverse events associated with topical application of tazarotene include drying, burning, pruritus, erythema, and peeling.[22,24] Tazarotene has not been found to be associated with contact sensitization, phototoxicity, photoallergic reactions, mutagenicity, or carcinogenicity.[28] The pharmacokinetic profile of tazarotene ensures minimal exposure to the drug and its metabolites. Specifically, there are three pharmacokinetic features that suggest that the post-treatment plasma levels of tazarotene and its metabolites are comparable to those of the endogenous retinoids, thereby greatly reducing the likelihood of teratogenic effects. First is the limitation of percutaneous penetration, with less than 6% of the applied drug being absorbed into the bloodstream. Second, tazarotene is rapidly metabolized and these metabolites are not lipophilic. Third, tazarotene and its metabolites are rapidly eliminated in the urine and feces.[28]

Adapalene

Adapalene is a synthetic retinoid that affects keratinization and epithelial tissue differentiation, like the other retinoids, but offers the advantages of increased chemical and light stability and high levels of lipophilicity.[29,30] Adapalene has selective affinity to RAR beta and RAR gamma and has considerable anti-inflammatory activity.[29,31]

Adapalene has been found to be at least as effective as tretinoin for the treatment of acne vulgaris.[30,32–34] Moreover, several studies have suggested that adapalene is better tolerated than either tretinoin, the most widely used treatment for acne, or isotretinoin.[30] A recent study by Ionnides et al. found that although adapalene was as effective as isotretinoin in reducing non-inflammatory and inflammatory lesion counts, adapalene was better tolerated, producing significantly less skin irritation.[30]

Interestingly, a meta-analysis reported by Czernielewski and associates reported that adapalene may be especially effective in skin of color.[35] Their evaluation of five randomized U.S. and European studies concluded that the efficacy of adapalene in reducing the number of inflammatory lesions was significantly greater in black patients than in whites. The percentage reductions in total inflammatory and noninflammatory lesions were similar in each group. Black patients were less likely than white patients to experience erythema or scaling, and a smaller percentage of black patients experienced moderate or severe drying than white patients. Additionally, Zhu and associates reported that adapalene was also effective in the treatment of acne in Chinese patients and that adapalene was more effective and better tolerated than tretinoin gel.[36]

RETINOL

All-*trans*-retinol, as known as vitamin A1, is the predominant circulating retinoid in human tissue.[37] Although retinol is believed to be a precursor of other retinoids, the metabolic pathways of the physiologic and pharmacologic effects are not well understood. Retinols are generally recognized as a safe ingredient in the United States and are widely used in cosmetics and toiletries, most often at a concentration of 0.1% to 1.0%.[37,38]

In a clinical trial, Kang and associates compared the clinical, histological, and molecular responses of normal human skin to topical retinol with that of a topical retinoid.[37] Application of the retinol produced trace erythema (that was not significantly different from the vehicle), whereas retinoic acid produced erythema and epidermal thickening. The authors suggest that these data are compatible with the idea that retinol may be a prohormone of retinoic acid. Retinol-based products appear to be well tolerated in darker racial/ethnic groups.[39]

NIACINAMIDE

Niacinamide (nicotinamide, 3-pyridinecarboxamide) is the physiologically active amide of niacin (vitamin B_3). Studies have suggested that niacinamide may have various dermatologic properties: it acts as an anti-inflammatory agent in the treatment of acne,[40] as an antioxidant,[41] in prevention of photoimmunosuppression and photocarcinogenesis,[42] and in increasing intracellular lipid synthesis.[43]

Recently, it has been suggested that niacinamide is an effective skin-lightening compound. Hakozaki and associates evaluated the effects of melanogensis *in vitro* and on facial hyperpigmentation and skin color *in vivo* in Asian women.[44] In this study, niacinamide reduced melanosome transfer by 35%–68% and reduced cutaneous pigmentation *in vitro*. *In vivo*, niacinamide significantly decreased hyperpigmentation and increased skin lightness after 4 weeks of use. These findings suggest that niacinamide effectively lightens skin by inhibition of melanosome transfer from melanocytes to keratinocytes.

BENZOYL PEROXIDE

Benzoyl peroxide-based products, some of the most commonly used products for the treatment of acne vulgaris, have extensively demonstrated efficacy.[45] Benzoyl peroxide has marked bactericidal activity against *Propionbacterium acnes*, microbes that are commonly implicated in the pathogenesis of acne,[46] and is highly lipophilic.[47,48] Several studies have demonstrated that combination therapy with benzoyl peroxide and topical antimicrobial products containing clindamycin or erythromycin is more effective than monotherapy with any component when treating acne.[49-51] Moreover, several studies have demonstrated that the development of antibiotic resistance, which is becoming increasingly important in the treatment of acne, can be reduced by the concomitant use of benzoyl peroxide and an antibiotic.[52-55] The most commonly reported side effects of topical benzoyl peroxide therapy are dry skin and postinflammatory hypopigmentation and hyperpigmentation.[55] Uncommonly, some patients develop allergic contact dermatitis to benzoyl peroxide. In darker racial/ethnic groups, side effects can be controlled or avoided by initiating therapy with low concentrations of the drug and gradually increasing the concentration and frequency of use of the formulation. Benzoyl peroxide formulations include gels, lotions, and cream. Maximal efficacy is usually associated with gel-formulations.

ANTI-INFECTIVE THERAPY

Topical Antibiotics

In recent years, the use of topical antibiotics in dermatology has greatly expanded. The benefits of topical therapy include reduced risk of systemic side effects, the avoidance of resistance selection in the gut microflora, higher concentration of antibiotic at the site of action, and overall usage of less drug.[56]

The macrolide antibiotics, including clindamycin and erythromycin, are among the topical antibiotics most often used in dermatology. Macrolides are xenobiotics, produced by soil fungi, which have immunosuppressive properties.[57] Although both clindamycin and erythromycin have been available as hydroalcoholic solutions for more than 20 years, newer formulations including hydrophilic gels and lotions have been developed that reduce irritation.[58]

Clindamycin and erythromycin have both been shown to effectively reduce colonization of *P. acnes*, the causative agent in most cases of inflammatory acne, and they may also possess direct anti-inflammatory effects via suppression of neutrophil chemotaxis.[59,60] A study by Thomas and associates reported that clindamycin and erythromycin were therapeutically equivalent for the treatment of acne.[60]

Several fixed-combination gels are also available for the treatment of acne. Interestingly, several clinical studies have demonstrated that combination products containing either erythromycin or clindamycin plus benzoyl peroxide have been found to be superior to concomitant use of their individual components.[49,50,61]

These agents, in general, are well tolerated in pigmented skin. Lotions may be less irritating when compared to cream and gel formulations. Cream formulations of topical antibiotics are less common. Erythromycin cream formulations are available. However, gels are frequently associated with enhanced efficacy.

Systemic Antibiotics

Systemic therapy for dermatologic conditions is most often indicated for moderate to severe forms of acne, rosacea, and other difficult-to-treat conditions that may not be treated topically. In the case of acne, systemic therapy is most often prescribed for patients at high risk for scarring. Effective oral therapies for acne include tetracycline, minocycline and doxycycline, erythromycin, azithromycin, and trimethoprim alone or in combination with sulfamethoxazole.[62]

The most notable side effects associated with systemic therapies include: phototoxicity with tetracycline and related compounds (especially doxycycline), dizziness from minocycline, and gastrointestinal upset from erythromycin administration. Tetracycline-related phototoxic reactions do not appear to be more common in darker racial/ethnic groups. However, when such reactions develop in pigmented skin, significant postinflammatory hyperpigmentation may ensue. Further, systemic antibiotic therapy may increase the incidence of *Candida* infections in women.[58]

Recent evaluations of the safety of minocycline indicate that the use of this compound may be associated with an increased likelihood of rare adverse events, including hypersensitivity reactions, serum-sickness-like reactions, drug-induced lupus, and organ failure.[63]

TOPICAL CORTICOSTEROIDS

Topical glucocorticosteroids are the most frequently prescribed drugs in dermatological practice[64] and are commonly indicated for conditions such as eczema, psoriasis, rosacea, and seborrheic dermatitis. These drugs are also frequently used intralesionally for a variety of inflammatory disorders, including acne vulgaris.

The mechanism of action of corticosteroids is influenced by their molecular structure and is believed to be mediated via binding to nuclear receptors and activation of gene expression.[65] Corticosteroids enter the cells and combine with steroid receptors in the cytoplasm. This combination molecule then enters the nucleus and functions to control protein synthesis as well as vital cell activities. Corticosteroids cause the formation of a protein that inhibits phospholipase A2, a necessary element to regulate the supply of arachidonic acid, which is essential to the formation of inflammatory mediators. Corticosteroids also alter the ion permeability of cell membranes and can modify the production of neurohormones.[65,66]

The therapeutic effects of corticosteroids are derived primarily through their anti-inflammatory and immunosuppressive properties. Importantly, the therapeutic efficacy of corticosteroids is limited by their absorption by the skin. Percutaneous absorption of topical steroids is affected by the molecular structure of the agent, the vehicle into which the drug is incorporated, and the permeability of the skin itself.[65]

Although much progress has been made over the years in increasing the potency and tolerability of topical corticosteroids, the use of these agents is associated with a number of side effects, especially over the long term. Side effects include skin atrophy, striae, telangiectasia, acneiform lesions, and rosacea-like eruptions. In general, topical steroids are tolerated well in dark skin. However, prolonged use of mid- to high-potency nonfluorinated preparations can be associated with significant hypopigmentation. Prolonged use of even low-potency nonfluorinated preparations can induce rosacea-like eruptions of facial skin. In recent years, a trend toward an increased incidence of steroid-induced dermatological disturbances has been noted.[67] Many types of steroid-induced skin lesions and skin atrophy can occur by such mechanisms as the suppression of cell proliferation, immunosuppression, or hormonal activity. Moreover, systemic side effects have also been documented.[67] The likelihood of adverse events is directly related to the potency of the corticosteroid, and clinicians should use these drugs carefully to maximize their therapeutic benefits while minimizing their side effects. When evaluating this balance between efficacy and risk of side effects, the clinician should consider at least the following four variables: the specific diagnosis, which will allow for the selection of the most appropriate agent; strength of the compound needed for control of the disease, selecting the lowest strength possible; length of therapy; and choice of vehicle adequate to the skin lesion.[68]

Intralesional steroids are a mainstay for treatment of acne vulgaris and keloids. Concentrations of 1–3 mg/ml are often used for acne cysts and papules. Use of higher concentrations on the face can increase the risk of atrophy and hypopigmentation, which usually resolves in several months. Higher doses are essential for keloids. Concentrations are usually 20 to 40 mg/ml. Side effects include atrophy and hypopigmentation. These changes usually clear with discontinuation of steroid use. In some instances however, atrophy and hypopigmentation can take 6 months or longer to clear.

VITAMIN C

The regulation of antioxidant capacity in the skin, including the maintenance of adequate levels of antioxidant compounds and enzymes, must be tightly controlled in order to diminish or prevent the damaging effects of UVB.[69] L-ascorbic acid, commonly known as Vitamin C, has been the focus of extensive study in recent years and is an essential requirement and nutrient for humans. Ascorbic acid has been shown to protect against sunburn, delay the onset of skin tumors, and reduce ultraviolet-B-radiation-induced skin wrinkling.[70–73]

Ascorbic acid displays potent antioxidant properties and is the primary water-soluble nonenzymatic biologic antioxidant in human tissues.[74–78] Vitamin C is necessary for the normal formation and maintenance of collagen and is a cofactor for several hydroxylating enzymes.[79–81] The topical application of vitamin C has been suggested in order to maximize its antioxidant properties and stimulate collagen production, as oral administration is believed incapable of generating adequate tissue ascorbic acid levels for these tissue effects.[71] The efficacy of various topical vitamin C preparations has been extensively evaluated and has been found to significantly improve photodamage and stimulate new collagen formation.[82] Ascorbyl palmitate, a fat-soluble synthetic ester of vitamin C, has also been shown to reduce redness associated with sunburn 50% more quickly than areas on the same patient that were left untreated.[83] The apparent dual antioxidant and anti-inflammatory properties of ascorbyl palmitate have also been shown to be beneficial for the treatment of other dermatological conditions with an inflammatory component of the disease process, such as psoriasis and asteototic eczema.[84]

Vitamin C formulations are typically non-irritating when applied topically and have also been shown to improve cholasma and postinflammatory hyperpigmentation.[85] In general, Vitamin C products are well tolerated in darker skin types.[86]

HYDROQUINONE

Hydroquinone is a highly efficacious bleaching agent and is commonly used in the treatment of melasma and postinflammatory hyperpigmentation, lentigines, and freckles. Hydroquinone acts by inhibiting tyrosinase and preventing the conversion of tyrosine to dopa. This agent is used worldwide for treatment of disorders characterized by hyperpigmentation. It can prevent the synthesis of melanin and initiate the decomposition of already-formed melanin. With repeated application, hydroquinone may cause destruction of melanosomes, melanocyte organelles, and melanocyte necrosis.[87] Mild reversible hypopigmentation in the form of a halo around the treated area of hyperpigmentation is often seen in patients with skin types V and VI.

In the United States, concentrations range from 2% (over-the-counter) to 4% (by prescription). Higher concentrations can be compounded by pharmacists for stubborn cases of hyperpigmentation. Multiple studies have documented the efficacy of hydroquinone formulations for hyperpigmentation.[88] Recently, a new combination formulation containing hydroquinone 4%, tretinoin 0.05%, and fluocinolone was FDA approved for treatment of melasma (Tri-Luma). This formulation was based on the Willis–Kligman formula.[88] In addition, other new hydroquinone drugs contain 4% hydroquinone plus retinol (EpiQuin and Alustra).

Complications of hydroquinone therapy include acute and chronic reactions. Common acute reactions are irritant and allergic contact dermatitis and postinflammatory hyperpigmentation. Lesional and perilesional hypopigmentation may occur. This is usually a temporary complication. The major long-term concern regarding the use of hydroquinone is ochronosis. This condition is most often observed in African-American patients who have used products containing high concentrations of hydroquinone for prolonged periods.[88–90] In contrast, cases in the United States are rare and are predominantly associated with the use of hydroquinone 2%. Clinically, ochronosis is characterized by reticulated, sooty hyperpigmentation of the face. Ochronosis is often considered permanent. However, some cases may respond to use of topical retinoids and topical corticosteroids combined with a series of superficial salicylic acid chemical peels.[91]

TOPICAL IMMUNOMODULATORS

Topical nonsteroidal immunomodulatory agents have been extensively tested and are now approved for treatment of atopic dermatitis. These agents include tacrolimus and pimecrolimus. Multiple studies have documented the efficacy and safety of these agents in children and adults.[92,93] Recently, tacrolimus has also proven to be efficacious in the treatment of vitiligo. Tacrolimus was well tolerated in darker-skinned patients.[94,95]

The precise mechanism of action of tacrolimus and pimecrolimus in atopic dermatitis is unknown. However, data suggest that both drugs inhibit T-cell activation of proinflammatory cytokines. Specifically, these drugs inhibit calcineurin, which prevents the dephosphorylation and translocation of the nuclear factor of activated T cells, hence inhibiting the formation of interleukin-2, gamma interferon, and other cytokines. Compared to topical steroids, these drugs offer several advantages. Tacrolimus and pimecrolimus can be used for prolonged periods without induction of steroid-related side effects such as atrophy, striae, and telengiactasias of the skin.

REFERENCES

1. Kang S, Leyden JJ, Lowe NJ, et al. Tazarotene cream for the treatment of facial photodamage. *Arch Dermatol* 2001; 137: 1597–1604.
2. Chandraratna RAS. Tazarotene: first of a new generation of receptor-selective retinoids. *Br J Dermatol* 1996; 135: 18–25.
3. Levin AA, Sturzenbecker LJ, Kazmer S, et al. 9-cis retinoic acid stereoisomer binds and activates the nuclear receptor RXR alpha. *Nature* 1992; 355: 359–361.
4. Grimes PE, Stockton TC. Pigmentary abnormalities in blacks. *Dermatol Clin* 1988; 6(2): 271–281.
5. Kakita LS, Lowe NJ. Azelaic acid and glycolic acid combination therapy for facial hyperpigmentation in darker-skinned patients: a clinical comparison with hydroquinone. *Clin Ther* 1998; 20: 960–970.
6. Webster GF, Berson D, Stein LF, Fivenson DP, Tanghetti EA, Ling M. Efficacy and tolerability of once-daily tazarotene 0.1% gel versus once-daily tretinoin 0.025% gel in the treatment of facial acne vulgaris: a randomized trial. *Cutis* 2001; 67: 4–9.
7. Kligman AM, Grove GL, Hirose R, Leyden JJ. Topical tretinoin for photoaged skin. *J Am Acad Dermatol* 1986; 15: 836–859.
8. Fisher GJ, Wang ZQ, Datta SC, et al. Pathophysiology of premature skin aging induced by ultraviolet light. *N Engl J Med* 1997; 13: 1419–1428.
9. Weinstein GD, Nigra TP, Pochi RE, et al. Topical tretinoin for treatment of photoaged skin. *Arch Dermatol* 1991; 127: 659–665.
10. Griffiths CE, Russman AN, Majmudar G, et al. Restoration of collagen formation in photodamaged human skin by tretinoin (retinoic acid). *N Engl J Med* 1993; 329: 530–535.
11. Nyriady J, Bergfeld W, Ellis C, et al. Tretinoin cream 0.02% for the treatment of photodamaged facial skin: a review of 2 double-blind clinical studies. *Cutis* 2001; 68: 135–142.

12. Bhawan J, Gonzalez-Serva A, Nehal K, et al. Effects of tretinoin on photodamaged skin. A histologic study. *Arch Dermatol* 1991; 127: 666–672.
13. Griffiths CEM, Finkel LJ, Ditre CM, Hamilton TA, Ellis CN, Voorhees JJ. Topical tretinoin (retinoic acid) improves melasma. A vehicle-controlled, clinical trial. *Br J Dermatol* 1993; 129: 415–421.
14. Weiss JS, Ellis CN, Headington IT, et al. Topical tretinoin improved photoaged skin: a double-blind, vehicle-controlled study. *JAMA* 1988; 259: 527–532.
15. Rafal ES, Griffiths CEM, Ditre CM, et al. Topical tretinoin (retinoic acid) treatment for liver spots associated with photodamage. *N Engl J Med* 1992; 126: 368–374.
16. Griffiths CEM, Goldfarb MT, Finkel LJ, et al. Topical tretinoin (retinoic acid) treatment of hyperpigmented lesions associated with photoaging in Chinese and Japanese patients: a vehicle-controlled trial. *J Am Acad Dermatol* 1994; 30: 76–84.
17. Tadaki T, Watanabe M, Kumasaka K, et al. The effect of topical tretinoin on the photodamaged skin of the Japanese. *Tohoku J Exp Med* 1993; 169; 131–139.
18. Bulengo-Ransby SM, Griffiths CEM, Kimbrough-Green CK, et al. Topical tretinoin (retinoic acid) therapy for hyperpigmentation lesions caused by inflammation of the skin in black patients. *N Engl J Med* 1993; 328: 1438–1443.
19. Tzaneva S, Seeber A, Honigsmann H, Tanew A. A comparison of psoralen plus ultraviolet A (PUVA) monotherapy, tacalcitol plus PUVA and tazarotene plus PUVA in patients with chronic plaque-type psoriasis. *Br J Dermatol* 2002; 147: 748–753.
20. Green L, Sadoff W. A clinical evaluation of tazarotene 0.1% gel, with and without a high- or mid-high-potency corticosteroid, in patients with stable plaque psoriasis. *J Cutan Med Surg* 2002; 6(2): 95–102.
21. Guenther LC. Topical tazarotene therapy for psoriasis, acne vulgaris, and photoaging. *Skin Ther Lett* 2002; 7: 1–4.
22. Webster GF, Guenther L, Poulin YP, Solomon BA, Loven K, Lee J. A multicenter, double-blind, randomized comparison study of the efficacy and tolerability of once-daily tazarotene 0.1% gel and adapalene 0.1% gel for the treatment of facial acne vulgaris. *Cutis* 2002; 69: 4–11.
23. Tanghetti EA. An observation study evaluating the treatment of plaque psoriasis with tazarotene gels, alone and with an emollient and/or corticosteroid. Tazarotene Stable Plaque Trial Study Group. *Cutis* 2000; 66: 4–11.
24. Leyden JJ, Tanghetti EA, Miller B, Ung M, Berson D, Lee J. Once-daily tazarotene 0.1% gels versus once-daily tretinoin 0.1% microsponge gel for the treatment of facial acne vulgaris: a double-blind randomized trial. *Cutis* 2002; 69: 12–19.
25. Draelos ZD, Tanghetti EA. Optimizing the use of tazarotene for the treatment of facial acne vulgaris through combination therapy. Tazarotene Combination Leads to Efficacious Acne Results (CLEAR) Study Group. *Cutis* 2002; 69: 20–29.
26. Grimes PE, Calendar V. Tazarotene cream for facial post inflammatory hyperpigmentation associated with acne vulgaris. *Cutis* 2005 (in press).
27. Sefton J, Kligman AM, Kopper SC, Lue JC, Gibson JR. Photodamage pilot study: a double-blind, vehicle-controlled study to assess the efficacy and safety of tazarotene 0.1% gel. *J Am Acad Dermatol* 2000; 43: 656–663.
28. Menter A. Pharmacokinetics and safety of tazarotene. *J Am Acad Dermatol* 2000: 43:S31–S35.
29. Bernard BA. Adapalene, a new chemical entity with retinoid activity. *Skin Pharmacol* 1993; 6: 61–69.
30. Ioannides D, Rigopoulos D, Katsambas A. Topical adapalene gel 0.1% vs. isotretinoin gel 0.05% in the treatment of acne vulgaris: a randomized open-label clinical trial. *Br J Dermatol* 2002; 147: 523–527.
31. Redfern CRF. Molecular markers of retinoid activity in the skin. *J Invest Dermatol* 1994; 102: 11–12.
32. Verschoore M, Langner A, Wolska H, et al. Efficacy and safety of CD 271 alcoholic gels in the topical treatment of acne vulgaris. *Br J Dermatol* 1991; 124: 368–371.
33. Shalita A, Weis JS, Chalker DK, et al. A comparison of the efficacy and safety of adapalene gel 0.1% and tretinoin gel 0.025% in the treatment of acne vulgaris: a multicenter trial. *J Am Acad Dermatol* 1996; 34: 482–485.
34. Cunliffe WJ, Caputo R, Dreno B, et al. Clinical efficacy and safety comparison of adapalene gel and tretinoin gel in the treatment of acne vulgaris. Europe and US multicenter trials. *J Am Acad Dermatol* 1997: 36: S126–S134.
35. Czernielewski J, Poncet M, Mizzi F. Efficacy and cutaneous safety of adapelene in black patients versus white patients with acne vulgaris. *Cutis* 2002; 70: 243–248.

36. Zhu XJ, Tu P, Zhen J, Duan YQ. Adapalene gel 0.1%: effective and well tolerated in the topical treatment of acne vulgaris in Chinese patients. *Cutis* 2001; 68(4 Suppl): 55–59.
37. Kang S, Duell EA, Fisher GJ, et al. Application of retinol to human skin *in vivo* induces epidermal hyperplasia and cellular retinoid binding proteins characteristic of retinoic acid but without measureable retinoic acid levels or irritation. *J Invest Dermatol* 1995; 105: 549–556.
38. Cosmetic Ingredient Review. Final report on the safety assessment of retinyl palmitate and retinol. *J Am Coll Toxicol* 1987; 6: 279–320.
39. Grimes PE. Author's personal database.
40. Shalita AR, Smith JG, Parish LC, et al. Topical nicotinamide compared with clindamycin gel in the treatment of inflammatory acne vulgaris. *Int J Dermatol* 1995; 34: 434–437.
41. Bowes J, Piper J, Thiermermann C. Inhibitors of the activity of poly (ADP-ribose) synthetase reduce the cell death caused by hydrogen peroxide in human cardiac myoblast. *Br J Dermatol* 2000; 143: 524–531.
42. Gensler HL. Prevention of photoimmunosuppression and photocarcinogenesis by topical nicotinamide. *Nutr Cancer* 1997; 29: 157–162.
43. Tanno O, Oya Y, Kitamura N, et al. Nicotinamide increases biosynthesis of ceramides as well as other stratum corneum lipids to improve the epidermal permeability barrier. *Br J Dermatol* 2000; 143: 524–531.
44. Hakozaki T, Minwalla L, Zhuang J, et al. The effect of niacinamide on reducing cutaneous pigmentation and suppression of melanosome transfer. *Br J Dermatol* 2002; 147: 20–31.
45. Leyden JJ. Therapy for acne vulgaris. *N Engl J Med* 1997; 336: 1156–1162.
46. Borglund E, Osten H, Nord CE. Impact of topical clindamycin and systemic tetracycline on the skin and colon microflora in patients with acne vulgaris. *Scand J Infect Dis* 1984; 43(suppl): 76–81.
47. Decker LC, Deuel DM, Sedlock DM. Role of lipids in augmenting the antibacterial activity of benzoyl peroxide against *Propionibacterium acnes*. *Antimicrob Agents Chemother* 1989; 33: 326–330.
48. Nacht S, Yeung D, Beasley JN, et al. Benzoyl peroxide: percutaneous penetration and metabolic disposition. *J Am Acad Dermatol* 1981; 4: 31–37.
49. Lookingbill DP, Chalker DK, Lindholm JS, et al. Treatment of acne with a combination clindamycin/ benzoyl peroxide gel compared with clindamycin gel, benzoyl peroxide gel and vehicle gel: combined results of two double-blind investigations. *J Am Acad Dermatol* 1997; 37: 590–595.
50. Chalker DK, Shalita AR, Smith JG, Swann RW. A double-blind study of the effectiveness of a 3% erythromycin and 5% benzoyl peroxide combination in the treatment of acne vulgaris. *J Am Acad Dermatol* 1983; 9: 933–936.
51. Tucker SB, Tausend R, Cochran R, Flannigan SA. Comparison of topical clindamycin phosphate, benzoyl peroxide, and a combination of the two for the treatment of acne vulgaris. *Br J Dermatol*. 1984; 110(4): 487–492.
52. Harkaway KS, McGingley KJ, Foglia AN, et al. Antibiotic resistance patterns in coagulase-negative staphylococci after treatment with topical erythromycin, benzoyl peroxide, and combination therapy. *Br J Dermatol* 1992; 126: 586–590.
53. Eady EA, Farmery MR, Ross JI, et al. Effect of benzoyl peroxide and erythromycin alone and in combination against antibiotic-sensitive and -resistant skin bacteria from acne patients. *Br J Dermatol* 1994; 131: 331–336.
54. Eady Ea, Bojar RA, Jones CE, et al. The effects of acne treatment with a combination of benzoyl peroxide and erythromycin on skin carriage of erythromycin-resistant propionibacteria. *Br J Dermatol* 1996; 134: 107–113.
55. Tschen EH, Katz HI, Jones TM, et al. A combination benzoyl peroxide and clindamycin topical gel compared with benzoyl peroxide, clindamycin phosphate, and vehicle in the treatment of acne vulgaris. *Cutis* 2001; 67: 165–169.
56. Eady EA, Cove JH. Topical antibiotic therapy: current status and future prospects. *Drugs Exp Clin Res* 1990; 16(8): 423–433.
57. Marsland AM, Griffiths CEM. The macrolide immunosuppressants in dermatology: mechanisms of action. *Eur J Dermatol* 2002; 12: 618–622.
58. Bershad SV. The modern age of acne therapy: a review of current treatment options. *Mt Sinai J Med* 2001; 68: 279–286.

59. Cunliffe WJ, Topical erythromycin in clinical and laboratory studies. In: Mark SR (Ed) *Topical Antibiotics in Acne*. London: Martin Duritz, 1989.
60. Thomas DR, Raimer S, Smith EB. Comparison of topical erythromycin 1.5 percent solution versus topical clindamycin phosphate 1.0 solution in the treatment of acne vulgaris. *Cutis* 1982; 29: 628–632.
61. Chu A, Huber FJ, Plott RT. The comparative efficacy of benzoyl peroxide 5%/erythromycin 3% gel and erythromycin 4%/zinc 1.2% solution in the treatment of acne vulgaris. *Br J Dermatol* 1997; 136: 235–238.
62. White GM. Acne therapy. *Adv Dermatol* 1999; 14: 29–58.
63. Shapiro LE, Knowles SR, Shear NH. Comparative safety of tetracycline, minocycline, and doxycycline. *Arch Dermatol* 1997; 133: 1224–1230.
64. Brazzini B, Pimpinelli N. New and established topical corticosteroids in dermatology: clinical pharmacology and therapeutic use. *Am J Clin Dermatol* 2002; 3(1): 47–58.
65. Chan HL. The effects of topical corticosteroids on human skin. *Ann Acad Med Singapore* 1991; 20: 133–138.
66. Priestley GC, Brown JC. Effects of corticosteroids on the proliferation of normal and abnormal human connective tissue cells. *Br J Dermatol* 1980; 102(1): 35–41.
67. Takeda K, Arase S, Takahashi S. Side effects of topical corticosteroids and their prevention. *Drugs* 1988; 36: 15–23.
68. Sterry W. Therapy with topical corticosteroids. *Arch Dermatol Res* 1992; 284: S27–S29.
69. Suzuki S, Miyachi Y, Niwa Y, Isshiki N. Significance of reactive oxygen species in distal flap necrosis and its salvage with liposomal SOD. *Br J Plast Surg* 1989; 42: 559–564.
70. Bissett DL, Chatterjee R, Hannon DP. Photoprotective effect of superoxide-scavenging antioxidants against ultraviolet radiation-induced chronic skin damage in the hairless mouse. *Photodermatol Photoimmunol Photomed* 1990; 7: 56–62.
71. Darr D, Combs S, Dunston S, Manning T, Pinnel S. Topical vitamin C protects porcine skin from ultraviolet radiation-induced damage. *Br J Dermatol* 1992; 127: 247–253.
72. Black HS. Potential involvement of free radical reactions in ultraviolet light mediated cutaneous damage. *Photochem Photobiol* 1987; 46: 213–221.
73. Eberlein-Konig B, Placzek M, Pryzbilla B. Protective effect against sunburn of combined systemic ascorbic acid (vitamin C) and d-alpha-tocopherol (vitamin E). *J Am Acad Dermatol* 1998; 38: 45–48.
74. Colvin RM, Pinnell SR. Topical vitamin C in aging. *Clin Dermatol* 1996; 14: 227–234.
75. Bachowski GJ, Girotti AW. Light-stimulated formation of hydrogen peroxide and hydroxyl radical in the presence of uroporphyrin and ascorbate. *Free Radic Biol Med* 1988; 5: 3–6.
76. Bacq ZM, Fischer P. The action of various drugs on the suprarenal response of the rat to total-body x-irradiation. *Radiat Res* 1957; 7: 365–372.
77. Frei B, England L, Amos B. Ascorbate is an outstanding anti-oxidant in human blood plasma. *Proc Natl Acad Sci USA* 1989; 86: 6377–6381.
78. Koch CJ, Biaglow JE. Toxicity, radiation sensitivity modification, and metabolic effects of dehydroascorbate and ascorbate in mammalian cells. *J Cell Physiol* 1978; 94: 299–306.
79. Bartlett MK, Jones CM, Ryan AE. Vitamin C and wound healing: II. Ascorbic acid content and tensile strength of healing wounds in human beings. *N Engl J Med* 1942; 226: 474–481.
80. Padh H. Cellular functions of ascorbic acid. *Biochem Cell Biol* 1990; 68: 1166–1173.
81. Abt AF, von Schurching S. Catabolism of L-ascorbic-1-C acid as a measure of its utilization in the intact and wounded guinea pig on scorbutic maintenance, and saturation diets. *Ann NY Acad Sci* 1961; 92: 148–158.
82. Fitzpatrick RE, Rostan EF. Double blind, half-face study comparing topical vitamin C and vehicle for rejuvenation of photodamage. *Dermatol Surg* 2002; 28: 231–236.
83. Perricone NV. The photoprotective and anti-inflammatory effects of topical ascorbyl palmitate. *J Geriatr Dermatol* 1993; 1: 5–10.
84. Perricone NV. Topical vitamin C ester (ascorbyl palmitate). *J Geriatr Dermatol* 1997; 5: 162–170.
85. Hayakawa R, Ueda H, Nozaki T, et al. Effects of combination treatment with vitamins E and C on chloasma and pigmented contact dermatitis. A double blind controlled clinical trial. *Acta Vitaminol Enzymol* 1981: 31–38.
86. Pandya AG. Pharmacological agents in skin of color. *Cosmet Dermatol* 2003; 16; 49–52.

87. Jimbow K, Obata H, Pathak MA, et al. Mechanism of depigmentation by hydroquinone. *J Invest Dermatol* 1974; 62; 436–449.
88. Grimes PE. Melasma: In: *Dermatology: Cutaneous Medicine and Surgery in Primary Care*. Harcourt, Brace, and Co., 1997; 151–153.
89. Findlay GH, Morrison JG, Simson IW. Exogenous ochronosis and pigmented colloid milium from hydroquinone bleaching creams. *Br J Dermatol*. 1975; 93(6): 613–622.
90. Mahe A, Ly F, Aymard G, Dangou JM. Skin diseases associated with the cosmetic use of bleaching products in women from Dakar, Senegal. *Br J Dermatol* 2003; 148(3): 493–500.
91. Grimes PE. Author's personal database.
92. Kang S, Paller A, Soter N, Satoi Y, Rico MJ, Hanifin JM. Safe treatment of head/neck AD with tacrolimus ointment. *J Dermatol Treat* 2003; 14(2): 86–94.
93. Eichenfield LF, Lucky AW, Boguniewicz M, Langley RG, Cherill R, Marshall K, Bush C, Graeber M. Safety and efficacy of pimecrolimus (ASM 981) cream 1% in the treatment of mild and moderate atopic dermatitis in children and adolescents. *J Am Acad Dermatol* 2002; 46(4): 495–504.
94. Grimes PE, Soriano T, Dytoc MT. Topical tacrolimus for repigmentation of vitiligo. *J Am Acad Dermatol* 2002; 47(5): 789–791.
95. Grimes PE, Morris R, Avaniss-Aghajani E, Soriano T, Meraz M, Metzger A. Topical tacrolimus therapy for vitiligo: therapeutic responses and skin messenger RNA expression of proinflammatory cytokines. *J Am Acad Dermatol* 2004; 51: 52–61.

12 Cosmetic and Dermatologic Surgery for Pigmented Skins

Pearl E. Grimes and Brooke A. Jackson

INTRODUCTION

Cosmetic procedures including chemical peels, microdermabrasion, and botulinum toxin injections have become increasingly popular among darker racial ethnic groups including Asians, Native Americans, Hispanics, and blacks. Data from the American Society of Plastic and Reconstructive Surgery shows that cosmetic procedures among darker-skinned patients increased from 12% of all patients in 1992 to 20% in 1998. Of those, 8% were African-American (up from 4%), 8% were Hispanic (up from 5%), and 4% were Asian (up from 3%).

Serial superficial peeling agents and microdermabrasion offer substantial benefits for the dyschromias, acne, oily skin, and texturally rough skin in darker racial ethnic groups. In light of the labile responses of melanocytes of darker-complexioned individuals, the clinician must always weigh the indication/necessity and risk/benefit ratios of any resurfacing procedure. These techniques should be performed with care and caution. Current data also suggest that botulinum toxin injections for glabellar lines are well tolerated in darker racial/ethnic groups.

REJUVENATION IN ETHNIC SKIN

Intrinsic factors such as gravity and other external factors (e.g., pollution) that are unrelated to sun exposure contribute to the cutaneous aging process; however, 95% of the visible signs of aging are caused by sun exposure, which begins in infancy and accumulates throughout life.[33] Fine perioral and periorbital lines, seen as early as the second decade in white patients, tend not to occur in the patient with ethnic skin. Not only do the manifestations of the cutaneous aging process in ethnic skin occur 10–20 years later than those in age-matched white counterparts, but they also tend to occur in the deeper muscular layers of the face rather than within the skin, thus minimizing rhytide formation.

Ethnic patients, particularly African-Americans, have a tendency toward midface aging, along with sagging of the malar fat pads toward the nasolabial folds, upper lid laxity, and jowl formation.[34] Because of the pervasive cultural attitude that facial plastic surgery conflicts with a healthy sense of racial identity, in addition to the increased risk of keloid and hypertrophic scar formation, African-American patients are much less likely to undergo facial plastic surgery. Whereas the traditional facelift is so pervasive in the white population, African-Americans will opt instead for body-recontouring procedures such as liposuction and breast augmentation. For those patients with ethnic skin who do choose facial rejuvenation procedures, many minimally invasive procedures are chosen. These include botulinum toxin injections and soft tissue augmentation, which are ideally suited for those with midface aging who do not need a more drastic lifting procedure.[35]

BOTULINUM TOXIN

Botulinum A exotoxin injections are commonly used to improve facial aesthetics. Different strains of the bacterium *Clostridium botulinum* produce serologically distinct types of botulinum toxins.

Seven serotypes of botulinum neurotoxin have been identified: A, B, C1, D, E, F, and G.[1] All of the botulinum neurotoxins produce chemodenervation and atrophy of skeletal muscles by blocking acetylcholine release from motor neurons at the neuromuscular junction. The neurotoxin serotypes differ in their cellular mechanisms of action, however, and their clinical profiles also vary.[2]

Type A botulinum toxin was the first to be developed for clinical use. Botulinum toxin type A is manufactured and distributed by Allergan, Inc. under the brand name BOTOX® Cosmetic. Speywood Pharmaceuticals Ltd. also markets botulinum A toxin under the brand name Dysport®. Although the active agent in each formulation is botulinum A toxin, the two preparations have different clinical properties that might be due to differences in the vehicle, formulation, or manufacturing process.[3]

Botulinum toxin injections are highly successful in smoothing hyperdynamic lines (glabellar lines, horizontal frown lines, and "crow's feet") in the upper face.[4–6] Although several recent studies have evaluated the efficacy of Botox for hyperfunctional facial lines in Asian patients,[7,8] there is minimal published data regarding the efficacy and dosing of botulinum toxin in African-Americans. In view of basic structural and morphological differences in black and white skin,[9] one could postulate that dosing might differ. There were 21 African-American women included in the phase III botulinum toxin study for FDA drug approval for treatment of glabellar lines.[10] Grimes et al.[11] compared these African-American women to the overall group of 405 patients in this double-blind, multi-center, placebo-controlled study. A total of 20 units of botulinum toxin was injected for glabellar lines. There were no significant differences between groups in ratings of severity scores or global improvement post-treatment. Botulinum toxin was well tolerated and without side effects in the 21 African-American women included in the aforementioned study (Figure 12.1). In a 4-month randomized, double-masked dosing study for treatment of glabellar lines in women with skin types V and VI, both 20 U and 30 U doses of botulinum toxin A were well tolerated.[12]

The effects of botulinum A toxin injections are usually apparent within a day or two and typically last for 3 or 4 months, but they may last for 6 months or longer. With repeated injections, there is a tendency for later injections to provide aesthetic improvement that lasts longer.[13,14] The reason for this is unknown, but it is possible that over the course of treatment, individuals alter their habitual use of muscles that cause expression lines.

Side effects of botulinum toxin injections are ptosis, headache, diplopia, and edema and bruising at the injection site. Contraindications for botulinum toxin injections include pregnancy, breast-feeding, myasthenia gravis, and Lambert–Eaton Syndrome.

CHEMICAL PEELS

Peeling Agents

Chemical peels are often performed for the treatment of photodamage, actinic keratoses, rhytides, scarring, acne, and dyschromias.[15] Historically, chemical peels were most frequently performed in patients with lighter skin (Fitzpatrick skin types I, II, and III). In the past, clinicians were often reluctant to offer these therapies to patients with darker skin, in particular, Fitzpatrick skin types V and VI. This hesitation was due to concerns regarding the induction of dyschromias and scarring.[16] However, multiple recent reports have demonstrated that chemical peels can be safely performed in patients with skin of color.[16–22]

Prior to commencing a peeling procedure in patients with darker skin types, it is important to consider that the indications for peeling procedures differ in darker skin types and include melasma and postinflammatory hyperpigmentation unresponsive to topical bleaching agents, texturally rough skin, oily skin, and acne vulgaris. Peeling procedures may also improve pseudofolliculitis barbae and keratosis pilaris.

Chemical peeling agents are classified as superficial, medium-depth, or deep peels. Superficial peels targeting the stratum corneum to the papillary dermis include glycolic acid, salicylic acid,

Cosmetic and Dermatologic Surgery for Pigmented Skins

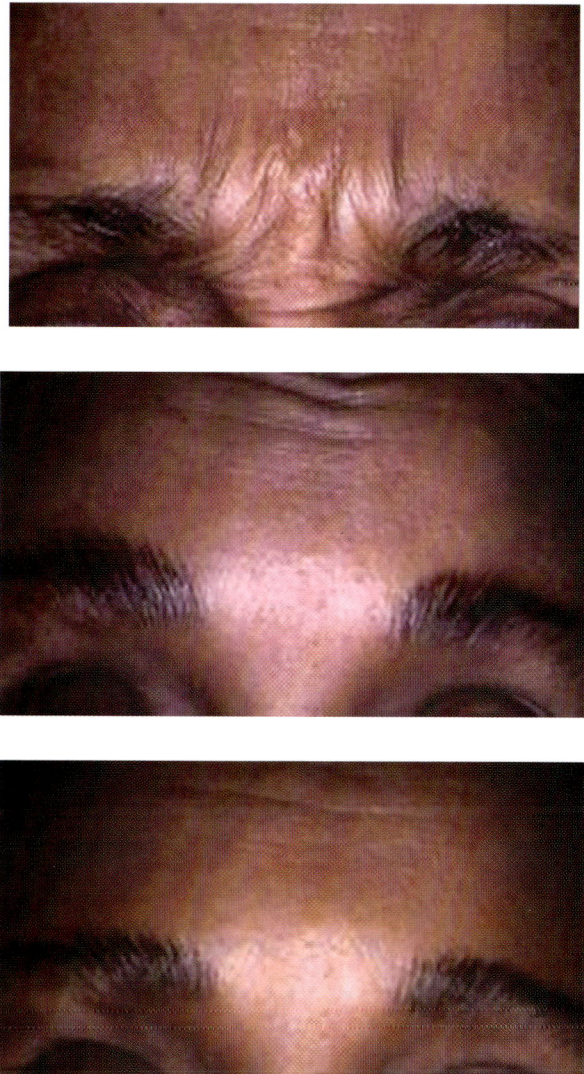

FIGURE 12.1 Before and after Botox injections (30–90 days). A total of 20 units was used for glabellar lines.

Jessner's solution, and trichloroacetic acid (TCA) in concentrations ranging from 10% to 30%. Medium-depth peels penetrate to the upper reticular dermis and include TCA (35%–50%) and phenol 88%. Deep chemical peels utilize the Baker–Gordon formula and penetrate to the midreticular dermis.

Peeling Protocol

Despite studies that have documented the efficacy and safety of superficial peeling agents in darker racial/ethnic groups, there is indeed variability in the reactivity and responses to chemical peeling agents. Superficial chemical peels can cause hyperpigmentation and scarring. The initial peel should be performed at the lowest concentration of the peeling agent to assess the patient's sensitivity and reactivity. The standard protocol for Grimes[16,19] involves initial pretreatment with bleaching agents for 1–2 weeks prior to peeling. Such agents include hydroquinone 4%, azelaic acid, or kojic acid formulations. In pigmented skin, retinoid-based products should be discontinued 1–2 weeks prior to peel. Tretinoin often increases the depth of peeling, which can cause epidermolysis and post-peel hyperpigmentation. Peels are performed at 2–4-week intervals. A series of four to six glycolic acid or salicylic acid peels are routinely performed. TCA peels are usually administered at 1-month intervals for a total of three peels. Post-peel care includes the use of bland cleansers and moisturizers until peeling and irritation subside.

GLYCOLIC ACID

Glycolic acid is an alpha-hydroxy acid (AHA). AHAs are organic carboxylic acids that have one hydroxyl group attached to the alpha position of the carboxylic carbon atom. These compounds occur naturally in sugar cane juice, sour milk, grapes, and apple and tomato juice.

Glycolic compounds for skin peeling include buffered, partially neutralized, and esterified products. Typically, concentrations of glycolic acid in these formulations range from 20% to 70%. The efficacy of glycolic acid peels has been demonstrated in patients with darker skin. In a split-face comparison, Lim and Tham treated ten Asian women with melasma and fine wrinkles with 2% hydroquinone and 10% glycolic acid applied to both sides of the face.[18] A series of 20%–70% glycolic acid peels were performed on the other side for comparison. Greater improvements were noted on the side of the face that underwent the glycolic acid peels.

Burns et al. treated 19 black patients with postinflammatory hyperpigmentation.[18] A control group was treated with 2% hydroquinone/10% glycolic acid twice per day and tretinoin 0.05% at bedtime, whereas the treatment group received the same regimen plus a series of six glycolic acid peels. Although not statistically significant, greater improvement was noted in the patients in the chemical peel group.

Side effects of glycolic acid peels in darker racial ethnic groups may be minimized by initiating therapy using the lower-strength peeling agents and gradually titrating to the higher strengths (Figure 12.2). Lower-concentration glycolic acid peels (20%–35%) are less irritating and produce less epidermolysis than the lower-concentration salicylic acid peels. In contrast, a 70% glycolic acid peel is more aggressive compared with a 30% salicylic acid peel.

SALICYLIC ACID

Salicylic acid is commercially available as a superficial peeling agent in a hydrethanolic vehicle solution at concentrations of 20% and 30%. Salicylic acid is a hydroxyl derivative of benzoic acid

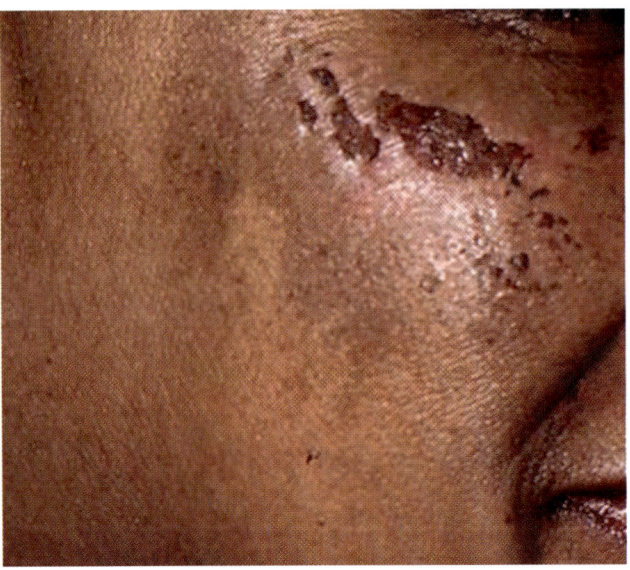

FIGURE 12.2 Crusting following a 35% glycolic acid peel.

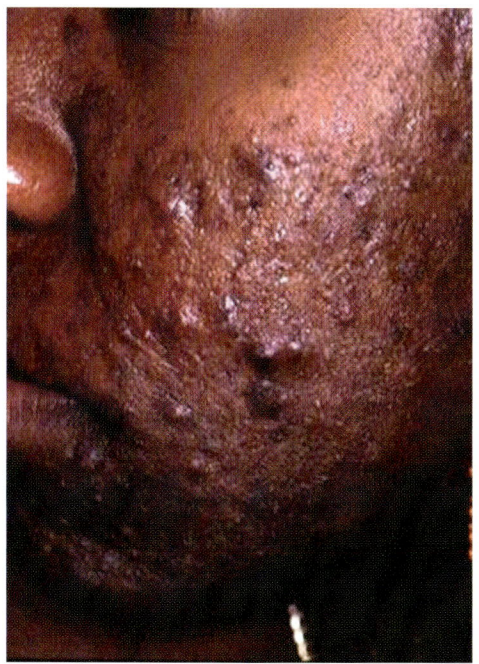 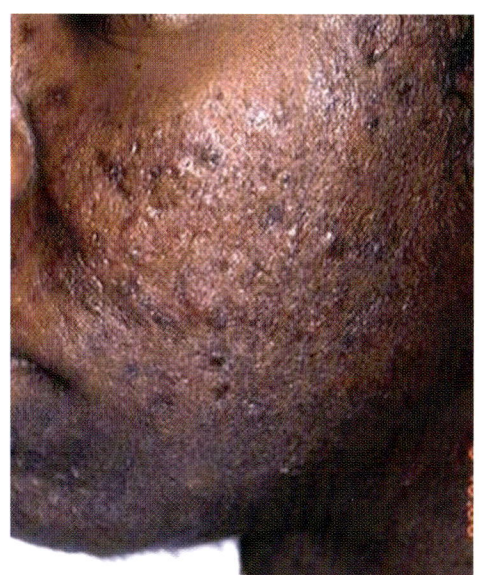

FIGURE 12.3 Before and after a series of five salicylic acid peels.

and is a lipophilic agent that produces desquamation of the upper lipophilic layers of the stratum corneum. Its efficacy as a peeling agent is well established.[23,24] In a recent evaluation, 25 patients with skin types V and VI were treated with a series of five salicylic acid peels.[19] Conditions treated included acne vulgaris; postinflammatory hyperpigmentation; texturally rough, oily skin; and melasma. Patients were treated with hydroquinone 4% for 2 weeks, followed by a series of two 20% and three 30% salicylic acid peels performed biweekly. Moderate to significant improvement was noted in 88% of the treated patients, with minor side effects reported in 16% (Figure 12.3). Three patients experienced hyperpigmentation that resolved in less than 2 weeks.

In addition, the efficacy of a series of five salicylic acid peels and five glycolic acid peels was assessed in 90 and 75 patients, respectively. Ninety percent of patients in salicylic acid groups had moderate to significant improvement compared with 82% for glycolic acid patients. Both peels were well tolerated, with minimal side effects.

TRICHLOROACETIC ACID

TCA peels have long been considered the gold standard by which the efficacy of other peels is measured. Superficial peeling is usually accomplished with concentrations of 10%–35%. TCA precipitates epidermal proteins, causing sloughing and necrosis of the treated areas in a concentration-dependent manner. Although TCA may be safely used in darker skin, there is a smaller margin of safety compared with glycolic acid and salicylic acid peels. The incidence of post-peel hyperpigmentation is significantly more common in darker skin and may best be left for use only in patients in which severe pigmentation and wrinkles are a major issue of cosmetic concern.

JESSNER'S SOLUTION

Jessner's solution contains 14% resorcinol, 14% salicylic acid, and 14% lactic acid. The Jessner's chemical peel has been used to treat moderate to severe facial dyschromias, acne, oily skin, texturally rough skin, fine wrinkles, and pseudofolliculitis. Jessner's solution is used alone for superficial peeling. It is often combined with 35% trichloroacetic acid for medium-depth peeling. When Jessner's solution was used as a superficial peeling agent in a subgroup of patients,[25,26] the peel was well tolerated in individuals with skin types V and VI.

MEDIUM AND DEEP PEELS

Medium and deep peels utilize TCA concentrations of 40% or greater, or phenol combinations. Medium-depth peels also utilize glycolic acid 70% or Jessner's solution in a combination with 35% TCA. These peels are most often used to treat moderate to severe photodamage. The best results are achieved in patients with skin types I and II. Appropriate patient selection is essential.

Pierce and Brown[27] reported the use of deeper peeling procedures in African-Americans. However, clinicians should be acutely aware that deeper peels carry substantial risks of inducing scarring and hypopigmentation in darker-skinned racial/ethnic groups.

MICRODERMABRASION

Microdermabrasion has become one of the most popular forms of superficial resurfacing. The technique of microdermabrasion was first developed in Italy in 1985. Most units for microdermabrasion are closed-loop, negative-pressure systems that pass aluminum oxide crystals onto the skin while simultaneously vacuuming the crystals. Another system utilizes sodium chloride and positive pressure for resurfacing. Other crystals used include magnesium oxide and sodium bicarbonate. Indications for microdermabrasion include acne, acne scarring, hyperpigmentation, textural changes, and striae.

According to 2002 data from the American Society for Aesthetic Plastic Surgery, 1,032,417 microdermabrasion procedures were performed in 2002. Microdermabrasion showed the highest one-year gain of all the nonsurgical cosmetic procedures, surpassing chemical peels, fillers, and botulinum toxin injections. Tsai et al.[28] reported the first series of patients treated with microdermabrasion in 1995. The authors reported good to excellent results in 41 patients treated with microdermabrasion for facial scarring. Subsequent studies have documented the efficacy of microdermabrasion for improvement of acne, hyperpigmentation, texturally rough skin, and photodamage.[29–32]

Skin barrier changes induced by microdermabrasion have also been studied.[32] The investigators assessed transepidermal water loss, capacitance (hydration), skin pH, and sebum production at 24 h and again at 7 days post-microdermabrasion. Both aluminum oxide and sodium chloride microdermabrasion at 7 days enhanced skin hydration and decreased transepidermal water loss. Other mechanisms of action include exfoliation, decreased epidermal melanization, increased epidermal thickness, and increased elastin production.[30,31]

The skin depth of the microdermabrasion procedure is determined by the rate of movement of the handpiece, strength of the flow of crystals, and the number of passes per anatomic area. Slow movement of the handpiece, increased flow of crystals, and increased passes increase the depth of the microdermabrasion procedure.

In general, microdermabrasion is extremely well tolerated in skin of color (Figure 12.4). However, if the procedure is performed aggressively, hyperpigmentation, purpura, streaking, and telangiectasia can occur (Figure 12.5).

INJECTABLE FILLING AGENTS

Although cosmetic correction of the upper third of the face is largely the domain of botulinum toxin, dermal fillers are the agents of choice for the nonsurgical correction of the mid- and lower-face. The ideal filling agent is easily used, natural in appearance, well tolerated, nonmigratory,

Cosmetic and Dermatologic Surgery for Pigmented Skins

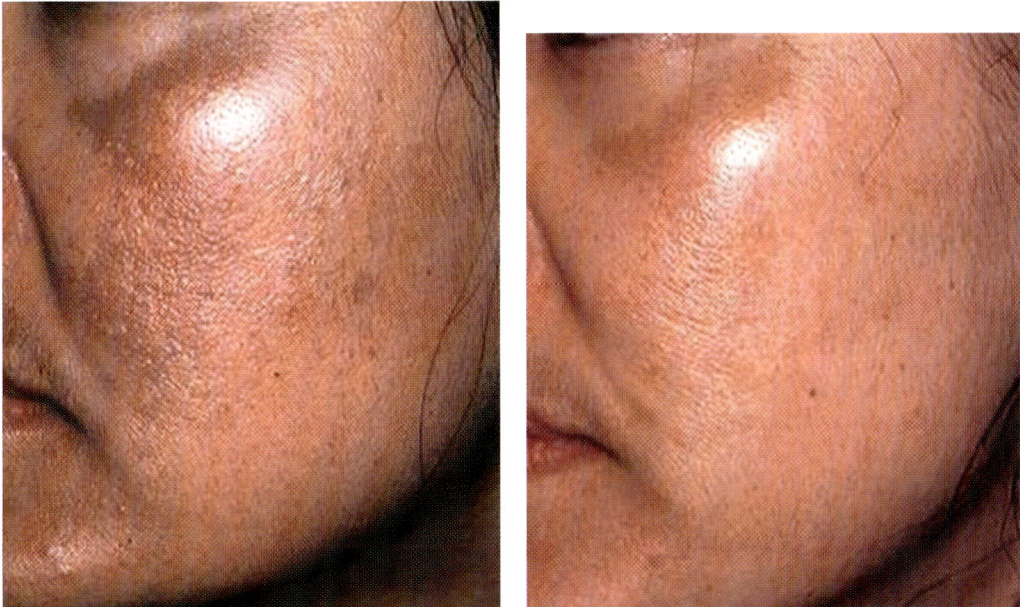

FIGURE 12.4 Before (left) and after (right) six microdermabrasion treatments for melasma.

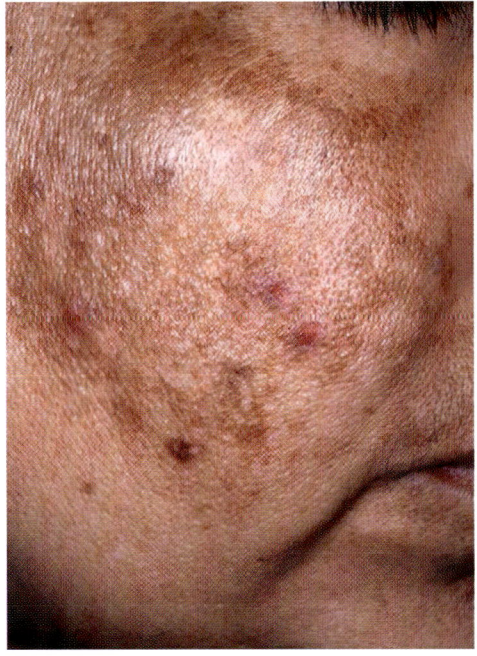

FIGURE 12.5 Hyperpigmentation secondary to aggressive microdermabrasion.

nonimmunogenic, and permanent; however, the permanent nature of some implants can be problematic not only for the physician with poor technique but also for the patient who changes his or her mind of what is ideal. Although no currently available injectable agent fulfills all of these criteria, there are many that are safe and provide high patient satisfaction (Table 12.1).

TABLE 12.1
FDA-Approved Injectable Filling Agents

Product	Material	Company
Zyderm/Zyplast	Bovine collagen	Inamed Aesthetics
Cosmoderm/Cosmoplast	Human-based collagen	Inamed Aesthetics
Perlane	Hyaluronic acid	Medicis
Radiance	Calcium hydroxylapatite	BioForm

COLLAGEN

With an estimated 1.5 million treatments performed to date in the United States,[36] bovine collagen (available as Zyderm and Zyplast; Inamed Aesthetics, Santa Barbara, CA) injection in the lower two thirds of the face is well tolerated with good patient satisfaction and was, for many years, the gold standard for the correction of acne scars and rhytides. The major disadvantage of this product is the need for pretreatment skin testing and the short duration of correction, lasting from 8 to 20 months in the treatment of acne scars and less time in areas of increased motion such as the nasolabial folds.[37] Cosmoderm or Cosmoplast (Inamed Aesthetics) is a bioengineered form of human collagen, producing similar results to Zyderm and Zyplast but, because of its origin, obviating the need for pretreatment testing,[40] making it a more appealing and immediate therapeutic option for those seeking cosmetic correction.

HYALURONIC ACID

Hyaluronic acid (HA), a gylcosaminoglycan component of the extracellular matrix, along with collagen and elastin, is one of the building blocks of the skin. HA binds collagen and elastin into the matrix, giving skin its supportive structure. HA also draws water into the skin, giving it volume and fullness, such that loss of HA with age results in dermal dehydration and rhytid formation.[41] Restylane is a nonanimal stabilized HA (NASHA) product prepared in bacterial cultures of equine streptococci that is cross-linked, forming an injectable gel. Although rare, the presence of bacterial proteins can cause a hypersensitivity reaction in one in 5000 patients.[42] Because of its hydrophilic nature, lack of need for pretreatment allergy testing, and longer results lasting up to 8 months,[43] restylane is a potentially useful same-day treatment alternative for midface aging in ethnic skin.

HYDROXYLAPATITE

Radiance (BioForm; Franksville, WI) is composed of microspheres of calcium hydroxylapatite (CaHA) in an inert, aqueous gel. A synthetic compound, CaHA is identical to the chemical structure of calcium naturally present in the body. After injection, this filling substance is thought to last 3–5 years, which can be problematic if injected improperly. The radiopaque nature of CaHA may also interfere with proper interpretation of dental x-rays, making the use of this substance less desirable until more information is available. Long-term and animal studies are not available.

BODY IMAGE AND BODY-CONTOURING PROCEDURES

Although the desire for the perfect body image affects both men and women of all cultural backgrounds, there are distinct cultural differences with what is perceived as the ideal body image. White and Hispanic Americans foster more weight-related body image distortion than Asian and African-Americans,[44–46] who report the greatest body image satisfaction. These findings support not only a higher incidence of eating disorders seen in white women but also the higher demand for cosmetic procedures in this same demographic group.

TUMESCENT LIPOSUCTION

Developed in 1985 by Klein,[47] tumescent liposuction offers localized body contouring without the need for, or risk of, general anesthesia, providing high patient satisfaction. Large volumes of very dilute lidocaine with epinephrine are infiltrated into the subcutaneous space, followed by suction-assisted lipectomy. The technique and procedure are discussed exhaustively elsewhere.[48]

Although the technique does not vary between ethnic groups, cultural preference does exist regarding ideal body contours, particularly in the hip, thigh, and buttock areas, which should be discussed with the patient in the preoperative consultation.[49] While much has been written in the medical literature and in the lay press on the safety of liposuction as an in-office procedure and the performance of this procedure by dermatologists, the significant contributions made by dermatologists in the field of liposuction have made this procedure, when performed by properly trained dermatologic surgeons, a safe in-office procedure.[50]

REFERENCES

1. Jankovic J, Hallett M (Eds) *Therapy with Botulinum Toxin*. New York: Marcel Dekker, 1994.
2. Eleopra R, Tugnoli V, Rossetto O, De Grandis D, Montecucco C. Different time courses of recovery after poisoning with botulinum neurotoxin serotypes A and E in humans. *Neurosci Lett* 1998; 256: 135–138.
3. Sampaio C, Ferreira JJ, Simoes F, et al. DYSBOT: a single-blind, randomized parallel study to determine whether any differences can be detected in the efficacy and tolerability of two formulations of botulinum toxin type A — Dysport and Botox assuming a ratio of 4:1. *Mov Disord* 1997; 12: 1013–1018.
4. Carruthers A, Carruthers J. Cosmetic uses of botulinum A exotoxin. In: Klein AW (Ed) *Tissue Augmentation in Clinical Practice: Procedures and Techniques*. New York: Marcel Dekker, 1998; 207–236.
5. Blitzer A, Binder WJ, Aviv JE. The management of hyperfunctional facial lines with botulinum toxin: a collaborative study of 210 injection sites in 162 patients. *Arch Otolaryngol Head Neck Surg* 1997; 123: 389–392.
6. Carruthers A, Carruthers J. Botulinum toxin type A: history and current cosmetic use in the upper face. *Semin Cutan Med Surg* 2001; 20(2): 71–84.
7. Ahn KY, Park MY, Park DH, Han DG. Botulinum toxin A for the treatment of facial hyperkinetic wrinkle lines in Koreans. *Plast Reconstr Surg* 2000; 205: 778–784.
8. Lew H, Yun YS, Lee SY, Kim SJ. Effect of botulinum toxin A on facial wrinkle lines in Koreans. *Ophthalmologica* 2002; 216: 50–54.
9. Montagna W, Carlisle K. The architecture of black and white facial skin. *J Am Acad Dermatol* 1991; 24(6 Pt 1): 929–937.
10. Carruthers JA, Lowe NJ, Menter MA, et al. A multicenter, double-blind, randomized, placebo-controlled study of the efficacy and safety of botulinum toxin type A in the treatment of glabellar lines. *J Am Acad Dermatol* 2002; 46(6): 840–849.
11. Grimes PE. Botox: beyond the female Caucasian patient. Hawaii Dermatology Seminar, Skin Disease Education Foundation. Maui, Hawaii, February 2003.
12. Grimes PE. A four-month randomized, double-masked evaluation of the efficacy of Botulinum toxin type A for the treatment of glabellar lines in women with skin types V and VI. Poster presentation submitted for American Academy of Dermatology annual meeting, Washington DC, 2004.
13. Ahn MS, Catten M, Maas CS. Temporal brow lift using botulinum toxin A. *Plast Reconstruct Surg* 2000; 105: 1129–1135.
14. Carruthers JDA, Carruthers JA. Treatment of glabellar frown lines with *C. botulinum*-A exotoxin. *J Dermatol Surg Oncol* 1992; 18(1): 17–21.

15. Brody HJ. *Chemical Peeling.* New York: Mosby Year Book, 1992; 23–50.
16. Grimes PE. Agents for ethnic skin peeling. *Dermatol Ther* 2000; 13: 159–163.
17. Lim JT, Tham SN. Glycolic acid peels in the treatment of melasma in Asian women. *Dermatol Surg* 1997; 20: 27–34.
18. Burns RI, Provost-Blank PC, Lawry MA, et al. Glycolic acid peels for post inflammatory hyperpigmentation in black patients: a comparative study. *Dermatol Surg* 1997; 23: 171–174.
19. Grimes PE. The safety and efficacy of salicylic acid chemical peels in darker racial-ethnic groups. *Dermatol Surg* 1999; 25: 18–22.
20. Sarkar R, Kaur C, Bhalla M, Kanwar AJ. The combination of glycolic acid peels with a topical regimen in the treatment of melasma in dark-skinned patients: a comparative study. *Dermatol Surg* 2002; 28(9): 828–832.
21. Javaheri SM, Handa S, Kaur I, Kumar B. Safety and efficacy of glycolic acid facial peel in Indian women with melasma. *Int J Dermatol* 2001; 40(5): 354–357.
22. Grimes PE. Glycolic acid peels in blacks. In: Moy R, Luftman D, Kakita L (Eds) *Glycolic Acid Peels.* New York: Marcel Dekker, 2002; 179–185.
23. Kligman D, Kligman AM. Salicylic acid as a peeling agent for the treatment of acne. *Cosmet Dermatol* 1997; 10: 44–47.
24. Kligman D, Kligman AM. Salicylic acid peels for the treatment of photoaging. *Dermatol Surg* 1998; 24: 325–328.
25. Lawrence N, Cox SE, Cockerell CJ, Freeman RG, Cruz PD Jr. A comparison of the efficacy and safety of Jessner's solution and 35% trichloroacetic acid vs. 5% fluorouracil in the treatment of widespread facial actinic keratoses. *Arch Dermatol* 1995; 131(2): 176–181.
26. Lawrence N, Cox SE, Brody HJ. Treatment of melasma with Jessner's solution versus glycolic acid: a comparison of clinical efficacy and evaluation of the predictive ability of Wood's light examination. *J Am Acad Dermatol* 1997; 36(4): 589–593.
27. Pierce HE, Brown LA. Laminar dermal reticulotomy and chemical face peeling in the black patient. *J Dermatol Surg Oncol* 1986; 12: 69–73.
28. Tsai R, Wang C, Shan H. Aluminum oxide crystal microdermabrasion: a new technique for treating facial scarring. *Dermatol Surg* 1995; 21: 531–542.
29. Hernandez-Perez E, Ibiett EV. Gross and microscopic findings in patients undergoing microdermabrasion for facial rejuvenation. *Dermatol Surg* 2001; 27(7): 637–640.
30. Shim EK, Barnette D, Hughes K, et al. Microdermabrasion: a clinical and histopathologic study. *Dermatol Surg* 2001; 27(6): 524–530.
31. Tan MH, Spencer JM, Pires LM, Ajmeri J, Skover G. The evaluation of aluminum oxide crystal microdermabrasion for photodamage. *Dermatol Surg* 2001; 27(11): 943–949.
32. Rajan P, Grimes PE. Skin barrier changes induced by aluminum oxide and sodium chloride microdermabrasion. *Dermatol Surg* 2002; 28: 390–393.
33. Matory WE. Skin care. In: Matory WE (Ed) *Ethnic Considerations in Facial Aesthetic Surgery.* Philadelphia: Lippincott-Raven, 1998; 100.
34. Matory WE. Aging in people of color. In Matory WE (Ed) *Ethnic Considerations in Facial Aesthetic Surgery.* Philadelphia: Lippincott-Raven, 1998; 151–170.
35. Jackson BA. Cosmetic considerations and nonlaser cosmetic procedures in ethnic skin. *Dermatol Clin* 2003; 21: 703–712.
36. Klein AW, Elson ML. The history of substances for soft tissue augmentation. *Dermatol Surg* 2000; 26: 1096–1115.
37. Robinson JK, Hanke CW. Injectable collagen implant: histopathologic identification and longevity of correction. *J Dermatol Surg Oncol* 1985; 11: 124–130.
38. Elson ML. The role of skin testing in the use of collagen injectable materials. *J Dermatol Surg* 1989; 15: 301–303.
39. Moody BR, Sengelmann RD. Topical tacrolimus in the treatment of bovine collagen hypersensitivity. *Dermatol Surg* 2001; 27: 789–791.
40. Alter T, West T. New options for soft tissue augmentation. *Skin Aging* 1998; 6: 32–36.
41. Feldman SG. In: Klein AW (Ed) *Tissue Augmentation in Clinical Practice.* New York: Marcel Dekker, 1998; 293–306.

42. Friedman PM, Mafong EA, Kauvar AN, Geronemus RG. Safety data of injectable nonanimal stabilized hyaluronic acid gel soft tissue augmentation. *Dermatol Surg* 2002; 28: 491–494.
43. Duranti F, Salti G, Bovani B, Calandra M, Rosati ML. Injectable hyaluronic acid gel for soft tissue augmentation. A clinical and histological study. *Dermatol Surg* 1998; 24: 1317–1325.
44. Altabe M. Ethnicity and body image: quantitative and qualitative analysis. *Int J Eat Disord* 1998; 23: 153–159.
45. Miller KJ, Gleaves DH, Hirsch TG, et al. Comparisons of body image dimensions by race/ethnicity and gender in a university population. *Int J Eat Disord* 2000; 27: 310–316.
46. Demarest J, Allen R. Body image: gender, ethnic and age differences. *J Soc Psychol* 2000; 140: 465–472.
47. Kelin JA. The tumescent technique for liposuction surgery. *Am J Cosmetic Surg* 1987; 4: 263–267.
48. Coleman WP, Lillis PJ. Liposuction. *Dermatol Clin* 1999; 17: 723–727.
49. Lack EB, Contouring the female buttocks. *Dermatol Clin* 1999; 17: 815–822.
50. Fischer G. Liposculpture: the "correct" history of liposuction: part 1. *J Dermatol Surg Oncol* 1993; 19: 1129.

13 Hair Transplantation for Pigmented Skins

Valerie D. Callender

INTRODUCTION

More women suffer from hair loss than is commonly thought. Racial differences in hair morphology and hair-grooming practices can impact the incidence and severity of alopecia. In African-American women in particular, curly hair and the related use of damaging hair chemicals and tight braiding techniques may be associated with especially high levels of severe scarring alopecias. Although medical treatment and education on hair care practices remain the core of therapy for most women with alopecia, new tailored approaches to hair transplantation are emerging as options for carefully selected women with significant permanent hair loss.

In recent years, the techniques of hair transplantation surgery have improved and the understanding of hair loss burden, pathology, and repair in women has spread. Responding to changing demographics, many clinicians have also recently honed their sensitivity to the special management requirements related to ethnic hair.[1–3] In this chapter, after general descriptions of alopecia in women and racial variations in hair morphology and grooming, the proper role of hair transplantation in women will be reviewed. Because their curly hair and distinctive grooming practices make them susceptible to the scarring and traction alopecias that often result in hair transplantation, African-American women are the natural focus of this chapter. Although several specific surgical transplantation techniques will be described here, the chapter is not intended as a step-by-step guide for the aesthetic surgeon. Many excellent reviews of current transplantation techniques are available in the literature.[4–6] Instead, this chapter is meant as a general guide for dermatologists and internists who are advising female patients about their full range of options for dealing with alopecia. Because they are female, and because they are black, African-American patients have acquired a "double-minority" status in the world of hair transplantation. The background and recommendations reviewed here will help the clinician optimize care for this special and often underserved group.

While it may seem obvious, clinicians first need to remind themselves that hair loss in women is a culturally different phenomenon than hair loss in men. In men, hair loss is considered normal. It is an accepted fact of life for about 50% of the male population over age 50.[7] It sustains an American mini-industry of medications (e.g., minoxidil, finasteride), surgical techniques, home remedies, and late-night infomercials. Treated or not treated, men with androgenetic alopecia can still walk the streets without causing heads to turn. Hair loss in women, on the other hand, is still considered abnormal, a cultural oddity. However, about 30% of women over the age of 50 have significant hair loss, and this incidence increases with age.[7] Although the pattern of this alopecia in women is typically more diffuse and less glaring — literally — than in the male, the cultural double take engendered by any degree of female hair loss increases the propensity toward self-consciousness and lowered self-esteem. Studies have documented what most dermatologists know intuitively: women have a greater emotional and psychological reaction to hair loss than men.[7–9] In one study of women with female pattern hair loss, about 75% manifested negative self-esteem and half experienced social problems.[10] Another recent study reported that the quality of life in women with alopecia was as low as that in patients with severe psoriasis.[11]

Whereas styling, coloring, wigs, hairpieces, and over-the-counter "cures" are familiar remedies for women, the opposite side of the tendency toward self-treatment in women is the relative lack of professional clinical attention for their alopecia. In fact, in the quality-of-life study just mentioned,[11] 40% of women said they were dissatisfied with the way their current doctor managed their hair loss. Such attitudes may explain why for most women with significant hair loss, the wig, adoption of a disguising hairstyle, or frequent consultations with hair stylists have been the solutions rather than targeted medical therapy or hair transplantation. In 2002, the latest year for which statistics are available, only 864 (4.9%) of the total 18,120 hair transplantation procedures in the United States were performed on women.[12]

Historically, African-American women have been dissuaded from hair transplantation due to difficulties with hair harvesting from curved follicles and concerns over hypertrophic and keloidal scarring.[13] Race-based differences in the perceived need to correct alopecia also have been proposed[14] but never substantiated. One could even argue that the increased attention to hair care required by those of African origin[15,16] would heighten a black woman's sensitivity to alopecia, but formal comparisons of hair loss perception in white and black women have never been reported.

More generally, hair transplantation in women has been limited by the perceived inability of traditional standard punch grafts to produce aesthetically satisfying results.[17] These procedural limitations with the older, outdated methods have in many men and women resulted in disappointing, if not disfiguring, results (e.g., large "plug-like" grafts, hair placed in the wrong direction, unrealistic attempts at coverage, scarring in recipient area). A legacy of poorly planned and executed grafts is the growing demand for more artful corrective procedures.[18,19] These cosmetic defects may also account, along with the increasing use of minoxidil and finasteride, for an overall slowing of enthusiasm for hair transplantation. One large survey even showed a sharp drop in overall hair transplantation procedures performed between 1997 and 2002 (−70% overall and −92% in women).[12] However, there are no consistent national estimates of the number of hair transplants performed annually. The American Academy of Cosmetic Surgery, for example, reports that hair transplantation is still the fourth most commonly performed invasive procedure among its surveyed members.[20]

Although the exact number of hair transplants done every year remains in question, the relative frequency of these procedures in men and women is clear: only about 5% to 15% are currently done in women.[12,20] This may be changing, however, as evidenced by the growing number of educational sessions at national dermatology meetings now devoted to hair transplantation in women. As awareness of alopecia in women grows, and as American women age, hair transplantation in women will become more common.

The key to allowing more women to benefit from hair transplantation, and to avoiding the need for repairs, is a meticulous surgical technique that is individualized to mimic each patient's original hair distribution and pattern.[19] This requires that dermatologists tailor their advice and care for African-American women who may benefit from hair transplant surgery. Subtle modifications in hair transplantation techniques for black women can produce substantial improvements in outcomes and patient satisfaction. Thus, whereas the principles of hair transplant surgery cross lines of gender and race, the successful practice of this cosmetic technique still depends on the clinician's ability to understand and adapt to every patient's distinguishing characteristics — including gender and race.

RACIAL VARIATIONS IN HAIR MORPHOLOGY

Although there are no major biochemical differences among black, Caucasian, and Asian hair types, there are obvious differences in hair morphology among these racial groups (Table 13.1).[1,2,15,21–23] Most notably, black hair appears tightly coiled, helical, or spiraled. In cross section it is elliptical or flattened. It must be mentioned, of course, that African-American hair is highly heterogeneous and some black individuals will even have nearly straight hair. In general, however, African-American hair is curly. By contrast, Caucasian hair is straight, wavy, or helical and it is usually

TABLE 13.1
Racial Differences in Hair Morphology

	Blacks (African, African-American, Afro-Caribbean)	Caucasians	Asians (Japanese, Chinese, Koreans, Filipinos, Indians)
Hair structure	Tightly coiled, helical, or spiraled	Straight, wavy, or helical	Straight
Cross section	Elliptical, flattened	Round or oval	Round, greater diameter
Hair follicle	Curved	Straight	Straight
Follicular units/mm^2*	0.6	1	1 (0.7 Chinese)
Average density hairs/mm^2*	1.6	2	1.7 (1.4 Chinese)
Predominant hair grouping*	Three	Two	Two (Two Asian)
Hair density (mean) # follicles/4 mm**	21.4	35.5	
# Terminal follicles**	18.4	30.4	
# Average hairs**	17.3	28.8	

* *Source:* Bernstein R.M. The aesthetics of follicular transplantation. *Dermatol. Surg.*, 23(9), 785–799, 1997.

** *Source:* Sperling L.C. Hair density in African Americans. *Arch. Dermatol.*, 135, 656–658, 1999.

round or oval in cross section. Asian hair is typically straight, round in cross section, and larger in diameter than hair of the other groups. In terms of hair transplantation, one main implication of the unique curly morphology of African-American hair is that the surgeon may be able to "do more with less." Fewer donor hairs will be required to create the impression of fullness and increase density. The other relevant difference in morphology involves the follicle, which is curved in each black hair and straight in Caucasians and Asians. This curved hair follicle in black patients accounts for the challenge of hair donor harvesting and dissection into follicular units during hair transplant surgery and will be discussed later (Figure 13.1).

In addition to fundamental differences in shape, the density of hairs and follicles also varies among the races. In particular, density and diameter are lower in African-Americans than whites.[23]

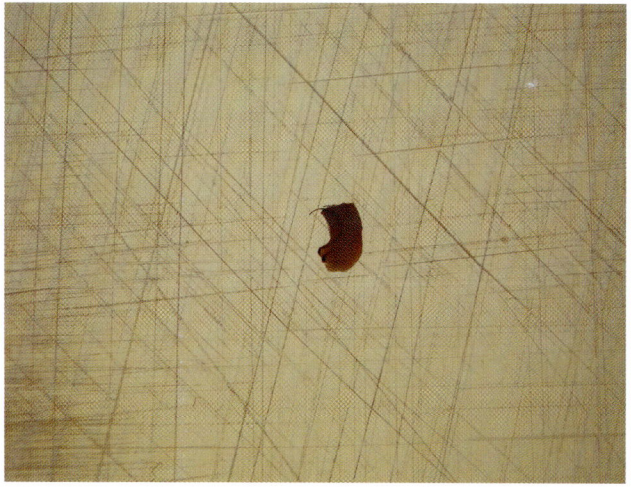

FIGURE 13.1 Black hair. Tightly curled with a curved hair follicle.

For example, when scalp biopsies from 22 African-Americans were compared to those from 12 Caucasians, Sperling found a reduced overall hair density (21.4 vs. 35.5 follicles per 4 mm^2), reduced number of terminal follicles (18.4 vs. 30.4), and reduced number of anagen hairs (17.3 vs. 28.8).[24] These and other published estimates of racial variation in hair density (Table 13.1) show that clinicians need to consider not only the qualitative but also the quantitative race-based differences in hairs and follicles when planning hair transplant surgery.[5,25,26] On balance, the low follicular density that is typical of black hair is more than compensated for by the curliness of the hair and by the tendency for each follicular unit to contain more hairs. This is why black patients often achieve better cosmetic results with hair transplantation than white patients — especially if the patient has very dark skin, which visually fills in the gaps between black hairs.[5] This lack of contrast between skin and hair creates an "illusion of density" that can be used to great advantage by the surgeon.

Several structural features of African black hair predispose the hair to breakage, knotting, and general "unmanageability."[15,16,27] Black hair also tends to grow more slowly than white hair.[28] Furthermore, due to the decreased ability of sebum to coat the hair, curly black hair also has less shine and often appears dry.[29] These inherent fallibilities of fragility and dryness in curly black hair help explain why black women typically spend so much time on hair straightening (with chemicals or heat), moisturizing, braiding, and weaving — all aggressive and relatively race-specific hair grooming techniques that place them at elevated risk of alopecia and hair shaft fragility.

INDICATIONS FOR HAIR TRANSPLANTATION IN AFRICAN-AMERICAN WOMEN

Although there are no recent epidemiological data addressing the true incidence of alopecia in black females, Halder et al. reported alopecia as the fifth most common dermatosis in African-Americans seen in private dermatology practices; traction and chemical alopecia were cited as the predominant causes.[30] In my private dermatology practice in the Washington, DC area, alopecia is the third most common presenting disorder, after acne and postinflammatory hyperpigmentation. Although there are several underlying causes of alopecia, this chapter will focus on the two identified by Halder et al. as most relevant to the black female patient: traction alopecia and "chemical" alopecia, now called central centrifugal cicatricial alopecia (CCCA). These are also two of the most frequent indications for hair transplantation surgery in black women. In general, the approach to the female patient with other types of alopecia (e.g., female pattern hair loss, alopecia areata, telogen effluvium, seborrheic dermatitis) is similar to those for Caucasian patients.

The cause of hair loss can be investigated with a thorough history and physical examination. A full medical workup will help rule out any causes of alopecia that can be treated medically.[4,31] The duration and pattern of hair loss, as well as the patient's diet, medications, medical conditions, and family history, are important factors; the scalp should be examined for the presence or absence of inflammation and follicular units.[32,33] Rare underlying causes such as elevated testosterone, hypothyroidism, infections, iron or zinc deficiencies, and postpregnancy hormonal changes can be ruled out with diagnostic biopsies or laboratory tests.[31,33–35] Episodes of emotional or physical stress (e.g., extreme diets, surgery) that may produce transitory hair loss should also be ruled out.[4]

The most common cause of hair loss in all women is female pattern hair loss. According to one recent estimate, it occurs in about 20% of American women overall, ranging from an incidence of 16% in those aged 30–49 years to 28% in those aged 50–69 years.[36] Researchers using different criteria have previously reported even higher rates of significant hair loss in older women due to androgenetic alopecia.[37,38] Androgenetic alopecia in women, which is now usually called female pattern hair loss, rarely requires hair transplantation. In early-onset or advanced cases not responding to medical treatment with minoxidil,[31,39] however, clinicians should be aware that follicular grouping (minigrafts) or follicular unit (micrografts) techniques now deliver cosmetically satisfying

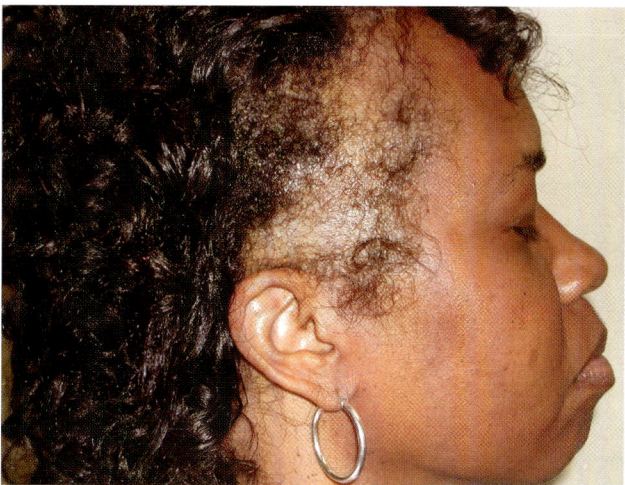

FIGURE 13.2 Traction alopecia. Mechanical loosening of the hairs from the follicle — often caused by tight braiding, ponytails, or hair weaves — can lead to permanent alopecia.

results.[17,35,40] One key in evaluating women with female pattern hair loss for hair transplantation is the degree of thinning in donor and recipient areas; those women with diffuse thinning on all scalp areas may not be suitable candidates.[4,31] Also, because women tend to develop iatrogenic hair loss in the recipient region more frequently than men, in some cases the use of larger grafts may still be required.[35] This is a strategy, as described later, that is especially appropriate in hair transplantations performed in black women with scarring alopecia.

TRACTION ALOPECIA

Traction alopecia is associated with the chronic use of tight braids, cornrows, ponytails, hair rollers, and hair weaves[41–43] (Figure 13.2). Although these natural styling techniques are low maintenance and allow the hair to rest from chemical straightening processes, overly tight or prolonged braiding can lead to a mechanical loosening of the hairs from the follicle and subsequent perifolliculitis. Steady tension on the hair often leads first to erythema and pustules, sometimes accompanied by a seborrhea-like hyperkeratosis; eventually, terminal hairs are lost and only vellus hairs remain. Acute traction alopecia is normally considered reversible and, like androgenetic alopecia, "non-scarring." But if the tension is sustained, it can result in scarring and permanent alopecia.[44] Adding synthetic or human hair fibers — known as hair weaving — is a variation on braiding that may also produce traction alopecia. Allergic reactions to hair glue used in hair weaving have also been reported.[45,46] In rare cases, the weight of long "dreadlocks" may cause traction alopecia. Treatment of traction alopecia requires immediate discontinuance of the hairstyle that produces tension or pulling of the hair. Antibiotics or corticosteroids may be necessary to treat inflammatory folliculitis.[1] Hair transplantation is an option in those cases in which the chronic hair tension has produced well-defined areas of serious follicular loss[47] (Figure 13.3).

CENTRAL CENTRIFUGAL CICATRICIAL ALOPECIA (CCCA)

Over the past several decades, various names have been assigned to the distinctive inflammatory and scarring alopecia often seen in black women who straighten their hair with chemicals (Figure 13.4). These names have included hot comb alopecia,[48] pseudopelade,[49] chemically induced alopecia,[50] follicular degeneration syndrome,[51] and central centrifugal cicatricial alopecia (CCCA).[44,52] The underlying pathological cause of this primary scarring alopecia is unknown and probably

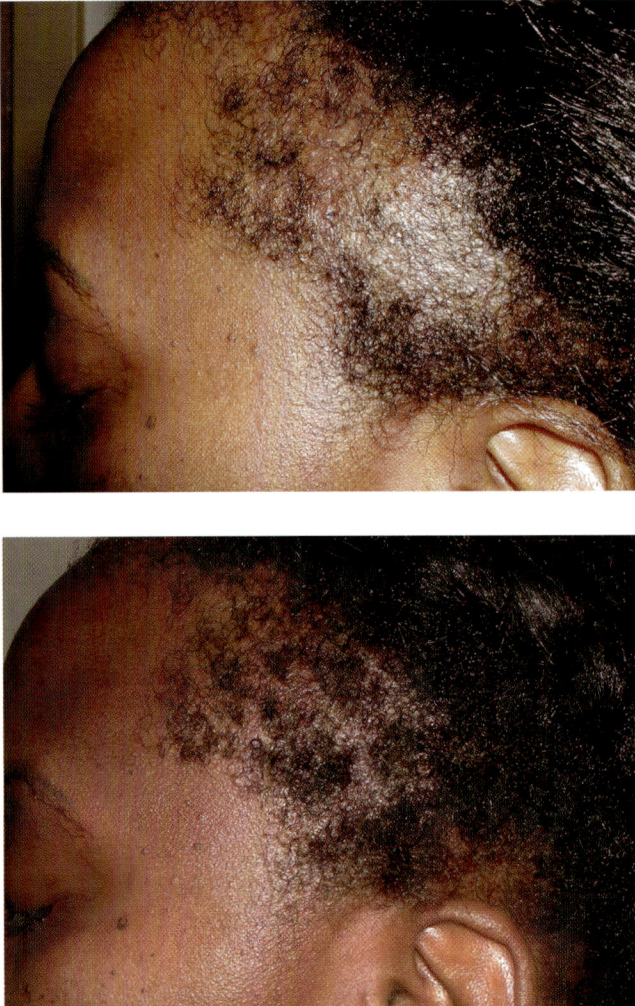

FIGURE 13.3 Hair transplant surgery for traction alopecia: before (top) and after (bottom) one session.

involves a combination of genetic predisposition and environmental factors.[52] In general, the condition has been associated with use of hot combs, hair chemicals to relax or curl the hair, and bonding glues.[1] However, before the majority of black women now use some form of chemicals to straighten their hair, deciphering the exact roles of various styling agents in this form of permanent hair loss is difficult. Because the cause remains unexplained, the broader and more neutral term of cicatricial (meaning scarring) alopecia is now employed to describe any hair loss with marked loss of follicular units. When the scarring and hair loss start on the central scalp and progress centrifugally, the classification of CCCA is applied[44,52] (Figure 13.4). Further investigations into the etiology of CCCA in black women are needed.

Terminology aside, the practical clinical distinction to make in black women with significant hair loss is between nonscarring temporary alopecia and scarring alopecia with permanent follicular loss. The scarring and irreversible follicle destruction that define CCCA make medical treatment extremely difficult and challenging. Therapy is aimed at controlling symptoms and slowing progression rather than reversing hair loss. The first step in management is discontinuing use of hair chemicals or extreme heat and then substituting alternative hairstyling methods. Discussions involving camouflage techniques, natural hairstyles, decreasing the frequency of chemical relaxing, the

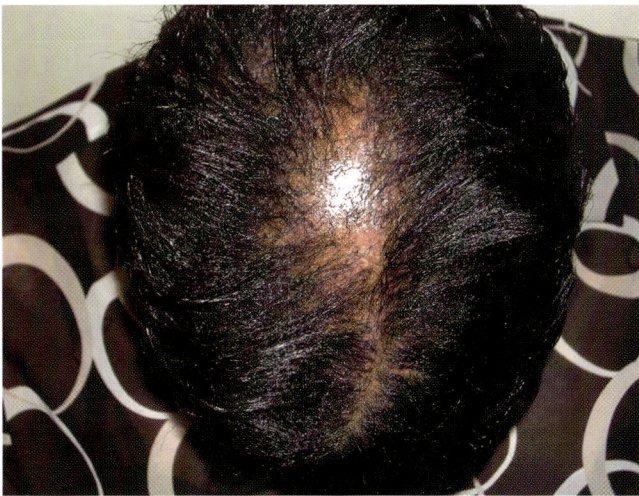

FIGURE 13.4 Central centrifugal cicatricial alopecia. Hair loss starting at the vertex, with gradual expansion, broken hairs, loss of follicular ostia, and dyspigmentation.

use of milder chemical relaxers, basing the entire scalp prior to chemical relaxing, and taking a "relaxer holiday" by wearing braids for several months should be undertaken for all black females with hair loss. Medications used with varying success for cicatricial hair loss have included oral antibiotics, topical and intralesional corticosteroids, antifungals, and even antimalarials.[1,2,53] Medical management for CCCA by aggressive anti-inflammatory agents can be effective in some patients if treatment is initiated early on in the course of this disease. In those cases in which the CCCA progression can be stabilized for at least 6 months, hair transplant surgery can be considered to restore hair to the areas of permanent loss.

HAIR TRANSPLANTATION: SPECIAL CONSIDERATIONS FOR BLACK WOMEN

When considering hair transplantation for alopecia in black women, clinicians and surgeons may need to adjust a few assumptions and biases built on years of treating mainly Caucasian males with androgenetic alopecia. The surgical techniques are essentially the same, but the selection and application of the techniques, the use of concomitant medications, and the pre- and post-procedure counseling may all require subtle modifications based on gender or race differences previously discussed (Table 13.2).

WHY LARGER GRAFTS MAY BE PREFERRED IN CCCA

The first assumption that must be reconsidered involves the whole concept of historical progress in hair transplantation. Cosmetic surgeon Norman Orentreich pioneered the punch-grafting technique of hair transplantation in the 1950s.[54] This procedure involved transplanting round grafts or "hair plugs" (typically 4-mm clusters of 15–20 hairs) from the occipital area of the scalp (donor site) to the area of hair loss (recipient area), usually the anterior/vertex area in male patients with androgenetic alopecia. In the 1980s, surgeons began using smaller "mini-" and "micrografts" to reduce the "plug-like" look.[55] In 1995, Bernstein et al. developed follicular unit transplantation (FUT), which involves transplanting the "natural" follicular units rather than the larger round grafts.[56] Follicular units were defined by Headington as consisting of small bundles or units of 1–4 hairs, surrounded by a fine adventitial sheath.[57] A goal of these progressively smaller grafts was to allow for a more natural-appearing anterior hairline.

TABLE 13.2
Racial Differences in Hair Transplant Surgery

	Blacks	Caucasians	Asians (Japanese, Koreans, Filipinos, Indians)
Indication	TA, CCCA ♀, and AGA ♂	AGA ♀ and ♂	AGA ♂
Adjunctive medical therapy	Topical corticosteroids, Minoxidil, Finasteride ♂	Minoxidil, Finasteride ♂	Minoxidil, Finasteride ♂
Hair line design	Less important (TA, CCCA) in ♀	Very important AGA ♂	Very important AGA ♂
Whorl pattern (males)*	Diffusion	"S"	"S"
Graft site	Follicular groupings (larger graft)	FU	FU
Donor harvesting	More difficult (curved hair & hair follicle)	Less difficult	Less difficult
Recipient sites	Larger	Smaller	Smaller
Keloid risk	High	Low	Moderate
Hair grooming practices	Extremely important	Not as important	Not as important

TA = traction alopecia; CCCA = central centrifugal cicatricial alopecia; FU = follicular units; AGA = androgenic alopecia; ♂ = male; ♀ = female.

* Ziering, C. and Krenitsky, G. The Ziering whorl classification of scalp hair. *Dermatol. Surg.*, 29, 8, 2003.

Notwithstanding other refinements in hair transplant technique (e.g., strip harvesting of the donor area and use of slits or laser ablation for the recipient area), the clear driving force in the evolution of hair transplantation surgery over the past several decades has been the move from plug grafts to finer follicular units or follicular groupings. For most patients today, including women,[40] the state-of-the-art transplant technique leading to the most aesthetically pleasing results is the FUT with 1–4 hairs. For many black women with CCCA, however, this mantra of "the smaller the graft, the better the transplant" does not apply. In these African-American patients, a larger standard round graft or minigraft may still be preferred.

What explains this apparent rejection of transplantation's central dogma? One reason for larger graft selection is the difficulty in harvesting individual follicular units from the donor tissue in black patients with curly hair. Even for skilled hair transplant surgeons in a procedure on white patients, transection of the hair follicle is a limiting factor in the procedure. In African-Americans, the curliness of the hair follicles makes this dissection particularly challenging, and magnification is essential. Harvesting larger grafts (i.e., minigrafts or follicular groupings) rather than follicular units decreases the risk of transecting the curved follicles. Thus, the punch-graft technique can also be used to optimize follicle survival in black patients with scarring alopecia. The donor punch grafts are typically 3 or 4 mm and the recipient sites are approximately 2.5 or 3.5 mm, respectively. Moving the punch in a gradual arc as the donor incision is made (i.e., angling the punch to follow the curve of the hair follicle) may limit transections and increase the number of intact follicles per graft.[13] As mentioned earlier, an inherent advantage of using these curved hair follicles is that the associated curly hairs provide better coverage than with straight hairs. Thus, the usual objections related to use of larger plugs (e.g., an unnatural pluglike) are more likely to be camouflaged in black women. The plugs are also less visible because CCCA usually calls for hair transplantation at the vertex rather than the anterior hairline. If needed, the smaller minigrafts harvested from the donor tissue can be reserved for the hairline (Figure 13.5).

Another reason thicker grafts are often preferred in African-Americans is that these patients are more often being treated for CCCA or other inflammatory disorders in which the scalp tissue is scarred and the blood supply is limited. Compared to a normal 90%–95% survival rate of hairs

Hair Transplantation for Pigmented Skins

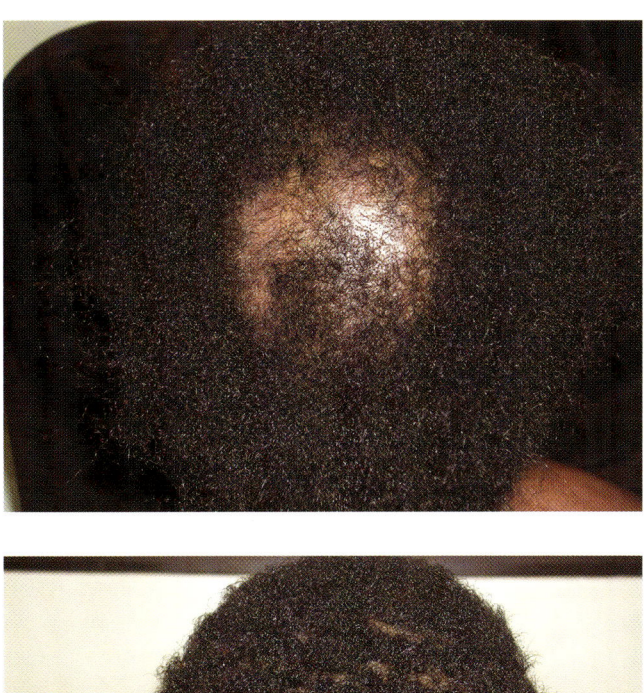

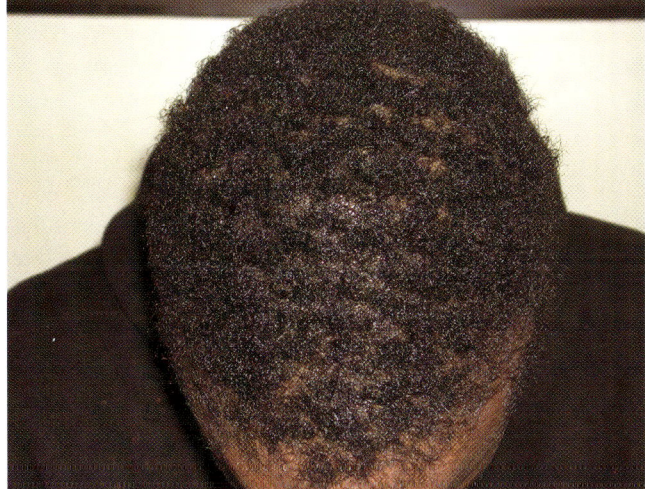

FIGURE 13.5 Hair transplant surgery for central centrifugal cicatricial alopecia: before and after.

in nonscarred areas, the survival rate in scarred areas has been estimated at only 50%–70%.[7,35] A larger graft essentially imports more of its own healthy perifollicular tissue and blood supply and thereby encourages better uptake. Deeper incisions in recipient sites may also promote neovascularization at these scarred sites. Use of larger grafts has also been recommended in some women with female pattern hair loss in order to minimize iatrogenic loss.[35] In patients with global diffuse thinning, the larger grafts (3–4 mm) may also appear more acceptable because the donor grafts themselves have a wide interfollicular distance and, again, the tightly curled African-American hair will provide excellent scalp coverage.[7] In general, careful hairline design involving small graft placement is less critical in women than in men, and it is even less so in black women because of the curliness of their hair.

In patients with traction alopecia, the FUT procedure with a few modifications may be most appropriate. Harvesting may occur via the strip technique with an elliptical strip (e.g., 1 × 8 cm), the size of which is calculated based on the number of hairs to be transplanted to cover the recipient area. The strip is then cut into follicular units and follicular groupings that typically contain 2–4 hairs. Again, because of the technical challenge in isolating individual follicular units when the follicles are curved, these grafts from black patients are generally larger than those harvested from Caucasian or Asian patients. The dissected follicular units are placed into recipient incisions created with an 18-gauge NoKor needle, Spearpoint 90 or 91 blades, and, in some cases, 1 or 2 mm punch.

HOW TO REDUCE THE RISK OF SCARRING

Dark-skinned individuals have a tendency to develop keloids — irregularly shaped and elevated spreading scars that probably result from abnormal collagen synthesis and fibroblast growth following traumatic or inflammatory events.[3,58] Postinflammatory hyperpigmentation (PIH) is another common skin disorder in African-Americans[30] that may be triggered by any cutaneous injury,[3,59] such as that induced by a hair transplantation procedure. Although keloidal scars and postoperative hyperpigmentation are not a widespread problem immediately following hair transplant surgery in African-Americans, these adverse events may develop postoperatively.[60] For this reason, all black patients should be warned of the possibility of hypertrophic keloidal scarring and PIH before their procedure. If keloids are present during the physical exam preoperatively or if the patient has a strong history of keloids, the procedure should not be undertaken.

The donor site is probably the most common area for the development of keloids, but they may occur at the recipient sites as well (Figure 13.6). Some surgeons recommend test grafting prior to transplant in all black patients.[13] In this test session, 1–5 punch grafts are placed on the fringe of the planned recipient area and survival and growth are observed for at least 3 months before proceeding. Any evidence of scarring in the test area is a contraindication for hair transplantation.

To reduce these surgical risks in black patients with a suspected propensity toward hypertrophic or keloidal scarring, surgeons may also use prophylactic corticosteroids. Preventive treatment with a twice-a-day compound containing a midpotency topical corticosteroid plus a topical antibiotic can be initiated at the donor site immediately after the procedure and continued for 2 weeks (Table 13.3). When the sutures are removed, at about day 14, regardless of the technique used for harvesting, a high-potency topical corticosteroid may be used for another 2 weeks. In patients with CCCA, topical or intralesional corticosteroid therapy may be started at the first signs of any cobblestoning at the recipient punch-graft sites. Postsurgical inflammation and scarring is less likely to occur at the recipient site in black patients with traction alopecia who are receiving smaller follicular unit or follicular grouping hair transplants.

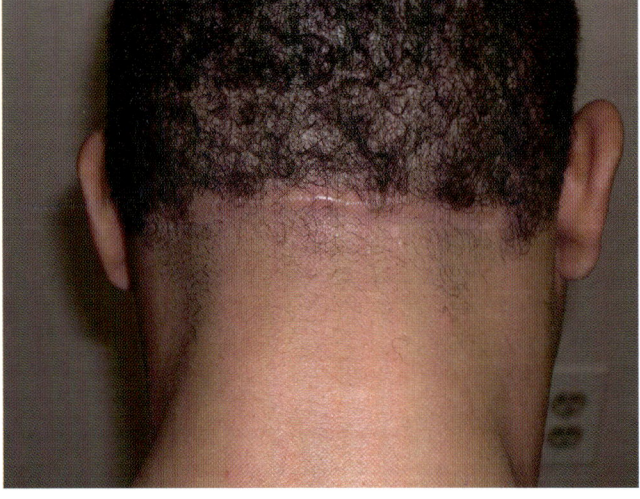

FIGURE 13.6 Keloidal scarring of the donor site area following hair transplantation.

TABLE 13.3
Improving Transplantation Success in African-American Patients: Focus on Preventing Hypertrophic Scars and Keloids

Preoperative Care
1. Obtain patient history of keloids
2. Examine patient for evidence of keloids or postinflammatory hyperpigmentation
3. Perform test grafting prior to hair transplantation

Postoperative Care
1. Day 1: Begin mid-potency topical corticosteroid + bacitracin compound twice a day to donor site and continue for 2 weeks
2. Day 14: Apply high-potency topical corticosteroid to donor site post-suture removal and continue for 2 weeks
3. In patients with hypertrophic scars or keloids, perform intralesional corticosteroid therapy (20–30 mg/ml), every 2–4 weeks, until flat

THE IMPORTANCE OF PHYSICIAN–PATIENT COMMUNICATION

Before surgery is attempted, all patients with CCCA should be under medical management for at least 6 months. A scalp biopsy should be taken prior to the hair transplant procedure to ensure the resolution of the inflammation. This waiting period also provides an opportunity to assess the rate of alopecia progression and the degree of irreversibility of the hair loss. Perhaps most importantly, the built-in wait period also allows the clinician time to assess patient desires, expectations, and willingness to comply with changes in hair styling techniques. All of these behavioral factors are critical in determining the ultimate success of the procedure.

In their presurgical assessments of black female patients, clinicians should realize that women in general might be harder to please and have higher expectations for hair restoration than male patients.[7] This higher potential for dissatisfaction with the eventual result should further the need for proper patient selection and education.[4] If a black woman with extensive CCCA has an expectation of quickly regaining a full head of thick hair with minimal detectability, further counseling may be required to set more realistic goals. If a woman with alopecia is eager for surgery so she can return to the very hair style (e.g., tight cornrow braids) or hair grooming practice (e.g., chemical straightening) implicated in her hair loss, more discussion is needed to ensure that aesthetic gains provided by hair transplantation are not eroded.

SUMMARY

Hair transplantation can play an important second-line role in the management of alopecia in men and women. There are several racial differences in hair transplant surgery, due mainly to the curved hair follicle and curly hair of African-Americans. In African-American women, the curly hair and associated cosmetic and hair-grooming practices often lead to traction alopecia and CCCA. These forms of alopecia are often more visible and more permanent than the nonscarring androgenetic forms. Although prevalent among African-American women, these distinctive alopecias have also been overlooked as a surgically correctable condition. Concerns about naturally low hair density and risks of keloidal scarring in this population should not prevent the aesthetic surgeon from considering hair transplantation in appropriately selected African-American men and women. In fact, the natural curliness in black hair provides greater scalp coverage, camouflaging any remaining areas of thinning. Essentially, the hair transplant surgeon can "do more with less" in African-American patients. At the same time, several special management practices must be considered, including educating patients on alternative hair care practices, selecting the surgical technique (e.g., perhaps even use of minigrafts rather than follicular units) that is best suited to the natural curvature of the black hair follicle, and reducing the risk of keloidal scarring with patient screening and use of corticosteroids.

REFERENCES

1. McMichael, A.J. Hair and scalp disorders in ethnic populations. *Dermatol. Clin.*, 21, 629, 2003.
2. McMichael, A. Ethnic hair update: past and present. *J. Am. Acad. Dermatol.*, 48, S127, 2003.
3. Taylor, S.C. Skin of color: biology, structure, function, and implications for dermatologic disease. *J. Am. Acad. Dermatol.*, 46 (2 Suppl), S41, 2002.
4. Unger, W.P. and Unger, R.H. Hair transplanting: an important but often forgotten treatment for female pattern hair loss. *J. Am. Acad. Dermatol.*, 49, 853, 2003.
5. Bernstein, R.M. and Rassman, W.R. The aesthetics of follicular transplantation. *Dermatol. Surg.*, 23, 785, 1997.
6. Bernstein, R.M. and Rassman, W.R. Follicular transplantation — patient evaluation and surgical planning. *Dermatol. Surg.*, 23, 771, 1997.
7. Vogel, J.E. Hair transplantation in women: a practical new classification system and review of technique. *Aesthetic Surg. J.*, 22, 247, 2002.
8. Cash, T.F., Price, V.H. and Savin, R.C. Psychological effects of androgenetic alopecia on women: comparisons with balding men and with female control subjects. *J. Am. Acad. Dermatol.*, 29, 568, 1993.
9. Girman, C.J., et al. Patient-perceived importance of negative effects of androgenetic alopecia in women. *J. Women's Health Gend. Based Med.*, 8, 1091, 1999.
10. Van Der Donk, J., et al. Quality of life and maladjustment associated with hair loss in women with alopecia androgenetica. *Soc. Sci. Med.*, 38, 159, 1994.
11. Williamson, D., Gonzalez, M. and Finlay, A.Y. The effect of hair loss on quality of life. *J. Eur. Acad. Dermatol. Venereol.*, 15, 137, 2000.
12. American Society for Aesthetic Plastic Surgery. Cosmetic Surgery National Data Bank: 2002 Statistics. www.surgery.org. Accessed January 2004.
13. Unger, W.P. Hair transplantation in blacks. In: Unger, W.P. *Hair Transplantation*, 3rd Edition. New York: Marcel Dekker, 1995, 281–285.
14. Pierce, H.E. The uniqueness of hair transplantation in black patients. *J. Dermatol. Surg. Oncol.*, 3, 533, 1977.
15. Holloway, V.L. Ethnic cosmetic products. *Dermatol. Clin.*, 21, 743, 2003.
16. Grimes, P.E. Skin and hair cosmetic issues in women of color. *Dermatol. Clin.*, 18, 659, 2000.
17. Halsner, U.E. and Lucas, M.W. New aspects in hair transplantation for females. *Dermatol. Surg.*, 21, 605, 1995.
18. Bernstein, R.M., et al. The art of repair in surgical hair restoration — part I: basic repair strategies. *Dermatol. Surg.*, 28, 783, 2002.
19. Bernstein, R.M., et al. The art of repair in surgical hair restoration — part II: the tactics of repair. *Dermatol. Surg.*, 28, 873, 2002.
20. American Academy of Cosmetic Surgery. 2003 Procedural Census. LeeveResearch, p. 4, 2004.
21. Lindelof, B., et al. Human hair form. *Arch. Dermatol.*, 124, 1359, 1988.
22. Rook, A. Hair II: racial and other genetic variations in hair form. *Br. J. Dermatol.*, 92, 599, 1975.
23. Richards, G.M., Oresajo, C.O. and Halder, R.M. Structure and function of ethnic skin and hair. *Dermatol. Clin.*, 21, 595, 2003.
24. Sperling, L.C. Hair density in African-Americans. *Arch. Dermatol.*, 135, 656, 1999.
25. Tsai, R.Y., Lee, S.H. and Chan, H.L. The distribution of follicular units in the Chinese scalp: implications for reconstruction of natural appearing hairlines in orientals. *Dermatol. Surg.*, 28, 500, 2002.
26. Lee, H.J., et al. Hair counts from scalp biopsy specimens in Asians. *J. Am. Acad. Dermatol.*, 46, 218, 2002.

27. Khumalo, N.P., et al. What is normal black African hair? A light and scanning electron-microscopic study. *J. Am. Acad. Dermatol.*, 43, 814, 2000.
28. Loussouarn, G. African hair growth parameters. *Br. J. Dermatol.*, 145, 294, 2001.
29. Johnson, B.A. Requirements in cosmetics for black skin. *Dermatol. Clin.*, 6, 489, 1988.
30. Halder, R.M., et al. Incidence of common dermatoses in a predominantly black dermatologic practice. *Cutis*, 32, 378, 1983.
31. Olsen, E.A. Female pattern hair loss. *J. Am. Acad. Dermatol.*, 45, S70, 2001.
32. Thiedke, C.C. Alopecia in women. *Am. Fam. Phys.*, 67, 1007, 2003.
33. Shapiro, J., Wiseman, M. and Lui, H. Practical management of hair loss. *Can. Fam. Physician*, 46, 1469, 2000.
34. Drake, L.A., et al. Guidelines of care for androgenetic alopecia. American Academy of Dermatology. *J. Am. Acad. Dermatol.*, 35, 465, 1996.
35. Epstein, J.S. Hair transplantation in women. *Arch. Facial Plast. Surg.*, 5, 121, 2003.
36. Norwood, O.T. Incidence of female androgenetic alopecia (female pattern alopecia). *Dermatol. Surg.*, 27, 53, 2001.
37. Venning, V.A. and Dawber, R.P. Patterned androgenic alopecia in women. *J. Am. Acad. Dermatol.*, 18, 1073, 1988.
38. Hamilton, J.B. Patterned loss of hair in man: types and incidence. *Ann. N.Y. Acad. Sci.*, 53, 708, 1951.
39. Jacobs, J.P., Szpunar, C.A. and Warner, M.L. Use of topical minoxidil therapy for androgenetic alopecia in women. *Int. J. Dermatol.*, 32, 758, 1993.
40. Avram, M.R. Hair transplantation in women. *Semin. Cutan. Med. Surg.*, 18, 172, 1999.
41. Sleyan, A.H. Traction alopecia. *Arch. Dermatol.*, 78, 395, 1958.
42. Rudolph, R.I., Klein, A.W. and Decherd, J.W. Corn-row alopecia. *Arch. Dermatol.*, 108, 134, 1973.
43. Sperling, L.C. Traction alopecia. In: *An Atlas of Hair Pathology with Clinical Correlations*. New York: Parthenon Publishing Group, 2003; 51–57.
44. Sperling, L., Solomon, A. and Whiting, D. A new look at scarring alopecia. *Arch. Dermatol.*, 136, 235, 2000.
45. Cogen, F.C. and Beezhold, D.H. Hair glue anaphylaxis: a hidden latex allergy. *Ann. Allergy Asthma Immunol.*, 88, 61, 2002.
46. Wakelin, S.H. Contact anaphylaxis from natural rubber latex used as an adhesive for hair extensions. *Br. J. Dermatol.*, 146, 340, 2002.
47. Earles, R.M. Surgical correction of traumatic alopecia marginalis or traction alopecia in black women. *J. Dermatol. Surg. Oncol.*, 12, 78, 1986.
48. Lopresti, P., Papa, C.M. and Kligman, A.M. Hot comb alopecia. *Arch. Dermatol.*, 98, 234, 1968.
49. Dawber, R. What is pseudopelade? *Clin. Exp. Dermatol.*, 17, 305, 1992.
50. Nicholson, A.G., et al. Chemically induced cosmetic alopecia. *Br. J. Dermatol.*, 128, 537, 1993.
51. Sperling, L. and Sau, P. The follicular degeneration syndrome in black patients: hot comb alopecia, revisited and revised. *Arch. Dermatol.*, 128, 68, 1992.
52. Olsen, E.A., et al. Summary of North American Hair Research Society (NAHRS)–sponsored workshop on cicatricial alopecia, Duke University Medical Center, February 10 and 11, 2001. *J. Am. Acad. Dermatol.*, 48, 103, 2003.
53. Scott, D.A. Disorders of the hair and scalp in blacks. *Dermatol. Clin.*, 6, 387, 1988.
54. Orentreich, N. Autografts in alopecias and other selected dermatological conditions. *Ann. N.Y. Acad. Sci.*, 83, 463, 1959.
55. Marritt, E. Single-hair transplantation for hairline refinement: a practical solution. *J. Dermatol. Surg. Oncol.*, 10, 962, 1984.
56. Bernstein R.M., et al. Follicular transplantation. *Int. J. Aesth. Restor. Surg.*, 3, 119, 1995.
57. Headington, J.T. Transverse microscopic anatomy of the human scalp. A basis for a morphometric approach to disorders of the hair follicle. *Arch. Dermatol.*, 120, 449, 1984.
58. Kelly, A.P. Keloids: pathogenesis and treatment. *Cosmet. Dermatol.*, 16, 29, 2003.
59. Grimes, P.R. and Stockton, T. Pigmentary disorders in blacks. *Dermatol. Clin.*, 6, 271, 1988.
60. Brown, M.D., Johnson, T. and Swanson, N.A. Extensive keloids following hair transplantation. *J. Dermatol. Surg. Oncol.*, 16, 867, 1990.
61. Ziering, C. and Krenitsky, G. The Ziering whorl classification of scalp hair. *Dermatol. Surg.*, 29, 8, 2003.

14 Laser Therapy for Pigmented Skins

Lori M. Hobbs and Eliot F. Battle

INTRODUCTION

HISTORICAL ASPECTS OF LASER SURGERY

In 1917, Einstein published the Quantum Theory of Radiation that described the basic principles and concepts that led to the development of lasers today.[1] Based on this principle, in 1958 Townes and Schawlow produced the first MASER (Microwaves Amplification for the Stimulated Emission of Radiation), which generated monochromatic infrared radiation with alkali vapor as the active medium.[2] The first functional laser, the ruby laser, was made in 1960 by Maiman. It utilized a synthetic ruby crystal to emit a red laser light at 694 nm. Maiman coined the term LASER (Light Amplification byStimulated Emission of Radiation). Later, Leon Goldman, the father of lasers in dermatology, published reports on the effects of the ruby laser on the skin.[4] Thereafter, continuous-wave argon and carbon dioxide lasers were developed, followed by multiple highly target-specific laser devices.

Prior to the late 1990s, lasers were less than satisfactory for the treatment of dermatological disorders in darker phototypes. Lasers surgeons were fraught with concerns of cutaneous side effects such as scarring, textural irregularities, and dyspigmentation. However, it was not until 1999, with the principles developed from laser-assisted hair removal research performed at the Wellman Laboratories headed by Battle and Anderson, that we were able to treat a variety of cutaneous disorders on pigmented skin. The Wellman group found that longer wavelengths and pulse durations, coupled with efficient cooling devices, were efficacious in treating of darker skin types. Through this research, we are not limited to the treatment of hair disorders, but a variety of other disorders of pigmented skins also being treatable.

LASER PRINCIPLES

Based upon Einstein's Quantum Theory of Radiation, atoms or molecules are normally in a resting state. With the absorption of light, they become excited and move from a stable state to an unstable excited state. The unstable excited molecule must return to its stable state. As it does, the molecule spontaneously emits the previously absorbed energy as a photon of light. This process is called spontaneous emission of radiation. If that photon collides with an excited atom that has previously absorbed another photon of light, it emits two photons of light as it returns to its stable state. These two photons of light are the same wavelength and frequency that were previously absorbed. This process is called the stimulated emission of radiation and is the basic principle of laser physics.

Lasers are composed of a power source, an active media, and an optical resonator with mirrors. The power source is the energy needed for the atoms or molecules to achieve an excited state. The flashlamp is an example of the power source used in the pulsed dye laser. The active medium can be gaseous, liquid, or solid (CO_2, fluorescent dyes, and ruby, respectively). The source of the laser radiation supplies the electrons needed for the stimulated emission of radiation. The wavelength is determined by the distinctive energy transition of the active medium. The optical resonator is the cavity where excitation takes place. It houses the active medium. When most of the atoms are in an excited state, there is an increased chance that photons of light will be emitted. These photons of light will collide with other excited atoms and produce stimulated emission of radiation. To help amplify this process, there are mirrors at either end of the optical cavity. The mirrors reflect the light energy and promote amplification by allowing photons to bounce back and forth. At one end of the optical cavity, there is partially reflective mirror that allows 5%–10% of light to travel out in the form of a laser beam.

Unlike sunlight or light from a lamp, laser light is coherent (aligned with each other traveling in phase), collimated (parallel bands of light), and monochromatic (emitting light in a single wavelength). This allows high-intensity light to be delivered to a small spot size area. The laser light can be continuous, pseudocontinuous, or pulsed. The carbon dioxide, argon, and krypton lasers are examples of continuous-wave lasers. Continuous-wave lasers emit a constant beam of light with little or no variation in intensity. The copper vapor laser is an example of a quasi-continuous laser in which the pulses are so rapidly fired that they appear by the tissue to be continuous. The pulsed lasers produce bursts of light energy within a limited time period. They can be divided into long-pulsed laser systems with pulse durations in the millisecond domain and short-pulsed laser systems with pulse durations in the nanosecond or microsecond domain. The pulsed dye laser is an example of a long-pulsed laser producing quick bursts of light, with pulse durations typically in the millisecond domain. The Q-switched ruby laser is an example of a short-pulsed laser device producing high energy of light between 25 and 50 nanoseconds.

The Grothus–Draper law states that light must be absorbed by tissue to bring about a clinical effect.[5] The rate at which light energy is absorbed on the skin during a single pulse is termed irradiance or power density. Irradiance describes the rate of energy output from continuous-wave lasers. It is measured in watts per square centimeter (W/cm^2). One watt is one joule per second (J/s).

The energy absorbed or the capacity to do work is measured in joules. Joules measure the energy in a single pulse from pulsed laser systems. The amount of energy delivered per square centimeter is called fluence. Fluence, or energy density, is inversely proportional to the square radius of the spot size. For example, halving the spot size increases the energy density by a factor of four. For the same energy density with one-half the diameter of the spot size, the laser energy output would have to be reduced by a factor of four.

The principle of laser surgery is to use a wavelength of light that can be fully and selectively absorbed by a component or target of the skin to produce a desired tissue response. The cutaneous target is called a chromophore (light-absorbing compound). A chromophore comprises a group of atoms that can impart color to a substance and absorbs a specific wavelength of light. There are two main chromophores of the skin: oxygenated hemoglobin and melanin. Oxyhemoglobin has three main absorption peaks: 418, 542, and 577 nm. Melanin, on the other hand, absorbs over a very broad range within the visible and infrared wavelengths. Water is another component of the skin, though not a true chromophore, that has laser tissue interactions within the infrared region of the electromagnetic spectrum (Figure 14.1). In addition, chromophores can be endogenous or exogenous. Oxyhemoglobin, melanin, and water are endogenous chromophores. Tattoo ink is an example of an exogenous chromophore.

Laser light is absorbed by the chromophore, which then undergoes an intense thermal reaction to destroy the absorbing tissue. For this thermal reaction to be contained within the target or chromophore without dissipating heat to the surrounding structures, it needs to follow the theory of selective photothermolysis.[6] This theory states that by choosing an appropriate wavelength, pulse duration, and fluence, thermal injury can be confined to the target chromophore. In efforts to assure that selective damage occurs only to the target, the exposure time of the laser must be equal to or less than the thermal relaxation time of the target. The thermal relaxation time is based on the size of the target and varies directly with the square of its diameter. Smaller objects cool faster than larger objects. The thermal relaxation time is defined as the time required for an object to cool by 50% without conducting heat to the surrounding tissue. If laser light exposure is longer than the

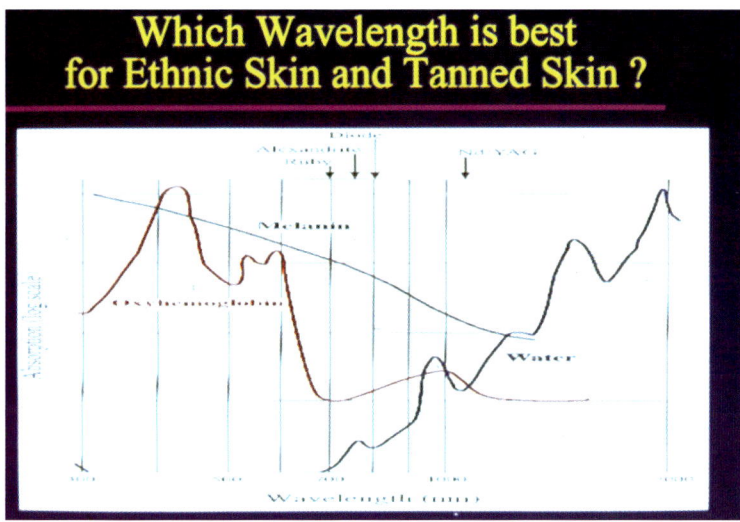

FIGURE 14.1 Absorption spectrum chart.

thermal relaxation time of the target, thermal damage will occur not only to the target but also to the surrounding tissues. Therefore, by choosing a wavelength that is specifically absorbed by the target, coupled with the appropriate fluence and pulse duration, there is selective destruction of the intended target with thermal confinement and sparing of thermal injury of adjacent tissue.

LASER PRINCIPLES IN PIGMENTED SKIN

The main challenge in treating darker skin is the high degree of melanization within the epidermis, which acts as a competitive chromophore. The laser light becomes absorbed within the pigmented epidermis and is converted to epidermal heat, which can create side effects such as blistering and dyspigmentation. In addition, the competition of the epidermal melanin absorption causes less laser light to reach its intended chromophore. This reduces the efficacy of lasers for persons with darker skin types. By exploiting laser parameters such as wavelengths and pulse durations and using efficient cooling devices, darker skin can be treated safely and efficaciously.

Melanin absorbs laser light over a wide range of wavelengths, from ultraviolet to near infrared. It has an absorption spectrum between 250 and 1200 nm. Therefore, any laser device with a wavelength between 250 and 1200 nm emits light that can become preferentially absorbed by the chromophore melanin within the epidermis before reaching its intended dermal target. However, as the wavelength increases, the absorption by melanin decreases. Thus, longer wavelengths allow a greater depth of penetration. Therefore, there is less melanin absorption within the epidermis and greater depth of penetration. This allows less epidermal injury, making it possible to treat patients with darker ethnic skin.

Longer pulse durations allow for more efficient cooling of the epidermis. These longer pulse durations slowly and gently heat, and concomitantly slowly cool, the targeted chromophore and, indirectly, nontargeted smaller chromophores. This hypothesis is based upon the fact that the slower the deposition of light energy into the skin, the slower the laser light is absorbed by the chromophore melanin. This slow deposition of heat allows the epidermis to heat up more slowly, thereby making the cooling of the skin more efficient. Thus, there will be little to no thermally related side effects of the epidermis if heat can be effectively removed and not reach damaging thresholds. This principle is related to the theory of thermokinetic selectivity.[7] It states that smaller structures (e.g., epidermal melanin) will lose heat more quickly than larger structures (e.g., dermal hair follicles). The quicker dissipation of heat of the epidermal melanocytes in comparison to larger dermal targets serves as a protective mechanism for the epidermis.

In addition to longer wavelengths and longer pulse durations, cooling devices are crucial to minimize thermal damage. Cooling devices can be contact or noncontact. Contact cooling devices directly touch the skin. Noncontact cooling devices cool the skin by emitting a coolant-type spray, air or gas. However, over-exuberant cooling devices on pigmented skin can produce unwanted side effects such as blistering and dyspigmentation.

TYPES OF LASERS COMMONLY USED FOR PIGMENTED SKINS

There are many different lasers available to treat a wide range of dermatological disorders. However, the most commonly used lasers in pigmented skins will be reviewed. These lasers and light sources are categorized according to their most common clinical use. There are four main categories: vascular, pigmented, ablative and non-ablative, and laser-assisted hair-removal devices.

Vascular Lasers and Light Sources

The majority of lasers to treat vascular lesions emit wavelengths in the visible spectrum. There are three absorption peaks for oxyhemoglobin: 418, 542, and 577 nm. Vascular lasers emitting a longer wavelength are capable of penetrating deep within the skin. To selectively destroy blood vessels, the laser light must be of an appropriate wavelength for absorption of oxyhemoglobin, and the pulse duration must be equal to or less than the thermal relaxation time of blood vessels. For example, for blood vessels of 10–100 μm in diameter, the thermal relaxation time should be between 1 and 10 ms.

Port wine stains (PWS), hemangiomas, and telangiectasias are less common in darker-skinned individuals. The difficulty in treating vascular lesions with lasers in darker skin tones is due to epidermal melanin acting as a competing chromophore against hemoglobin. This causes potential side effects such as permanent or transient dyspigmentation, vesiculation, and scarring, especially if high fluences, short pulse durations, and inefficient cooling devices are utilized.

The response rate for the treatment of vascular lesions in pigmented skins is not known. For PWS, the rate is presumably lower than reported in the literature, which varies but has been published in the range from 36.5% to 78.8% for more than 50% clearing.[8,9] Parameters that portend a better clearance with laser treatment are young age, facial location, smaller-sized lesions, and lighter-colored lesions. Variables that portend a negative response rate are PWS located on the distal extremities, those occurring in phototypes above IV, large lesions, purplish color, and those subjects older than 50 years of age.[10]

The flashlamp pulsed dye laser, with longer wavelengths and deeper penetration, is safe to use on pigmented skins for facial telangiectasias, hemangiomas, and PWS. The flashlamp pulsed dye laser emits a yellow beam of light. Depending upon the manufacturer, it produces a wavelength between 585 and 595 nm, with pulse durations ranging from 0.45 to 40 ms. It is generally thought that pulse durations of 1.5 ms can treat blood vessels typically found within the PWS that range from 30 to 150 μm in diameter. Shorter pulse durations ranging from 0.45 to 10 ms produce transient purpura lasting 3–14 days (the longer the pulse duration, the less intense purpura, the shorter duration of purpura). Little to no purpura is seen with longer pulse durations of 20–40 ms. It is generally agreed that some degree of purpura is necessary to obtain a faster clinical resolution.[11]

In treating pigmented skins, the pulsed dye laser systems with longer wavelengths and longer pulse durations are ideal. However, shorter pulse durations of 0.45–1.5 ms may be safely utilized with longer wavelengths of 595 nm if low to modest fluences are chosen. The 595-nm pulse dye laser, with its variable pulse durations, is safe to use on darker skin types and allows for the treatment of larger deeper vessels. Nevertheless, when determining the appropriate fluence and pulse duration, tissue response is crucial. Moderate to intense purpura is usually seen in lighter phototypes (I–III) when appropriate fluence and pulse durations are chosen. However, intense purpura in darker phototypes is not the typical clinical tissue response seen in darker phototypes (IV–VI). For the same fluences and pulse duration, mild to modest purpura is seen in phototypes IV–VI, depending upon the degree of competition of the epidermal melanin. When treating pigmented skin, there should be no grayish discoloration, vesiculation, or crusting seen during or immediately after treatment. These are indicators that the fluence will need to be adjusted downward and/or the pulse duration lengthened.

In treating darker skin for vascular lesions, epidermal cooling is imperative. Ho et al. found that Chinese patients were less responsive to PWS laser treatment with a higher complication rate, especially when cryogen spray was not utilized.[12] Cryogen spray cooling enhances efficacy and allows higher fluences to be used without an increase in complications.[13,14] Cryogen spray and cooling parameters are important. More complications are seen without the use of cryogen spray.[15] Chui et al. found that having a short cryogen spray (20 ms) with a longer delay (30 ms) between pulses allowed for adequate epidermal cooling. In addition, Chiu theorized that cryogen spray cooling with a longer delay than spray time allows a gradual deposition of heat into the vessels that is greater than the heat that is lost by heat diffusion between pulses. This allows for a gentle increase in heating of the vessels within the PWS to cause significant thermal damage while protecting the epidermis.[15]

With low to modest fluences and intermediate to long pulse durations, side effects are generally not encountered. Multiple treatments are necessary with fluences starting on the low to modest threshold, increasing to moderate fluences with each additional treatment depending upon the clinical response and tissue interaction. Treatments can be performed every 6–8 weeks, with multiple treatments necessary. Partial clearing is usually the norm with PWS.[12,13,15] Postinflammatory altered pigmentation, textural changes, vesiculation, and scarring are potential side effects, with dyspigmentation infrequent and, if encountered, usually transitory. With the beam emitting a Gaussian-like curve, pulses are placed with a slight overlap by 25%–30% to prevent a cobblestoning effect.

The frequency-doubled Nd:YAG (532-nm) laser may be used to treat facial telangiectasias and vascular lesions. However, with the shorter wavelength, there is more competition with epidermal melanin. Ho et al., in their retrospective study of 107 Asian patients with PWS, compared the treatment of pulsed dye laser and the variable pulse width frequency-doubled Nd:YAG 532-nm laser. He found 14% of patients experienced altered pigmentation regardless of the type of vascular laser. None of the patients had complete clearance. Twenty-three percent of patients experienced clearance of more than 50%. The average number of treatments was six.[12]

However, due to the strong epidermal melanin competition resulting in the high risk of cutaneous side effects, the frequency-doubled Nd:YAG laser (532 nm) is less than ideal for the use of telangiectasias in phototype V. It should be used cautiously in phototype VI. If chosen, lower fluences should be initiated and tissue response is crucial.

For the treatment of leg veins, the Nd:YAG (1064 nm) long-pulse laser potentially can be used for the treatment of vascular lesions in darker skin types. However, the high fluences (100–150 J/cm^2) necessary to achieve adequate clearance is fraught with difficulty in the treatment of leg veins on pigmented skins. Nevertheless, sclerotherapy remains the gold standard for the treatment of leg veins.[16] Therefore, lasers are an option based on the practitioner's comfort level and the patient's willingness for an alternative therapeutic modality. Lasers are chosen over sclerotherapy for those patients who are needle-phobic, for those in which sclerotherapy was unsuccessful, and for those patients in which there is postsclerotherapy matting. However, in the pigmented skin patient, laser treatment of leg veins with the long-pulse Nd:YAG, coupled with the need of using high fluences, is an undesirable option. Currently, there are no published reports in the literature of these lasers for the treatment of leg veins in darker skin types.

With the gold standard for the treatment of leg veins being sclerotherapy, lighter- and paler-complexioned ethnic patients can be treated cautiously with the 595-nm as well as with the long-pulse Nd:YAG. The patient should not be tanned and should be as pale as possible. Purpura with the 595-nm may exist for several weeks to months, and there is a great risk of dyspigmentation and an inherent risk of scarring. Lower than the usual fluences should be implemented. A test spot should be performed. The laser surgeon should take great care not to double-pulse. Explicit disclosure of the risks and benefits should be explained. Careful follow-up is prudent. Patient selection is the key.

THE INTENSE PULSE LIGHT SYSTEMS

The intense pulse light (IPL) emits a polychromatic band of light, typically from 515 to 1200 nm, and is thus not considered a laser (monochromatic light source). This system uses cutoff filters to maximize wavelengths that are produced beyond the filters. In general, for lighter-complexioned patients, shorter cutoff filters are chosen, and for darker complexions, longer cutoff filters are used. Because of the various wavelengths, both vascular and pigmented lesions are targets as well as the chromophore water. These light sources have been used to treat conditions including skin rejuvenation, vascular ectasias, pigmentary disorders and trichologic disorders. Side effects are dyschromia, scarring, and textural irregularities.

There are limited reports in the literature of the use of IPL on pigmented skin. Negishi et al. conducted a study on Asian skin with the IPL and found that there was an 83% improvement of telangiectasias. Cutoff filters of shorter wavelengths were utilized.[17] Chan et al. experienced more side effects with shorter-wavelength cutoff filters and utilized longer filters to avoid unwanted cutaneous side effects.[18] It is our opinion that longer cutoff filters rather than shorter ones are safer to use on pigmented skin. Mild erythema is seen during treatment. However, darker phototypes V and VI may not exhibit any true erythema. More research needs to be conducted with the use of the IPL on phototypes V to VI to determine its true efficacy and safety profile.

LASERS FOR PIGMENTED LESIONS

Patients of darker skin tones have a great concern with pigmentary dermatologic conditions. Melasma, postinflammatory altered pigmentation, lentigines, dermatosis papulosis nigra, nevus of Ota, and tattoo removal are common dermatologic disorders for which patients seek laser treatment. However, not all are amenable to laser treatment. Some of these conditions may be treated with lasers, whereas others are best treated with conventional therapies.

The target chromophore for most endogenous pigmented dermatologic disorders is the melanosome. Melanin has an absorption spectrum from 250 to 1200 nm. Melanosomes are approximately 1 μm in diameter. Pulse durations on the order of 1 μs or shorter can selectively damage melanosomes without producing damage to the surrounding tissue.

Currently, Q-switched lasers have been shown to effectively treat both epidermal and dermal pigmented lesions in a safe and reproducible fashion. Of the Q-switched systems (Q-switched ruby, Alexandrite, Nd:YAG [1064 nm], and frequency-doubled [532-nm] Nd:YAG), when there is a choice, the longer-wavelength lasers are the safest in darker skin tones. However, all can be used depending upon the phototype of the patient, fluence, and tissue response.

The Q-switched ruby (694 nm) is one of the oldest laser systems. It emits a visible red light at 694 nm with a pulse duration between 25 and 50 ns. The active medium is a ruby (aluminum oxide) crystal. The 694-nm wavelength is selectively absorbed by melanin. The short pulses of the Q-switched ruby induce microscopic photodistribution to melanosomes.[19] Treatment with this laser causes immediate whitening that fades in 20 min. A thin crust may occur, taking 10–14 days to disappear. If there is marked splattering of the epidermal debris during treatment, the fluence is too high. Transient dyspigmentation is common when treating darker skin types. The Q-switched ruby is used frequently to treat lentigines, nevus of Ota, and black tattoo ink. It can be used safely on phototype IV and with caution in phototype V. It is not ideal for phototype VI.

The Q-switched Alexandrite laser emits a 755-nm wavelength with a pulse duration of 50–100 ns. Immediately upon contact with the chromophore, there is a whitish crust that can occur. Like the Q-switched ruby, crusting can last for a several weeks. Dyspigmentation is the most common side effect. This laser can be used safely on phototype IV and with caution on the darker phototypes.

It is best suited for treatment of lentigines, nevus of Ota, and brightly colored tattoo ink such as purple and teal as well as darker-colored tattoo ink.

The Q-switched Nd:YAG laser emits a wavelength of near-infrared light at 1064 nm with a pulse duration of 10 ns. This laser has an yttrium aluminum garnet doped with 1%–3% neodynium ions. It penetrates to a depth of 3.7 nm and is poorly absorbed by melanin and hemoglobin. The poor melanin absorption makes this laser ideal in darker-skinned individuals. When the laser light is delivered onto the skin, pinpoint bleeding can occur, especially when smaller spot sizes such as 2 mm are used. This laser is ideal in treating dark-colored tattoos on pigmented skin and dermal melanocytic conditions such as nevus of Ota.

The frequency-doubled (532-nm) Q-switched Nd:YAG works well for lentigines on phototypes I–IV. A whitish discoloration may be seen immediately. Crusting develops and usually dissipates over 1–3 weeks. Transient dyspigmentation is common and can last for several weeks.

The IPL is a light source that can be used for the treatment of pigmentary disorders, most commonly lentigines. It is well suited to treat facial lentigines in phototypes I–III and has been used in Asian skin. However, dyspigmentation is a risk when treating phototypes III–IV. The IPL in general requires more treatment than the Q-switched systems for lentigines. The Q-switched systems clear lentigines in 1–2 treatments on average, with the IPL sessions being more numerous.

SPECIFIC PIGMENTED DISORDERS COMMON TO ETHNIC SKIN TYPES

Melasma

Melasma is a commonly acquired hypermelanosis that occurs most frequently on the faces of females with darker phototypes. The Q-switched lasers for the treatment of melasma are generally considered ineffective. More specifically, the Q-switched ruby laser has been used unsuccessfully. Histologically, the laser produces immediate rupture of the melanosomes, with fluence-related injury to the pigment-containing cells found in the epidermis and dermis. There is pigment incontinence and repackaging of the melanosomes, which may contribute to the refractory nature of the laser-treated melasma.[20] Clinically, patients may experience an initial clearing with ensuing altered hyperpigmentation. Therefore, the Q-switched systems are not used in the treatment of melasma.

Ablative lasers have been cautiously used in the treatment of melasma in pigmented skin. Both the Erbium:YAG and CO_2 laser have been evaluated. The difficulty with ablative lasers is the side effects of transient hyperpigmentation and, more devastatingly, the possibility of permanent hypopigmentation. Manaloto and Alster resurfaced ten female patients of phototypes II–V with the Erbium:YAG laser.[21] All patients showed improvement and all experienced transient postinflammatory hyperpigmentation. The authors concluded that the Erbium:YAG laser should be considered only for refractory melasma. In addition, Nouri et al., in a small series of four patients of phototypes IV–VI, compared the pulsed CO_2 laser with the pulsed CO_2 laser followed by the Q-switched Alexandrite laser.[22] The combination-treatment group was designed for treatment of the epidermal as well as the dermal component of melasma. Complete resolution was seen in the combination group. In the CO_2 treatment group alone, at 4–6 weeks follow-up, there was peripheral hyperpigmentation. Nouri et al. hypothesized that in persons with an underlying aberrant melanocytic disorder such as melasma, the low energy used at the edges in the CO_2 treatment group caused enough cutaneous injury to induce postinflammatory hyperpigmentation.[22] Another small pilot study enrolled six Thai females with melasma. This study compared the CO_2 laser followed by the Q-switched Alexandrite laser and the Q-switched Alexandrite laser alone. The bilateral split study showed a statistically significant improvement with the combination group; however, there were more side effects of dyspigmentation. The authors noted that the darker phototypes IV–V in the combination group developed postinflammatory hyperpigmentation, requiring the use of hydroquinones.[23] It is evident from these two studies that future laser studies for the treatment of melasma may form a dual therapeutic approach: the use of ablative laser to remove the aberrant epidermal melanin in the epidermis and the Q-switched Alexandrite laser to remove the dermal component of melasma. Nevertheless, conventional therapies are recommended and remain the gold standard for the treatment of melasma. Due to the ontoward side effects with ablative lasers in darker phototypes, non-ablative devices, especially the 1064 nm lasers, have been utilized to help diminish the dyschromia of melasma. These laser treatments are best used in conjunction with topical medications and/or exfoliating type of peels. Several treatments are necessary. There is little downtime. Side effects are rare. The clinical response is variable depending upon the type of melasma.

Postinflammatory Hyperpigmentation

The self-limiting disorder of postinflammatory hyperpigmentation is a major concern for most persons with darker skin tones. In a study conducted by Halder et al., postinflammatory hyperpigmentation was the third most common presenting diagnosis in persons of phototypes IV–VI.[24] Postinflammatory hyperpigmentation can be categorized as superficial or deep. Q-switched lasers and ablative lasers are not effective in the treatment of postinflammatory hyperpigmentation for similar reasons as stated above with melasma. Because of the high risk of pigmentary alteration with laser treatment and the self-limiting nature of this disorder, conventional topical hydroquinone therapies are the gold standards for treatment. However, there has been unpublished data of non-ablative lasers to aid in the improvement of post-inflammatory hyperpigmentation. Sunscreens, topical hydroquinones, and/or exfoliating modalities are continued with lasers as an adjunct. Multiple treatments are needed with the resulting outcome variable.

Lentigines

Lentigines mark the sign of aging and photodamage for persons of color, especially Asians. They are often seen on sun-exposed areas. Q-switched lasers are effective for treating lentigines. The Q-switched ruby laser is safe to use on phototype IV but is not advised for use on phototypes V–VI due to the strong risk of hypopigmentation, which may be transient or permanent. When used to treat lentigines, the Q-switched systems, especially the ruby, alexandrite, and double-frequency Nd:YAG (532 nm), produce an immediate whitening and subsequent crusting at the treated site that typically lasts 7–14 days. Postinflammatory hyperpigmentation occurs often, with reported rates in the literature ranging from 4% to 25%.[25,26] In our experience transient hyperpigmentation is mostly seen when using the shorter-wavelength lasers (Q-switched ruby and double-frequency Nd:YAG 532 nm) and less commonly with the longer-wavelength lasers (Q-switched 755 and 1064 nm). Nevertheless, the changes of hyperpigmentation can last for several months. For the treatment of lentigines, one to two treatments is the average.

The intense pulse light systems can treat lentigines in darker phototypes. There have not been many published studies in the literature on phototypes IV–VI, but published reports on phototype IV exist. In general, longer cutoff filters with multiple treatments are necessary. There are few adverse effects, with transient hyperpigmentation being the most common in phototypes IV.

Lentigines are not as commonly encountered in darker phototypes V and VI. Thus, to our knowledge there are no published studies to date on the treatment of lentigines with intense pulse light in darker phototype VI. For this reason, the safety and efficacy for the treatment of lentigines in phototype VI with intense pulse light have not been established.

Dermatosis Papulosis Nigra (DPN)

Dermatosis papulosis nigra (DPN) can be treated with the 532-nm double-frequency Nd:YAG lasers. However, conventional electrodesiccation is the preferred treatment. If the 532-nm double-frequency Nd:YAG is utilized, the laser surgeon should use the lowest possible fluence to obtain the desired popping sound with the lesion appearing somewhat darker in color. The lesion then crusts and sloughs over 1–2 weeks. DPNs respond in 1–2 treatments. The spot size should cover the lesion completely. The side effect is postinflammatory altered pigmentation.

NEVUS OF OTA

To date the Q-switched lasers are the best treatment modality for nevus of Ota. Lighter-complexioned ethnic phototype IV can safely use the Q-switched ruby. Darker phototypes V–VI should use the longer-wavelength Q-switched systems (Q-switched alexandrite and Q-switched Nd:YAG). The Q-switched Nd:YAG (1064 nm) is the ideal system to use for darker phototypes such as V and VI. Multiple treatments are necessary, with the ideal interim between treatments of 2 months or longer. From observation, the longer the interval between treatments, the fewer number of treatments are needed over time. There is usually transient dyspigmentation. Thereby, strict sun avoidance is the rule to decrease the degree of hyperpigmentation. Transient hyperpigmentation may last for several months. Infrequently encountered side effects are textural irregularities and scarring. Overall, the complication rate is generally low.

With the Q-switched ruby, superficial punctate erosions immediately appear with the development of edema, which can last for several days. The fluence is generally too high if there is marked epidermal splattering. The Q-switched Nd:YAG, depending upon the spot size and fluence, can produce pinpoint bleeding, tissue splattering, and edema.

It is theorized that the Q-switched systems lighten the nevus of Ota through an inflammatory neutrophilic response, with subsequent removal of the melanin by laser-affected melanosomes that are removed by macrophages to the regional lymph nodes.[27,28] It is further believed that the tissue splattering that is seen with the Q-switched Nd:YAG system promotes a transepidermal elimination of melanin in addition to the removal of melanosomes via macrophages to the regional lymph nodes.[29]

All Q-switched laser systems work well for nevus of Ota. It is well established that the Q-switched ruby laser is efficacious in treating nevus of Ota in phototype IV.[27] Chan et al. found the Q-switched alexandrite laser was more tolerable than the Q-switched Nd:YAG laser, with no true difference in efficacy.[29] Tse et al. showed a slight improvement with the Q-switched ruby laser in comparison with the double-frequency Q-switched Nd:YAG laser.[30] Nevertheless, lighter-skinned individuals fare better with shorter wavelengths, and darker-skinned individuals fare better with slightly longer wavelengths. Postinflammatory hypopigmentation is expected more with the shorter wavelengths. Postinflammatory hyperpigmentation is seen in darker-skinned patients.

Recurrence of nevus of Ota has been reported to range from 0.6% to 1.2%.[31] The mechanism is unclear. It is not known if there is incomplete clearance with reactivation or if it is laser dependent. There have been limited reports in the literature regarding this issue. It is prudent to have patients undergo periodic follow-up to pick up those patients with recurrences so that there is early intervention with laser treatments.

TATTOOS

Tattoos in darker skin are no longer a problem for laser tattoo removal. In fact, for persons of pigmented skin, laser tattoo removal is the treatment of choice. Surgical modalities, salabrasion, mircosanding, and re-tattooing have more untoward effects of scarring and dyspigmentation than laser-assisted tattoo removal.

The Q-switched Nd:YAG laser is an excellent choice for treating dark tattoo ink in persons of color[32] (Figure 14.2). Compared with the Q-switched alexandrite and the Q-switched ruby lasers, there is less risk of dyspigmentation and scarring. The longer wavelength of 1064 nm has less competition with epidermal melanin than the other Q-switched devices. Brightly colored tattoos such as purple and teal are best treated with the Q-switched alexandrite laser (Figure 14.3). Red tattoos are best treated with the 532-nm Q-switched Nd:YAG laser. On pigmented skin, this wavelength has a greater risk of hypopigmentation because of the strong competition with melanin.

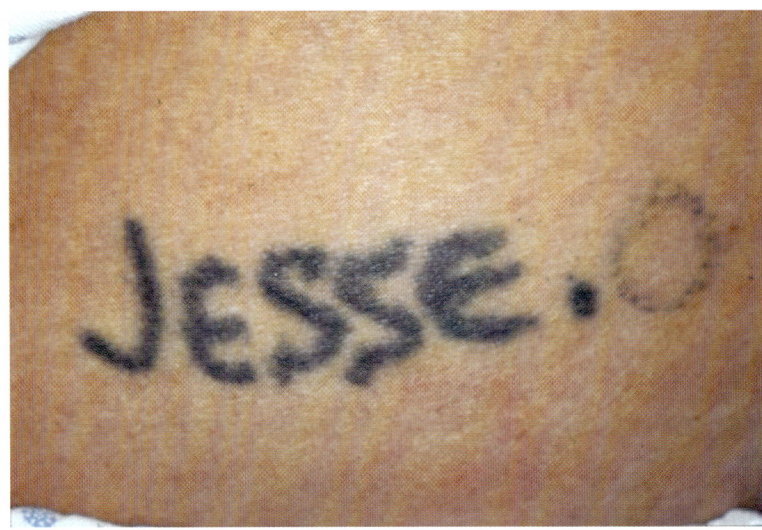

FIGURE 14.2 Eight weeks after a test spot to the letter "O" with the Q-switched 1064-nm Nd:YAG. Excellent clearance noted at the test spot compared with the nontreated site. A 3-mm test spot at 3.8 J/cm^2.

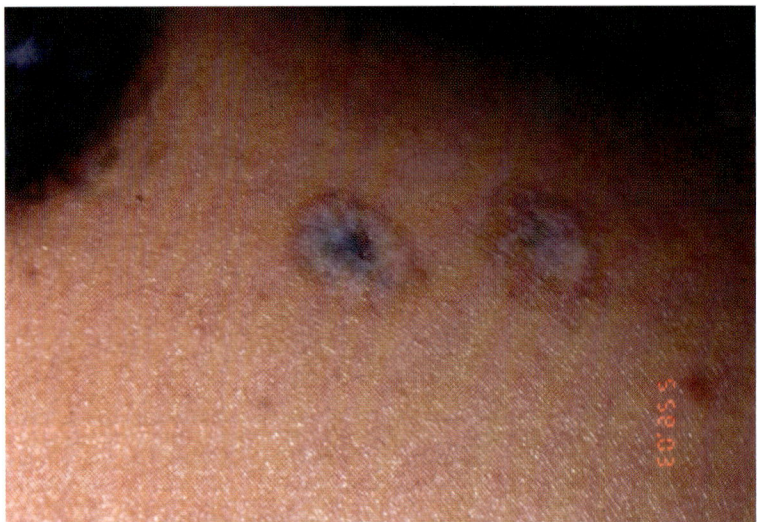

FIGURE 14.3 Tribal tattoo on the back with a teal color plant extract. Treated first with the 1064-nm Q-switched Nd:YAG laser unsuccessfully. The 755-nm Q-switched alexandrite was used to clear the teal color. Postinflammatory hypopigmentation resulted after three treatments.

Flesh-tone tattoos are generally not treated with the Q-switched systems because of immediate pigment darkening. Persons with allergic responses to tattoo ink should never be treated with the Q-switched systems. These tattoos should be ablated due to the possibility of anaphylaxis.

Multiple treatments are necessary. On average, 8–12 treatments may be required with a minimum of 6–8 weeks between treatment sessions. Longer durations beyond 8 weeks may decrease the number of treatment sessions over time. Amateur tattoos require fewer treatments than professional tattoos.[33] There is rarely 100% clearance with most tattoos, even after several treatments. Nevertheless, the results are generally consistently cosmetically acceptable to the patient.

It should be noted that for large multicolored decorative tattoos on darker skin, it is advisable to discuss the possibility of incomplete clearance. The brighter-colored inks necessitate shorter wavelengths that compete with the chromophore melanin. Hypopigmentation may ensue. Cosmetically, the treated outcome may be worse than the original decorative tattoo.

Side effects of laser tattoo removal on pigmented skin are transient dyspigmentation, hypopigmentation, and scarring. These side effects can generally be avoided by starting at low fluences and evaluating the tissue response. Typical initial settings for phototype V with the Q-switched Nd:YAG laser are a spot size of 3 mm and fluence of 3.6–3.8 J/cm^2. For phototype VI, lower fluences are used. With some small variation between laser devices, the best indicator for the ideal fluence is tissue response. With additional treatments, the fluence should be adjusted upward to accommodate for the clearance of pigment (or less amount of chromophore needing a higher fluence). Initial whitening and subsequent crusting are typical tissue responses. The crusting resolves over 2 weeks. Tissue splattering and pinpoint bleeding are seen with the smaller spot size of 2 mm. Edema and erythema can be seen and last for a few hours.

Intense pulsed light sources provide promise for tattoo removal in pigmented skin. However, to date there are no specific reports on such use on pigmented skin.

MISCELLANEOUS DISORDERS

Keloids and Hypertrophic Scars

There is no effective treatment for keloids. Surgical modalities are often temporary and discouraged because of a high rate of recurrence. Intralesional steroids, interferon, radiation therapy, silicone dressings, and lasers are common therapeutic options. Hypertrophic scarring, unlike keloids, responds better to the use of intralesional steroids. Nevertheless, keloids and hypertrophic scarring can be both a symptomatic concern and a cosmetic issue for most patients.

The pulsed dye laser (PDL), with its known histologic remodeling of collagen, is the laser of choice for both keloids and hypertrophic scarring.[34,35] The PDL is effective in reducing erythema, decreasing symptomatology, decreasing size, and improving pliability.[34,35] By selectively targeting the scar, there is decreased blood supply to the growing aberrant fibroblast within the keloidal tissue. Collagen remodeling can then ensue, creating a softer and less erythematous keloid or hypertrophic scar.

The PDL can be used in combination with other treatments. Intralesional steroids injected after PDL treatment are helpful in decreasing the height of the scar and improving erythema and symptomatology. Injection after the PDL treatment is often easier and its facilitation is due to the softer and more edematous tissue occurring after laser treatment.[36] In a study comparing 5-fluorouracil, 5-fluorouracil and intralesional steroids, and PDL alone, the results were equivocal overall. However, it was noted that the PDL group had a statistically significant decrease in the height of scars.[37]

For pigmented hypertrophic scars, the 532-nm Q-switched Nd:YAG laser may be helpful to decrease the amount of hyperpigmentation.[38] This study was not conducted in phototype VI. Enrolled in this small pilot study were six patients of phototypes II–V. Further research needs to be conducted to determine the true efficacy of the 532-nm Q-switched Nd:YAG and its role in persons with darker phototypes.

Nevertheless, for keloids and hypertrophic scars, the laser of choice in pigmented skin is the PDL. The earlier the intervention with treatment of these scars with the PDL, the better the clinical outcome. It is suggested that PDL treatment begin on the day of suture removal.[39] Multiple treatments are necessary. A combination approach with lasers and medication should be considered.

Psoriasis Vulgaris

Psoriasis is a common skin disorder affecting 2.6% of the U.S. population.[40] There is a host of therapeutic options available to control psoriasis. Ablative lasers have yielded variable responses and, for the most part, have lost favor as a good viable laser therapeutic option. Vascular lasers have been helpful in the treatment of psoriasis due to the increased blood flow and increased vasculature of the psoriatic lesion. Hence, the 585-nm PDL has been employed with often-promising results. Multiple treatments are necessary. Pulse durations of 450 and 1500 ms did not show a statistically significant difference in clinical outcome.[41] Interestingly, it appears that lesions with vertically oriented vessels, opposed to those vessels that were more tortuous, improved the best.[42] Clearly, more studies will need to be conducted.

The excimer laser is another type of laser that has shown potential in the treatment of psoriasis. In 1997, Bonis et al. was the first to use the excimer laser in psoriasis.[42] The laser cleared psoriasis in 7–11 treatments with lower cumulative doses in comparison to the conventional NBUVB (narrow-band UVB).[42] With multiple treatments, clinical remission may be as long as several months. To our knowledge, there have been no published studies specifically performed on ethnic skin types.

NEWER APPLICATIONS FOR LASERS

Acne Vulgaris

Light sources are now available to help control acne vulgaris. This mechanism is based upon the principle of photodynamic therapy. The visible light, in the blue range and perhaps the red range, aids in reducing the bacterium *Propionibacterium acnes*. This bacterium produces endogenous porphyrins. When exposed to blue light in the 400–420-nm range (the Soret band), these porphyrins release a singlet oxygen that aids in killing the bacteria. Thus, acne is reduced. Multiple treatments are necessary. The results are variable and, if successful, can last for a few months post-treatment. Patients should be off all oral photosensitizers. Patients should be off all oral photosensitizers. Topical retinoids do not pose a problem and need not be stopped before light treatment. This is a good therapeutic option to offer those patients in whom conventional medications are not amenable.

With blue light, no photosensitizer is required to treat acne vulgaris. For recalcitrant severe acne, a topical photosensitizer, aminolevulinic acid, has been used with blue light and red light devices. Lighter-skinned phototypes I–III and sometimes IV are able to undergo this treatment. However, the safety has not been established with darker-skinned phototypes with the use of aminolevulinic acid as a topical photosensitizer and light devices in the treatment of acne vulgaris.

In addition to the porphryins released by *P. acnes*, inflammatory acne lesions have much vascularity. Newer broadband light sources with wavelengths between 400 and 600 nm are now being tested with or without a topical photosensitizer to aid in the control of the vascular as well as the bacterial component seen in inflammatory acne vulgaris. Additional studies will need to be conducted in all phototypes to determine their efficacy.

Vitiligo

The specific 308-nm device, is a therapeutic option for the treatment of vitiligo. Treatment is done two times weekly starting with a low exposure time and increasing as tolerated with additional treatments. As with UV light, burning is discouraged. Repigmentation can be seen as early as 1 to 2 months. Facial areas treated seem to respond better than those in the trunk and extremities.[43]

Laser-Assisted Hair Removal

Prior to the late 1990s, laser-assisted hair removal was performed on light-skinned and dark-haired individuals. From research conducted at the Wellman Laboratories at the turn of the 21st century, the ideal patient is no longer fair skinned with dark hair. Now we are able to treat all skin types, provided that the hair color is dark.

Unlike other techniques such as electrolysis, waxing, and plucking, which can be tedious, laborious, and temporary, laser hair removal is fast, is efficacious, and results in a permanent reduction of hair. Multiple treatments, approximately 5–6, are necessary, depending upon body site. When laser-assisted hair removal is done correctly, there is no down time. The hair becomes carbonized and is expelled by the body, usually in 1–2 weeks. With each treatment, there is a resulting finer and lighter-colored hair, with an approximately 20% decrease in amount of hair.

The follicular melanin is the targeted chromophore in laser-assisted hair removal. The epidermal melanin is the unintended chromophore in darker phototypes. Melanin has an absorption spectrum ranging from 250 to 1200 nm; hence, the longer the wavelength, the less melanin absorption. In addition, the longer the wavelength, the deeper its penetration. Thus, the longer wavelengths penetrate deep to the intended chromophore, i.e., the hair follicle. Therefore, longer-wavelength laser-assisted hair-removal devices are best when treating darker skin types.

The diode laser (810 nm) and the Nd:YAG laser (1064 nm) are both FDA approved for the treatment of laser-assisted hair removal in phototypes IV–VI. These longer wavelengths allow a greater depth of penetration to the intended follicular melanin chromophore with less absorption within the epidermis. Cooling devices are imperative to protect the epidermis from heat-related injuries, which can result in scarring, dyspigmentation, and blistering. Both of these lasers have either a contact cooling device or a noncontact cooling device. In addition to the longer wavelengths and adjunctive cooling devices, longer pulse durations allow gentle heating of the intended chromophore, i.e., follicular melanin, with parallel cooling of the unintended chromophore, i.e., epidermal melanin. This allows for added protection of the epidermis.

With the use of longer-wavelength devices, adjunctive cooling devices, and long pulse durations, there are few to no side effects with laser-assisted hair removal on ethnic skin.[44–46] Side effects such as blistering, crusting, and dyspigmentation are usually encountered when fluences are too high and/or improper cooling of the epidermis occurs.

The authors believe that the long-pulsed Nd:YAG systems provide the best safety profile on pigmented skin with good efficacy. Lighter ethnic phototypes III, IV and V can be treated with both the long-pulsed diode and Nd:YAG laser-assisted hair-removal devices with little to no side effects (Figures 14.4–14.7).

Hirsutism and hypertrichosis are the most commonly treated hair disorders with the laser-assisted hair-removal devices. Multiple treatments are necessary, which can be performed monthly to every 2 months. It is important to closely shave or clip the hair prior to treatment. When treating the upper lip, it is important to protect the enamel of the teeth. This can be achieved by simply

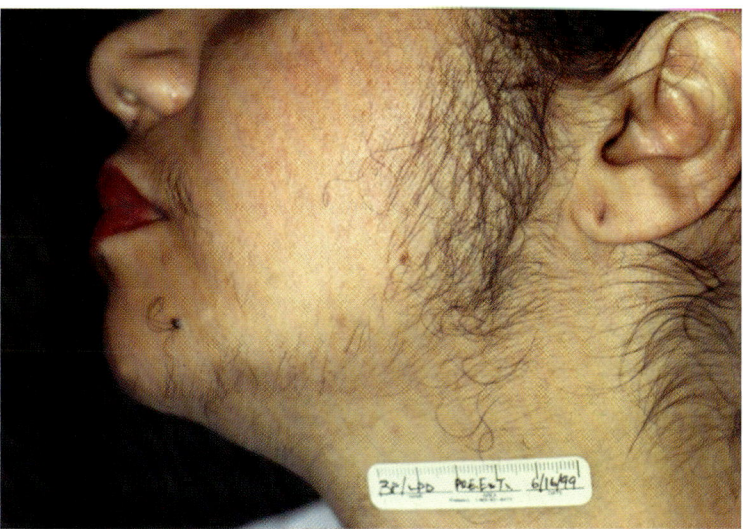

FIGURE 14.4 Hirsutism in a female patient with skin type V before laser-assisted hair removal.

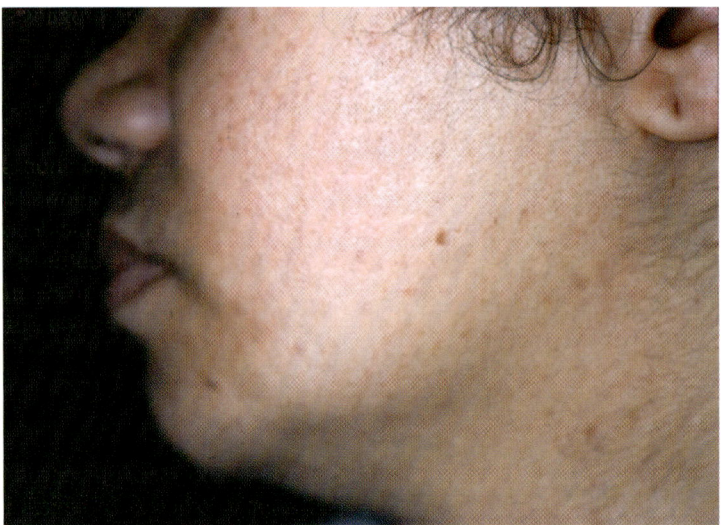

FIGURE 14.5 Three months after three treatments with the long-pulsed diode laser at 100-ms pulse duration and 25 J/cm^2.

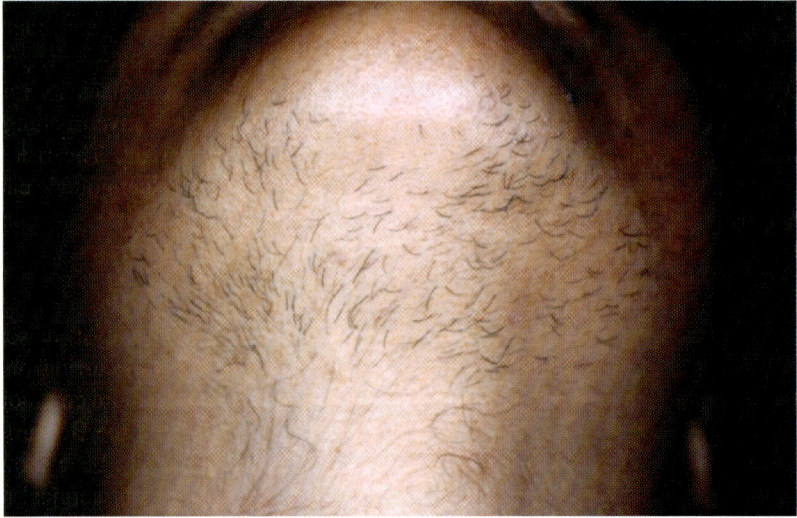

FIGURE 14.6 Hirsutism in a female patient with skin type V before laser treatment.

having the patient place his or her tongue over the teeth or using a protective covering such as a dental roll.

Pseudofolliculitis barbae (PFB) occurs in both men and women. Laser-assisted hair removal is a successful treatment for PFB.[46,47] It is our opinion that laser-assisted hair removal should be considered the gold standard for the treatment of PFB. The laser-assisted hair removal for PFB, depending upon the number of treatments, will either temporarily or permanently remove the hair or leave a finer-textured hair. By altering the nidus (the hair) of PFB, this will dramatically improve this skin condition while improving texture and postinflammatory hyperpigmentation.

In treating the bearded area of men, it is important to inform the patient that laser-assisted hair removal could be permanent. If the risk of creating a "bald" look in the bearded area is not cosmetically appealing to the patient, laser-assisted hair removal should not be done. However,

Laser Therapy for Pigmented Skins

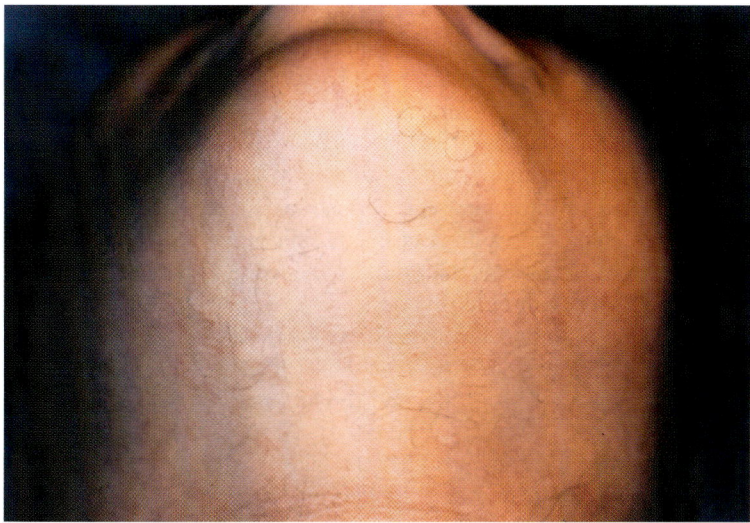

FIGURE 14.7 Four months after three treatments with the 1064-nm long-pulsed Nd:YAG laser at 40-ms pulse duration and 40 J/cm².

using lower fluences, longer pulse durations, and fewer treatments allows for hair growth delay with a finer hair that will help to manage the therapeutic approach of PFB. It should be noted that in treating the bearded area in men, lower fluences are mandatory secondary to the bridging effect in which the thickness of the hair shaft and the density of the hair cause a heat sink that can potentially lead to scarring. However, for females the desired outcome for PFB is permanent hair removal at the affected sites. Thus, multiple treatments, higher fluences appropriate for laser-assisted hair removal, and long pulse durations are appropriate.

ACNE KELOIDALIS NUCHAE

With laser-assisted hair removal, the goal is to destroy the tuftlike hair that acts as a foreign body in the hope of decreasing further scarring. Early lesions that are not as thick or indurated have the best potential for improvement with laser-assisted hair removal. Chronic large plaques and nodules are not as amenable. The clinical outcome at best, especially for the chronic cases, is not as satisfactory. For acne keloidalis nuchae, both medicinal and laser-assisted hair removal need to be implemented to increase the chance of improving this condition.

NONABLATIVE LASERS

For facial rejuvenation, nonablative lasers are ideally suited for ethnic skin. With its limited role, ablative laser resurfacing is extinct with its considerable downtime and inherent risks of permanent dyspigmentation, scarring, and textural abnormalities. This technique should be reserved for the experienced laser surgeon and performed on those patients for whom the risks outweigh the benefits. Nevertheless, the nonablative techniques work and are helpful in reducing acne scarring and mild rhytides while providing skin rejuvenation.

The 1320- and 1064-nm nonablative lasers are suitable devices in treating ethnic skin types. It is important to note that other lasers such as the pulsed 595-nm have been used for photofacials and skin rejuvenation on ethnic skin as well. Zelickson et al. demonstrated dermal collagen contraction, fibroblast stimulation, and prolonged neocollagenesis using the pulsed dye laser.[48] Although there is noted histopathologic improvement, the clinical effect of these changes is not dramatic. Therefore, multiple treatments are necessary and patient selection is crucial.

The nonablative lasers work best on those patients who have mild to slightly moderate facial rhytides and mild acne scarring. In comparison with the ablative technique, the ablative lasers will help reduce acne scarring between 30% and 50%, with a higher percentage of improvement for facial rhytides. Thus, the nonablative techniques, even after multiple treatments, have a drastically less optimal improvement in comparison with the ablative lasers for acne scarring and facial rhytides. The exact percentage of improvement is unknown and is variable from patient to patient, depending upon the degree of the underlying dermatologic condition. In general, patients with severe rhytides will not demonstrate a great cosmetic improvement. Hence, the nonablative techniques are best suited for those patients with mild to moderate rhytides, with the most noticeable improvement in those patients with mild rhytides.

In general, there is no downtime when using these lasers. The 595-, 1064-, and 1320-nm lasers remodel collagen, thus enhancing the quality of the skin. These lasers can be used for dermatological conditions including rhytides, acne scarring, and dyschromia. As stated, multiple treatments are necessary and can be performed monthly if necessary. A series of 5–6 treatments is usually the norm, with continued improvement months after the final treatment.

The broadband light source, the intense pulse light system (IPL), has wavelengths ranging from 550 to 1200 nm (visible to near infrared). Filters are used to block unwanted wavelengths. These lasers have the capacity to treat not only rhytides but also erthyema, telangiectasias, lentigines, acne scarring, and hair. Remodeling of the collagen has been demonstrated histologically.[49] Multiple treatments are necessary to achieve the desired outcome. The IPL works best on lighter phototypes but can be used on phototypes IV and V with caution and experience.

CONCLUSION

By combining new laser technology with revised and improved techniques based on clinical experience, we are able to safely treat a multitude of dermatological conditions in darker phototypes. However, there is still a limitation on the current laser devices available. To continue advancing the field of "color-blind" lasers, dedicated and continued research is warranted. This will assure that we will continue to be able to offer our darker-skinned patients better and more efficacious therapeutic laser modalities.

REFERENCES

1. Einstein A. Zur quantentheorie der strahlung. *Physik Z* 1917; 18: 121–128.
2. Schawlow AL, Townes CH. Infra-red and optical masers. *Physiol Rev* 1958; 112: 1940–1941.
3. Maiman T. Stimulated optical radiation in ruby. *Nature* 1960; 187:493–494.
4. Goldman L, Blaney DJ, Kindel DJ, Franke EK. Effect of the laser beam on the skin: preliminary report. *J Invest Dermatol* 1963; 40: 121–122.
5. Fitzpatrick T. *Dermatology in General Medicine*, Vol. 1. New York: McGraw Hill, 1993; 1629–1630.
6. Anderson RR, Parrish JA. Selective thermolysis: precise microsurgery by selective absorption of pulsed radiation. *Science* 1993; 220: 524–527.
7. Fuchs M. Thermokinetic selectivity — a new highly effective method for permanent hair removal: experience with the LPIR alexandrite laser. *Derm Prakt Dermatol* 1997; 5: 1.
8. Yohn JJ, Huff JC, Aeling JL, Walsh P, Morelli JG. Lesion size is a factor for determining the rate of port wine stain clearing following pulsed dye laser treatment in adults. *Cutis* 1997; 59: 267–270.
9. Katugampola GA, Lanigan SW. Five years experience of treating port wine stains with the FLPD laser. *Br J Dermatol* 1997; 137: 750–754.
10. Morelli JG, Weston WL, Huff JC, Yohn JJ. Initial lesion size as a predictor factor in determining the response of port wine stains in children treated with pulsed dye laser. *Arch Pediatr Adolesc Med* 1995; 149: 1142–1144.

11. Alam M, Dover JS, Arndt KA. Treatment of facial telangiectasia with variable-pulse high fluence pulsed-dye laser: comparison of efficacy with fluences immediately above and below the purpura threshold. *Dermatol Surg* 2003; 29(7): 681–685.
12. Ho WS, Chan HH, Ying SY, Chan PC. Laser treatment of congenital facial port wine stains: long term efficacy and complication in Chinese patients. *Lasers Surg Med* 2002; 30(1): 44–47.
13. Chang CJ, Nelson JS. Cryogen spray cooling and higher fluence pulsed dye laser treatment improve port wine stain clearing while minimizing epidermal damage. *Dermatol Surg* 1999; 25: 767–72.
14. Chang CJ, Kelly KM, van Gemert MJC, Nelson JS. Comparing the effectiveness of 585 nm vs 595 nm wavelength pulsed dye laser treatment of port wine stains in conjunction with cryogen spray cooling. *Lasers Surg Med* 2002; 31: 352–358.
15. Chui CH, Chan H, Ho WS, et al. Prospective study of pulsed dye laser in conjunction with cryogen spray cooling for treatment of port wine stain in Chinese patients. *Dermatol Surg* 2003; 29(9): 909–915.
16. Lupton JR, Alster TS, Romero P. Clinical comparison of sclerotherapy versus log pulsed Nd:YAG laser treatment for lower extremity telangiectases. *Dermatol Surg* 2002;28(8):694–697.
17. Negishi K, Tezuka Y, Kudshikata N, Wakamatsu S. Photorejuvenation for Asian skin by intense pulsed light. *Dermatol Surg* 2001; 27; 627–632.
18. Chan HH, Alam M, Kono T, Dover JS. Clinical application of lasers in Asians. *Dermatol Surg* 2002; 28: 556–563.
19. Ohshiro T, Maruyanma V, Makajima H, et al. Treatment of pigmentation of the lips and oral mucosa in Peutz–Jeghers syndrome using ruby and argon lasers. *Br J Plast Surg* 1980; 33: 346–349.
20. Taylor CR, Anderson RR. Ineffective treatment of refractory melasma and post inflammatory hyperpigmentation by Q switched ruby laser. *J Dermatol Surg Oncol* 1994; 20: 592–597.
21. Manaloto RM, Alster TS. Erbium:YAG laser resurfacing for refractory melasma. *Dermatol Surg* 1999; 25: 121–123.
22. Nouri K, Bowles L, Chartier T, Romagosa R, Spencer J. Combination treatment of melasma with pulsed CO_2 laser followed by Q switched Alexandrite laser; pilot study. *Dermatol Surg* 1999; 25: 494–497.
23. Angsuwarangsee S, Polnikorn N. Combined ultrapulse CO_2 laser and Q switched Alexandrite laser compared with the Q switched Alexandrite alone for refractory melasma: split face design. *Dermatol Surg* 2003; 29: 59–64.
24. Halder RM, Grimes PE, McLaurin CL, et al. Incident of common dermatoses in a predominantly black dermatologic practice. *Cutis* 1983; 32: 388–390.
25. Murphy MJ, Huang MY. Q switched ruby laser treatment of benign pigmented lesions in Chinese skin. *Ann Acad Med Singapore* 1994; 23: 60–66.
26. Jang KA, Chung EC, Choi JH, Sung KJ, Moon KC, Koh JK. Successful removal of freckles in Asian skin with a Q switched alexandrite laser. *Dermatol Surg* 2000, 26. 231–234.
27. Watanabe S, Takahashi H. Treatment of nevus of Ota with the Q switched ruby laser. *N Engl J Med* 1994; 331: 1745–1750.
28. Hakozaki M, Musuda T, Oikawa H, Nara T. Light and electron microscopic investigation of the process of healing of the naevus of Ota by Q switched alexandrite laser irradiation. *Virchows Arch* 1997; 431: 63–71.
29. Chan HH, Ying SY, Ho WS, Kono T, King WW. An *in vivo* trial comparing the clinical efficacy and complications of Q switched 755 nm alexandrite and Q switched 1064 nm Nd:YAG lasers in the treatment of nevus of Ota. *Dermatol Surg* 2000; 26: 919–922.
30. Tse Y, Levine VJ, McClain S, Ashinoff R. The removal of cutaneous pigmented lesions with the Q switched ND:YAG laser. *J Dermatol Surg Oncol* 1994; 20: 795–800.
31. Chan HH, Lam LK, Wong DS, et al. Nevus of Ota: a new classification based upon the response to laser treatment. *Lasers Surg Med* 2001; 28: 267–272.
32. Jones A, Roddey P, Orengo I, Rosen T. Q switched Nd:YAG laser effectively treats tattoos in darkly pigmented skin. *Dermatol Surg* 1996; 22: 999–1001.
33. Stratigos AJ, Alora MB, Urioste S, Dover JS. Cutaneous laser surgery. *Curr Probl Dermatol* 1998; 10(4): 127–174.
34. Alster T, Williams CM. Treatment of keloid sternotomy scars with 585 nm flashlamp-pumped pulsed dye laser. *Lancet* 1995; 345(8959): 1198–2000.

35. Berman B, Flores F. Treatment of hypertrophic scars and keloids. *Eur J Dermatol* 1998; 8: 595–595.
36. Connell PG, Harland CC. Treatment of keloid scars with pulsed dye laser and intralesional steroid. *J Cutan Laser Ther* 2000; 2(3): 147–150.
37. Manuskiatti W, Fitzpatrick RE. Treatment response of keloidal and hypertrophic sternotomy scars: comparison among intralesional corticosteroid, 5-FU and 585 FLPD laser treatments. *Arch Dermatol* 2002; 138(9): 1149–1155.
38. Bowles LE, Nouri K, Berman B, et al. Treatment of pigmented hypertrophic scars with the 585 nm pulsed dye laser and the 523 nm frequency doubled Nd:YAG laser in the Q switched and variable modes: a comparative study. *Dermatol Surg* 2002; 28(8): 714–719.
39. Nouri K, Jimenez GP, Harrison-Balestra C, Elgart GW. 585 nm pulsed dye laser in the treatment of surgical scars starting on the suture removal day. *Dermatol Surg* 2003; 29: 65–73.
40. Koo JY. Current consensus and update on psoriasis therapy: a perspective from the US. *J Dermatol* 1999; 26: 723–733.
41. Zelickson BD, Mehregan DA, Wendelschfer-Crabb G, et al. Clinical and histologic evaluation of psoriatic plaques treated with a flashlamp pulsed dye laser. *J Am Acad Dermatol* 1996; 35: 64–68.
42. Motley RJ, Lanigan SW, Katugampola GA. Videomicroscopy predicts outcome in treatment of port wine stains. *Arch Dermatol* 1997; 133: 921–922.
43. Spencer JM, Nossa R, Ajmeri J. Treatment of vitiligo with the 308-nm excimer laser: a pilot study. *J Am Acad Dermatol* 2002; 46: 727–731.
44. Greppi I. Diode laser hair removal of the black patient. *Laser Surg Med* 2001; 28; 150–155.
45. Adrian RM, Shay KP. 800 nm diode laser hair removal in African American patients: a clinical and histologic study. *J Cutan Laser Ther* 2000; 2: 183–190.
46. Ross EV, Cooke LM, Timko AL, et al. Treatment of pseudofolliculitis barbae in skin types IV, V, and VI with the long pulsed Nd:YAG laser. *J Am Acad Dermatol* 2001; 47: 263–270.
47. Ross EV, Cooke LM, Overstreet KA, et al. Treatment of PFB in very dark skin with a long pulsed Nd:YAG laser. *J Natl Med Assoc* 2002; 94(10): 888–893.
48. Zelickson BD, Kilmer SL, Bernstein E, et al. Pulsed dye laser therapy for sun damaged skin. *Laser Surg Med* 1999; 25; 229–239.
49. Zelickson BD, Kist D. Effect of pulsed dye laser and intense pulsed light sources on the dermal extracellular matrix remodeling. *Laser Surg Med* 2000; 17 (suppl 12): abstract 68.

15 Cosmetics, Hair Care Products, and Personal Care Products for Pigmented Skins

Victoria L. Holloway

INTRODUCTION

The field of cosmetics is an important one for the dermatologist to understand. Patients including men, women, and children each apply several different cosmetic products to the hair, face, and body every day. These patients may consult their physicians for suggestions on specific products or brands, particularly if they have an underlying skin disease. Occasionally, patients have dermatological reactions to their cosmetics, and the physician must be able to diagnose and treat these conditions. Also, the misuse of cosmetic products can cause hair and skin problems, so the dermatologist must be aware of not only the specific products but also their appropriate use.

Within the field of cosmetics, there is the ethnic product market. This market has traditionally been known for products developed specifically for the tightly curled hair that is characteristic of most African-Americans. Although hair care is still the cornerstone of the ethnic market, specialized skin care and color cosmetics are also available. According to the U.S. Bureau of the Census, 30% of this country's population is nonwhite, and 80% of the world's population is from Africa, Asia, Latin America, and the Caribbean.[1,2] It is reasonable to expect to see a broadening of the concept of "ethnic" products to reflect the increasing diversity of the population in the United States and the predominance of people of color around the world. In addition, "mainstream" cosmetics products are now being formulated with a more diverse consumer base in mind.

This chapter offers a review of the cosmetic products that are of particular significance to people of color, including people of African descent, people of Asian descent, and Hispanics.

HAIR CARE

UNIQUE CHARACTERISTICS OF ETHNIC HAIR

The need for ethnic-specific products is based largely on some of the unique properties of ethnic hair. Asian hair tends to grow very straight, African hair is tightly curled, and Caucasian hair may fall anywhere on the spectrum but is usually in between these two extremes. Asian hair is generally round in cross section, whereas African hair has the shape of a flattened ellipse, with Caucasian hair in between the two. African hair routinely has several small twists along the length of the hair shaft, and neither the fiber diameter nor the cuticle diameter is consistent along its length. This means that there are several fragile points along the length of African hair, and hair breakage is a particular concern in this population, even in virgin hair that has not been chemically treated.[3] In addition, research has demonstrated that African hair is less dense and tends to grow more slowly than Caucasian hair.[4] Thus, with the significant fragility of virgin hair, the chemical processes discussed below, and slower regrowth, alopecia is a major concern for many African-American women in particular.

Hair Relaxers

History

Chemical hair straightening dates back to the 1940s. African-American men gave rise to a process called the congalene, or "conk." A homemade mixture of potatoes, eggs, and lye was combed though the hair until the burning sensation could no longer be tolerated and was then rinsed out. Commercially available products soon followed. In 1954, the chemist George Johnson revolutionized chemical straightening by putting the lye in a petrolatum base. The lye-based relaxer dominated the industry until 1978, when Mario de la Guardia invented the first no-lye relaxer. Both lye and no-lye relaxers are still in use today, not only by African-Americans but also by people of African descent around the world, including many Hispanics.[5]

Chemistry

Most relaxers use caustic alkalis to straighten the hair. Although the exact mechanism of action is not known, lanthionine formation does result and is generally believed to be responsible for the straightening of the hair. The disulfide bonds are broken as follows:

$$\underset{\text{Cystine}}{K-S-S-K} + \underset{\text{Hydroxide}}{OH^-} \rightarrow \underset{\text{Lanthionine}}{K-S-K} + OH^- + S^{2-}$$

The alkalis are divided into two categories. Lye relaxers contain sodium hydroxide as the active ingredient, whereas no-lye relaxers contain guanidine, lithium, or potassium hydroxide. Guanidine hydroxide is not stable and must be prepared immediately prior to use. Two-component no-lye kits contain calcium hydroxide and guanidine carbonate that are mixed to form guanidine hydroxide and calcium carbonate.[6] Most relaxers have a pH of 12–14. Acidic neutralizing shampoos follow the application and rinsing of the relaxer.

Use of the term "no-base relaxer" should not be confused with the term "no-lye relaxer." "Basing" refers to the application of a petrolatum-based protectant to the hairline and scalp. In this manner, the relaxer is prevented from coming into contact with the scalp and the chance of irritation is reduced. Basing is used prior to the application of sodium hydroxide relaxers and prior to the application of any relaxer to a person known to have a sensitive scalp. The term "no base" does not suggest that the product is not an alkali.

Proper Use

Hair relaxers may be applied either in hair salons by professional stylists or at home by consumers. Professional products may contain either sodium hydroxide or guanidine hydroxide as the active ingredient. Because sodium hydroxide is more irritating to the scalp, only guanidine hydroxide products are available in home-use kits. The benefit of sodium hydroxide relaxers is that they are the most effective straighteners and require the shortest application time. Although the guanidine relaxers are less irritating, they do not leave the hair as straight as sodium hydroxide relaxers and they sometimes leave a calcium residue on the hair. Choice of the type of relaxer one uses is a matter of personal preference and tolerance. Specific lye and no-lye relaxers are listed in Table 15.1.

Because the effects of the relaxer on the hair are permanent, patients should be instructed to apply the product only to the new hair growth. These "touch-ups" should occur not more than every 6 to 8 weeks. Patients often mistakenly comb the product through the entire length of the hair, leading to overprocessing of already relaxed hair. This activity should be discouraged. It is also important to note that immediately following the application and thorough rinsing of a hair

TABLE 15.1
Hair Relaxer Brands and Companies

Professional Products (Sodium Hydroxide)	Home Use Kits (Guanidine Hydroxide)	Children's Products
Affirm (Avlon)	Africa's Best	Beautiful Beginnings (Soft Sheen Carson)[a]
Dudley	African Pride	Just for Me
Mizani[a]	Dark & Lovely (Soft Sheen Carson)[a]	Motions for Kids
Motions	Gentle Treatment (Johnson Products)[b]	
	Optimum Care (Soft Sheen Carson)[a]	
	Realistic (Revlon)	
	TCB	

[a] A L'Oréal Company.
[b] A Proctor and Gamble Company.

relaxer, an acidic neutralizing shampoo must be used to help restore the normal pH of the hair. These special shampoos are routinely provided in the relaxer kit.

Many people use hair dye in addition to hair relaxer. Use of permanent dye should follow the use of the relaxer by at least 2 weeks. This reduces the chance of overprocessing by the two chemicals. However, temporary and semipermanent dyes are able to be used in the same day as relaxers without overprocessing the hair. This allows maximum penetration of the dye following alteration of the cuticle caused by the relaxer.

Adverse Events

The actual incidence of relaxer-related adverse events is not known. Alopecia and contact dermatitis have been reported in the literature.[7] Clinical experience suggests that these outcomes occur frequently from product misuse or chemical overprocessing of the hair, but many consumers do not mention these problems to their physicians or hairdressers. There also has been one report of a staphylococcal infection resulting from a relaxer-induced irritant contact dermatitis.[8]

Particularly concerning was the outbreak of alopecia that followed the introduction of the Rio Hair Naturalizer System and Rio Hair Naturalizer System with Color Enhancer onto the market in 1994. Complaints were so numerous that the FDA issued a warning against the products in December of that year.[9] Swee et al. analyzed data from 464 patients who complained to the FDA between 1994 and 1995 and subsequently returned their questionnaires. They found that the most common complaint was hair breakage or hair loss, with three quarters of the patients reporting loss of 40% or more of their hair. Nine percent of the respondents had no regrowth up to 2 years after the incident. Unlike all other available relaxers that are strong bases, the average pH of these products was found to be 1.39 for the relaxer kit and 2.82 for the kit with the color enhancer.[10] These products are no longer available.

The most serious adverse event is the accidental ingestion of hair relaxer. This is generally seen when the product is not stored appropriately in the home and children access the product. Mucosal injury may result.[11,12] Current literature suggests that endoscopy is not necessary for these patients if they present to the emergency room.[13,14]

THIOGLYCOLATES FOR PERMANENT WAVES, "CURLS," AND THERMAL RECONDITIONING

Salts of thioglycolic acids such as ammonium thioglycolate and calcium thioglycolate have historically been used to permanently curl the straight hair of Caucasians, Asians, and Latinos. In the

1980s, these same permanents became popular for African-Americans as an alternative look to relaxer hair, a style known as the "curl." These products are currently making a resurgence for African-Americans.

Thioglycolates reduce disulfide bonds, converting cystine to cysteine. Once this has been done, the hair is set on rods and treated with a neutralizer that oxidizes the cysteine and reforms cystine, locking the hair in the new curl formation. Because of the resulting dryness of the hair, African-Americans use high-content glycerin products to keep the hair moisturized. These same thyoglycolates are used in the newly popular "thermal reconditioning" process, also know as Japanese hair straightening. In this process, the thiol product is applied to reduce cystine. Rather than curling the hair with rods, the hair is straightened with a heated flat iron. The hair is then neutralized to re-form cystine and allows the hair to maintain its new straightened arrangement.

HAIR BLEACH AND HAIR COLOR

Hair decolorizing solutions, or "bleaches," are used to dissolve the hair's melanin granules, facilitating removal of color from the hair. Key ingredients are the hydrogen peroxide that facilitates protein degradation, the ammonia that serves as an alkalizer to achieve the needed pH, and ammonium or potassium persulfates as the color "booster."[15] Bleaching alters the structural integrity of the hair, so patients should be very cautious when combining bleaching with other strong chemical treatments such as relaxers due to the risk of overprocessing the hair.

There are three main types of hair color. Temporary colorants coat the hair cuticle but do not penetrate it. Semipermanent and demipermanent dyes act by diffusion of dye molecules into the cortex, but no changes to the natural melanin occur. All of these products are safe to use at the same time as a relaxer treatment. Permanent hair dyes, including the progressive (gradual) colorants, work by oxidation using hydrogen peroxide that decolorizes the hair and induces coupling of the aromatic amines and phenols that provide color. This active chemical process should not be combined with relaxing in the same session and is best carried out at least 2 weeks after hair relaxing to minimize damage.

SHAMPOOS, CONDITIONERS, AND STYLING PRODUCTS

Shampoos are used to remove sebum, other soil, and product build-up from the hair. They are generally composed of surfactants, foam boosters, thickening agents, and preservatives as well as other ingredients to impart desired fragrance, color, and conditioning. Most deep-cleansing shampoos use high-level anionic surfactants, whereas milder and baby formulations generally use a lower-level anionic surfactant in combination with the milder amphoteric surfactants.[16]

Selection of a shampoo is largely a matter of personal preference. However, African-American women must achieve a delicate balance. The already dry, fragile, and sometimes chemically treated hair is even more prone to breakage when it is wet and during the initial styling that is undertaken immediately after it is washed. As a result, most African-American women wash their hair once a week, with some washing more frequently but many washing only every other week in an attempt to prevent excess dryness and breakage. However, there may be a significant amount of product build-up during the time interval between shampoos, so the milder shampoos may require more than one application. Conditioning shampoos are useful, but for added softness and detangling, the use of a conditioner is usually desired.

Conditioners serve to reduce the frictional force generated by combing the hair and to counteract the cuticle damage that is caused by grooming, chemical agents, thermal styling, and the environment. Most commercially available conditioners contain several conditioning agents. There are hundreds of different agents available, but they are broadly divided into two categories. Cationic conditioners include surfactants and polymers. Nonionic conditioners include silicones, esters, and oils.

Hair styling aids are found in many forms, including sprays, gels, mousses, lotions, creams, and pomades. They serve many purposes, including providing hold, shine, or moisturization. There are a few points regarding styling products that are salient for African-Americans in particular. Oils, sheen sprays, holding sprays, and gels are often used, sometimes on a daily basis. However, because the hair is generally not shampooed daily, the products may build up. Some patients with already dry, fragile hair will find that these products exacerbate their problem. These patients should be instructed to look for products that do not contain alcohol and hence are less drying.

Pomade is used more frequently by African-Americans than by people of other ethnicities. The waxy substance has many uses, including coating and protecting the hair, relieving dry scalp, and conducting heat for thermal appliance styling such as hot combing or curling ironing. As such, pomade acne is a condition that is commonly seen in this population. For many patients with this condition, simply ceasing pomade use may be difficult given their hair dryness and styling needs. These patients should be instructed to wear styles with hair off the face.

Depilatories

Chemical depilatories are commonly used by African-American men to remove unwanted facial hair. The use of these products is prevalent because of the high percentage of African-American men who suffer from pseudofolliculitis barbae (PFB). Studies estimate the incidence of this condition in this population to be between 43% and 83%.[17,18] Whereas shaving leaves the end of the hair shaft with a sharp edge which is able to pierce the skin and exacerbate PFB, depilatories leave the end of the shaft with a dull edge and helps to prevent PFB. In one study of patients presenting with PFB, 17% of men and 20% of women reported depilatory use as one of their methods of hair removal.[19]

Depilatories remove hair by swelling and degrading the hair shaft followed by the mechanical removal of the degraded hair. In mainstream depilatory products, calcium thioglycolate or sodium thiogylcolate are the commonly used active ingredients. However, African-American men often require products that are stronger than the mainstream products because of the relative coarseness of their beard hair. Sodium hydroxide, potassium hydroxide, strontium sulfide, and barium sulfide have all been used with much greater prevalence in ethnic products. Although these agents are much more effective at bond breakage, they can also be more irritating to the skin and must be used with care.

SKIN CARE

The skin care category is composed of a vast array of products. The skin type of the individual determines the optimal combination of products used. In general, products address one of four skin types: normal, dry, oily, or combination. Although there is no difference in the distribution of skin types between Caucasian people and people of color, both dry skin and oily skin are more apparent on darker backgrounds. Thus, dryness and oiliness are both particular concerns for people of color.

In addition to addressing skin types, many products address specific skin problems. For example, there are products for acne-prone skin, aging skin, and sensitive skin. Because hyperpigmentation is a particular concern for ethnic populations, two categories of cosmetics significant to people of color are discussed below: skin bleaches and brighteners that fade affected areas, and the sunscreens that can sometimes prevent the condition.

Skin Lightening and Brightening Products

Dermatologists are accustomed to diagnosing and managing the pigmentary disorders that are prevalent in ethnic populations, including postinflammatory hyperpigmentation and melasma. Dermatologists have a number of effective modalities available to safely treat hyperpigmentation in

TABLE 15.2
Skin Bleaching and Brightening Agents Commercially Available in the United States

Cosmetics
Arbutin
Bearberry extract
Burner root extract
Calcium D-pantetheine-S-sulfonate
Kojic acid
Kojic acid dipalmitate
Licorice extract
Melanostat
Mulberry extract
Scutellaria extract
Vitamin C and derivatives
Vitamin B_3

Over-the-Counter Drug
Hydroquinone up to 2%

people of color, including hydroquinone alone or compounded with tretinoin and/or topical steroids, alpha-hydroxy acid and beta-hydroxy acid chemical peels, and laser use. However, many people first attempt to treat themselves with over-the-counter preparations before seeking medical treatment. In the United States, bleaching agents are considered drugs because they suppress melanin formation, either due to melanocytotoxicity or by inhibiting tyrosinase. As such, over-the-counter preparations are covered under the FDA's Tentative Final OTC Drug Monograph. Only hydroquinone 1.5%–2% is recognized by this monograph and may be sold to consumers as an over-the-counter product. Of course, dermatologists may prescribe any one of numerous brands of hydroquinone 4% products or have it compounded up to 10% or higher on rare occasion, with patients being followed carefully.

The use of hydroquinone is a well-known cause of exogenous ochronosis.[20] Other adverse effects include irritant and allergic contact dermatitis and colloid milia.[21,22] Because of these risks, the cosmetics industry has actively pursued the development of other agents to lighten the skin. Because these ingredients are not listed in the FDA monograph, they cannot be sold as "skin bleaches" or "skin lighteners" and must be sold as "skin brighteners" or "skin toners." Although they vary in effectiveness, a list of ingredients available in the United States is listed in Table 15.2.

Physicians are concerned with helping their patients achieve an even complexion. However, when reviewing the subject of bleaching creams, it is important to note that there are complex historical and social factors that affect some people's perceptions about skin color and skin bleaching. Although a discussion of these issues is outside the scope of this paper, the dermatologist must recognize the potential for misuse of these products in some people of color. In other countries, particularly in many African countries, hydroquinone, topical steroids, and mercury are readily available to consumers without a prescription. Published reports of skin lightener use range from 36% to 77%.[23,24]

SUNSCREENS

The role of sunscreens for fair-skinned patients in the prevention of skin cancer and photoaging is well recognized and heavily promoted by dermatologists to patients. People of color do have a

TABLE 15.3
Sunscreen Actives Approved by the FDA

Chemical Name	Trade Name(s)	Maximum Percent	Spectrum
Avobenzone	Parsol 1789	3	UVA
Dioxybenzone	Benzophenone-8	3	UVA
Menthyl anthranilate	Neo Heliopan MA	5	UVA
Oxybenzone	Neo Heliopan BB Uvinul MS 40	6	UVA
p-aminobenzoic acid	PABA Pabanol	15	UVB
Cinoxate	—	3	UVB
Homosalate (homomenthyl salicylate)	Eusolex Heliophan Kemester HMS	15	UVB
Octyl methoxycinnamate (ethylhexyl methoxycinnamate)	Escalol 557 Neo Heliopan AV Parsol MCX	7.5	UVB
Octyl salicylate (ethylhexyl salicylate)	Escalol 587	5	UVB
Padimate O	Escalol 507	8	UVB
Phenylbenzimidazole sulfonic acid	Eusolex 232 Parsol HS	4	UVB
Trolamine salicylate	—	12	UVB
Octocrylene	Escalol 597 Neo Heliopan 303 Uvinul N539	10	UVA/UVB
Titanium dioxide	—	25	UVA/UVB
Sulisobenzone	Syntase 230 Uvinol MS 40	10	UVA/UVB
Zinc oxide	—	25	UVA/UVB

lower incidence of skin cancer than fair-skinned patients and less photoaging. Although the role of sunscreens for skin cancer prevention in these populations has not been well studied, their role in the prevention and treatment of pigmentary disorders such as melasma is well known. Also, although there is little published research on sunscreen use in people of color, in one study of high school students by Hall et al., black and Hispanic students showed less frequent sunscreen use than whites.[25] It is important that dermatologists stress the importance of sunscreen use to people of color with pigmentary disorders.

Sunscreens may be either UV blockers or UV absorbers. UV blockers, which include titanium dioxide and zinc dioxide, offer excellent protection against both UVA and UVB. Traditionally, they have been particularly unpopular with ethnic patients, however, because of their obvious chalkiness against the dark skin. This is less of a problem with the newer, micronized formulations.

Chemical absorbers may be effective against either UVA or UVB. Because the effects of UVA have become clearer to dermatologists over the past few years, patients should be encouraged to look for products that protect against both forms of radiation. These products are generally very cosmetically elegant. A list of active ingredients currently approved by the FDA is listed in Table 15.3. Not listed is Mexoryl SX, an effective UVA filter that is currently available in Canada and Europe but not in the United States at the time of publication.

Allergic contact dermatitis, photoallergic contact dermatitis, and contact urticaria may be seen in patients allergic to the active ingredient in sunscreens. Several studies report the presence of sunscreen allergy in photosensitive patients; prevalence ranges from 7.4% to 20% in these reports.[26–28] Oxybenzone and PABA (*p*-aminobenzoic acid) and its derivatives are widely recognized common allergens. In these studies, other reported allergens included avobenzone, octyl methoxycinnamate, and phenylbenzimidazole sulfonic acid. Patients allergic to sunscreens should be reminded to check ingredient listings on facial moisturizers, lip balms, and shampoos. These cosmetic products may contain sunscreens.

It is important to note that there has been some controversy in the literature regarding whether sunscreen actually increases the risk of malignant melanoma. Although some small studies have suggested such, two recent meta-analyses found no increased risk of melanoma with sunscreen use.[29,30]

COLOR COSMETICS

Women wear makeup for a variety of reasons. Some like the way it creates a polished, finished appearance. Others like to "re-create" themselves through experimentation with different colors, formulations, and application techniques. Many women use products to enhance their best natural attributes, and others seek to conceal imperfections. Whatever the personal reason for choosing to wear color cosmetics, there have never been more choices of product than there are today.

There are many types of color cosmetics and they are broadly defined by function. Concealers, foundation, and pressed and loose face powders are used to even the complexion. Blush is used to color and contour the face. Eyeliner, eye shadow, mascara, and eyebrow pencil are used to define the eyes. Lip pencil, lipstick, and lip gloss add color to the lips. Products may be liquids, creams, or powders. Factors influencing the consumer's selection of cosmetics include color, aspects of performance such as being waterproof or long lasting, formulation appropriate to skin type, and price point.

Women of color tend to be particularly concerned about the color of the cosmetics. Frequent complaints include makeup lines that do not include colors that are vast enough or intense enough to complement darker skin. In addition to wanting a greater range of shades, women find it difficult to tell how a shade will look on them once they get it home. The actual color of a product on the skin varies, based on the skin color background on which it is placed. Makeup brands marketed specifically to people of color are listed in Table 15.4.

Adverse reactions from color cosmetics are relatively infrequent. Allergic contact dermatitis usually results from either the fragrance or the preservatives within the products. Irritant contact dermatitis may also occur. Microbial contamination of product may occur. Comedogenesis may occur from the oils used to give products the appropriate amount of spreadability. Most cosmetic

TABLE 15.4
Color Cosmetics and Skin Care Brands Marketed Specifically for People of Color

	General Ethnic	African-American	Latino	Asian
Department store/boutique	Iman Interface	Fashion Fair		Shiseido
Mass	Iman	Black Opal Black Radiance Milani Posner Tropez Zuri		
Online/other	Sacha Cosmetics Universal Colors	Elissia Cosmetics and Skin Care Great Face Café	Zalia	Zhen Beauty

products can be patch tested directly. Products with volatile compounds, such as mascaras and liquid eyeliner, should be allowed to dry before being occluded.

A specific category of product that dermatologists should be familiar with is the "camouflage cosmetic" or "corrective cosmetic." These products are specifically formulated to conceal visible skin lesions such as port wine stains, nevi, discoid lupus erythematosis, vitiligo, scars, and other lesions that may be troubling to patients. As such, they are more opaque than other foundations, smudge resistant, and waterproof. There is a psychological component for the patient that compels him or her to want to use corrective cosmetics, and the dermatologist must be sensitive to this.[31,32] Proper application techniques are important to achieve the desired effect.[33] These techniques can be taught by a medical aesthetician or by trained personnel at the cosmetics counter where the products are sold.

CONCLUSION

Based both on actual differences in the hair and skin and on cultural desire, people of color do have special considerations for cosmetic products. As the experts in hair and skin, it is incumbent upon dermatologists to understand the needs of a diverse patient base, to be knowledgeable about the products that patients need and desire, and to be aware of possible adverse effects related to product use or misuse. Further research is needed both to continue to understand the needs of the hair and skin of people of color and to understand the effects of products on ethnic hair and skin.

REFERENCES

1. U.S. Bureau of the Census. Census Redistricting Data (P.L. 94–171). Summary File for States and Census 2000 Redistricting Summary File for Puerto Rico, Tables PL1 and PL2. Available at: www.census.gov. Accessed April 26, 2004.
2. U.S. Bureau of the Census. Report WP/98, World Population 1998. Washington: U.S. Government Printing Office; 1999.
3. Kamath YK, Hornby SB, Weigman HD. Mechanical and fractographic behavior of Negroid hair. *J Soc Cosmet Chem* 1984; 35: 24.
4. Loussouarn G. African hair growth parameters. *Br J Dermatol* 2001; 145(2): 294–297.
5. Byrd AD, Tharps LL. *Hair Story: Untangling the Roots of Black Hair in America*. New York: St. Martin's Press; 2001.
6. Reiger MM. *Harry's Cosmeticology*, 8th ed. New York: Chemical Publishing, 2000.
7. Miller JJ. Relaxer-induced alopecia. *Am J Contact Dermat* 2001; 12(4): 238–239.
8. Kaur BJ, Singh H, Lin-Greenberg A. Irritant contact dermatitis complicated by deep-seated staphylococcal infection caused by a hair relaxer. *J Natl Med Assoc* 2002; 94(2): 121–123.
9. Stone B. FDA warns against use of "Rio" hair relaxer. Dec 21, 1994. http://origin.www.fda.gov/bbs/topics/ANSWERS/ANS00620.html. Accessed April 26, 2004.
10. Swee W, Klonz KC, Lambert LA. A nationwide outbreak of alopecia associated with the use of a hair-relaxing formulation. *Arch Dermatol* 2000; 136(9): 1104–1108.
11. Forsen JW, Muntz HR. Hair relaxer ingestion: a new trend. *Ann Otol Rhinol Laryngol* 1993; 102(10): 781–784.
12. Rauch DA. Hair relaxer misuse: don't relax. *Pediatrics* 2000; 105(5): 1154–1155.
13. Cox AJ, Eisenbeis JF. Ingestion of caustic hair relaxer: is endoscopy necessary? *Laryngoscope* 1997; 107(7): 897–902.
14. Ahsan S, Haupert M. Absence of esophageal injury in pediatric patients after hair relaxer ingestion. *Arch Otolaryngol Head Neck Surg* 1999; 125(9): 953–955.
15. Brown KC. Hair coloring. In: Johnson DH (Ed) *Hair and Hair Care*. Cosmetic Science and Technology Series, Vol. 17. New York: Marcel Dekker, 1997.
16. Wong M. Cleansing of hair. In: Johnson DH (Ed) *Hair and Hair Care*. Cosmetic Science and Technology Series, Vol. 17. New York: Marcel Dekker, 1997; 43–52.

17. Alexander AM, Delph WI. Pseudofolliculitis barbae in the military. A medical, social and administrative problem. *J Natl Med Assoc* 1974; 66: 459–479.
18. Edlich RF, Haines PC, Nichter LS, Silloway KA, Morgan RF. Pseudofolliculitis barbae with keloids. *J Emerg Med* 1986; 4: 283–286.
19. Perry PK, Cook-Bolden FE, Rahman Z, Jones E, Taylor SC. Defining pseudofolliculitis barbae in 2001: a review of the literature and current trends. *J Am Acad Dermatol* 2002; 46(2): S113–S119.
20. Kramer KE, Lopez A, Stefanato CM, Phillips TJ. Exogenous ochronosis. *J Am Acad Dermatol* 2000; 42(5 Pt 2): 869–871.
21. Findlay GH, Morrison JGL, Simson IW. Exogenous ochronosis and pigmented colloid milium from hydroquinone bleaching creams. *Br J Dermatol* 1975; 93: 613–622.
22. Grimes PE, Davis LT. Cosmetics in blacks. *Dermatol Clin* 1991; 9(1): 53–68.
23. Del Giudice P, Yves P. The widespread use of skin lightening creams in Senegal: a persistent public health problem in West Africa. *Int J Dermatol* 2002; 41(2): 69–72.
24. Adebajo SB. An epidemiological survey of the use of cosmetic skin lightening cosmetics among traders in Lagos, Nigeria. *West Afr J Med* 2002; 21(1): 51–55.
25. Hall HI, Jones SE, Saraiya M. Prevalence and correlates of sunscreen use among US high school students. *J Sch Health* 2001; 71(9): 453–457.
26. Szczurko C, Dompmartin A, Michel M, Moreau A, Leroy D. Photocontact allergy to oxybenzone: ten years of experience. *Photodermatol Photoimmunol Photomed* 1994; 10(4): 144–147.
27. Journe F, Marguery MC, Rakotondrazafy J, El Sayed F, Bazex J. Sunscreen sensitization: a 5-year study. *Acta Derm Venereol* 1999; 79(3): 211–213.
28. Schauder S, Ippen H. Contact and photocontact sensitivity to sunscreens. Review of a 15-year experience and of the literature. *Contact Dermatitis* 1997; 37(5): 221–232.
29. Huncharek M, Kupelnick B. Use of topical sunscreens and the risk of malignant melanoma: a meta-analysis of 9067 patients from 11 case-control studies. *Am J Public Health* 2002; 92(7): 1173–1177.
30. Dennis LK, Beane Freemman LE, VanBeek MJ. Sunscreen and the risk for melanoma: a quantitative review. *Ann Intern Med* 2003; 139(12): 966–978.
31. Westmore MG. Makeup as an adjunct and aid to the practice of dermatology. *Dermatol Clin* 1991; 9(1): 81–88.
32. Roberts NC. Corrective cosmetics — need, evaluation and use. *Cutis* 1988; 41(6): 439–441.
33. Draelos ZK. Cosmetic camouflaging techniques. *Cutis* 1993; 52(6): 362–364.

Part II

16 Dermatologic Disease in Asians

Chai Sue Lee, Hiok-Hee Tan, Mark Boon-Yong Tang, Chee-Leok Goh, and Henry W. Lim

Little research has been performed on the incidence and special concerns of skin disease in the sizeable Asian community in the United States even though Asian-Americans constitute 4.2% of the U.S. population according to the most recent U.S. Census.[1] As a result, the information contained in this chapter is derived from the handful of articles addressing specific skin conditions in Asians as well as from peer and personal experiences from the United States and Singapore.

DERMATOSES COMMON OR UNIQUE IN ASIANS

ACNE VULGARIS

Introduction

Acne vulgaris is a common, multifactorial, inflammatory disease of the pilosebaceous follicle commonly seen in young Asians.

Incidence/Prevalence

Acne vulgaris affects almost all adolescents at some point in time.[2] Although epidemiological data suggest that acne affects 40 to 50 million individuals in the United States,[3] there is scant information concerning the incidence and prevalence of acne among Asians. In a recent survey done in multiracial Singapore, acne affected more than 75% of schoolgoing children at one time or another in their lives.

Clinical Manifestations

In Asians, the clinical manifestation of acne vulgaris lesions includes noninflammatory (Figure 16.1) and inflammatory (Figure 16.2) lesions. The earliest clinical expression of acne is that of noninflammatory comedones in the midline areas of the face. Inflammatory lesions manifest as papules, pustules, and, in more severe cases, nodules and cysts (Figure 16.3). Pitted or hypertrophic scars may be present (Figure 16.4). In Singapore, 79% of patients with acne presented with facial lesions only, 5% had lesions confined to the trunk only, and 23% of patients had lesions on the face and trunk.

In a review of acne patients in Singapore's Asian population, the average age of patients presenting with acne vulgaris was 23 years.[4] The age of onset was 20 years, and most did not seek treatment until after 2 years of having the acne. In a recent survey of a multiracial Asian clinic population in Singapore, acne occurred with equal frequencies in male and female (46% vs. 54%) and predominantly among Chinese (82%) vs. Malays (8%), Indians (6%), and others (4%).

It is not uncommon to see Asian patients with severe inflamed lesions, as many patients do not seek treatment early, believing that acne is part of adolescence and growing up and that the condition

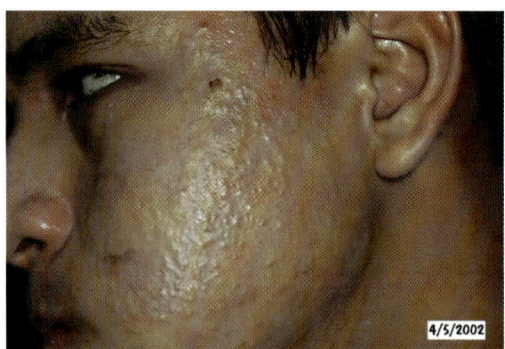

FIGURE 16.1 Acne vulgaris in a Chinese man. (Courtesy of National Skin Centre, Singapore.)

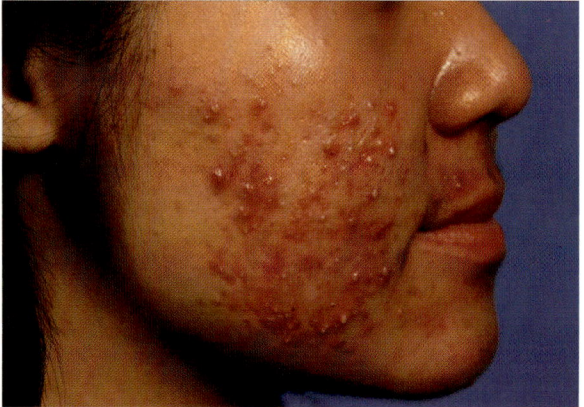

FIGURE 16.2 Inflammatory acne vulgaris in a Chinese teenager. (Courtesy of National Skin Centre, Singapore.)

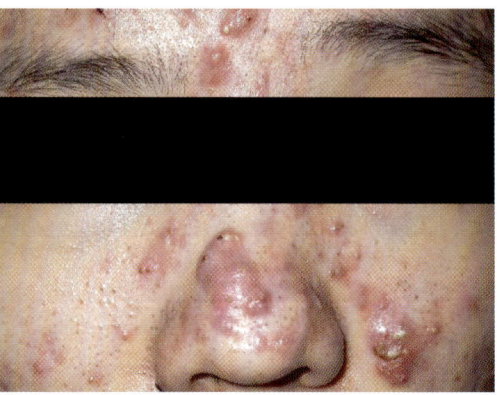

FIGURE 16.3 Severe nodulocystic acne in a Chinese man. (Courtesy of National Skin Centre, Singapore.)

will pass over a period of time. A survey of school children in Singapore indicated that more than 50% of children did not seek treatment for their acne. It is therefore important to counsel Asian patients to seek treatment early to prevent complications, especially severe scars.

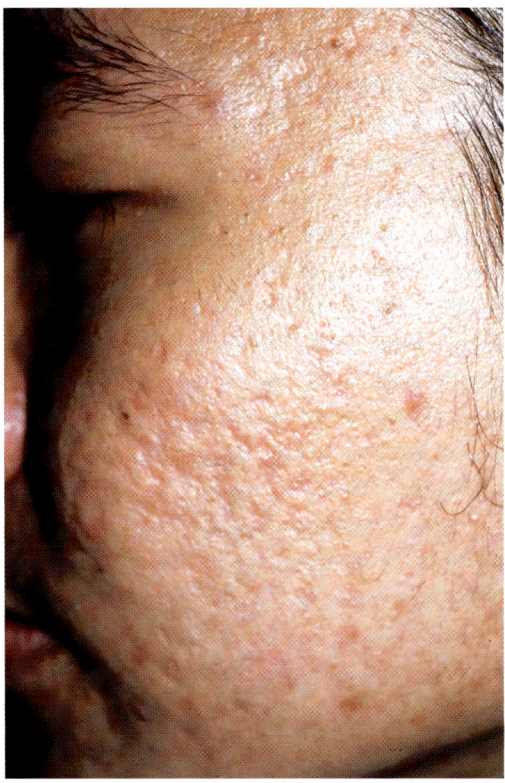

FIGURE 16.4 Post-acne scarring in a Chinese man. (Courtesy of National Skin Centre, Singapore.)

Histology

A comedone contains keratinized cells, sebum, and some microorganisms. The pigmentation seen on closed comedones or "blackheads" is due to melanin. Inflamed lesions result from inflamed pilosebaceous units, with the sebaceous glands and follicular lumens infiltrated with polymorphs.

Pathophysiology

Sebum production, abnormal follicular hyperkeratinization, action of *Propionibacterium acnes*, and inflammation are important factors that contribute to the pathogenesis of acne.[2] Inflammation in acne can be a direct or indirect result of the proliferation of *P. acnes*.[5] It produces lipases that hydrolyze triglycerides to glycerol and free fatty acids, which have proinflammatory and comedogenic properties.[6]

Therapy

Treatment of acne vulgaris in Asians is similar for all races. For mild acne, topical treatment may be adequate. The treatment of choice for comedone-predominant acne includes topical benzoyl peroxide, tretinoins, and resorcinol-containing preparations.

Inflamed lesions are more effectively treated with topical antibiotics, e.g., erythromycin and clindamycin lotion or gel. Combination comedolytic/antibiotic agents are available, but they tend to be more expensive. Patients with moderately severe or severe acne vulgaris should be treated with systemic antibiotics or oral isotretinoin where indicated.

In Asia, oral doxycyline is the treatment of choice for acne. Based on our experience, photosensitivity from doxycycline is rare in Asians. Pigmentation on inflamed lesions may rarely occur with doxycycline and minocycline therapy. Minocycline, which is more expensive than doxycyline, is the alternative to doxycycline. Tetracycline hydrochloride is seldom prescribed, as it has to be taken on an empty stomach and is often associated with dyspepsia. The second line of antibiotics is oral erythromycin base. Erythromycin ethylsuccinate is an expensive alternative in patients who experience dyspepsia from the base. Oral sulfamethoxazole is occasionally used for patients who failed oral tetracyclines and erythromycin, but the response rate is generally poor.

Oral treatment often has to be extended for several months, and patients must be counseled that initial improvement may be slow. Patients must be convinced to continue the oral antibiotics until the acne clears, and there is a often a cultural belief that long-term use of antibiotics is harmful to the body.

Oral isotretinoin is a useful drug for severe nodulocystic acne. A study in Singapore's Asian population showed that increasing total cumulative doses of isotreinoin was associated with lower rates of relapse and confirmed that a minimum cumulative dose of 120 mg/kg was required to achieve long-term remission.[4]

Antiandrogens in oral contraceptives may be effective in late-onset acne vulgaris in females, especially in patients with hormonal abnormalities such as polycystic ovarian syndrome.

An emerging issue with the use of antibiotics is the increasing levels of antibiotic resistance in *P. acnes*.[7] First detected in the United States,[8] *P. acnes* resistance has become more widespread[9] and has been detected in Europe, Australia, Japan, and, lately, Singapore.[10,11]

Atopic Dermatitis

Introduction

Atopic dermatitis is a common, chronic, pruritic eruption that occurs primarily in infants and children. It is often associated with a personal or family history of atopy, such as asthma, allergic rhinitis, and atopic dermatitis.

Incidence/Prevalence

There is a clinical impression among many dermatologists and pediatricians that the incidence of atopic dermatitis is disproportionately high among Asian infants. Current evidence is somewhat conflicting, however. Atopic dermatitis has been reported to be more common at least among the Chinese population. Mar et al.[12] compared the 12-month cumulative incidence of atopic dermatitis in Chinese, Vietnamese, and Caucasian infants born in Melbourne, Australia. Atopic dermatitis developed in 44% of Chinese, 17% of Vietnamese, and 21% of Caucasian infants. The researchers suggest that the high incidence of atopic dermatitis in Chinese compared with Caucasian infants tends to reflect genetic differences between the two populations, whereas the difference in incidence between the Chinese and Vietnamese infants possibly reflects more the environmental contribution to disease expression. These findings are in agreement with a study from 1962, which found that atopic dermatitis occurs much more frequently in Chinese than in Caucasian infants in San Francisco (27% vs. 11%) and Honolulu (23% vs. 3%).[13]

A study from Leicester, United Kingdom, found a significant increase in the number of referrals of atopic dermatitis from the Asian community to the dermatology department.[14] However, a follow-up study showed that although there are more Asian referrals, the incidence is, in fact, the same in Asian and non-Asian groups.[15] In addition, a history of eczema in a first-degree relative was found to be 14% in Asians but as high as 35% in non-Asians. The researchers suggest that a lack of familiarity with atopic dermatitis may have resulted in the high referral rate for Asians.

Dermatologic Disease in Asians

Clinical Manifestations

The clinical findings of atopic dermatitis are often divided into acute, subacute, and chronic lesions. In the acute phase, the involved skin presents as intensely pruritic, erythematous papules and vesicles that become excoriated and exudative (Figure 16.5). These areas commonly become secondarily infected. In the subacute phase, the involved skin has excoriated, erythematous, scaling papules and plaques. As the lesions become more chronic and are continually scratched by the patient, the eczema becomes leathery and dry (Figure 16.6). Chronic eczema is characterized by changes secondary to repeated rubbing and scratching called lichenification, in which the skin is thickened with accentuated skin lines.

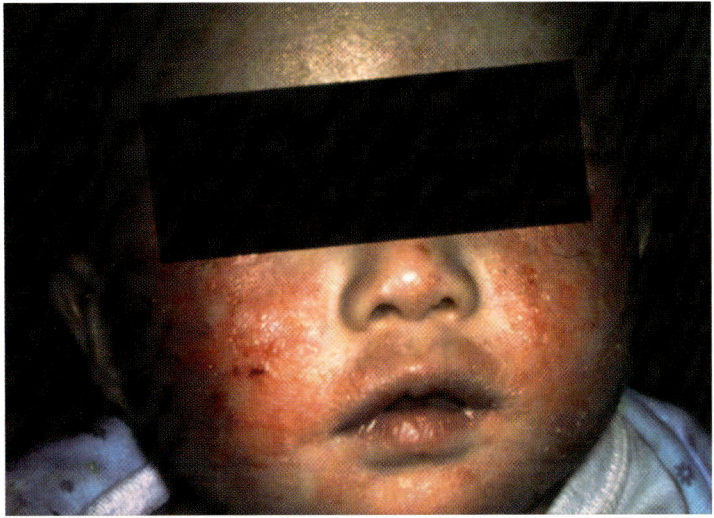

FIGURE 16.5 Erythema, excoriations, and erosions on cheeks of an 8-month-old Chinese girl.

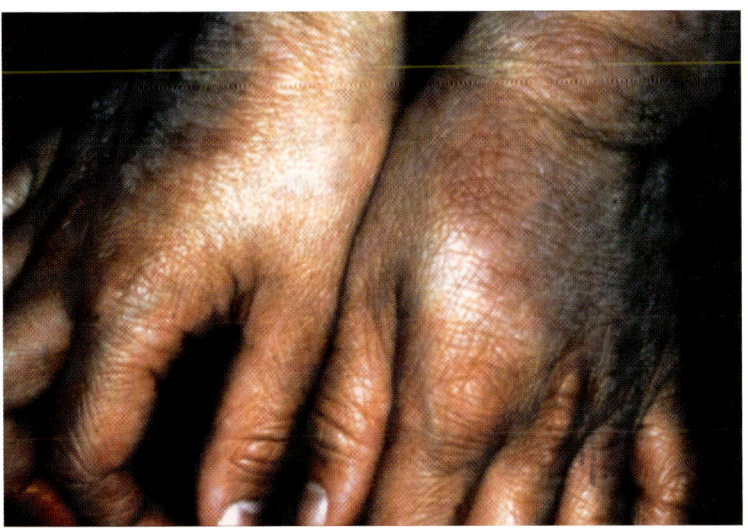

FIGURE 16.6 Lichenification and fine scales on dorsal surface of hands and forearms of a Chinese man (Courtesy of Xue-Jun Zhu, M.D., Peking University, Beijing, China.)

The distribution of the rash in atopic dermatitis changes depending on the patient's age. In infancy and early childhood, the face is the most common site of involvement. In later childhood, adolescence, and adulthood, a shift occurs from the face to the flexural surfaces, mainly affecting the neck, antecubital and popliteal fossae, wrists, and ankles.

Histology

In early phases, there is spongiosis, papillary dermal edema, and a sparse perivascular and interstitial lymphoeosinophilic infiltrate. With time, the changes may be those of lichen simplex chronicus.

Pathophysiology

The cause of atopic dermatitis is unknown. There appears to be a genetic predisposition for atopic dermatitis that can be affected by a number of factors, including food or aeroallergens, wool clothing, extremes of temperature or humidity, and anxiety or emotional stress.

Patients with atopic dermatitis exhibit a number of immunologic abnormalities. They tend to have an overactivity of T cells, specifically T-helper type 2 (Th_2) cells as opposed to as T-helper type 1 (Th_1) cells. Th_2 cells are associated with increasing or encouraging the humoral immune system to elaborate immunoglobulin E (IgE), so elevated IgE levels are common in these patients.

Therapy

Management is similar to that used in the non-Asian population. This includes proper skin care, moisturizers, topical corticosteroids, topical tacrolimus ointment (Protopic®), pimecrolimus cream (Elidel®), ultraviolet-based therapy (broad-band and narrow-band UVB, PUVA, and UVA1), and oral antihistamines for pruritus.

XEROSIS, NUMMULAR DERMATITIS, AND DYSHIDROTIC ECZEMA

Introduction

Xerosis, nummular dermatitis, and dyshidrotic eczema are common, chronic, pruritic, eczematous eruptions with distinctive clinical findings.

Incidence/Prevalence

It is our impression that in the United States xerosis, nummular dermatitis, and dyshidrotic eczema are significantly more common among Asians, especially those whose professions require frequent hand washing. The lack of knowledge about proper skin care, the lack of use of moisturizers in the winter, the cultural habit of taking hot and long showers in order to "treat" itchy skin, and the constant exposure to water for many who work in the restaurant business all contribute to the development of these cutaneous conditions.

Clinical Manifestations

Xerosis (asteatotic dermatitis or dry skin) occurs with a frequency from 48% to 98% in patients with atopic dermatitis, although it can certainly occur in patients without history of atopy. It presents as fine-scaled, noninflammatory areas of skin that have a rough texture, often with perifollicular accentuation.

Nummular dermatitis is characterized by coin-shaped, eczematous patches, mainly affecting the extensor extremities, although they may be seen on the trunk (Figure 16.7).

Dyshidrotic eczema (*pompholyx*) is characterized by recurrent eruptions of clear vesicles or bullae affecting the palms, soles, and the volar aspects and sides of the digits.

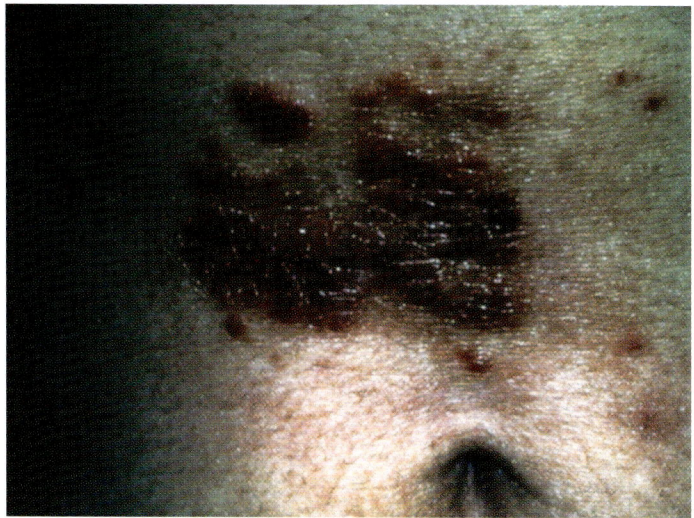

FIGURE 16.7 Erythematous excoriated papules and plaques on abdomen of an Asian woman.

Histology

In general, eczematous diseases, which include xerosis, nummular dermatitis, and dyshidrotic eczema, are distinguished clinically rather than histologically. Nevertheless, the histopathologic hallmark of eczematous diseases is spongiosis. It is often difficult to distinguish histologically each specific type of spongiotic dermatitis. There are no consistent distinguishing features in xerosis. Nummular dermatitis may have more crusting and spongiosis. Dyshidrotic eczema may have more spongiosis or vesicles.

Pathophysiology

The etiology of these entities is unknown.

Therapy

Management is similar to that used in the non-Asian population. This includes proper skin care, moisturizers, and topical corticosteroids.

CONTACT DERMATITIS

Introduction

Dermatitis is the most common skin disorder seen in dermatology clinics. In Singapore 30% of outpatient clinic attendances are for dermatitis. Contact dermatitis is one of the common causes. Irritant contact dermatitis is more prevalent than allergic contact dermatitis in the Asian community. The common contactants are different from those seen in Caucasians.

Incidence/Prevalence

In a retrospective study in 1990 in Singapore, 34.1% of 25,448 new patients who attended the clinics presented with dermatitis. Among these, 13.7% were diagnosed to have contact dermatitis, of which 39% were irritant contact dermatitis and 11% were allergic contact dermatitis; the remainder were unclassified.[16]

Irritant contact dermatitis is often seen in people engaged in wet work, including housewives and unskilled workers in industry who are exposed to solvents and cutting fluids.

Asians tend to self-medicate, especially with topical traditional medication, many containing counter-irritants that are contact irritants. Topical traditional Chinese medicine is still widely used, especially by those of Chinese descent, in many countries.[17] In a report from Hong Kong, where there is a predominantly Chinese population, the most common causative agents for contact dermatitis were soap (22.0%) and traditional Chinese medicine (17.3%); the latter was a more common cause of contact dermatitis than Western medicine (9.0%) or metals (13.4%).[18] When managing Asian patients with dermatitis, dermatologists should have a high index of suspicion about traditional medications and should patch-test with the suspected substance when patients give a history of use.

In a report from China, it was found that the most common causes of contact dermatitis from Chinese medicinal materials were topical analgesics and anti-inflammatory agents. The report indicated that fragrance, colophony, and ammoniated mercury were common sensitizers in the topical analgesics and anti-inflammatory agents.[19]

Clinical Manifestation

Contact dermatitis presents as an eczematous reaction. In acute dermatitis the hallmarks are erythema, edema, and vesiculation or bullae formation. In chronic eczema, it presents with lichenification, scaliness, pigmentary changes and fissuring. Subacute eczema presents with mild features of acute eczema, and chronic eczema with mild erythema, edema, occasional vesicles, and mild scaliness.

It is often not possible to ascertain the cause of contact dermatitis (irritant, allergic, or endogenous) from physical examination alone. A detailed history, physical examination, relevant patch test, and, occasionally, relevant laboratory tests are necessary to come to a definitive diagnosis.

However, the cause of some contact dermatitis may manifest with characteristic telltale features; e.g., in Asians, contact dermatitis to Chinese counter-irritant plaster (containing medicaments or colophony) tends to produce dermatitis with angulated outlines (outline of plaster) (Figure 16.8). Phytodermatitis tends to produce streaky dermatitis (Figure 16.10).

Rarely, a noneczematous contact reaction may occur, e.g., urticarial papules, plaque eruptions (erythema multiforme-like), lichen planuslike eruptions, purpura (Figure 16.9), and pigmented contact dermatitis. However, in these conditions a positive eczematous patch test reaction to the causative agent can usually be elicited.

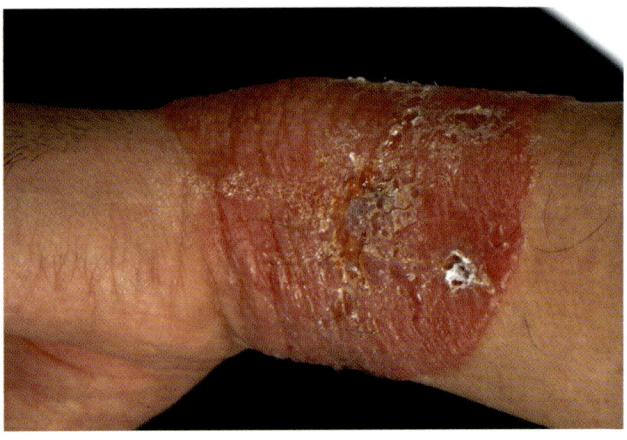

FIGURE 16.8 Allergic contact dermatitis from colophony from medicated plaster for sprained ankle. Note angulate margin. (Courtesy of National Skin Centre, Singapore.)

Dermatologic Disease in Asians

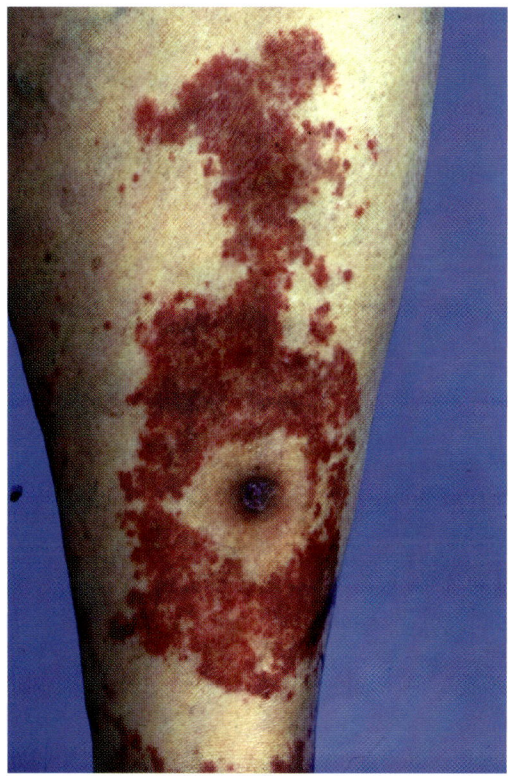

FIGURE 16.9 Purpuric allergic contact dermatitis from self-medication from proflavin. (Courtesy of National Skin Centre, Singapore.)

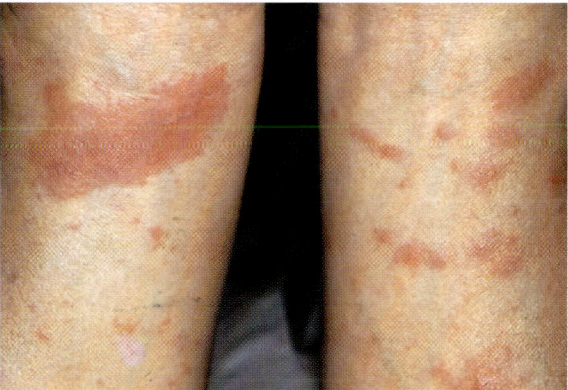

FIGURE 16.10 Phytodermatitis. Note streaking dermatitis characteristic of phytodermatitis. (Courtesy of National Skin Centre, Singapore.)

Dyshydrotic eczema presents with vesiculation on the palms and soles and may be a manifestation of contact dermatitis.

Pathophysiology

Common Causative Contact Allergens

The most common contact allergens in Asian countries include metals, fragrance, medicaments, colophony, and rubber chemicals. Less common contact allergens include preservatives and dyes.

A high proportion of patients reacts to thimerosal and gold salt but the majority were of unknown relevance.

Nickel has always been the most common contact allergen in Singapore. Nineteen percent of patients patch-tested had positive patch test reaction to the metal. The most common sources include costume jewelry, watch straps, belt buckles, jean studs, and metallic spectacle frames.[20]

The prevalence of *chromate* allergy in Singapore has declined from about 6% in the early 1980s to less than 3% over the last few years. This is probably the result of the decline in construction activities and automation in the construction industry. Other sources of chromate include chrome tanned leather shoes and watch straps, welding fumes, and electroplating fluids.

Fragrance-mix, which contains the eight common fragrances, is a common contact allergen in Singapore. The prevalence of fragrance-mix has declined from about 13% in the 1980s to about 6% in 1996 in the patch-test clinic in Singapore. Most positive reactions were relevant and were due to sensitization from cosmetics, toiletries, and medicaments.

Colophony allergy occurs in 3% of patients attending the contact clinic in Singapore. The main source of sensitization is medicated plasters used typically among Asians to relieve pain and aches. Other sources include medicament, papers, and fluxes.

Rubber chemical allergies occur in about 2% of patients attending the patch-test clinic in Singapore. The most common sensitizers are the thiuram-mixes (1.7%), carba-mix (0.1%), and PPD-mixes (0.2%). Contact allergy to naphthyl mixes are uncommon nowadays. The main source of rubber chemical allergies are rubber apparels including rubber gloves, rubber boots, and, occasionally, rubber linings of underwear.

Preservatives (e.g., parabens, formaldehyde, famaldehyde releasers, Kathon CG, Euxyl K 400) allergies are uncommon.

Para-phenylenediamine (PPD) is a common contact allergen in Singapore. Of our patch-tested patients, 3.6% had positive patch-test reactions to PPD. The most common source of PPD allergy is hair dyes. Rarely, PPD leached from dyed clothing may cause textile dermatitis. PPD dermatitis is occasionally referred to as "mourner's" dermatitis because of the Chinese custom of wearing freshly dyed black clothing when they are mourning.

Medicament allergy is not uncommon among older Asians. Common contact allergens here include neomycin (3%) and clioquinol (positive patch-test rates of 3% and 0.3%, respectively, in Singapore). Concomitant contact allergy to lanolin in lanolin-containing topical medicament is not uncommon (1.4%). Patients with stasis eczema are the at-risk group, for which more than half of patients are found to have one or more positive patch-test reactions. Proflavine, used as an antiseptic in Asian countries, is also a common contact allergen (positive patch-test rate has declined from about 7% in the 1980s to 3.3% in 1995).[21,22]

Traditional Chinese medicaments (unknown allergens) are a common cause of medicament contact dermatitis. Mastic and myrrh, natural gum resins widely used in traditional Chinese medicine to relieve pain and swelling due to trauma, have been identified as putative allergens in three Asian patients.[23]

Many topical traditional Chinese medicaments are contact irritants. In a report in which 11 common herbal topical medicaments in Hong Kong were selected for patch testing, many were found to cause skin irritation, especially when used under occlusion. The authors recommended that patients should be warned about their irritant properties.[24] Similarly, a Chinese herbal medicine containing *Venenum bufonis*, used for treating boils and other skin infections, can cause irritant contact dermatitis.[25]

Photocontact Allergens

Among the photocontact allergens, the sunscreens are now the most common photosensitizers, replacing musk ambrette and salicylanilide, which were the common photosensitizers in the 1980s and 1960s, respectively, in Asian countries. Occasional cases of photoallergy to nonsteroidal anti-inflammatory drugs (NSAIDs) are observed, with sensitization often resulting from use of topical NSAIDs for musculoskeletal aches and pain.

Contact Urticaria

Contact urticaria is seen occasionally, especially among food handlers and hospital workers. The most common causes of contact urticaria are proteinacious foodstuff and, recently, natural rubber latex. The prevalence of patients with contact urticaria is unknown but probably low at present.

Contact Irritants

In Asian countries, water, solvents, and cutting fluids are common contact irritants prompting patients to seek treatment. Housewives, chefs, hotel cleaners, factory operators, and especially cutting fluids workers form the largest proportion of patients with irritant contact dermatitis.

Therapy

Treatment of contact dermatitis is carried out as follows.

1. *Diagnosis* — The management of contact dermatitis depends on an accurate diagnosis. The etiologic agent must be ascertained. A good history, thorough physical examination, and patch test will often enable the investigating physician to arrive at a correct diagnosis. When managing Asians, it is important to inquire about self-medication, especially with topical traditional herbal medication.
2. *Specific treatment* — This depends on the diagnosis. If the dermatosis is severe, the worker should be removed from the causative agent immediately. Severely affected patients should be given medical leave or hospitalized.

Dermatitis is treated according to its severity. Acute dermatitis should be treated with a wet compress. Normal saline or potassium permanganate (1:10,000) lotions should be used until the lesion dries up. Chronic dermatitis should be treated with topical steroid cream or ointment. Only steroids of mild to moderate potency (e.g., hydrocortisone, betamethasone valerate, fluocinide) should be used to minimize side effects. Potent steroids (e.g., clobetasol dipropionate) should be avoided or used for short periods only because of their side effects. It is advisable to avoid steroids, antibiotics, and antifungal preparations, as they risk sensitization. Sensitization to neomycin and quinolines in such preparations is not uncommon. Oral antibiotics should be administered where secondary bacterial infection is suspected. Oral antihistamines to relieve pruritus should also be given if pruritus is a problem.

PIGMENTED CONTACT DERMATITIS

Introduction

Pigmented contact dermatitis was first reported by Osmundsen in 1969, when he studied seven patients who developed a pronounced and bizarre hyperpigmentation[26] attributable to contact allergy to Tinopal (CH3566), an optical whitener.

Pigment contact dermatitis is a characteristic allergic contact dermatitis reaction manifesting as macular pigmentation on contact sites. Patients often observe brownish to gray pigmentation on the face after using cosmetics containing azo-dyes (as contaminants) or fragrances. The allergic nature of the skin lesion can be confirmed by patch-testing with the incriminating allergens.

Incidence/Prevalence

Pigmented contact dermatitis is rare in Caucasians but not uncommon in Asians. In the early 1980s pigmented contact dermatitis due to Naphthol AS in Japanese garments was reported, presenting as pigmented contact dermatitis of the covered areas of the skin.[27] The most common cause of hyperpigmentation due to contact dermatitis was pigmented cosmetic dermatitis affecting the face of Asian women.[28]

An outbreak of pigmented contact dermatitis from cosmetics was reported in Japan, Korea, India, Taiwan, and China in the 1970s. Fragrances and Sudan I (an impurity in Brilliant Lake Red) were the causative allergens. The sources of these contact allergens are usually found in cosmetics that are produced by small cosmetics manufacturers where there is little product quality control.

Clinical Manifestations

The signs of pigmented cosmetic contact dermatitis are diffuse or reticular black or dark brown hyperpigmentation of the face that cannot be cleared by topical corticosteroids (Figures 16.11 and 16.12). The border of the pigmented cosmetic dermatitis is neither sharp as in lichen planus or melasma nor spotlike as in nevus of Ota.

Mild dermatitis is occasionally seen with hyperpigmentation, or dermatitis may precede hyperpigmentation. Patients may experience slight erythema and itch before the onset of pigmentation. Unlike melasma, the pigmentation clears upon avoidance of the causative allergen.

The neck, chest, and back may be involved and in a few exceptional cases, hyperpigmentation may extend to the whole body.

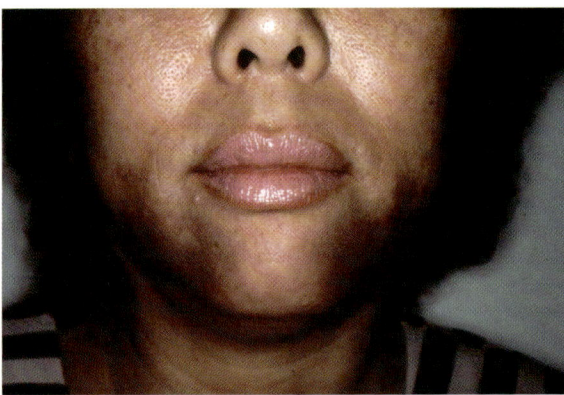

FIGURE 16.11 Pigmented contact dermatitis from fragrance in cosmetic. (Courtesy of National Skin Centre, Singapore.)

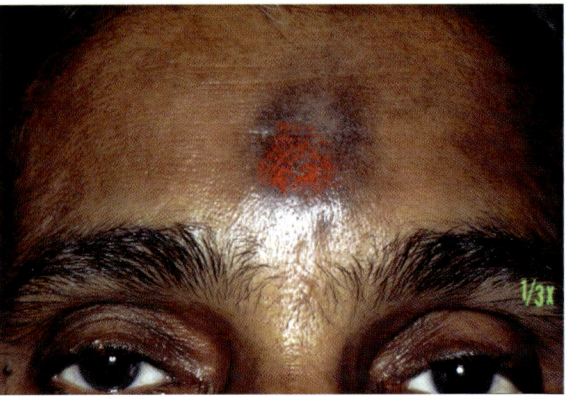

FIGURE 16.12 Pigmented allergic contact dermatitis from Sudan 1 in a red cosmetic (kumkum) applied by married Hindu female as a cultural necessity. (Courtesy of National Skin Centre, Singapore.)

Histology

Basal liquefaction degeneration of the epidermis and incontinence of pigment are observed histologically. The epidermis is often atrophic, presumably the effect of frequently applied corticosteroid for itchy dermatitis of the face, and cellular infiltrates of lymphocytes and histiocytes are seen perivascularly, as is often seen in ordinary allergic contact dermatitis.

Pathophysiology

In Asian countries, pigmented contact dermatitis from fragrances in cosmetics and Sudan I has been reported. Another common cause of pigmented contact dermatitis is seen in Hindu women who present with pigmentation on their mid-forehead due to allergens (usually Sudan I) in the red dyes applied on their foreheads for cultural reasons.[29]

Discovered sensitizers include mainly fragrance materials and pigments including jasmine absolute, ylang-ylang oil, canaga oil, benzyl salicylate, hydroxycitronellal, sandalwood oil, artificial sandalwood, geranoil, geranium oil, D&C Red 31, and Yellow No. 11.[28,30,31]

Therapy

Identification of causative allergens in pigmented contact dermatitis is necessary to eradicate the pigmentation. It is essential that the use of textiles and washing powders containing strong contact sensitizers be avoided in order to prevent contact dermatitis and pigmented contact dermatitis of the areas that come into contact with the fabric and washing powders or softening agents that remain on them, even after rinsing.

For cosmetic pigmented contact dermatitis, avoidance of the causative cosmetic allergens followed by the exclusive use of soaps and cosmetics that were completely allergen-free for such patients (designated the allergen control system) produced dramatic effects. It usually takes about 1–2 years for a patient to regain normal nonhyperpigmented facial skin.

PRURIGO NODULARIS, ACTINIC PRURIGO, AND PRURIGO PIGMENTOSA

Introduction

Prurigo nodularis is a characteristic chronic dermatosis of unknown etiology, presenting with extremely itchy nodules, usually on the extremities. There are several dermatological conditions that present with pruritic pruriginous eruptions, namely: (a) prurigo nodularis — of unknown etiology, often following insect bite reactions presenting as persistent pruritic nodules on the extremities, sometimes on the trunk; (b) actinic prurigo — a rare photodermatosis among Asians but not infrequently affecting young American Indian girls; and (c) prurigo pigmentosa — a rare dermatosis of unknown etiology, characterized by severely pruritic red papules, that coalesce to form a reticulate, mottled pigmentation, mostly reported in Japanese.

Incidence/Prevalence

There is little epidemiological data available on these conditions. Prurigo nodularis is not uncommon, but detailed information on its prevalence is lacking. Actinic prurigo is reported as a rare familial photodermatosis that mostly affects young American Indian girls,[32] but it has also been reported in Chinese and Malay patients in Singapore[33] as well as in Japan.[34] The clinical features of Asians in Singapore differ from the classical description in that they occur predominantly among male Chinese, with onset between 20 and 62 years of age.[35] Prurigo pigmentosa is rare and has been reported mostly from Japan,[36] with some cases reported from Taiwan[37] and isolated cases in Caucasian patients,[38] and Turkey.[39]

Clinical Manifestations

Prurigo nodularis

Prurigo nodularis is readily diagnosed clinically. It is characterized by intensely pruritic papules and nodules scattered on the extremities. The papules and nodules are discrete, firm and often hyperkeratotic, appearing mainly on the extensor aspects of the limbs (Figures 16.13 and 16.14). The condition may be associated with atopic disorders.[40] Prurigo nodularis has two subsets, namely early-onset prurigo which is associated with atopy and late-onset prurigo which is not associated

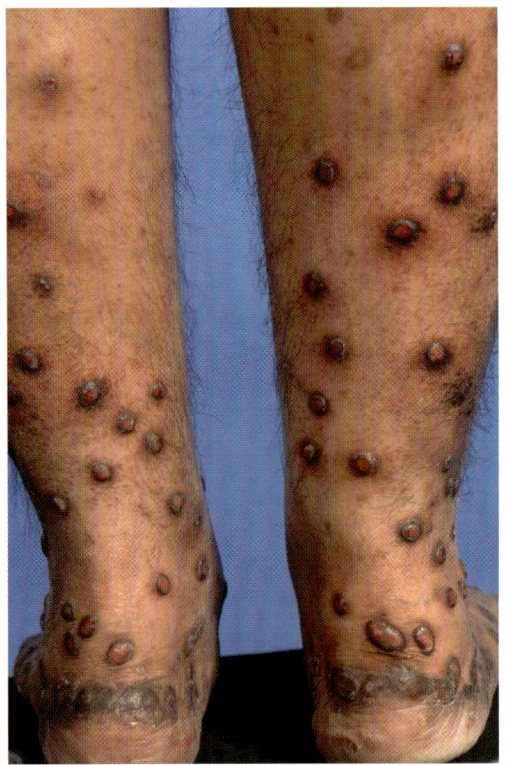

FIGURE 16.13 Prurigo nodules following insect bites on the leg of a Chinese man.

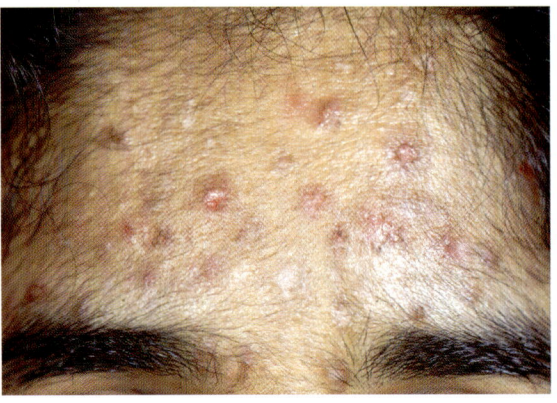

FIGURE 16.14 Multiple excoriated prurigo nodules on the leg of a Chinese patient with renal failure.

with atopic disorders.[41] Insect bites have been reported to be an important causative factor. A report from the United Kingdom indicated that 19% of incidents with prurigo nodularis followed an insect bite.[42]

Actinic Prurigo

Actinic prurigo presents primarily with papules and nodules and eczematous patches on sun-exposed parts of the body (Figures 16.15 and 16.16). The lesions are usually excoriated. Occasionally, covered areas of the body are also affected. Some patients have been reported to have cheilitis and conjunctivitis.[43] Unlike chronic actinic dermatitis, the lesions are more discrete, less confluent, and not as infiltrative. Distinction from polymorphous light eruption includes the appearance of irritable pruriginous eruptions that persist until winter, presence of conjunctivitis and cheilitis, and a positive family history. Classical actinic prurigo almost always has its onset before puberty, although a study of Asian patients in Singapore revealed patients with onset predominantly in adulthood.[35]

Prurigo pigmentosa

Prurigo pigmentosa is characterized by an inflammatory phase with pruritic erythematous papules and a resolution phase with reticulated pigmentation.[36] There is a tendency for recurrent attacks, and the chest, back, and neck are the main sites affected, although occasionally the face and limbs are also involved.[39]

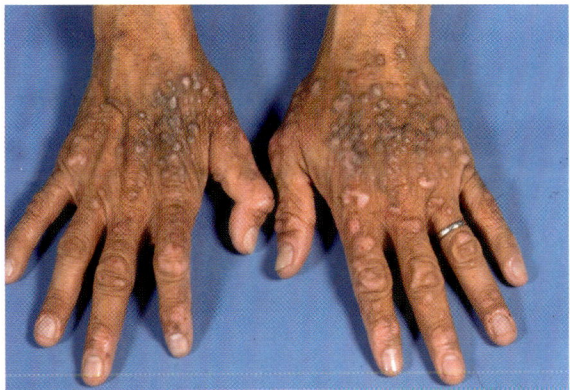

FIGURE 16.15 Actinic prurigo — multiple lesions on the dorsum of the hands.

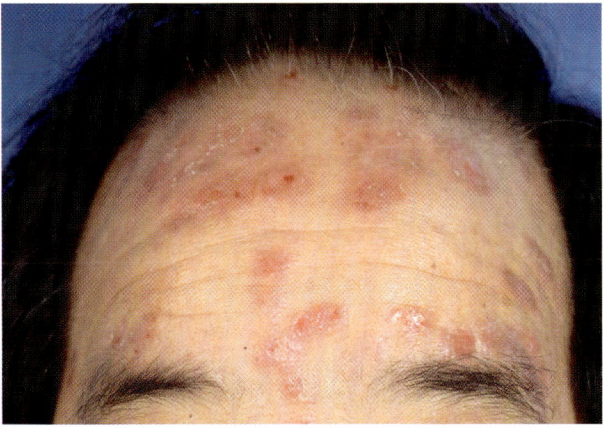

FIGURE 16.16 Actinic prurigo — involvement of the upper limb. (Courtesy of National Skin Centre, Singapore.)

Histology

Prurigo Nodularis

There is pronounced hyperkeratosis and acanthosis, with the dermis showing a nonspecific inflammatory infiltrate. The finding of neural hyperplasia is regarded as a diagnostic feature, and S100 staining may be useful to detect this.[44]

Actinic Prurigo

Nonspecific changes of acanthosis, exocytosis, epidermal spongiosis, and crusting, as well as perivascular lymphocytic infiltrate, are found. Lymphoid follicles have been shown in biopsy specimens from the lip.[43]

Prurigo Pigmentosa

Features are nonspecific, consisting of spongiosis, necrotic keratinocytes, exocytosis, vacuolar alteration of the basal layer, papillary dermal edema, and superficial perivascular lymphocytic inflammation.

Pathophysiology

The pathophysiology of prurigo nodularis and prurigo pigmentosa is unknown. Prurigo nodularis may be associated with atopy and insect bites, as mentioned earlier. It has also been linked to systemic diseases such as gluten enteropathy,[45] uremia,[46] and Hodgkin's disease.[47] Contact sensitivity to metals, fragrances, or chemical compounds has also been implicated in its pathogenesis.[48] Prurigo pigmentosa has been linked with fasting, diabetes mellitus, and pregnancy.[49] Exogenous factors such as physical trauma,[38] friction,[50] and acupuncture[51] have also been implicated as possible triggers.

In actinic prurigo, there is an abnormal response to UV radiation in most patients, with the action spectrum for erythema in actinic prurigo in both UVA and UVB. There has been genetic susceptibility reported in association with HLA A28 and HLA B39,[52] HLA DR4,[53] HLA A24,[54] and HLA CW4.[55]

Therapy

Topical corticosteroids are frequently used in the treatment of prurigo nodularis. Intralesional steroid injections may be useful. Systemic antihistamines may partially alleviate the itch. Phototherapy has also been used with some improvements for some patients. In severe recalcitrant cases oral cyclosporin[56] and thalidomide have been used.[57] The treatment of prurigo pigmentosa is not well defined. Most patients respond poorly to topical steroids and antihistamines. Dapsone has been used with some success,[58] as have systemic antibiotics such as minocycline[37] and doxycycline.[39]

The treatment of actinic prurigo includes sun protection, emollients, and topical corticosteroids. Intralesional corticosteroid injections, systemic corticosteroids, narrow-band UVB, psoralen plus UVA (PUVA) phototherapy,[59] azathioprine,[43] and thalidomide[60] have also been used.

PRIMARY CUTANEOUS AMYLOIDOSIS

Introduction

Primary localized cutaneous amyloidosis is a benign primary cutaneous disorder commonly seen in Asians. It often presents as pigmented macular or papular (lichen amyloidosis) or mixed forms (macular and lichen amyloidosis) or, rarely, nodular cutaneous lesions. There is an abnormal extracellular tissue deposition of amyloid material in the dermal papillae. The amyloid material is composed predominantly of a fibrillary protein component and amyloid P component, a glycoprotein.[61]

Incidence/Prevalence

Primary cutaneous amyloidosis is a skin disease commonly seen in Asians. It has been reported in Taiwan[62] and other Asian countries including Singapore,[63] Indonesia,[64] and Thailand.[65] It is also seen in South Asians (Indians and Pakistanis). Among the Asians, the Chinese race was noted to be predominantly affected.[66] Lichen amyloidosis appears to be more common in females, with a female:male ratio of 2.7:1 in Indonesia, 4.5:1 in Thailand, and 3:1 in Singapore.[66] Lichen amyloidosis is more commonly seen in Southeast Asia, accounting for between 69% and 80% of cases of primary cutaneous amyloidosis in series from Thailand[5] and Singapore,[67] respectively. Macular amyloidosis is more common among Middle Easterners[68] and Central and South Americans.[69] Biphasic amyloidosis is a term used to describe the coexistence of both macular and papular forms of amyloidosis and has been described in Thailand[70] and Singapore.[66] Nodular localized cutaneous amyloidosis is rare and has been reported in Japanese patients, in association with Sjogren's syndrome.[71]

Clinical Manifestations

Lichen amyloidosis is characterized by pruritic, brown or skin-colored, hyperkeratotic papules, which may coalesce into plaques. The lower anterior legs are the most commonly affected site (Figure 16.17). Other affected sites include the dorsum of the feet, thighs, extensor surface of the arms, and, rarely, the abdominal and chest walls.[62]

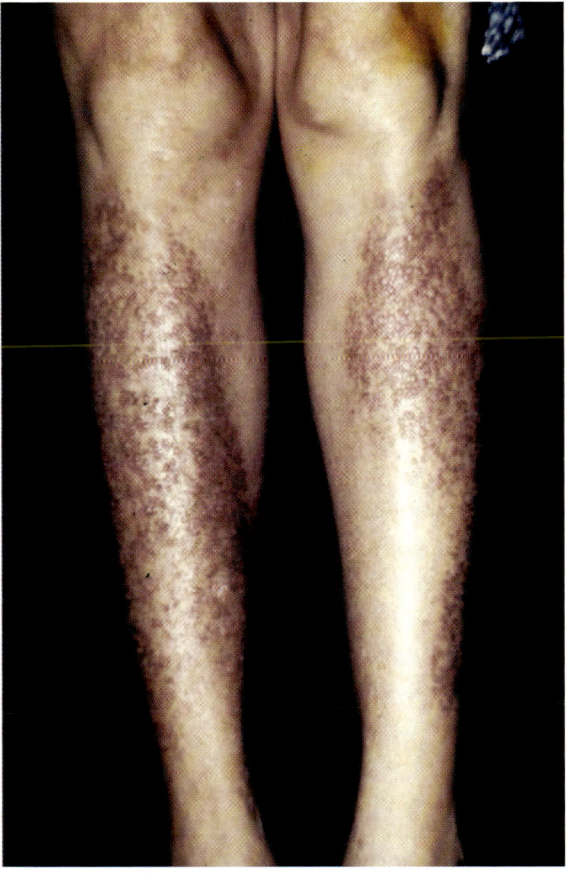

FIGURE 16.17 Lichen amyloidosis in a Chinese man. The shins are a common site of involvement. (Courtesy of National Skin Centre, Singapore.)

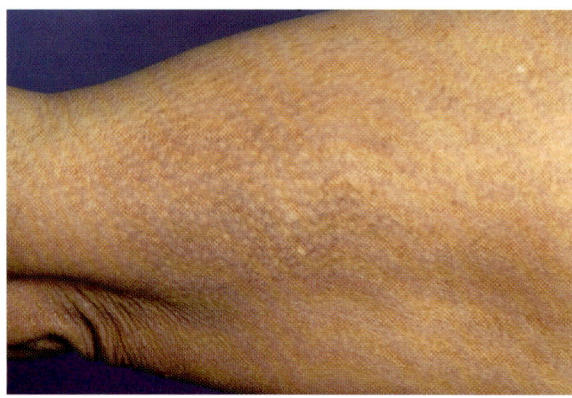

FIGURE 16.18 Macular amyloidosis on the forehead of a Chinese woman. (Courtesy of National Skin Centre, Singapore.)

Macular amyloidosis is characterized by moderately pruritic brownish macules with a characteristic reticulate or rippled appearance. It occurs most commonly in the interscapular area and less commonly on the chest and extremities (Figure 16.18).

Biphasic or mixed amyloidosis describes the coexistence of macular and lichen amyloidosis in an affected individual. Nodular amyloidosis typically presents as solitary or waxy nodules on the face, trunk, or genitalia. The nodules may measure from 1 to 3 cm in diameter and may be associated with systemic amyloidosis.[72]

Histology

Both lichen amyloidosis and macular amyloidosis are characterized histologically by deposits of amyloid materials localized in the dermal papillae. Lichen amyloidosis is also associated with epidermal changes such as acanthosis and hyperkeratosis, which are not present in the macular form. In nodular amyloidosis, there is an atrophic epidermis, beneath which are large masses of amyloid material.

The histological diagnosis of amyloid is based on its staining characteristics. Congo red imparts a pink or red color to amyloid deposits under ordinary light. Congo red-stained amyloid deposits also show a green birefringence under polarized light.

Pathophysiology

The pathogenesis of primary localized cutaneous amyloidosis has not been fully elucidated. Kumakiri and Hashimoto[73] suggest that it begins with focal epidermal damage, which then causes filamentous degeneration of keratinocytes. Apoptosis then occurs, and keratinocyte tonofilaments are converted into amyloid material in the papillary dermis. Another theory proposes that dermal fibroblasts and macrophages act to transform keratin present in the papillary dermis into amyloid because there is specific immunologic intolerance to the presence of keratin (colloid) bodies in the area.[74]

Therapy

There is no effective definitive treatment for macular or lichen amyloidosis. Treatment is mainly symptomatic. Emollients and topical steroids are the mainstay of treatment to relieve xerosis and itch. Sedative antihistamines taken at night help to relieve pruritus and scratching and further lichenification of the lesions.

Moderate-potency topical corticosteroids should be prescribed to relieve itch and pruritus. Topical corticosteroids under occlusion often result in clinical improvement of lichen amyloidosis, but the lesions tend to relapse on cessation of treatment and may result in skin atrophy.[75]

A pilot study on the use of calcipotriol ointment showed it to be as effective as betamethasone 17-valerate ointment in reducing roughness, hyperpigmentation, and pruritus in patients with lichen amyloidosis, but with a greater potential for irritation and at a higher cost.[76]

Other treatment modalities have been tried with variable results. Destructive therapy with carbon dioxide laser[77] and dermabrasion[78] has been reported in small series. Topical dimethyl sulfoxide (DMSO) showed positive results in some patients[79] but not in others.[80] Systemic therapy with etretinate[81] or acitretin[82] seems to benefit some patients, but long-term use of systemic retinoids has its drawbacks. Phototherapy with UVB has been reported anecdotally to reduce pruritus in macular amyloidosis,[83] and a small comparative study of broad-band UVB phototherapy and PUVA photochemotherapy showed the potential for these modalities to be useful alternatives in the treatment of primary cutaneous lichen amyloidosis.[84]

MELASMA

Introduction

Melasma is a commonly acquired hyperpigmentary skin disorder characterized by irregular, light to dark brown macules occurring in the sun-exposed areas of the face and neck. Etiologic factors and aggravating factors in melasma include genetic predisposition, exposure to ultraviolet light, pregnancy, and hormonal therapy.

Among Asians, melasma is as major a problem as any type of pigmentary disorder. It appears to have a social stigma that almost amounts to that of the dysmorphic syndrome.[87]

Incidence/Prevalence

Melasma is reported to be a common pigmentary disorder in Asians.[85] The exact prevalence of melasma in most countries is unknown. It is a very common skin disorder encountered by dermatologists, accounting for 0.25%–4% of patients seen in dermatology clinics in Southeast Asia.[86] The estimated prevalence of melasma is estimated to be as high as 40% in females and 20% in males.[86] In Singapore, melasma represented about 0.5% of new dermatological consultations seen.

Clinical Manifestation

Melasma is diagnosed clinically. It is defined as an acquired, light to dark brown, macular pigmentation of the face (predominantly over the cheeks and/or nose and/or forehead and/or jaws) where no obvious antecedent skin disorders, such as postinflammatory pigmentation, pigmented contact dermatitis, ashy dermatosis can be identified.

There appears to be a female predominance. There appears to be a higher proportion of Chinese with melasma than the other Asian races.

Melasma tends to occur during the fourth decade of life. Most patients seek treatment 3–5 years after the appearance of their melasma. Most melasmas recorded are light brown to brown or gray in color, and the majority is distributed on the malar areas. More than two thirds are of the epidermal type. Most patients have pigmentation confined to less than 10% of the total facial skin. Malar pigmentation (86%) appears to be the most common distribution for melasma. Centrofacial and mandibular pigmentation are relatively uncommon presentations.

As the pigmentation of most melasma is present in the epidermis, the intensity of the color contrast of melasma can be exaggerated by viewing with Wood's light (black light). Superficial pigmentation will bring about greater contrast. Pigmentation in the deeper layer of the epidermis

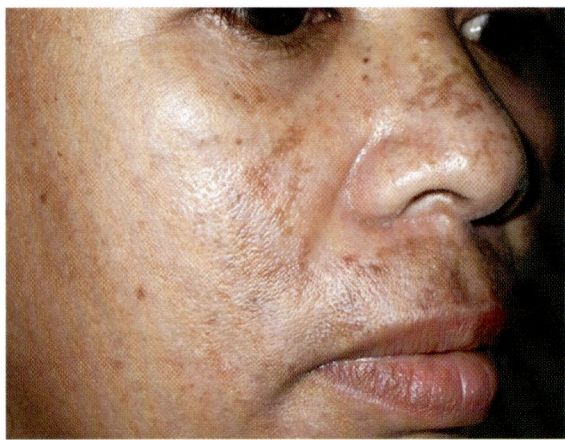

FIGURE 16.19 Epidermal melasma. (Courtesy of National Skin Centre, Singapore.)

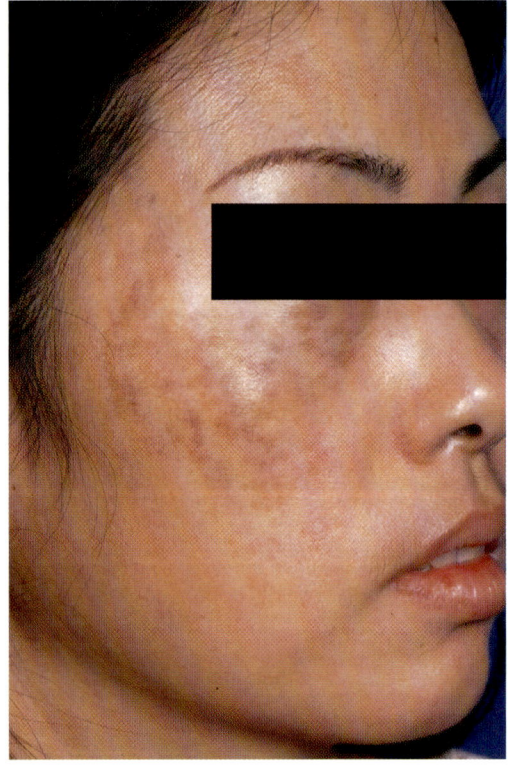

FIGURE 16.20 Dermal melasma. (Courtesy of National Skin Centre, Singapore.)

or in the upper dermis will not be accentuated by Wood's light. This has resulted in the classification of melasma into "epidermal" and "dermal" types in which accentuation of pigmentation is seen in the former and is absent in the latter (Figures 16.19 and 16.20). Some patients have a "mixed" pattern of melasma in which epidermal and dermal melasma is observed on different areas of the skin (Figure 16.21). Fitzpatrick[87] does not believe in the existence of dermal melasma, as he postulated that melasma in dark skin cannot be accentuated by Wood's light. Dermal melasma has not been observed in patients with skin types I and II. We noticed a significant difference in the

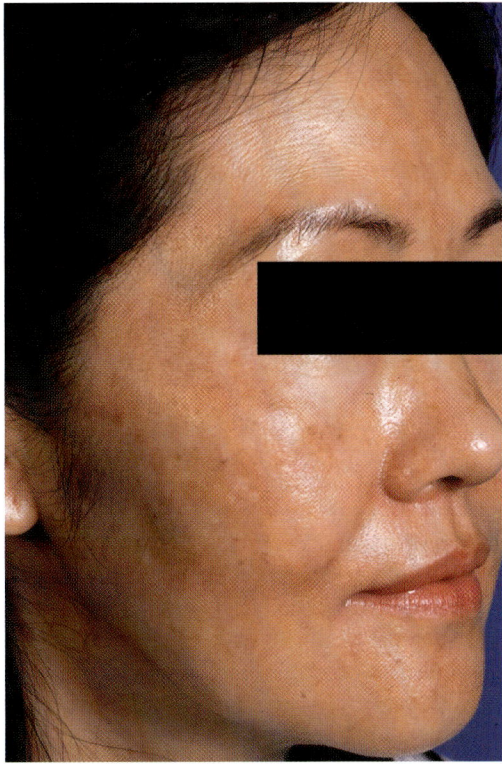

FIGURE 16.21 Mixed epidermal and dermal melasma. (Courtesy of National Skin Centre, Singapore.)

type of pigmentation using Wood's light. Clinically, there were definite features to suggest deep-seated epidermal or upper-dermal pigmentation (melanophages) in some of our patients with dermal melasma.

Histology

The epidermis and dermis are unremarkable except for an increase in melanin in keratinocytes, dermis, or, most commonly, both locations. Epidermal melanin is found in keratinocytes in the basal and suprabasal area. In most cases there is no increased number of melanocytes, but the melanocytes may appear slightly larger and more dendritic. Dermal melanin is found in the superficial and mid-dermis within macrophages, which often congregate around small, dilated vessels. Inflammation is sparse or absent.

Pathophysiology

Multiple causative factors have been implicated in the etiology of melasma, including ultraviolet light (sunlight), hormones (oral contraceptives), pregnancy, and genetic predisposition. In a report from Singapore,[89] of the 205 patients with melasma, 55 (26.8%) reported sun exposure, 25 (12.1%) reported pregnancy, and 27 (13.1%) reported oral contraceptives as precipitating factors. A positive family history of melasma was observed in 21 (10.2%) patients. Our figures were lower than those reported earlier.[90] There appears to be an increase in the number and activity of melanocytes in the epidermis in patients with melasma. The melanocytes appear to be functionally altered.[88] Pathak reported that oral contraceptive use is not the primary cause of melasma. He reported that only 20% of his melasma patients gave a history of infrequent use of oral contraceptives.[91] In a report from Thailand, 34% of women with melasma had taken oral contraceptives, but about half of them had melasma before they started taking oral contraceptive pills.[86] It would appear that contraceptive pills or even pregnancy may not be a significant contributing factor in melasma.

A report from Thailand[86] indicated that 72% of the patients studied reported sunlight aggravating their melasma. Pathak reported that sunlight exacerbated all melasma.[91]

A positive family history is observed in only 10.2% of our patients. This low rate is surprising, as genetic predisposition is considered to be an important factor in melasma. Melasma has been reported to be more prevalent in Asians than Caucasians.[85,88] Most of our patients with melasma were of skin types III and IV. This was also a reflection of the predominant skin types in Singapore. The high prevalence of patients with type III and IV skin in our study was not a reflection of a higher prevalence of melasma in dark-skinned individuals in our study. Fitzpatrick reported that melasma is a common problem in dark skin types, in particular types V and VI. Familial occurrence of melasma has been reported to vary from 20% to 70% in other studies.[90–92]

Therapy

Sunscreen in combination with topical bleaching cream forms the backbone in the treatment of melasma. It appears that epidermal-type melasma responds slightly better to treatment than dermal-type melasma. Our study indicated that half of our patients responded to treatment, although the majority improved only slightly. About half of our patients' melasma remained stable while on treatment.

However, response to treatment of melasma is generally unsatisfactory. Our findings indicated that some patients do benefit from the treatment although to a very limited extent. In a report from Singapore, 22% experienced reduction of pigmentation by more than 25% of baseline. Our findings indicate that patients with epidermal-type melasma responded marginally better than those with dermal-type.

Hydroquinone 2%–5% has been used in the treatment of melasma for many years.[93] A recent report indicated that epidermal-type melasma does respond well to topical hydroquinone. Improvements were observed in up to 70%–90% of treated patients.[94] Improvements have also been observed in using low-potency topical steroids, e.g., hydrocortisone 1% cream.[94]

Topical tretinoins at concentrations of 0.05% and 0.1% were reported to significantly reduce hyperpigmentation.[94,95] Griffiths et al. reported that 13 of 19 patients with melasma treated with 0.1% tretinoin improved, compared with 1 of 24 treated with the vehicle.[96] Improvements were not evident until the 24th week of treatment. Azelaic acid 20% cream used in the treatment of melasma has been reported to show a good response, with the majority of patients responding to treatment.[97–99]

Kligman and Willis proposed a combination of hydroquinone 5% with tretinoin 0.1% and dexamethasone 0.1% for the treatment of melasma and reported a good response to the combination treatment.[100] Pathak et al. obtained improvement with a formulation that did not include corticosteroids.[101] Sanchez et al. also reported improvement with combination hydroquinone 2% with retinoic acid 0.05%–0.1% without corticosteroids.[88] Various other combination regimens that have reported a good response include one containing hydroquinone 2% and tretinoin 0.05% or 0.1% in patients with epidermal melasma (in addition to sunscreens)[102] and another with a combination of tretinoin 0.05%, betamethasone valerate 0.1%, and hydroquinone 2% (65% improved).[102] A new cream consisting of the combination of fluocinolone (0.01%), hydroquinone (4%), and tretinoin (0.05%) has also been recently released in the United States. There are several new procedures including chemical peels, fruit acids, and various medications claiming to be effective, but they lack evidence-based scientific confirmation.

MONGOLIAN SPOT

Introduction and Clinical Manifestations

Mongolian spot is a congenital, blue-gray macular lesion commonly observed among Asian infants. It is generally located on the lumbosacral skin or on the buttocks (Figure 16.22). Aberrant Mongolian

Dermatologic Disease in Asians

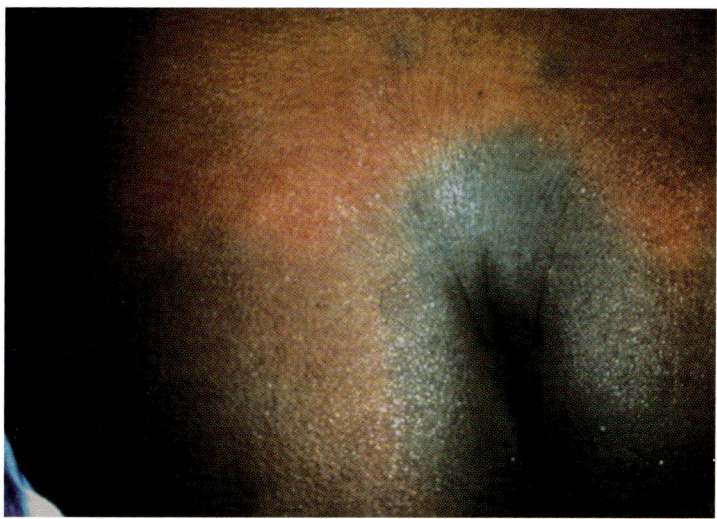

FIGURE 16.22 Mongolian spot in a 6-month-old boy.

spots refer to lesions that are present outside the lumbosacral area. Mongolian spot is often present at birth and usually disappears during childhood, although rarely it may persist into adulthood. The persistence of Mongolian spots into adult life was reported to occur in 4.6% of young Japanese adults.[103] No melanomas have been reported to occur in these lesions.

Histology

The diagnosis is based on the clinical morphology and, when in doubt, is confirmed by histopathologic examination of lesions. Histologically, Mongolian spot shows elongated melanocytes located deep in the dermis.

Pathophysiology

Melanocytes are not normally present in the dermis, and it is believed that these ectopic melanocytes represent pigment cells that have been interrupted in their migration from the neural crest to the epidermis.

Therapy

The parents may be reassured that the Mongolian spots usually disappear spontaneously during childhood.

NEVUS OF OTA AND NEVUS OF ITO

Introduction

Nevus of Ota and nevus of Ito are hamartomas of dermal melanocytes.

Incidence/Prevalence

The nevus of Ota is most commonly seen in Asians. It is said to occur in up to 0.8% of dermatological outpatients in Japan. It has also been reported in Chinese, East Indians, blacks, and, rarely, whites. Women are affected five times as frequently as men.

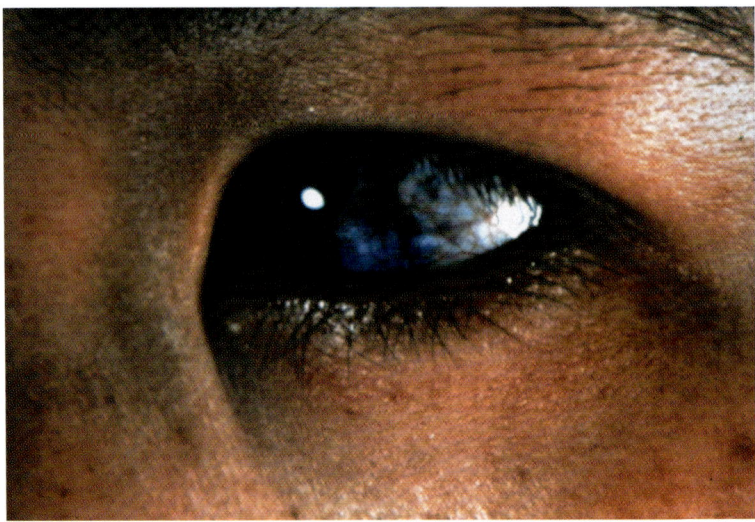

FIGURE 16.23 Bluish discoloration of the sclera. (Courtesy of Xue-Jun Zhu, M.D., Peking University, Beijing, China.)

Clinical Manifestations

The nevus of Ota, first described by Ota in 1939, is characterized by unilateral, irregularly patchy, bluish-gray discoloration of the skin of the face supplied by the first and second divisions of the trigeminal nerve, particularly the periorbital region, temple, forehead, malar area, and nose. Mucosa, conjunctivae, sclerae, and tympanic membranes may be involved (Figure 16.23). In about 5% of the cases, the nevus of Ota is bilateral.

Approximately 50% of lesions are congenital; the remainder generally appear during the second decade of life. Rarely the onset is later and may be associated with pregnancy. Unlike Mongolian spots, which tend to disappear with time, the nevus of Ota generally persists. Enlargement and darkening may be observed over time. Melanoma has been rarely reported in these lesions.

The nevus of Ito, first described by Ito in 1954, has the same features as the nevus of Ota except that the pigmentary changes occur in the distribution of the posterior supraclavicular and lateral cutaneous brachial nerves, involving the shoulder, supraclavicular areas, sides of the neck, upper arm, and scapular and deltoid regions. It may occur alone or be seen in conjunction with the nevus of Ota.

Histology

Histopathologic features of nevus of Ota and nevus of Ito show, similarly to Mongolian spots, elongated dendritic melanocytes scattered throughout the dermis. The melanocytes, however, frequently appear to be situated somewhat higher in the dermis than those seen in ordinary Mongolian spots.

Therapy

Selective photothermolysis with the Q-switched ruby laser is a safe and effective treatment. Multiple treatments increase the response rate. Watanabe and Takahasi[104] found that of the 35 patients who received four or five treatments, 33 had an excellent response (lightening of 70% of more).

Nonmelanoma Skin Cancer

Introduction

Nonmelanoma skin cancers include basal cell carcinoma (BCC), squamous cell carcinoma (SCC), and SCC *in situ,* Bowen's disease.

Incidence/Prevalence

Skin cancer is relatively uncommon in Asians. The incidence rates of BCC, SCC, and Bowen's disease in the American-Japanese population in Kauai, Hawaii, are 12, 4, and 11 times lower, respectively, than Caucasian Kauaiian rates.[1] The anatomical sites of BCC and SCC in Japanese Kauaiians are primarily the head and neck. The extremities are the most common anatomical sites for Bowen's disease. There does not appear to be a significant difference in working environment and recreational activities between resident Japanese and Caucasians. Therefore, it has been suggested that the Japanese skin type confers relative protection from UV light damage.

The incidence rates of nonmelanoma skin cancer including BCC, SCC, and Bowen's disease are at least 45 times higher in the Japanese residents of Kauai, Hawaii, than rates for the Japanese population in Japan.[105] Kauai's more intense year-round UV radiation and emphasis on outdoor activities probably contribute to these differing rates.

Clinical Manifestations

Kikuchi et al.[106] retrospectively examined 243 Japanese patients with BCC from Tokyo, Japan. Clinically, approximately 75% of the tumors showed a brown to glossy black pigmentation. The high incidence of pigmented BCC is the most characteristic feature of BCC in Japanese patients and probably in other Asians as well (Figure 16.24). Other clinical and histopathological features of BCC in Japanese are comparable to those in other races. Bowen's disease is also frequently pigmented in Asians (Figure 16.25).

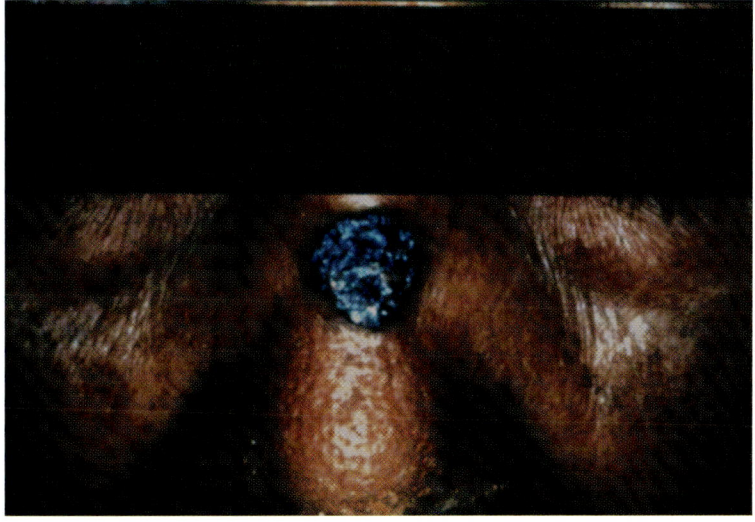

FIGURE 16.24 Pigmented basal cell carcinoma in a Thai man. (Courtesy of Krisada Duangurai, M.D., Pramongkutklao Hospital, Bangkok, Thailand.)

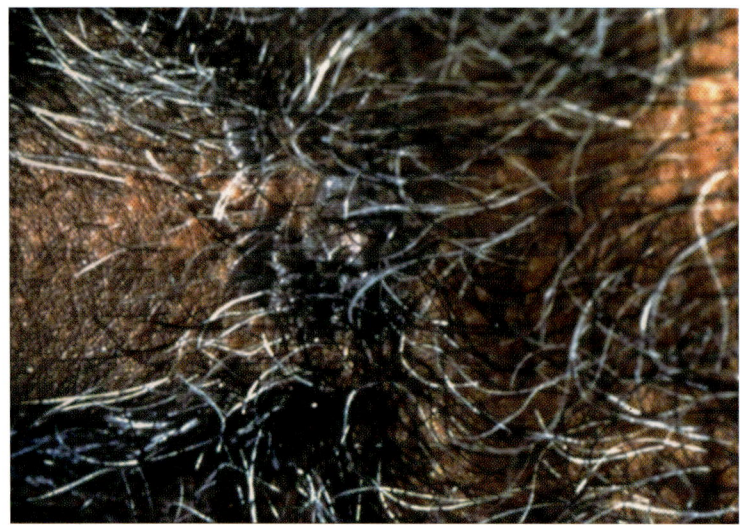

FIGURE 16.25 Pigmented Bowen's disease in suprapubic area of an Indian man.

Histology

BCCs are characterized histopathologically by the presence of basaloid tumor cells budding from epidermis or follicles, or within the dermis. SCCs are characterized histopathologically by the invasion of dermis by proliferation of atypical keratinocytes with hyperchromatism, pleomorphism, increased atypical mitoses, dyskeratosis, and loss of orderly maturation. Bowen's disease is SCC *in situ*.

Pathophysiology

Many etiological factors exist in the development of nonmelanoma skin cancers. Both SCC and BCC tend to occur more commonly in sun-exposed areas. The association of chronic sun exposure and SCC has been well established.[107] BCC has been found to be more likely to be associated with intermittent sun exposure.[108] In a study performed in Australia of 1383 subjects over a 4.5-year period, the use of sunscreen was found to decrease the incidence of SCC but not that of BCC.[109] Bowen's disease has been associated with arsenical exposure; it can occur in both sun-exposed and sun-protected areas.[110]

Therapy

Treatment is the same as that used in the non-Asian population. This includes curettage and electrodesiccation, excisional surgery, radiation, or Mohs micrographic surgery.

MELANOMA

Introduction

Melanoma among Asians differs in incidence, site distribution, stage at diagnosis, and histological type from melanoma among Caucasians.

Incidence/Prevalence

According to the California Cancer Registry 1988–1993,[111] incidence of cutaneous melanoma is highest among Caucasians, lowest among Asians and blacks, and intermediate among Hispanics.

The lower incidence of melanoma in Asians, blacks, and Hispanics most likely can be attributed to the protective effect of darker skin pigmentation.

Clinical Manifestations

In Asians, blacks, and Hispanics, melanoma was more likely to occur on the lower extremity, more likely to be acral lentiginous melanoma, and more likely to be diagnosed at a late stage when compared to Caucasians.[111] Acral melanoma is melanoma that occurs on the glabrous (hairless) skin of the palms of the hands, soles of the feet (Figure 16.26), fingers, toes, and nailbeds. Acral melanoma often is diagnosed at a later stage, with subsequently poorer survival than melanomas occurring on other sites.

Histology

Malignant melanomas are characterized histopathologically by asymmetrical proliferation of spindled or epithelioid melanocytes. Atypical melanocytes, often finely dusted with melanin, arise at the dermal/epidermal junction and invade the dermis.

Pathophysiology

Risk factors for melanoma among nonwhites have not been identified but are believed to be unrelated to sun exposure.[111] It has been suggested that acral melanomas may have an etiological agent other than direct sun exposure because acral melanomas occur with similar frequency at different latitudes and in different racial groups and because they occur on areas of the body usually protected from the sun by clothing and thick keratin.

At least among Caucasians, the risk of melanoma increases with increasing number of melanocytic nevi. The frequency of melanocytic nevi among nonwhite children and adults is substantially lower in comparison with whites.[2] Evaluation of pigmentation and solar-related factors in Asian children showed markedly different findings from Caucasians. In Asians, nevus density was not related to skin color or propensity to burn in the sun, and no association was seen with tanning and sunburn history.[112]

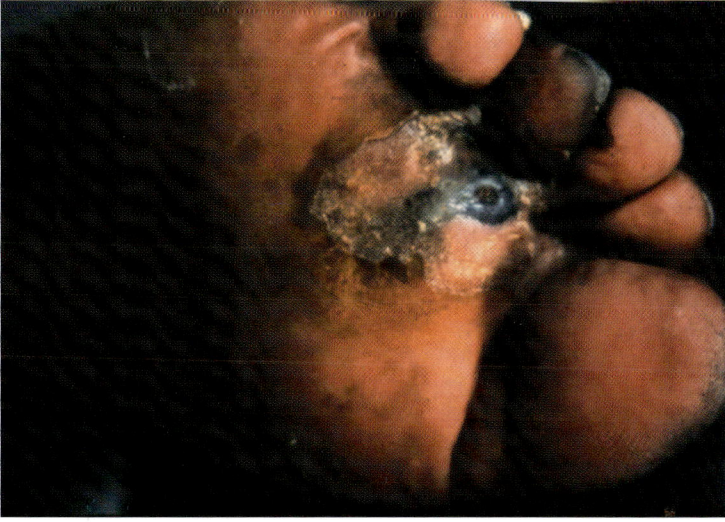

FIGURE 16.26 Acral lentiginous melanoma of the sole. (Courtesy of Xue-Jun Zhu, M.D., Peking University, Beijing, China.)

Therapy

Management of melanoma in Asians is similar to that in Caucasians. This includes surgery of the primary lesion, prognostic factors and staging, consideration of adjuvant therapy, and treatment of metastatic disease.

OFUJI'S DISEASE

Introduction

Ofuji's disease, or classic eosinophilic pustular folliculitis, was first described in Japan in 1970.[113] It is a rare inflammatory dermatosis characterized by recurrent crops of erythematous follicular papulopustules that coalesce to form annular plaques,[114] which occur mainly on the face, trunk, and extremities. The condition was first described in Japan and subsequently reported predominantly in Asians.

Incidence/Prevalence

Ofuji's disease has been reported mainly in Northern Asians, particularly in Japanese patients.[115,116] The peak incidence for onset of Ofuji's disease is between the third and fourth decades.[115,116] Most reports have reported a male preponderance, with a male-to-female ratio of approximately 5:1.[115,116] There is paucity of clinical data on Ofuji's disease in Southeast Asia. Cases have been reported from Thailand[117] as well as Singapore,[118] where it was observed that there was a marked predilection for the Chinese race.[118]

Clinical Manifestation

Erythematous patches with follicular papules and pustules characterize Ofuji's disease. The patches have a tendency toward central healing and peripheral extension (Figures 16.27–16.28).

Ofuji's disease has a chronic relapsing course, with periods of exacerbation and remission, but the patient is otherwise in good health. The disease is localized to the skin and is not associated with systemic manifestations. The skin lesion predominantly affects the seborrheic skin areas, namely the face (especially cheek areas) and extensor aspects of the upper arms and upper back.

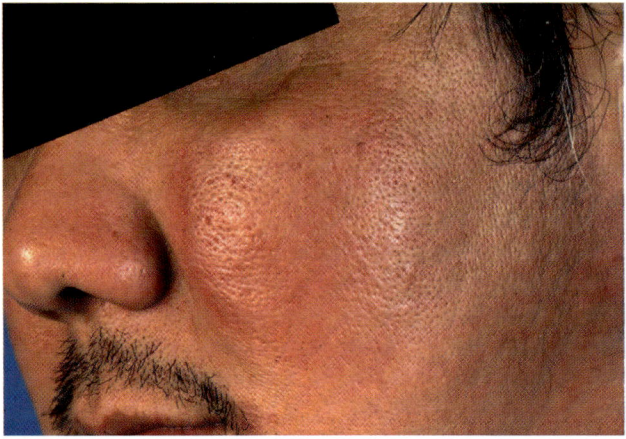

FIGURE 16.27 Ofuji's disease in a Chinese man. The cheeks are a common site of involvement. (Courtesy of National Skin Centre, Singapore.)

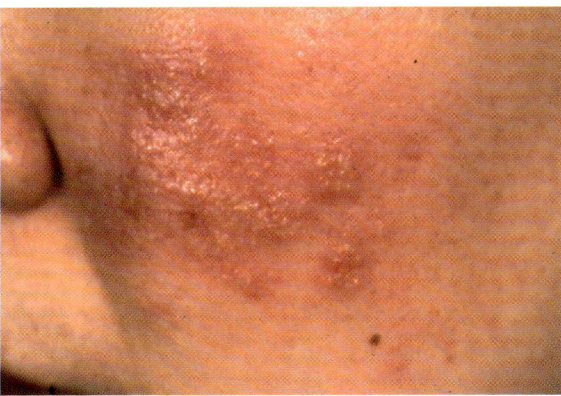

FIGURE 16.28 Ofuji's disease. Erythematous papules and pustules forming a plaque. (Courtesy of National Skin Centre, Singapore.)

Palmoplantar involvement may also be a presenting feature and has been reported in up to 20% of patients.[119] It is considered distinct from HIV-associated eosinophilic folliculitis[120] and pediatric eosinophilic pustular folliculitis.[121]

Patients may complain of pruritus[115] and mild peripheral blood eosinophilia may be present,[3] although this is not a constant feature.[118]

Histology

The key histological finding is the presence of a dense inflammatory infiltrate of eosinophils and mononuclear cells around the pilosebaceous unit.[122] Spongiotic degeneration and vesiculation of the outer root sheaths of the involved follicles may be seen in some cases. In addition, perivascular and dermal infiltrates of eosinophils and lymphocytes may be seen in the perifollicular areas.

Pathophysiology

The pathophysiology remains unclear. The condition is characterized by pilosebaceous follicular infiltrates with numerous eosinophils and some lymphocytes, but the pathomechanism of the accumulation of eosinophils and lymphocytes to pilosebaceous follicles is unknown.[123] It has been suggested that the efficacy of indomethacin in treating this condition is due to the reduction of the synthesis of an eosinophilic chemotactic factor by inhibition of cyclooxygenase activity.[124]

Treatment

Many therapeutic agents have been used to treat Ofuji's disease, including topical and oral corticosteroids,[115] minocycline,[125] isotretinoin,[126] ultraviolet B phototherapy,[127] interferon-gamma,[128] interferon-alpha,[129] and dapsone.[130] To date, the most effective agent used in the treatment of Ofuji's disease is oral indomethacin. Several case reports have described successful control of disease by oral indomethacin,[117,118,131] with one report giving a success rate of 92% of cases.[116] The effect of indomethacin can be remarkable, and this therapeutic response can distinguish Ofuji's disease from some of the conditions that it may resemble, such as acne vulgaris. Ketoprofen has also been used successfully,[118] as have topical piroxicam gel[117] and aspirin,[125] suggesting that the therapeutic efficacy may be a class effect for nonsteroidal anti-inflammatory drugs in general rather than restricted to indomethacin alone.

DERMATOSES OCCURRING IN ASIANS

VITILIGO

Introduction

Vitiligo is a depigmenting disorder characterized by loss of melanocytes from the epidermis, the mucous membranes, and other tissues.

Incidence/Prevalence

The incidence has been estimated to be 1%–2%. It affects both sexes equally. Although it can occur in all ethnic groups, the disease is much more noticeable in dark-skinned individuals, which has significant psychological impact and, in some cultures, social implications.

Clinical Manifestations

Typically, lesions of vitiligo are stark white with a well-demarcated border and no other skin changes. The sharp border of the lesions becomes apparent with Wood's light examination. Although vitiligo can affect any site, the face, joints, hands, and legs are most commonly affected. Follicular repigmentation frequently occurs as lesions respond to therapy (Figure 16.29).

Vitiligo has been reported to be associated with autoimmune disorders. Thyroid diseases (both hypothyroidism and hyperthyroidism as well as Graves' disease), diabetes mellitus, pernicious anemia, Addison's disease, multiglandular insufficiency syndrome, and alopecia areata may occur in patients with vitiligo. Family history is a factor in up to 30% of patients.

Histology

Vitiligo is caused by a loss of melanin from the epidermis, coupled with a decrease in the numbers of melanocytes in affected areas.

Pathophysiology

The etiology of vitiligo is unknown. Current hypotheses for the pathogenesis of vitiligo have been classified into two broad categories that include intrinsic melanocyte dysfunction and/or death and autoimmune-mediated destruction.[132]

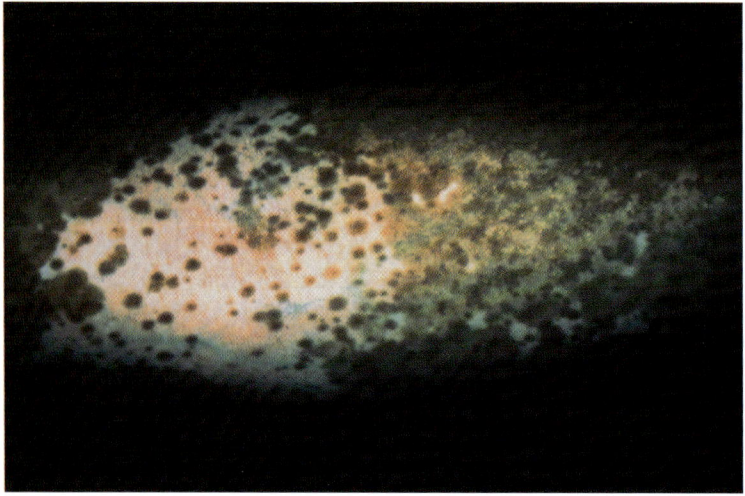

FIGURE 16.29 Vitiligo with follicular repigmentation.

Therapy

Although therapy for vitiligo is still unsatisfactory, several new treatment modalities have been described in the past few years.[133] Topical corticosteroids, topical tacrolimus ointment (Protopic),[134] phototherapy with narrow-band UVB,[135] photochemotherapy (PUVA), and combination of topical calcipotriene (Dovonex) with PUVA[136,137] or with narrow-band UVB phototherapy[138] have been shown to be effective in some patients. For patients with extensive depigmentation that involves more than half of the total body surface area, permanent depigmentation of the pigmented skin with monobenzylether of hydroquinone may be considered. All patients with vitiligo should use sunscreens to protect depigmented skin from sun damage. In addition, patients may choose to use makeup, dyes, and self-tanners (containing dihydroxyacetone) to cover the lesions. Makeup, applied properly, offers the best cosmesis, albeit a temporary one. Dyes and self-tanners usually produce less than satisfactory results.

CHRONIC ACTINIC DERMATITIS

Introduction

Chronic actinic dermatitis (CAD) encompasses entities previously described under other terminologies: actinic reticuloid, photosensitive eczema, photosensitivity dermatitis, and persistent light reactivity. The basic components of this disease are (1) a chronic, eczematous eruption on sun-exposed skin in the absence of exposure to known photosensitizers; (2) decreased minimal erythema dose to UVA, and/or UVB (required by some authors), and/or visible light; and (3) histology consistent with a chronic dermatitis with or without features of lymphoma.[139]

Incidence/Prevalence

Although CAD was initially reported to occur primarily in elderly white men, it is now clear that it can occur in all ethnic groups. CAD was the final diagnosis in 17% of patients evaluated in a photodermatology clinic in New York City[140] and in 5% of patients evaluated in Singapore.[141]

Clinical Manifestations

Clinically, the disease affects middle-aged or elderly men predominantly. Although the disease was initially reported to occur in white men, it has now been reported in all ethnic groups, including African-Americans and Asians.[139,142] Skin lesions consist of edematous, scaling, thickened patches and plaques that tend to be confluent. Lesions occur primarily or most severely on the exposed skin and may spare the upper eyelids, behind the ears, and skin folds (Figure 16.30). Involvement of unexposed sites may occurs.

The diagnosis of CAD is established by clinical and histological evaluations and phototesting. Phototesting results in abnormal response. A positive patch test to Compositae oleoresin extracts is strongly associated the United States with the disease in patients evaluated in Scotland,[143] less so in those in the United Kingdom,[143] and not associated in tested patients in the United States and Japan.

Histology

The histological changes vary with the severity of the disease and are consistent with a spongiotic dermatitis with superficial dermal perivascular lymphohistiocytic infiltrates. In some, atypical mononuclear cells may be present in the dermis and the epidermis.

Therapy

The treatment for CAD is difficult. Sun avoidance and broad-spectrum sunscreens are essential. Avoidance of relevant associated contact allergens or photocontact allergens is of equal importance.

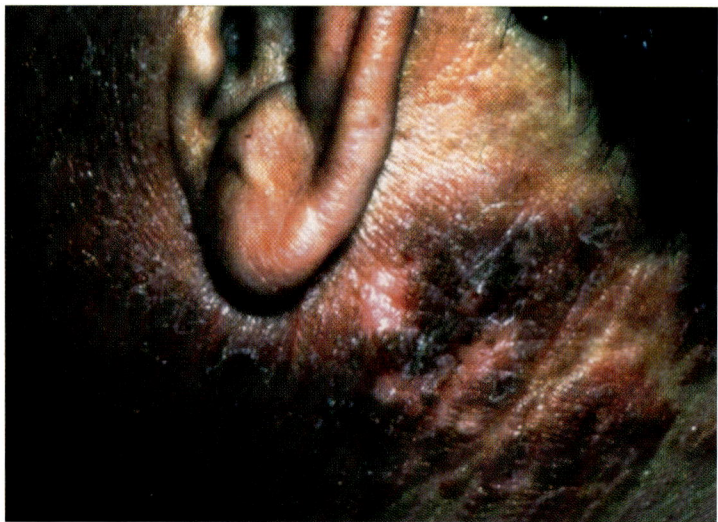

FIGURE 16.30 Lichenification, hyper- and hypopigmentation of sun-exposed area in an Asian man with chronic actinic dermatitis.

Topical corticosteroids are useful, especially in winter months when the disease activity is low. Preliminary open trials suggest that tacrolimus ointment (protopic) may be helpful in the treatment of CAD.[145] In many patients, it is necessary to use one or more of the following modalities: azathioprine, cyclosporine, systemic corticosteroids, PUVA, mycophenolate mofetil, and hydroxychloroquine.[139,146]

Erythropoietic Protoporphyria

Introduction

Erythropoietic protoporphyria (EPP) is an inherited disorder of porphyrin–heme metabolism with cutaneous and systemic manifestations arising from mutations of the ferrochelatase gene, resulting in an elevated level of protoporphyrin, a lipophilic, phototoxic precursor of heme.[147]

Incidence/Prevalence

EPP has been reported most often in whites but also has been observed in individuals of Asian, East Indian, and African origin.

Clinical Manifestations

EPP typically presents early in childhood (2–5 years of age), but presentation late in adulthood may occur. Patients usually complain of an immediate burning and stinging of the exposed skin following sun exposure. Infants cry when exposed to sunlight. Erythema, edema, urticarial lesions, and purpura may then develop; vesicles and scarring, although uncommon, may also occur. These lesions appear solely on sun-exposed areas, particularly on the nose, cheeks, and dorsal hands. With time, these areas develop atrophic, waxy scars. The skin over the knuckles may become thickened, wrinkled, and shiny, giving the appearance of aged hands (Figure 16.31).

EPP patients may have mildly elevated liver function tests. Cholelithiasis occurs in 10% of the patients, and hepatic failure occurs in 5%. A mild microcytic anemia is present in 25% of patients with EPP, but therapy with iron should be used only if iron deficiency is detected, because it may exacerbate symptoms.

Dermatologic Disease in Asians

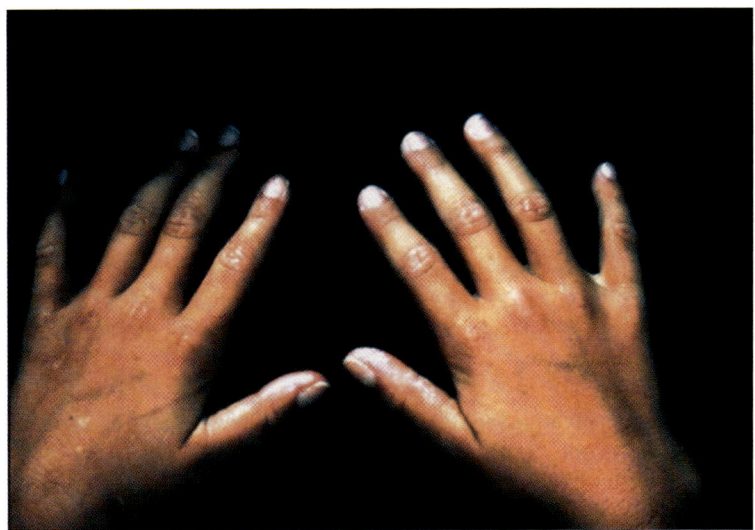

FIGURE 16.31 Waxy thickening of knuckles of a patient with EPP.

A diagnosis of EPP can usually be suspected on clinical grounds, especially if both the acute symptoms and chronic skin changes are found. The diagnosis is confirmed by finding elevated protoporphyrin levels in erythrocytes and plasma. Urinary porphyrin levels are normal.

Histology

Histologically, there is prominent ground glass, PAS-positive material in the upper dermis mostly perivascularly. On direct immunofluorescence, IgG and C3 may be found perivascularly and at the dermal epidermal junction.

Pathophysiology

EPP is a genodermatosis arising from mutations of the ferrochelatase gene, resulting in enzyme activity of only 30% of normal. A three-allele model of inheritance has been proposed, requiring the presence of a mutant allele and low-output "normal" allele for symptomatic expression of the disease.[148] More than 60 mutations of gene-encoding ferrochelatase have been reported.[149] Protoporphyrin, the substrate of ferrochelatase, becomes elevated. Phototoxicity occurs when protoporphyrin is exposed to its action spectra, the Soret band (400–410 nm).

Therapy

Therapy is primarily preventive, aimed at protecting the skin from ultraviolet and visible radiation with clothing and barrier sunscreens with titanium dioxide or zinc oxide. Beta carotene (Lumitene®), 30–300 mg daily, to maintain a serum level from 600 to 800 µg/100 ml, may be helpful.

DERMATOSES SECONDARY TO ASIAN CULTURAL MEDICAL PRACTICE

Introduction

Chinese medicine teaches that health is a state of spiritual and physical harmony with nature. The Asians believe that a healthy body is in a state of balance. Illness occurs when the balance is disrupted. Asians believe a balance is between "yin" and "yang." All things in the universe are primarily either yin or yang, including diseases, which may result from excess yin or yang, deficient yin, or deficient yang. Yin and yang are generally translated as hot (yang) and cold (yin); these refer to qualities, not temperatures.

The multiracial and multiethnic makeup of the Asian population accompanies various cultural beliefs and medical practices for treating diseases and the imbalance in "yin" and "yang." Some of these cultural medical procedures may cause bizarre dermatological signs that can baffle dermatologists and family practitioners managing their patients. It is therefore useful for practitioners to be familiar with some of the skin signs that result from some of these cultural medical procedures.

Coin rubbing

Coin rubbing ("Cao Gio" or Kuasha) is an ancient Vietnamese folk remedy that is practiced by many Southeast Asian ethnic groups. Coin rubbing is a dermabrasive therapy used to relieve symptoms in a variety of illnesses. This traditional health practice is said to release excess "wind" or energy considered responsible for illness. The skin is first lubricated with medical oils or balms and subsequently rubbed firmly and vigorously using the edge of a coin to produce parallel ecchymoses on the chest and the back. This procedure often generates skin eruptions in a pine-tree pattern, with two long vertical marks along either side of the spine and several lines paralleling the ribs (Figure 16.32). It is used to alleviate common symptoms of illness such as nausea, loss of appetite, headache, dizziness, and muscle aches. The back, neck, head, shoulder, and chest are common areas where the procedure is applied.[150–153]

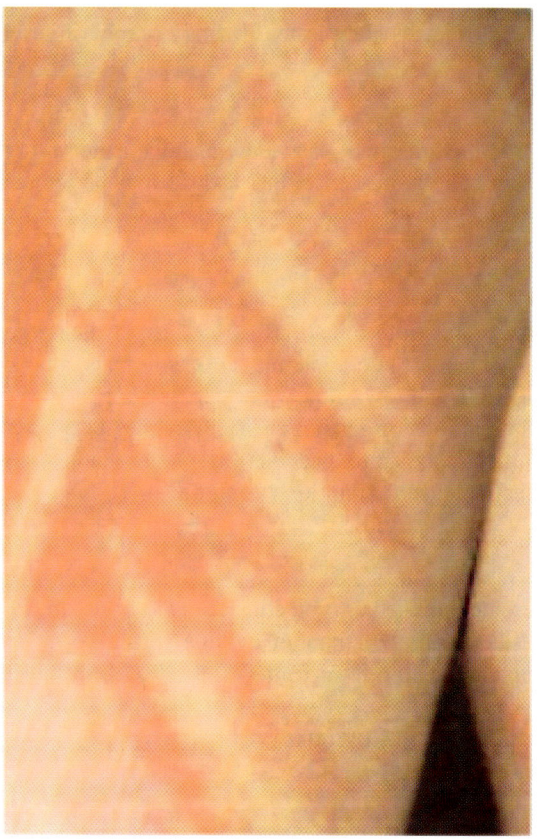

FIGURE 16.32 Coin rubbing. Linear streaky erythema. (Reproduced from *JAMA* 2002; 288: 45. With permission.)

There are few reported cases of serious complications from coin rubbing. Most of the complications have been minor frictional burns, but severe burns have also been reported.[154] To the untrained eyes, such skin signs may be mistaken for child abuse and torture.[155] Other common dermatological signs from coin rubbing include erythema, welts, and bruising. This practice may aggravate dermographism in persons with physical urticarias. There may be irritant or allergic contact dermatitis from ointment used preceding the coin-rubbing procedure.

Cupping

Cupping is a therapeutic procedure used by Traditional Chinese Medicine (TCM) practitioners in which a suction jar is attached to the skin surface to cause local congestion through a negative pressure. Suction is created by introducing heat into the jar. There is a variety of jars used, but they are usually made of bamboo or glass material. Cupping is frequently used as an auxiliary method of acupuncture and moxibustion.

The practitioner may apply one of two methods to induce suction.[156] The "fire throwing method" involves throwing a piece of ignited paper or an alcohol-soaked cotton ball into the cup, then rapidly placing the mouth of the cup firmly against the skin on the desired location. The burning flame creates a vacuum in the cup upon cooling. This method is applied to the lateral areas of the body to prevent the burning paper or cotton ball from coming into contact with the skin. The "fire twinkling" method involves placing an alcohol-soaked cotton ball in the cup, igniting it, and then taking it out immediately. The cup is then placed in the selected position. Generally, the cup is sucked in place for 10 minutes. The skin becomes congested with violet-colored blood stasis formation.

The skin will show changes from the suction effects created by negative pressure. There are circular ecchymotic areas. Blisters may be induced (Figure 16.33). The treated area develops a bruise that resolves in a few days. Bruising and purpura may be more severe in patients who have an underlying coagulation or platelet defect or in those on warfarin or with corticosteroid-induced cutaneous atrophy. Burns may be induced,[157] and the skin signs of treatment may be mistaken for child abuse[158] and other nonaccidental trauma.[159]

Moxibustion

Moxibustion is a method in TCM that treats and prevents diseases by applying heat to certain locations of the human anatomy. The material used is the herb *Artemesia vulgaris*, or wormwood, also known as "moxa-wool."[155] This is usually in the form of a cone or stick. The material is burned at specified points on or near the skin. Another variation of the technique involves transmitting the heat from the burning moxa indirectly onto the skin via acupuncture needles.

Treated areas of the skin will show erythema, and in more severe cases, different degrees of burns may occur.[156] Blistering may be induced, and there is a possibility of secondary infection and scarring.[157]

SUMMARY

In this chapter, common skin disorders in Asians are discussed along with the less common dermatoses that are usually seen in Asians, including Mongolian spot, nevus of Ota, nevus of Ito, primary cutaneous amyloidosis, pigmented basal cell carcinoma and Bowen's disease, acrolentigenous melanoma, and Ofuji's disease. Special considerations are given to dermatoses secondary to cultural practices such as coin rubbing, cupping, and moxibustion. Awareness of these dermatological disorders can be helpful, especially for clinicians who work in areas with a large Asian population.

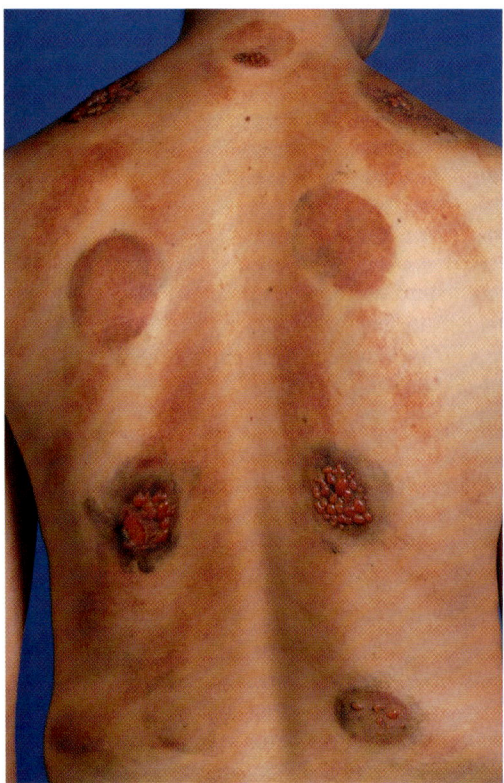

FIGURE 16.33 Cupping. Note circular purpuric blistering patches from suction effects of suction cup. (Courtesy of National Skin Centre, Singapore.)

REFERENCES

1. U.S. Census Bureau, Census 2000.
2. Kraning KK. Prevalence, morbidity, and cost of dermatological disease. *J Invest Dermatol* 1979; 73: 395–401.
3. White GM. Recent findings in the epidemiologic evidence, classification, and subtypes of acne vulgaris. *J Am Acad Dermatol* 1998; 39(3 pt 2): S34–S37.
4. Ng PPL, Goh CL. Treatment outcome of acne vulgaris with oral isotreinoin in 89 patients. *Int J Dermatol* 1999; 38: 207–216.
5. Thiboutot D. Acne: 1991–2001. *J Am Acad Dermatol* 2002; 47(1): 109–117.
6. Brown SK, Shalita AR. Acne vulgaris. *Lancet* 1998; 351: 1871–1876.
7. Shalita AR, Lee WL. Inflammatory acne. *Dermatol Clin* 1983; 1: 361–364.
8. Eady EA. Bacterial resistance in acne. *Dermatology* 1998; 196: 59–66.
9. Crawford WW, Crawford IP, Stoughton RB, et al. Laboratory induction and clinical occurrence of combined clindamycin and erythromycin resistance in *Corynebacterium acnes*. *J Invest Dermatol* 1979; 72: 187–190.
10. Ross JI, Snelling AM, Eady EA, et al. Phenotypic and genotypic characterization of antibiotic-resistant Propionibacterium acnes isolated from acne patients attending dermatology clinics in Europe, the USA, Japan and Australia. *Dermatology* 2001; 144: 339–346.
11. Tan HH, Goh CL, Yeo MGC, Tan ML. Antibiotic sensitivity of Propionibacterium acnes isolates from patients with acne vulgaris in a tertiary dermatological referral centre in Singapore. *Ann Acad Med Singapore* 2001; 30: 22–25.

12. Mar A, Tam M, Jolley D, et al. The cumulative incidence of atopic dermatitis in the first 12 months among Chinese, Vietnamese, and Caucasian infants born in Melbourne, Australia. *J Am Acad Dermatol* 1999; 40(4): 597–602.
13. Worth R. Atopic dermatitis among Chinese infants in Honolulu and San Francisco. *Hawaii Med J* 1962; 22(1): 31–34.
14. Sladden M, Dure-Smith B, Berth-Jones J, et al. Ethnic differences in the pattern of skin disease seen in a dermatology department. *Clin Exp Dermatol* 1991; 16(5): 348–349.
15. George S, Berth-Jones J, Graham-Brown R. A possible explanation for the increased referral of atopic dermatitis from the Asian community in Leicester. *Br J Dermatol* 1997; 136: 494–497.
16. Goh CL, Chua-Ty C, Koh SL. A descriptive profile of eczema in a tertiary dermatological referral centre in Singapore. *Ann Acad Med Singapore* 1993; 22: 307–315.
17. Ng SK. Topical traditional Chinese medicine. A report from Singapore. *Arch Dermatol* 1998; 134: 1395–1396.
18. Lee TY, Lam TH. Patch testing of 490 patients in Hong Kong. *Contact Dermatitis* 1996; 35: 23–26.
19. Li LF. A clinical and patch test study of contact dermatitis from traditional Chinese medicinal materials. *Contact Dermatitis* 1995; 33: 392–395.
20. Lim JT, Goh CL, Ng SK, Wong WK. Changing trends in the epidemiology of contact dermatitis in Singapore. *Contact Dermatitis* 1992; 26: 321–326.
21. Goh CL. Contact sensitivity to topical medicaments. *Int J Dermatol* 1989; 28: 25–28.
22. Ng SK. Common environmental contact allergens in Singapore. *Singapore Med J* 1990; 31: 616–618.
23. Lee TY, Lam TH. Allergic contact dermatitis due to a Chinese orthopaedic solution tieh ta yao gin. *Contact Dermatitis* 1993; 28: 89–90.
24. Lee TY, Lam TH. Patch testing of 11 common herbal topical medicaments in Hong Kong. *Contact Dermatitis* 1990; 22(3): 137–140.
25. Lee TY, Lam TH. Irritant contact dermatitis due to a Chinese herbal medicine lu-shen-wan. *Contact Dermatitis* 1988; 18: 213–218.
26. Osmundsen PE. Pigmented contact dermatitis. *Br J Dermatol* 1970; 83: 296–301.
27. Hayakawa R, Matsunaga K, Kojima S, et al. Naphthol AS as a cause of pigmented contact dermatitis. *Contact Dermatitis* 1985; 13: 20–25.
28. Nakayama H, Matsuo S, Hayakawa K, et al. Pigmented cosmetic dermatitis. *Int J Dermatol* 1984; 23: 299–305.
29. Goh CL, Kozuka T. Pigmented contact dermatitis from "Kumkum." *Clin Exp Dermatol* 1986; 11: 603–606.
30. Nakayama H. Perfume allergy and cosmetic dermatitis. *Jpn J Dermatol* 1974; 84: 659–667.
31. Nakayama H, Harada R, Toda M. Pigmented cosmetic dermatitis 1976; 15: 673–675.
32. Birt AR, Davis RA. Birt photodermatitis in North American Indians: familial actinic prurigo. *Int J Dermatol* 1971; 10: 107–114.
33. Khoo SW, Tay YK, Than SN. Photodermatoses in a Singapore skin referral centre. *Clin Exp Dermatol* 1996; 21: 263–268.
34. Aoki T, Fujita M. Actinic prurigo: a case report with successful induction of skin lesions. *Clin Exp Dermatol* 1980; 5: 47–52.
35. Lestarini D, Khoo SW, Goh CL. The clinical features and management of actinic prurigo: a retrospective study. *Photodermatol Photoimmunol Photomed* 1999; 15: 183–187.
36. Teraki Y, Shiohara T, Nagashima M, et al. Prurigo pigmentosa: role of ICAM-1 in the localization of the eruption. *Br J Dermatol* 1991; 125: 360–363.
37. Liu M, Wong CK. Prurigo pigmentosa. *Dermatology* 1994; 188: 219–221.
38. Joyce AP, Horn TD, Anhalt GJ. Prurigo pigmentosa. Report of a case and review of the literature. *Arch Dermatol* 1989; 125: 1551–1554.
39. Gurses L, Gurbuz O, Demircay Z, Kotiloglu E. Prurigo pigmentosa. *Int J Dermatol* 1999; 38: 916–925.
40. Miyachi Y, Okamoto H, Furukawa F, Imamura S. Prurigo nodularis — a possible relationship to atopy. *J Dermatol* 1980; 7: 281–283.
41. Tanaka M, Aiba S, Matsumara N, Aoyama H, Tagami H. Prurigo nodularis consists of two distinct forms: early-onset atopic and late-onset non-atopic. *Dermatology* 1995; 190: 269–276.
42. Rowland Payne CME, Wilkinson JD, McKee PH, Jurecka W, Black MM. Nodular prurigo — a clinicopathological study of 46 patients. *Br J Dermatol* 1985; 113: 431–439.

43. Hojyo-Tomoka T, Vega-Memije E, Granados J, Flores O, Cortes-Franco R, Teixeira F, Dominguez-Soto L. Actinic prurigo: an update. *Int J Dermatol* 1995; 34: 380–384.
44. Matilla JO, Vornenen M, Katila M. Histopathological and bacteriological findings in prurigo nodularis. *Acta Derm Venereol (Stockh)* 1997; 77: 49–51.
45. McKenzie AW, Stubbing DG, Elvy BL. Prurigo nodularis and gluten enteropathy. *Br J Dermatol* 1976; 95: 89–92.
46. Rien BE, Lemont H, Cohen RS. Prurigo nodularis — an association with uremia. *J Am Podiatr Assoc* 1982; 72: 321–323.
47. Fina L, Grimalt R, Berti E, Caputo R. Nodular prurigo associated with Hodgkin's disease. *Dermatologica* 1991; 182: 243–246.
48. Zelickson BD, McEvoy MT, Fransway AF. Patch testing in prurigo nodularis. *Contact Dermatitis* 1989; 20: 321–325.
49. Murao K, Urona Y, Uchido N, et al. Prurigo pigmentosa associated with ketosis. *Br J Dermatol* 1996; 134: 379–380.
50. Cotterill JA, Ryatt KS, Greenwood R. Prurigo pigmentosa. *Br J Dermatol* 1981; 105: 707–710.
51. Tanii T, Kono T, Katoh J, et al. A case of prurigo pigmentosa considered to be allergic contact to chromium in an acupuncture needle. *Acta Derm Venereol* 1991; 71: 66–67.
52. Hawk JLM. Cutaneous photobiology. In: Champion RH, Burton JL, Ebling FJG, et al. (Eds) *Textbook of Dermatology*, 5th ed. Oxford: Blackwell Scientific Publications, 1992; 849–866.
53. Dawe RS, Collins P, Ferguson J, et al. Actinic prurigo and HLA-DR4. *J Invest Dermatol* 1997; 108: 233–234.
54. Bernal JE, Duran MM, Ordonez CP. Actinic prurigo among the Chimila Indians in Colombia: HLA study. *J Am Acad Dermatol* 1990; 22: 1049–1051.
55. Sheridan DP, Lane PR, Irvine J, et al. HLA typing in actinic prurigo. *J Am Acad Dermatol* 1990; 22: 1019–1023.
56. Koblenzer CS. Treatment of nodular prurigo with cyclosporin (treat the disease, not just the symptoms). *Br J Dermatol* 1996; 135(2): 330–331.
57. Berger TG, Hoffman C, Thieberg MD. Prurigo nodularis and photosensitivity in AIDS: treatment with thalidomide. *J Am Acad Dermatol* 1995; 33 (5 pt 1): 837–838.
58. Sugawara H, Indaba S, Iojiima S. Three cases of so-called prurigo pigmentosa. *Jpn J Dermatol* 1973; 83: 111–112.
59. Duran MM, Ordonez CP. Treatment of actinic prurigo in Chimila Indian. *Int J Dermatol* 1996; 35: 413–416.
60. Ferguson J, Ibbotson, S. The idiopathic photodermatoses. *Semin Cutan Med Surg* 1999; 18: 257–273.
61. Glenner GG. Amyloid deposits and amyloidosis. The β-fibrilloses. *N Engl J Med* 1980; 302: 1283.
62. Wong CK. Lichen amyloidosis: a relatively common skin disorder in Taiwan. *Arch Dermatol* 1974; 110: 438–440.
63. Tay CH, Foo J, Leong YO, et al. Lichen amyloidosis in Singapore. *Int J Dermatol* 1971; 10: 156–158.
64. Harahap M, Hutapea NO. Lichen amyloidosis in Indonesia. *Int J Dermatol* 1970; 9: 114–118.
65. Piamphongsant T, Sittapairoachana D. Primary cutaneous amyloidosis. *J Med Assoc Thai* 1976; 59: 435–439.
66. Tan T. Epidemiology of primary cutaneous amyloidosis in Southeast Asia. *Clin Dermatol* 1990; 8(2): 20–24.
67. Tan T, Lee CT, Cheong WK. Epidemiology of primary localized cutaneous amyloidosis in Singapore. A retrospective study of epidemiology of 265 cases. *Proc World Cong Dermatol* 1987; 945–950.
68. Kurban AK et al. Primary localized macular cutaneous amyloidosis: histochemistry and electron microscopy. *Br J Dermatol* 1971; 85: 52.
69. Wolf M, Tolmach JA. Macular amyloidosis. *Arch Dermatol* 1969; 99: 373.
70. Piamphongsant T, Kullavanijaya P. Diffuse biphasic amyloidosis. *Dermatologica* 1976; 153: 243–248.
71. Kitajima Y et al. Partial amino acid sequence of an amyloid fibril protein from nodular primary cutaneous amyloidosis showing homology to λ immunoglobulin light chain of variable subgroup III (A λ III). *J Invest Dermatol* 1990; 95: 301.
72. Ann CC et al. Nodular amyloidosis. *Clin Exp Dermatol* 1988; 13: 20.
73. Kumakiri M, Hashimoto K. Histogenesis of primary cutaneous localized amyloidosis: sequential change of epidermal keratinocytes to amyloid via filamentous degeneration. *J Invest Dermatol* 1979; 73: 150.

74. Rune U, Orfanos CE. Amyloid production by dermal fibroblasts. Electron microscopic studies on the origin of amyloid in various dermatoses and skin tumours. *Br J Dermatol* 1977; 97: 155.
75. Tay CH, Dacosta JL. Lichen amyloidosis: clinical study of 40 cases. *Br J Dermatol* 1970; 82: 129–136.
76. Khoo BP, Tay YK, Goh CL. Calcipotriol ointment vs. betamethasone 17-valerate ointment in the treatment of lichen amyloidosis. *Int J Dermatol* 1999; 38: 539–541.
77. Truhan AP, Garden JM, Roenigk HH. Nodular primary localized cutaneous amyloidosis: immunohistochemical evaluation and treatment with carbon dioxide laser. *J Am Acad Dermatol* 1986; 14: 1058–1062.
78. Wong CK, Li WM. Dermabrasion for lichen amyloidosis: report of a long-term study. *Arch Dermatol* 1982; 118: 302–304.
79. Ozkaya BE, Baykal C, Kavak A. Local DMSO treatment of macular and papular amyloidosis. *Hautarzt* 1997; 48: 31–37.
80. Pandhi R, Kaur I, Kumar B. Lack of effect of dimethyl sulfoxide in cutaneous amyloidosis. *J Dermatol Treat* 2002; 13(1): 11–14.
81. Marschalko M, Daroczy J, Soos G. Etretinate for the treatment of lichen amyloidosis. *Arch Dermatol* 1988; 124: 657–659.
82. Hernandez-Nunez A, Dander E, Moreno de Vega MJ, Fraya J, Aragones M, Garcia-Diaz A. Widespread biphasic amyloidosis: response to acitretin. *Clin Exp Dermatol* 2001; 26(13): 256–259.
83. Hudson LD. Macular amyloidosis: treatment with ultraviolet B. *Cutis* 1986; 38: 61–62.
84. Goon ATJ, Ang P, Khoo LSW, Goh CL. Comparative study of phototherapy (UVB) vs. photochemotherapy (PUVA) vs. topical steroids in the treatment of primary cutaneous lichen amyloidosis. *Photodermatol Photoimmunol Photomed* 2001; 17: 42–43.
85. Jimbow M, Jimbow K. Pigmentary disorders in Oriental skin. *Clin Dermatol* 1989; 7: 11–27.
86. Sivayathorn A. Melasma in Orientals. *Clin Drug Invest* 1995; 10:(Suppl 2): 24–40.
87. Fitzpatrick TB. Pathophysiology of hypermelanosis. *Clin Drug Invest* 1995; 10 (suppl 2): 17–26.
88. Sanchez N, Pathak MA, Sato S et al. Melasma: a clinical, light microscopic, ultrastructural and immunofluorescence study. *J Am Acad Dermatol* 1981; 4: 698–710.
89. Annual Report 1996, National Skin Centre, Singapore.
90. Resnik S. Melasma induced by oral contraceptive drug. *JAMA* 1967; 199: 601–605.
91. Pathak MA. Clinical and therapeutic aspects of melasma: an overview. In: Fitzpatrick TB, Wick MM, Toda K (Eds) *Brown Melanoderma*. Tokyo: University of Tokyo Press, 1986; 161–172.
92. Vazquez M, Maldonado H, Benmaman C, et al. Melasma in men, a clinical and histologic study. *Int J Dermatol* 1988; 27: 25–27.
93. Arndt KA, Fitzpatrick TB. Topical use of hydroquinone as a depigmenting agent. *JAMA* 1965; 194: 965–967.
94. Ortonne JP, Bose SK. Pigmentation: dyscromia. In: Baron R, Maibach HI (Eds) *Cosmetic Dermatology*. London: Dunitz, 1994; 278–298.
95. Weinstein GD, Nigra TP, Pochi PE, et al. Topical tretinoin for treatment of photodamaged skin. *Arch Dermatol* 1991; 127: 660–665.
96. Griffiths CEM, Finkel LJ, Titre CM, et al. Topical tretinoin (retinoic acid) improves melasma. A vehicle controlled, clinical trial. *Br J Dermatol* 1993; 129: 415–421.
97. Nazzaro-Porro M. The use of azelaic acid in hyperpigmentation. *Rev Contemp Pharmacother* 1993; 4: 415–423.
98. Verallo-Rowell VM, Verallo V, Graupe K, et al. Double-blind comparison of azelaic acid and hydroquinone in the treatment of melasma. *Acta Derm Venereol (Suppl) (Stockh)* 1989; 143: 58–61.
99. Balina LM, Graupe K. The treatment of melasma — 20% azelaic acid versus 4% hydroquinone cream. *Int J Dermatol* 1991; 300: 893–895.
100. Kligman AM, Willis IA. New formula for depigmenting human skin. *Arch Dermatol* 1975; 11: 40–43.
101. Pathak MA, Fitzpatrick TB, Kraus EW. Usefulness of retinoic acid in the treatment of melasma. *J Am Acad Dermatol* 1986; 15: 894–899.
102. Haas AA, Arndt KA. Selected therapeutic applications of topical tretinoin. *J Am Acad Dermatol* 1986; 15: 870–877.
103. Hidano A. Persistent Mongolian spot in the adult. *Arch Dermatol* 1971; 103: 680–681.
104. Watanabe S, Takahashi H. Treatment of nevus of Ota with the Q-switch ruby laser. *N Engl J Med* 1994; 331: 1745.

105. Chuang T, Reizner G, Elpern D, et al. Nonmelanoma skin cancer in Japanese ethnic Hawaiians in Kauai, Hawaii: an incidence report. *J Am Acad Dermatol* 1995; 33: 422–426.
106. Kikuchi A, Shimizu H, Nishikawa T. Clinical histopathological characteristics of basal cell carcinoma in Japanese patients. *Arch Dermatol* 1996; 132(3): 320–324.
107. Franceschi S, Levi F, Randimbison L, La Vecchai C. Site distribution of different types of skin cancer: new aetiological clues. *Int J Cancer* 1996; 67(1): 24–28.
108. Kricker A, Armstrong BK, English DR, Heenan PJ. Does intermittent sun exposure cause basal cell carcinoma? A case-control study in Western Australia. *Int J Cancer* 1995; 60(4): 489–494.
109. Green A, Williams G, Neale R, et al. Daily sunscreen application and betacarotene supplementation in prevention of basal-cell and squamous-cell carcinomas of the skin: a randomized controlled trial. *Lancet* 1999; 354(9180): 723–729.
110. Thestrup-Pedersen K, Ravnborg L, Reymann F. Morbus bowen. A description of the disease in 617 patients. *Acta Derm Venereol* 1988; 68(3): 236–239.
111. Cress R, Holly E. Incidence of cutaneous melanoma among non-Hispanic whites, Hispanics, Asians, and blacks: an analysis of California Cancer Registry data, 1988–93. *Cancer Causes Control* 1997; 8: 246–252.
112. Gallagher R, Rivers J, Yang C, et al. Melanocytic nevus density in Asian, Indo-Pakistani, and white children: the Vancouver mole study. *J Am Acad Dermatol* 1991; 25: 507–512.
113. Ofuji S, Ogino A, Horio T, Ohseko T, Uehara M. Eosinophilic pustular folliculitis. *Acta Derm Venereol (Stockh)* 1970; 50: 195–203.
114. Burton JL, Holden CA. Eczema, lichenification and prurigo. In: Champion RH, Burton JL, Burns DA, Breathnanch SM (Eds) *Textbook of Dermatology*, Vol. 1, 6th ed. Oxford: Blackwell Science, 1998; 628–680.
115. Takematsu H, Nakamura K, Igarashi M, Tagami H. Eosinophilic pustular folliculitis. Report of 2 cases with a review of the Japanese literature. *Arch Dermatol* 1985; 121: 917–920.
116. Ota T, Hata A, Tanikawa A, Amagai M, Tanaka M, Nishikawa T. Eosinophilic pustular folliculitis (Ofuji's disease): Indomethacin as a first choice of treatment. *Clin Exp Dermatol* 2002; 46: 179–181.
117. Rattana AN, Kullavanijaya P. Eosinophilic pustular folliculitis: report of seven cases in Thailand. *J Dermatol* 2000; 27: 195–203.
118. Tang M, Tan E, Chua SH. Eosinophilic pustular folliculitis (Ofuji's disease) in Singapore: a review of 23 adult cases. *Australas J Dermatol* 2005; in press
119. Aoyoma H, Tagami H. Eosinophilic pustular folliculitis starting initially only with palmoplantar lesions. *Dermatology* 1992; 185: 276–280.
120. Rosenthal D, LeBoit PE, Klumpp L, Berger TG. Human immunodeficiency virus associated eosinophilic folliculitis. *Arch Dermatol* 1991; 127: 206–209.
121. Garcia-Patos V, Pujol RM, de Moraga JM. Infantile eosinophilic pustular folliculitis. *Dermatology* 1994; 189: 133–138.
122. Ishiguro N, Shishido E, Okamoto R, Igarashi Y, Yamada M, Kawashima M. Ofuji's disease: a report on 20 patients with clinical and histologic analysis. *J Am Acad Dermatol* 2002; 46: 827–833.
123. Teraki Y, Konohama I, Shiohara T, Nagashima M, Nishikawa T. Eosinophilic pustular folliculitis (Ofuji's disease): immunohistochemical analysis. *Arch Dermatol* 1993; 129: 1015–1019.
124. Takematsu H, Tagami H. Eosinophilic pustular folliculitis: studies on possible chemotactic factors involved in the formation of pustules. *Br J Dermatol* 1986; 114: 209–215.
125. Ofuji S. Eosinophilic pustular folliculitis. *Dermatologica* 1987; 174: 53–56.
126. Berbis P, Jancovici E, Lebreucil G, Benderitter T, Dubertret L, Privat Y. Eosinophilic pustular folliculitis (Ofuji's disease): efficacy of isotretinoin. *Dermatologica* 1989; 179: 214–216.
127. Porneuf M, Guillot B, Barneon G, Guilhou JJ. Eosinophilic pustular folliculitis responding to UVB therapy. *J Am Acad Dermatol* 1993; 29: 259–260.
128. Fushimi M, Tokura Y, Sachi Y, Hashizume H, Sudo H, Wakita H, Furukawa F, Takigama M. Eosinophilic pustular folliculitis effectively treated with recombinant interferon-gamma: suppression of mRNA expression of interleukin 5 in peripheral blood mononuclear cells. *Br J Dermatol* 1996; 134: 766–772.
129. Mohr C, Schutte B, Hildebrand A, Luger TA, Kolde G. Eosinophilic pustular folliculitis: successful treatment with interferon-alpha. *Dermatology* 1995; 191: 257–259.
130. Steffen C. Eosinophilic pustular folliculitis (Ofuji's disease) with response to dapsone therapy. *Arch Dermatol* 1985; 121: 921–923.

131. Kato H. Eosinophilic pustular folliculitis (Ofuji's disease) with response to indomethacin. *Dermatologica* 1989; 179: 217–218.
132. Fitzpatrick TB. Mechanisms of phototherapy of vitiligo. *Arch Dermatol* 1997; 133: 1591–1592.
133. Njoo MD, Spuls PI, Bos JD, et al. Nonsurgical repigmentation therapies in vitiligo. *Arch Dermatol* 1998; 134: 1532–1540.
134. Grimes PE, Soriano T, Dytoc MT. Topical tacrolimus for repigmentation of vitiligo. *J Am Acad Dermatol* 2002; 47(5): 789–791.
135. Scherschun L, Kim JJ, Lim HW. Narrow-band ultraviolet B is a useful and well-tolerated treatment for vitiligo. *J Am Acad Dermatol* 2001; 44(6): 999–1003.
136. Ermis O, Alpsoy E, Cetin L, Yilmaz E. Is the efficacy of psoralen plus ultraviolet A therapy for vitiligo enhanced by concurrent topical calcipotriol? A placebo-controlled double-blind study. *Br J Dermatol* 2001; 145: 472–475.
137. Ameen M, Exarchou V, Chu AC. Topical calcipotriol as monotherapy and in combination with psoralen plus ultraviolet A in the treatment of vitiligo. *Br J Dermatol 2001;* 145: 476–479.
138. Kullavanijaya, P, Lim, HW. Topical calcipotriene and narrowband UVB in the treatment of vitiligo. *Photodermatol Photoimmunol Photomed* 2004; 20: 248–251.
139. Lim HW, Morison WL, Kamide R, et al. Chronic actinic dermatitis. *Arch Dermatol* 1994; 130: 1284–1289.
140. Fotiades J, Soter NA, Lim HW. Results of evaluation of 203 patients for photosensitivity in a 7.3-year period. *J Am Acad Dermatol* 1995; 33: 597–602.
141. Khoo SW, Tay YK, Tham SN. Photodermatoses in a Singapore skin referral centre. *Clin Exp Dermatol* 1996; 21(4): 263–268.
142. Abe R, Shimizu T, Tsuji A, et al. Severe refractory chronic actinic dermatitis successfully treated with tacrolimus ointment. *Br J Dermatol* 2002; 147: 1273–1275.
143. du P Menagé H, Hawk JLM. Chronic actinic dermatitis/photosensitivity dermatitis/actinic reticuloid syndrome. In: KA Arndt, PE Leboit, JK Robinson, BU Wintroub (Eds) *Cutaneous Medicine and Surgery: An Integrated Programme in Dermatology*, Vol. 1. Philadelphia: Saunders, 1995.
144. Lim HW, Cohen D, Soter NA. Chronic actinic dermatitis: results of patch and photopatch tests with compositae, fragrances and pesticides. *J Am Acad Dermatol*. 1998; 38: 108–111.
145. Uetsu N, Okamoto H, Fujii K, et al. Treatment of chronic actinic dermatitis with tacrolimus ointment. *J Am Acad Dermatol* 2002; 47: 881–884.
146. Nousari HC, Anhalt GJ, Morison WL, et al. Mycophenolate in psoralen-UV-A desensitization therapy for chronic actinic dermatitis. *Arch Dermatol* 1999; 135: 1128–1129.
147. Cox TM, Alexander GJM, Sarkany RPE. Protoporphyria. *Semin Liver Dis* 1998; 18(1): 85–93.
148. Gouya L, Puy H, Lamoril J, Da Silva V, Grandchamp B, Nordmann Y, Deybach JC. Inheritance in erythropoietic protoporphyria: a common wild-type ferrochelatase allelic variant with low expression accounts for clinical manifestation. *Blood* 1999; 93: 2105–2110.
149. Rufenacht UB, Gregor A, Gouya L, Tarczynska-Nosal S, Schneider-Yin X, Deybach JC. New missense mutation in the human ferrochelatase gene in a family with erythropoietic protoporphyria: functional studies and correlation of genotype and phenotype. *Clin Chem* 2001; 47: 1112–1113.
150. Yeatman GW, Dang VV. Cao gio (coin rubbing). *J Am Med Assoc* 1990; 244: 2748–2749.
151. Amshel CE, Caruso DM. Vietnamese "coining": a burn case report and literature review. *J Burn Care Rehabil* 2000; 21(2): 112–114.
152. Hulewicz BS. Coin-rubbing injuries. *Am J Forensic Med Pathol* 1994; 15(3): 257–260.
153. Wang JX. A monograph on acupuncture and moxibustion. *J Tradit Chin Med* 1986; 6(1): 77–78.
154. Sagi A, Ben-Meir P, Bibi C. Burn hazard from cupping — an ancient universal medication still in practice. *Burns Incl Therm Inj* 1988; 4(4): 323–325.
155. Asnes RS, Wisotsky DH. Cupping lesions simulating child abuse. *J Pediatr* 1981; 99(2): 267–268.
156. Sandler AP, Haynes V. Nonaccidental trauma and medical folk belief: a case of cupping. *Pediatrics* 1978; 61(6): 921–922.
157. Lao L. Acupuncture techniques and devices. *J Altern Complement Med* 1996; 2(1): 23–25.
158. Conde-Salazar L, Gonzalez MA, Guimarens D, Fuente C. Burns due to moxibustion. *Contact Dermatitis* 1991; 25(5): 332–333.
159. Krishna G, Khanijow VJ. Nasal scarring by joss stick burns. *Med J Malaysia* 1994; 49(1): 90–92.

17 Dermatologic Disease in Blacks

Rebat M. Halder, Camille I. Roberts, Pavan K. Nootheti, and A. Paul Kelly

BASIC STRUCTURE OF BLACK SKIN AND HAIR

Information regarding cutaneous disease in the black races continues to evolve. It has not been until recently that differences in black skin structure and presentation were mentioned in most dermatologic, literature. Over the last few years controversy has ensued regarding the differences in structure and function of black skin compared to other skin types. (For the purposes of this chapter, the term "black" refers to those persons of African, African-American, and Afro-Caribbean descent.) It is well established, however, that one of the main differences in black skin occurs in the melanocytes. Although the number of melanocytes is the same regardless of a person's race, the difference occurs in the melanosomes. Melanosomes are larger and more individually arranged within the cytoplasm of keratinocytes in black skin, whereas in white skin the melanosomes are smaller and packed into membrane-bound aggregates.[1]

The difference in the thickness of black skin compared to white skin appears to be negligible, although black skin appears to be more compact, with more layers in the stratum corneum.[2] Black skin also appears to have a higher lipid content than white skin.[3] These factors may explain the greater cellular cohesion and resistance to stripping of the horny layer and the decrease permeability to certain chemicals of black skin.[4]

Researchers in the past have alluded to the fact that sebum secretion in black skin is increased when compared to sebum secretion in white skin. However, Pochi and Strauss quantified sebum production in black vs. white skin subsets and found that there was no consistent difference between the two races.[5]

The structure and function of black hair have been documented more clearly. Khumale et al. studied black hair vs. white and Asian hair.[6] In that study, virgin hair in black volunteers was studied. Subjects did not use chemical treatments but continued to use methods of daily grooming such as shampooing, combing, and hair drying. Hair was then studied using light microscopy. They found that black hair had a more tightly coiled and springlike structure compared to other skin types and had a more flattened cross-sectional appearance. There were also more longitudinal fissures and splits along the hair shafts compared to other ethnic groups.

CULTURAL ISSUES IN TREATING BLACKS FOR DERMATOLOGIC DISEASE

This section specifically emphasizes cultural issues in providing dermatologic care for African-Americans. There are many reasons why African-Americans receive insufficient dermatologic health care.[7] Thus, many individuals neglect the value of dermatologic care in this population. However, there are several prevalent dermatologic diseases in the African-American population that are associated with considerable morbidity.[7] Other patient-related risk factors for limited dermatologic care in African-Americans, when compared with other ethnic groups, include low income, lack of health insurance, and higher rates of poverty.[7] In fact, when compared with Hispanic and Caucasian populations, African-Americans are the largest ethnic group to state cost as an immense barrier to seeking dermatologic care.[8] African-Americans tend to have a fatalistic view toward cancer and are likely to be less knowledgable regarding skin cancer itself.[7,9] Upon discovering a dermatologic lesion, though they may want to perform a proper skin self-examination, African-Americans have less confidence than Caucasians to do so.[8,10] Folk medicine and home remedies may also contribute to decreased dermatologic visits, but African-Americans have actually been found to be less likely to use alternative therapies.[11] This may be due to lack of reporting or misinterpretation of the phrase "alternative therapies."

Several provider-related barriers to care in the African-American population also exist. Restricted appointment availability and clinic times can limit access to dermatologic health care, especially considering the rigidity in work schedules and limited time off in manual labor and unskilled jobs, which are more prevalent among African-Americans.[7] In addition, health insurance carriers and limited reimbursement may reduce access to dermatologic care.[7] More specifically, 50% of African-Americans are insured by Medicaid and many dermatologic providers do not accept this carrier secondary to its poor compensation.[12] Consequently, many individuals will instead visit their primary care provider for treatment of their dermatologic condition. This leads to suboptimal care for the patient. For example, one study showed that only 30% of patients who were treated by their primary care physician for a dermatologic lesion were content with their care.[13] Moreover, 87% of patients felt that direct access to dermatologic care was integral to their health care. Another important reason that African-Americans in particular should see a dermatologist for the primary evaluation of their skin lesions is because serious diseases in darker skin types can present differently than they would in lighter-complexioned individuals.[14] In fact, having direct access to a dermatologist can reduce the incidence of misdiagnosis and lag time before the initiation of treatment.[7]

There are several ways to improve access to dermatologic care for African-Americans. More large, prospective trials addressing cultural and psychological reasons for not seeking dermatologic care, addressing folk medicine and home treatments, and skin cancer education need to be conducted.[7] In addition, staff members should be educated about folk medicine and home treatments to avoid any cultural bias and misconceptions, and patients should be educated about skin cancer detection as well as prevention.[7] A few studies involving skin cancer education in African-Americans have been shown to be beneficial.[15] By implementing these studies and assessing the limitations mentioned above, African-Americans will have much improved dermatologic care.

NORMAL VARIANTS OF BLACK SKIN

In black skin there are variations in pigmentation that are considered normal. Some of these include hyperpigmentation and hypopigmentation.

Midline pigmentation is a condition that is seen in 30% of blacks.[16] This is characterized by discrete or linear hypopigmented macules and patches in the midsternal region of the chest. This hypopigmentation will occasionally track along the clavicles. Another variant in blacks is leukoderma, which is characterized by white patches, usually found on the buccal mucosa, that are not removed by scraping. They result from retained layers of parakeratotic cells.[17] Poor hygiene and cigarette smoking have been cited as etiologic factors. This condition is not premalignant. No treatment is necessary. In blacks, hyperpigmentation of the oral mucosa is also common. This hyperpigmentation occurs most commonly on the gingiva but may also occur on the buccal mucosa, hard palate, and tongue. This is seen in 75%–100% of black patients.[18] Pigmentary demarcation lines (Voight's line or Futcher's lines) are bilateral, sharp lines of pigmentation that correspond to underlying spinal nerves that occur along a dermatome. Five types are characterized, found on (1) the upper arms anteromedially, (2) the presternal area, (3) the bilateral aspect of the chest, (4) the posteromedial area of the spine, and (5) the posterior aspect of the lower limbs. Some cases are normal at birth and others become noticeable during pregnancy.

Hyperpigmentation of the palms and soles, commonly seen in blacks, must be differentiated from secondary syphilis, which is characterized by brown or dark brown macules of varying size and shape that have either sharp or distinct borders. Longitudinal melonychia is caused by an increase in melanin deposition in the nail plate and matrix.[18] This is seen more commonly with increasing age. Thumbs and index fingers are most commonly affected. This presents with a pigmented stripe along the vertical axis of the nail that may become more pronounced with age. The main differential diagnosis is malignant melanoma.

COMMON SKIN AND HAIR DISEASES

From a previous study by Halder et al., the ranking of common dermatologic diagnoses in blacks is given in Table 17.1 in order of frequency of disease seen.

Although it has been several decades since this study was published, the incidence of these dermatoses has not changed significantly; however, alopecias now have a higher incidence since 1982, particularly in black women. Common disorders of the skin seen in the black races, e.g., acne vulgaris, eczema, and fungal infections, are discussed in detail in Chapter 2. Pigmentary disorders are discussed in detail in Chapter 5 and alopecias in Chapter 4.

Seborrheic Dermatitis of Skin

Seborrheic dermatitis is a commonly encountered disorder with an occurrence rate of 2%–5% of the population.[19] It is a chronic, superficial, inflammatory condition of the skin. Seborrheic dermatitis is also common in the black population.

There is a wide range in presentation of seborrheic dermatitis in individuals, depending on the age, body site involved, and presence of any underlying disease. Seborrheic dermatitis may present as annular, erythematous, scaly lesions termed seborrhea petaloides, often seen in black patients (Figure 17.1). These types of annular lesions are typically confluent and usually located on the trunk, and they have been described as having a flowerlike contour. Such discrete lesions may provide a diagnostic challenge when present on the face on black patients. One postulated mechanism for the increased prevalence of annular lesions in black patients is that blacks have a higher tendency for fibroplasias.[20]

TABLE 17.1
Common Dermatologic Diagnoses in Blacks

1	Acne vulgaris	27.7%
2	Eczema	20.3%
3	Pigmentary disorders	9.0%
4	Seborrheic dermatitis	6.5%
5	Alopecias	5.3%
6	Fungal infection	4.3%
7	Contact dermatitis	3.1%
8	Warts	2.4%
9	Tinea versicolor	2.2%
10	Keloids	2.1%
11	Pityriasis rosea	2.0%

Source: Halder RM, Grimes PE, McLaurin CI, Kress MA, Kenney JA, Jr. Incidence of common dermatoses in a predominantly black dermatologic practice. *Cutis* 32: 388–390, 1983.

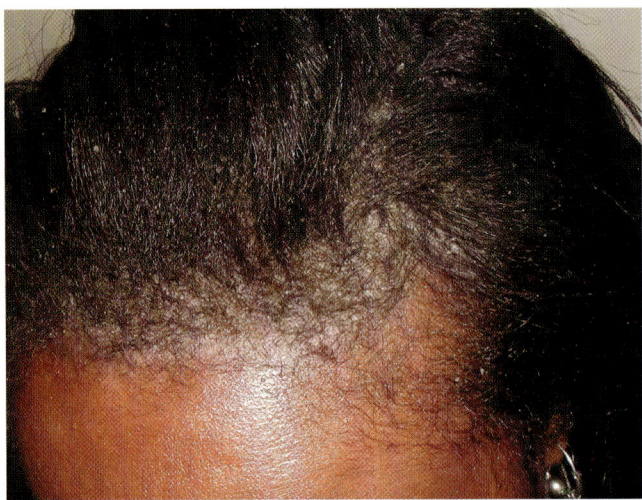

FIGURE 17.1 Annular seborrheic dermatitis in an African-American. (Courtesy of Valerie D. Callender, M.D.)

Tinea (Pityriasis) Versicolor

Tinea versicolor has a wide array of clinical presentations, including papulosquamous lesions, folliculitis, and inverse tinea versicolor.[21] The most commonly seen form is the scaly macular lesions, which vary in being hypo- or hyperpigmented. In darker-skinned individuals, tinea versicolor is thought to present more commonly with hypopigmented lesions. However, Aljabre et al. found no significantly increased prevalence of hypopigmented lesions in darker-skinned individuals.[22] The lesions likely appear more hypopigmented secondary to the marked contrast in individuals with darker skin.

Contact Dermatitis

Adverse Reactions to Hair-Coloring Products

Hair coloring has gained popularity. In the United States an estimated 46 million women use hair color products.[23] Although this data is not broken down by ethnic groups, black women use hair color for a variety of reasons, including highlighting, changing of hair color, and covering up gray hair. Although many classification systems are used, hair-coloring products can be simplified into three major categories: temporary, semipermanent, and permanent.

It has been estimated that true allergic reactions occur at the rate of about one in every 100,000 applications when using permanent hair color products.[24] However, DeLeo et al. report that black individuals displayed increased rates of sensitivity to para-phenylenediamine, which is commonly used in hair dyes.[25] This may be because darker shades of hair color are used by blacks. The best way to prevent allergic reactions to hair-coloring products is to perform a patch test before initial use of the product.

Trichorrhexis Nodosa

Trichorrhexis nodosa (TN) is best defined as a distinctive response of the hair shaft to injury. Trichorrhexis nodosa may occur in hair that has been inflicted with severe physical or chemical trauma, or it may occur with trivial trauma in hair that is abnormally fragile.[26] Fragility can be induced by conditions such as argininosuccinic aciduria, pili torti, Menke's syndrome, trichothiodystrophy,[27] Monilethrix, pseudomonilethrix, and trichorrhexis invaginata.[28] Some examples of physical trauma leading to damage of hair shafts include excessive brushing and combing, hair styles that put stress on the hair, heat, ultraviolet exposure, head rolling and banging, habit tics, trichotillomania, scratching and pulling, shampooing, hair setting, perming, and dyeing of hair. In particular, a number of grooming practices that are used by African-Americans tend to put stress on the hair.

One of the earliest pathological changes seen in TN is the disruption of cuticular cells causing the exposed cortical fibers to fray, leading to nodular swelling of the hair shaft. As the individual cortical fibers fracture, the classic appearance of two paintbrushes thrust into each other is observed.[28]

On clinical examination, single or multiple nodes are seen as whitish, grayish, or yellowish specks on the involved hair shaft. In the majority of cases, the distal portion of the hair shaft is involved, but the process may affect the proximal area as well. The propensity to fracture leads to areas of alopecia, which, depending on the severity, can be extensive. Although TN primarily affects the hair of the scalp, it may also involve hair in the pubic region, body hair, eyebrows, or eyelashes.[28]

Acquired TN is a condition that is secondary from physical and/or chemical trauma to the hair.[28] It is usually further subdivided into distal or proximal types, depending on where the pathology is located in the hair. Proximal TN occurs mostly in the African-American population. On examination, the hair is short in the affected area and TN is seen on microscopy.[26] This condition develops after many years of hair straightening with hot combs or permanent weaves. Proximal TN results in areas of alopecia and the patients present with brittle scalp hair that grows only a few inches before breaking off.

The treatment of distal TN is best accomplished by gentle hair care. This involves avoiding excessive physical trauma and manipulation of the hair and minimizing chemical irritation of the hair. Proximal TN is best treated by minimizing trauma and discontinuing grooming practices such as hot combing and permanent waving.[28]

Pseudofolliculitis Barbae

Pseudofolliculitis barbae (PFB) is a very common and distressing problem affecting almost exclusively black men who shave. Figures range from 45% to 83% for the prevalence of PFB among this population.[29,30–32] The etiology is a foreign-body inflammatory reaction surrounding an ingrown hair[29] secondary to the inherent properties of hair in many blacks. In kinky hair, a characteristic of many blacks, the hair follicles and shaft are curved. (The term "black hair" refers specifically to curved hair and follicles.) Pseudofolliculitis barbae has caused racial tensions in the military because of the requirement for a clean-shaven appearance.[30,33] In civilian life, PFB also causes tension in occupations in which the employers require a clean-shaven appearance, such as police and firemen, food service employees, and flight attendants.

Two major mechanisms that are related to the curved hair found in blacks are involved in the pathogenesis of PFB and are known as extrafollicular penetration and transfollicular penetration. In extrafollicular penetration, the hair grows out from the follicle, curves, and grows back toward the skin approximately 1 to 2 mm from the point of exit.[34] Kinky hair has a flattened elliptical shape.[35] Thus, when the hair is shaved, it develops a pointed tip, which causes invagination of the epidermis as it grows back toward the skin. The hair continues to grow downward, ruptures the epidermis, and eventually enters the dermis, where an inflammatory foreign-body reaction occurs.[5] In addition, as pointed out by Strauss and Kligman, the beard hair in blacks grows for a brief period initially parallel to the skin surface. Therefore, the hairs are cut at an oblique angle, causing an exaggerated pointed tip that penetrates the skin.[36] Pinkus described the phenomenon of a "loop hair" in PFB.[37] As a hair grows out of the skin in the extrafollicular pathway, it forms an arc or loop when it re-enters the skin. As the hair continues to grow, the loop becomes larger. The significance of this loop hair phenomenon will be discussed later, along with the treatment of PFB.

In contrast to extrafollicular penetration, transfollicular penetration usually does not occur spontaneously. Rather, it is the result of improper shaving techniques such as pulling the skin taut, which causes cut hair with its pointed tip to retract under the skin as the tension is released. Another common cause is plucking hair with tweezers, which can leave a fragment of hair below the skin line. In both cases, the curved hairs with sharp tips pierce the follicular wall and initiate an inflammatory foreign-body reaction.

Strauss and Kligman found foreign-body-type giant cells in the dermis in biopsies of PFB.[36] They also found leukocytes and micrococci in biopsies of papules and phagocytosing polymorphonuclear leukocytes in biopsies of pustules. Cultures of the occasional pustules in patients with PFB showed only normal flora. Among earlier studies, Greenbaum did not find leukocytes or bacteria.[38] Thus, bacteria are not implicated in the pathogenesis of PFB; they are seen only in secondary infection of the lesions.

Clinical Presentation

The diagnosis of PFB is not difficult to make. Lesions can occur on any bearded area of the face; however, the anterior neckline, mandibular areas, cheeks, and chin are most commonly involved (Figure 17.2). Interestingly, the moustache and nuchal areas are rarely affected.

Lesions appear as firm, flesh-colored to hyperpigmented papules. Although pustules or papulopustules are present, they are secondary lesions. Hairs can be seen within the papules but often must be gently teased from under the surface of a papule to become visible. Because hairs initially grow parallel and close to the skin, some individuals will develop grooves in the skin that are visible on examination.[39] The chronic irritation that develops from shaving over the papules can lead to postinflammatory hyperpigmentation. This change occurs most often on the neck.

The differential diagnosis of PFB includes acne vulgaris, sycosis barbae, and traumatic folliculitis. No comedonal lesions are found in PFB, and acne vulgaris affects other areas of the face in addition to the beard area. Pustules dominate acne vulgaris, whereas they are rare in PFB. In sycosis barbae, perifollicular pustules are the primary and predominant lesions. Lesions in pseudofolliculitis barbae are isolated, whereas in sycosis barbae they are confluent. Shaving improves sycosis barbae, whereas it makes PFB worse. "Razor burn," or traumatic folliculitis, occurs when shaving is done too closely. Lesions are erythematous, painful, small, follicular papules. These lesions disappear within 24–48 h after shaving. Pseudofolliculitis barbae persists for 1–2 weeks after cessation of shaving.

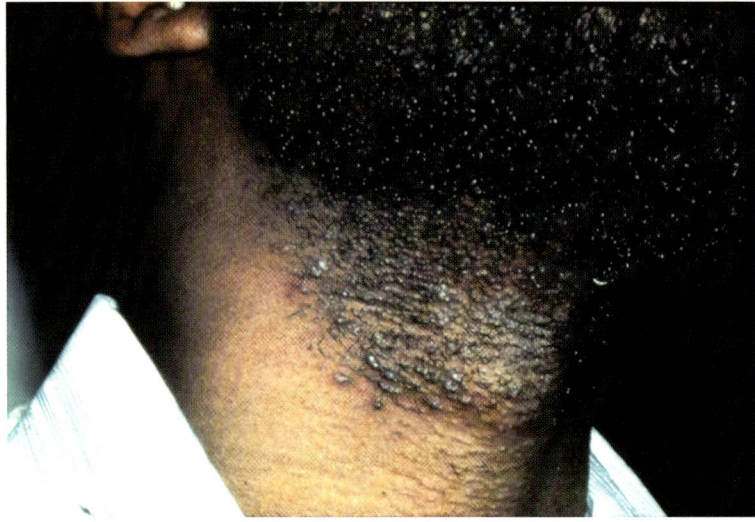

FIGURE 17.2 Pseudofolliculitis barbae in an African-American.

Dermatologic Disease in Blacks

Pseudofolliculitis Barbae in Women

Published reports of PFB in black women are rare,[40,41] probably because of a lack of interest in reporting this phenomenon. In actuality, PFB in black women is seen with some frequency. The most common areas of involvement are the axilla and pubis, which are shaved by some women. In hirsute women, PFB can occur on the face from either shaving or plucking hairs.

Treatment of PFB on the face in women does not differ from that for men. The preferred modality of treatment for PFB in the axilla and pubis is cessation of shaving. Facial PFB in women responds well to laser therapy, which is described later.

Acne Keloidalis Nuchae

Acne keloidalis nuchae is a chronic inflammatory process that occurs most often in black men on the nape of the neck. The etiology is unknown but, as in PFB, is related to the inherent curvature of the hair and follicle in blacks. Staphylococcal infection has been implicated in the pathogenesis, but repeated cultures from lesions are negative. Irritation from shirt collars may be a factor in the development of lesions, because they appear on the back of the neck. This disease may be associated with acne conglobata and dissecting cellulitis of the scalp.

Clinically, lesions appear as smooth, firm, skin-colored to translucent papules on the nape of the neck with occasional extension onto the occipital area. Pustule formation and coalescence of papules into keloidal plaques may eventually appear (Figure 17.3). Large cysts may develop and fuse to form sinus tracts. The vertex of the scalp and upper lip may also be involved.[42] Although primarily a disease of black men, it may certainly be seen in black women, particularly those who cut the hair close to the skin of the neck.[43]

Histologically a neutrophilic perifolliculitis with granulomatous changes and foreign-body giant-cell reaction occurs. This is followed by a plasma-cell infiltrate with replacement or engulfment of hair follicles by hypertrophic connective tissue.[44]

Dermatitis papillaris capillitii remains a therapeutic dilemma. As with PFB, no single therapy is effective in all patients. Intralesional steroids are effective for early papular lesions. Intralesional steroids are also helpful for sinus tracts. Electrodesiccation and shave excision of the papules have been used. Epilation by x-ray has had limited success. Epilation by electrolysis should be avoided because of the difficulty in destroying the root at the base of the curved follicle. Oral antibiotics

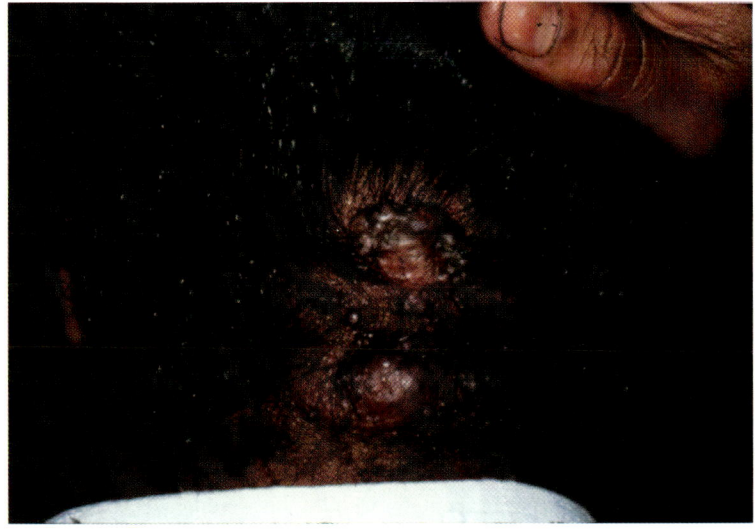

FIGURE 17.3 Acne keloidalis nuchae in an African-American.

such as tetracycline are used long term for pustular or cystic lesions. Applying a mixture of clindamycin powder (obtained from capsules) and a high-potency steroid cream is helpful for early lesions.[43] Severe cases with extensive keloid and scar formation may require local excision with grafting.[36] These extensive, scarred lesions may also benefit from the use of a tissue expander prior to excision and grafting.

Treatment of Pseudofolliculitis Barbae

One of the most effective treatments is to let the beard grow for 4 weeks, which allows ingrown hairs to erode the overlying epidermal covering and eventually come to the surface (the free end of each ingrown hair springs out of the skin). In the case of extrafollicularly buried hairs, this usually occurs after 10 days.[45] Strauss and Kligman[36] found that after approximately 1 month of beard growth, most papules resolve spontaneously. The natural tension of the hair is presumed to cause it to spring out of the area of foreign-body reaction spontaneously after it has grown to a length of 1 cm.[35] Not shaving can be an easy cure and the initial therapy for PFB,[1] but it is impractical for men who are required or prefer to shave.[46]

To control PFB, men can maintain their hair at an optimal length of 0.5 to 1 mm to prevent extrafollicular and transfollicular penetration. Use of triple "O" electric clippers have been successful in controlling PFB, but they leave the hair approximately 1 mm long, and patients may not like the look of this "stubble."[29]

Provided that correct techniques are used, both manual and electric razors can be used to control PFB. Patients should be advised to shave in the direction of hair growth. With manual razors, a new blade should be used for each shave (using a dull blade may mean having to shave a particular area repeatedly).[29] The skin should not be pulled taut because as the tension is released, cut hair goes below the skin surface, thereby leading to transfollicular penetration.[35]

The Bump Fighter® razor, designed with a single-edge blade, polymer coating, and a foil guard, is manufactured specifically for PFB and has been helpful in controlling the condition. The foil guard prevents 30% of the sharp edge from contacting the skin.[29] Applying benzoyl peroxide 3%–6% gel after shaving and 1% hydrocortisone cream at night may be helpful for mild PFB.[45] The mechanism of action of benzoyl peroxide in treating PFB is not fully understood. The antibacterial activity of benzoyl peroxide may prevent secondary infection in PFB. In addition, skin treated with benzoyl peroxide shows mild desquamation and a simultaneous reduction in lesions. Combination products containing both clindamycin and benzoyl peroxide in a gel formulation are effective.[47]

Low-dose systemic antibiotics are sometimes helpful, but their positive effects are often short-lived. Although bacteria are not the initiating factor in PFB, colonization by normal flora may worsen inflammation due to secondary infection. Low-dose systemic antibiotics such as tetracycline and erythromycin 250 mg twice daily may be used with topical antibiotics and may be effective in limiting the inflammatory process. Doxycycline 100 mg daily and minocycline 200 mg initially, followed by 100 mg twice daily, have also achieved similar results.

Topical tretinoin has been used with success in mild to moderate cases of PFB, but therapy is often discontinued because of resulting irritation. Topical tretinoin 0.05% solution or cream used daily may work by alleviating hyperkeratosis and hardening of the skin[45] and may be combined with a mild topical steroid to reduce irritation (Figures 17.1 and 17.2). Topical retinoids are more efficacious with straighter hair; they remove the thin film of epidermis covering the hair before the hair emerges from its follicle.

In an open study of a combination of topical tretinoin 0.025% cream applied once daily, the number of papules and hyperpigmented macules decreased after 8 weeks of use for mild to moderate PFB.[48] Adapalene 0.1% gel applied at bedtime has been effective in treating PFB in decreasing both the number of papules and hyperpigmented macules. Tazarotene gel 0.05%–0.1% applied daily has also been recently used and has shown a reduction in inflammatory lesions and postinflammatory hyperpigmented macules and overall improvement in PFB.[49] Tazarotene, however, can cause more irritation than tretinoin or adapalene.

Chemical depilatories (e.g., barium sulfide, calcium thioglycolate) are available in powder, lotion, cream, and paste vehicles. Use of these products, which cause lysis of disulfide bonds in the hair and make extrafollicular and transfollicular penetration less likely, produces softer, blunt- or feather-tipped hair. Use of depilatories also lengthens the time between shaves, thus reducing the chance of irritation. The technique involves moistening the bearded area with water, applying the depilatory, leaving it on for 5 min (barium sulfide) or 15 min (calcium thioglycolate), and then using a moistened wooden tongue depressor (scraping in the direction of hair growth) to remove the depillatory and hair. The face is then rinsed with water, and an emollient is applied. To limit skin irritation, depilatories should not be used more than every other day.[38]

Barium sulfide depilatories act rapidly, are convenient to use, and produce the smoothest shave. Their scent, however, is characteristically unpleasant. The mercaptan or sulfide odor of calcium thioglycolate depilatories can be masked with fragrances, but these depilatories do not leave the skin as smooth as barium sulfide products do. The patient should be informed of the potential for irritation, especially with barium sulfide. A patch test may be done before treatment to determine the potential for severe irritation.

Eflornithine hydrochloride cream, which recently became available in the United States, irreversibly inhibits the enzyme ornithine decarboxlyase (involved in hair cell division), decreasing the rate of hair growth and, thus, the need to shave as often. This cream is applied twice daily and is washed off after 4 h.[50] Currently, eflornithine hydrochloride cream is used to treat unwanted facial hair in women; it may be used with other hair-removal techniques to treat PFB.[51]

Adjuvant Treatment Measures

Various techniques and preventive practices are recommended for PFB. Washing the beard with an antibacterial soap and warm water in a circular motion for several minutes can be effective in releasing the hair before shaving. The soap helps to reduce the risk of secondary infection, and the heat from the water softens the hair, which makes it easier to manage and prevents a sharp edge from developing at hair tips after shaving.[52] Instrument type and shaving technique are important in prevention. The most important result, a less close shave, can be achieved (as mentioned) using electric clippers made with a protective gap.[52] Manually freeing ingrown hairs, a technique that can be used with other measures, may be effectively done with a toothpick. Using a toothbrush or a polyester scrub pad to brush the beard hairs free has also been helpful.[29]

Electrolysis

Electrolysis of beard hairs is not recommended for PFB. In addition to being painful, it is impractical and generally ineffective. The needle used in electrolysis may not reach the hair bulbs of a curved hair follicle; in fact, use of the needle may result in transfollicular penetration, which exacerbates PFB. Electrolysis may also cause hyperpigmentation at the site of needle insertion in patients with pigmented skin.[51]

Surgical Therapy

Chemical Peels

Pseudofolliculitis barbae treatment using glycolic acid peels is an effective and well-tolerated therapy. Although the mechanism of action of glycolic acid in PFB treatment is not clear, sulfhydryl bonds in the hair shaft are thought to be reduced by glycolic acid, resulting in straighter hair growth, which in turn reduces re-entry of the hair shaft into the epidermis or follicular wall. In recent clinical trials, daily application of topical glycolic acid lotion significantly reduced the number of

PFB lesions on the face and neck and allowed patients to shave daily, comfortably, and with minimal irritation.[50] Salicylic acid peels have also benefited some patients. The mode of action of these peels is similar to that of topical retinoids. Salicylic acid peels may also be effective in treating inflammatory lesions and decreasing hyperpigmented macules.[50]

Lasers

Laser therapy for PFB is also described in Chapter 14. Laser-assisted hair removal is effective in treating PFB. The Q-switched Nd:YAG laser with topical carbon suspension has a good safety record and is effective in removing hair and retarding hair growth.[46] Use of most hair-removal lasers depends on targeting melanin in the hair follicle. Topical carbon suspension, which surrounds the follicle, forms a target for the laser. In addition, the laser wavelength of 1064 nm has a greater affinity for carbon than for skin structures, leading to much less tissue damage.[46] In a study involving the Q-switched Nd:YAG laser (fluence 2.5 J/cm^2) with topical carbon suspension, 18 patients with PFB (3 with Fitzpatrick skin type II or III; 15 with types IV–VI) were enrolled. Nine patients completed the study and experienced a mean reduction of 56% in inflammatory lesions within 2 months after final treatment.[46] Ross et al. showed that a long-pulsed Nd:YAG laser coupled with a contact cooling window could be used to achieve safe hair removal in dark-skinned patients.[53] Elimination of hair shafts was associated with a reduction in the number of characteristic inflammatory lesions of PFB. Effects varied by skin type. No crusting or blistering occurred with skin type IV or V. For darker skin, type VI, 50 J/cm^2 was the highest fluence tolerated. Perifollicular crusting or hypopigmentation usually resulted from fluences of 80 J/cm^2 and higher in skin type VI.

A diode laser with a water-cooled sapphire tip lowers the temperature of the epidermis during treatment, thus limiting thermal damage to the epidermis. In a study of 10 patients with PFB, diode laser treatment improved acute and chronic changes of PFB in skin types I to IV.[54] In all 10 patients, inflammatory lesions of PFB decreased more than 50%, and hair growth was reduced.

In the treatment of the patient population most commonly affected by PFB — a population mostly with skin types IV to VI — protection of melanin is crucial. Hair removal depends on absorption of light by melanin in hair shafts and follicles. Eliminating targets without damaging surrounding tissue depends on selective photothermolysis, which is based on specific absorption of light by target chromophores.[55]

Summary — PFB

Pseudofolliculitis barbae is difficult to treat. The most important aspect of PFB management is keeping patients well informed regarding the cause of PFB and the consistency with which a regimen must be followed for treatment to be effective. Patients with PFB, particularly those who are required or prefer to shave, should be informed that the regimen for controlling the disorder may be time consuming.[29] The goal of management is to use a treatment strategy that will minimize both extrafollicular and transfollicular penetration, which in turn will eliminate an inflammatory reaction in the skin.

Permanent removal of hair follicles forms the basis for developing surgical therapies such as laser treatment and would be the only definitive treatment for PFB.[51] Lasers may be used to selectively destroy hair follicles and reduce hair density.[54]

Dermatosis Papulosa Nigra (DPN)

Dermatosis papulosa nigra (DPN) comprises small, darkly pigmented papules found most commonly on the faces of black patients. They may also occur on the neck and trunks of patients.[56] DPN is also seen in other darker-skinned races and is thought to be a variant of seborrheic keratosis (Figure 17.4). There have been theories that there is a genetic component to DPN. Patients usually present for cosmetic reasons, although some lesions of DPN based upon their location, can cause frequent irritation with clothing and jewelry and become inflamed. They are benign lesions and

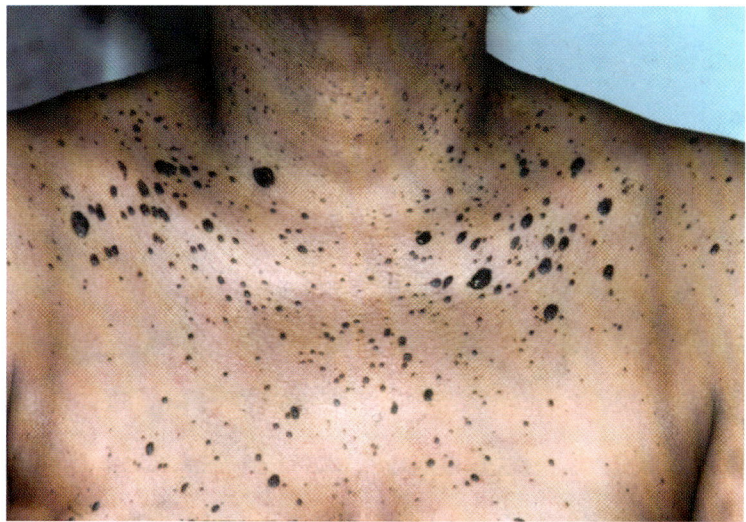

FIGURE 17.4 Extensive lesions of dermatosis papulosa nigra on the trunk of an African-American.

treatment is based upon patient preference. Treatment is best achieved by light electro-dessication or simple shave excision with or without local anesthesia.

PIGMENTARY DISORDERS

Vitiligo

Vitiligo is covered only briefly in this chapter, as it is extensively discussed in Chapter 5. Vitiligo is a disease caused by the loss of melanocytes leading to areas of amelanotic macules. It affects approximately 2% of the population, with an equal distribution among all races. However, the well-circumscribed depigmented macules are obviously more visible in individuals with darker skin such as blacks (Figure 17.5). Thus, it causes more of a cosmetic and psychological concern in darker-skinned individuals.

Although the exact etiology of vitiligo remains unknown, several hypotheses have been suggested. Vitiligo is also linked to a genetic component. It has been associated with numerous autoimmune diseases, and some think that an autoimmune component exists in the etiologic process of vitiligo.[57]

Clinically, there are several variants to the presentation of vitiligo. It can present as focal, segmental, generalized, acrofacial, or universalis type. Trichrome vitiligo is seen in areas where there are adjacent areas of normal skin, hypopigmented skin, and depigmented skin.[57]

Current treatments for the management of vitiligo include cosmetics, topical and intralesional corticosteroid therapy, phototherapy including both psoralen ultraviolet light therapy (PUVA) and narrow-band (311 nm) UVB treatment, surgical grafts, and melanocyte transplants.[58] New and emerging therapies may include the use of immunomodulators and laser therapy.

Melasma

Melasma (also discussed in detail in Chapter 5) is an acquired hypermelanosis of sun-exposed areas, especially involving the face. Although the exact etiology of melasma is unknown, many factors have been linked to the pathogenesis, such as genetics, UV radiation exposure, pregnancy, hormonal treatments, cosmetics, and phototoxic and seizure medications.[59] The pathogenesis and treatment of melasma in black individuals remain a challenge.[60] It has been stated that melasma seems to have a higher prevalence in both men and women from Ethiopia.[61]

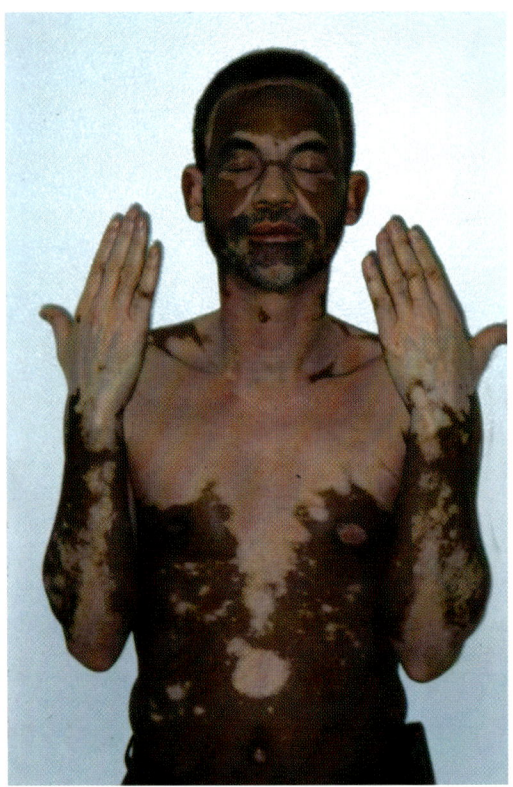

FIGURE 17.5 Generalized vitiligo in an African-American.

Clinically, melasma presents as areas of hyperpigmentation. These can range from light brown/gray to dark brown/gray macules and patches, usually in a symmetric pattern.[59]

Current treatment modalities include hypopigmenting agents, chemical peels, and lasers. Hypopigmenting agents may be divided into phenolic and nonphenolic compounds. The phenolic compounds include hydroquinone and hydroquinone-containing compounds. Nonphenolic compounds include tretinoin and azelaic acid. Kimbrough-Green et al. have reported the use of topical 0.1% tretinoin to lighten melasma in black patients with minimal side effects.[60] Breathnach reported the use of topical 20% azelaic acid to be superior to 2% hydroquinone and to be as effective as 4% hydroquinone, without the side effects of 4% hydroquinone. The study goes on to state that the use of azelaic acid in combination with tretinoin enhanced the effect of azelaic acid.[61] Although chemical peels have been shown to be useful in lighter-skinned individuals, they should be used with caution in darker-skinned patients to avoid further postinflammatory hyperpigmentation. Lasers have advanced the treatment of pigmentary disorders, but their application is still quite novel and requires careful assessment before being used to treat melasma.[59]

KELOIDS

Keloids are firm, erythematous, skin-colored papulonodules that form in response to trauma resulting from surgery, injury, insect bites, and ear piercing. There are also cases of spontaneous keloids that may occur in patients with a family history of keloidal lesions (Figure 17.6). Keloids are commonly found in blacks but have been described in people of all races. They result from increased activity of fibroblast growth factor that extends the growth cycle, allowing for prolonged growth.[63] As a result there is increased collagen disposition. Keloids may be tender or pruritic and, unlike

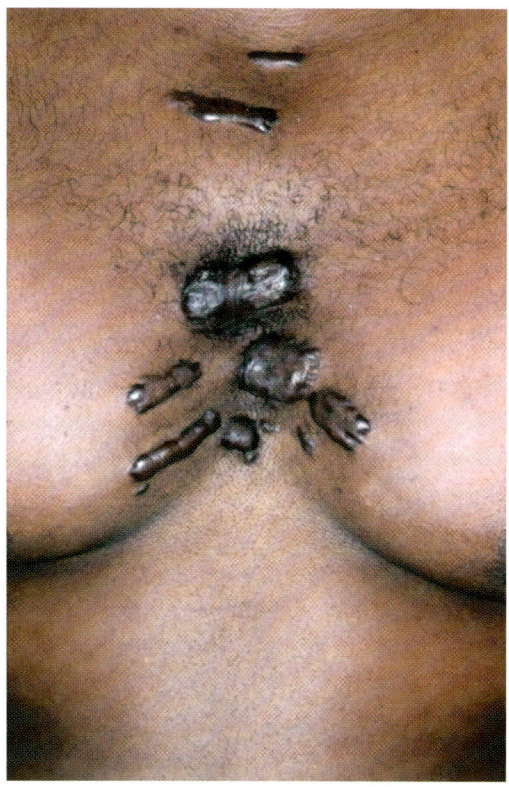

FIGURE 17.6 Spontaneous midsternal keloids in an African-American.

hypertrophic scars, may extend beyond the border of the primary lesion in a clawlike projection and be very disfiguring.

Treating keloids may be frustrating for both the patient and the physician. Nonsurgical techniques for treating keloids include topical and intralesional steroids, tretinoin, and pressure garments. Keloids may also be treated with steroids under occlusion. Treatments that may show promise in the future include interferon and transforming growth factor.[63] Surgical options include excision in combination with intralesional corticosteroids and radiation. Treatment with lasers such as pulsed dye and Nd:YAG in combination with other therapies is also possible.[64]

Medical Therapies

Steroid Injections

The most commonly used therapeutic modality is the intralesional (IL) injection of triamcinolone acetonide (10–40 mg/ml). Injected areas may become hypopigmented, and these areas may remain that way for 6–12 months. The needle should be inserted and triamcinolone injected into the papillary dermis, where collagenase is produced. The injected steroid should not be placed into subcutaneous tissue, because this may cause underlying fat atrophy. The corticosteroid inhibits alpha$_2$-macroglobulin, which itself inhibits collagenase. Once this pathway is blocked, collagenase is elaborated, thus enabling collagen degradation.[65] Keloid injections can be made easier and less painful if first treated with liquid nitrogen for a 10–15-second thaw time. This causes cutaneous edema, thereby allowing easier injection. To prevent post-IL corticosteroid clinical rebound, the injections should be given every 2–3 weeks. Prior to initiating IL triamcinolone therapy, patients should be warned that they may also develop atrophy and telangiectasias at and around the injection sites.

The use of pressure or silicone gel–sheeting therapy in conjunction with IL triamcinolone is more efficacious than when either modality is used as monotherapy.

Interferon Therapy

Interferon-alpha and -gamma inhibit types I and III collagen synthesis via a reduction in cellular messenger ribonucleic acid.[66] Berman and Flores reported an 18.7% recurrence rate when interferon alpha-2b injections were given after keloids excision vs. a 51% recurrence rate with excision alone and a 58% recurrence rate when treated with excision and postoperative IL triamcinolone.[64] One million units are injected into each linear centimeter of the skin surrounding the postoperative site immediately after surgery and 1–2 weeks later. For large excision sites, the patient should be premedicated with acetaminophen to help negate the flulike symptoms caused by the interferon. Interferon treatment is quite expensive for patients who undergo surgical excision for many keloids or large keloids.

5-Flurouracil Therapy

Intralesional 5-flurouracil (5-FU) has been used successfully to treat small isolated keloids.[67] Better results are obtained when 0.1 ml of triamcinolone acetonide (10 mg/ml) is added to 0.9 ml of 5-FU (50 mg/ml). This mixture is initially injected into the keloids three times per week, and the frequency is then adjusted according to the response. The average scar requires a total of 5–10 injections, usually given weekly. The major limiting factor in using 5-FU is the pain of injection. This leads to noncompliance for many patients.

Imiquimod Therapy

Imiquimod 5% cream induces local production of interferons at the site of application. Based on this information, Berman and Kaufman[68] applied imiquimod cream to the postoperative excision site of 12 patients who had a keloid removed surgically. Application of imiquimod should be started immediately after surgery and continued daily for 8 weeks. Berman's patients were evaluated 24 weeks postexcision and none had recurrence of their keloids. Most patients experience mild to marked irritation secondary to the daily application of imiquimod. Those with marked irritation will sometimes have to discontinue the medication for several days to a week and then resume therapy. Patients who have large surgical sites and wounds closed with flaps, grafts or tension should not start imiquimod cream therapy for 4–6 weeks postoperatively, because early application often causes the surgical site to splay or dehisce. More than 50% of the patients developed hyperpigmentation of the treated site.

Other Medical Therapies

Flurandrenolide tape applied to the keloid for 12–20 h per day will usually cause the keloid to slowly soften and become flatter. It will also usually eliminate the accompanying pruritus. Long-term use may cause cutaneous atrophy.

For small keloids, IL injection of bleomycin (1 mg/ml, 0.1–1 ml) has been reported to cause complete regression of some lesions.[69]

Clobetasol ointment or gel, applied twice a day, may soften and/or flatten keloids in addition to eliminating the accompanying pruritus, pain, and tenderness often associated with keloids. Long-term use will cause perilesional hypopigmentation, atrophy, and telangiectasia of the treated areas.

Tacrolimus is a new potential keloid therapy. Research by Kim et al. found increased expression of the *gli-1* oncogene in keloids but not in normal scar tissue.[70] Since tacrolimus may mute the *gli-1* oncogene, it has been used as a therapeutic alternative. Longer and larger studies are needed to determine its effectiveness.

When combined with surgical excision, methotrexate has been reported to prevent recurrences. Fifteen to 20 mg of methotrexate is given orally in a single dose every 4 days, starting a week prior to surgery and continued for 3 or 4 months after the postoperative site is healed.

Pentoxifylline (Trental) 400 mg three times a day has been somewhat successful in preventing recurrence of excised keloids. Its mechanism of action is not fully understood but may be a result of improved circulation, which, in turn, sweeps away fibroblast growth factors.

Colchicine has been used to treat and prevent recurrence of keloids via inhibition of collagen synthesis, microtubular disruption, and collagenase stimulation.[71]

Because topical zinc inhibits lysyl oxidase and stimulates collagenase,[72] it has been used to treat keloids but has had limited success. Topical tretinoin applied twice a day has been reported to alleviate pruritus and other keloid symptoms and may cause various degrees of regression.[73]

Other medications tried but found to have limited therapeutic success or a questioned risk–benefit ratio are IL verapamil,[74] cyclosporine,[75] methotrexate, D-penicillamine,[76] and Relaxin.[77]

Surgical Therapies

Before excising a keloid, the physician should be aware of the major risk factors associated with keloid recurrence:

- A family history of keloids
- An infected operative site
- Anatomical location (especially the midchest and shoulders)
- Type of participating injury (thermal or chemical burn)
- Tension of postoperative site
- Variation in recurrence rate from 50% to 80% for simple excision surgery of a keloid without postoperative adjunctive measures[78]

Primary Excision

The easiest and one of the most commonly performed procedures for keloid removal is surgical excision followed by IL corticosteroid injections.[79] Prior to excision, the operative site is anesthetized with a half-and-half mixture of 2% lidocaine with epinephrine and triamcinolone acetonide 40 mg/ml. For keloids with narrow bases (1 cm or less), a simple excision followed by undermining the base and closure with interrupted sutures is recommended. For keloids with wide bases, flaps and grafts may be required to close the postoperative site without tension. Most excised keloids need adjunctive therapy such as IL corticosteroids, pressure injections, pressure, silicone gel-sheeting, imiquimod cream, or interferon injections. Sutures need to stay for 10–14 days because the lidocaine/steroid mixture used to anesthetize the lesion will delay wound healing.

Therapy is more complex for large, nonpedunculated earlobe keloids and keloids with wide bases on other parts of the body. First, a half-moon or tonguelike piece of flap is made from the smoothest and flattest portion of the lesion, large enough to cover the base of the excised keloid. The tongue flap with 5-0 or 6-0 nylon sutures are left for 10–14 days in order to prevent wound dehiscence. The postoperative site is injected with 10–40 mg/ml of triamcinolone acetonide starting 1 week after suture removal (earlier injection, especially at the time of suture removal, may cause the wound to dehisce) and repeated every 3 weeks × 4 visits to help prevent keloid recurrence. Patients should be informed that the steroid injection sites may become hypopigmented and remain so for 6 months or more. Pressure garments and silicone gel-sheeting are usually important therapeutic adjuncts. For an earlobe keloid postoperative site, special pressure earrings with a silicone backing are available. They should not be applied until 2 weeks after suture removal because earlier use may cause the wound to dehisce.[79]

In cases in which an autograft is not possible to close the excised lesion, a tissue expander may be inserted under the keloid to be excised and closed primarily, without tension. For patients with large lesions or multiple lesions, a tissue expander may be inserted under the keloid and gradually expanded to enable the keloid to be excised and closed primarily, without tension.

As well, for patients with large lesions or multiple lesions, when primary excision is often not feasible, debulking the lesion(s) by shaving to the level of the surrounding clinically normal skin, followed by 8 weeks of topical imiquimod therapy, is sometimes successful. The postoperative site usually becomes hyperpigmented and does not match the texture of normal skin.

Cryosurgery

Freezing a keloid with liquid nitrogen causes cell and microvascular damage. The resulting anoxia causes tissue necrosis and sloughing, followed by tissue flattening.[80] A freeze–thaw time of greater than 25 seconds will usually result in hypopigmentation secondary to melanocyte destruction, especially for people with Fitzpatrick skin types IV–VI. Two 15–20-second thaw cycles on each visit every 3 weeks × 8–10 visits usually result in complete flattening in more than half of the cryotreated patients. When cryosurgery was used in combination with IL steroids, it resulted in an 84% positive response rate.[81] Many patients do not return for follow-up cryosurgery because of the postoperative pain, morbidity and slow healing. Also, the hypopigmentation may last for years. Cryofreezing may also be used to cause mild tissue edema, enabling easier injection of IL steroids.

Radiation Therapy

Radiation may be used as monotherapy or combined with surgery to prevent recurrence of keloids following excision. When used as monotherapy, radiation is not very effective (a recurrence rate of 50%–100%);[82] unless large doses are used, however, this may lead to squamous cell carcinoma of the skin of the treated sites 15–30 years later. A case of medullary thyroid carcinoma has been described in an 11-year-old boy 8 years after incision and postoperative radiation of a chin keloid.[83] Primary radiation is also successful in alleviating pruritus, pain, and tenderness of keloids.

Radiation is more effective if given either the first 2 weeks after excision, when fibroblasts are proliferating. The usual dose is 300 rad (3 Gy) q.o.d. × 4–5 days or 500 rad (5 Gy) q.o.d. × 3 days starting on the day of surgery. Young children with keloids should not be irradiated, but if it is the only viable option, the metaphyses should be shielded to prevent retardation of bone growth. Combined preoperative and postoperative radiation has no greater efficacy than postoperative radiation alone. Iridium-192 interstitial irradiation after surgical excision had a recurrence rate of 21% in 83 keloids.[63]

Because delivery of the radiation dose can be better targeted with brachytherapy than with external beam irradiation, high-dose rate (HDR) brachytherapy was used to treat keloids postexcision.[84] High-dose-rate brachytherapy was administered at a dose of 1200 cGy, delivered in four equal fractions over the first 24 h after surgery. Recurrence developed in eight patients (4.7%). This included 5 out of 147 patients (3.4%) who underwent surgical excision followed by HDR brachytherapy and 3 out of 22 patients who had been treated with HDR brachytherapy alone. Cosmetic results were good or excellent in 88%–94% of patients treated with excision plus HDR brachytherapy. All patients responded to HDR brachytherapy with a reduction in pruritus, redness, or burning. Thus, HDR brachytherapy combined with surgical excision seems to safely and effectively treat keloid scars and prevent their recurrence.

Physical Modalities for Treatment

Pressure

Pressure gradient garments are an adjunct for treating keloids postoperatively to prevent recurrence and are used to treat keloids after applying a potent topical steroid or flurandrenolide tape. The latter method enables reduction in the size and thickness of keloids by decreasing intralesional mast cells which are increased in keloids and decreasing histamine production, which is also increased in keloids. Pressure seems to decrease alpha-macroglobulins, which inhibit collagenase breakdown of collagen. Other possible mechanisms of pressure therapy are a decrease in scar hydration, resulting in mast cell stabilization, and a decrease in neovascularization and extracellular matrix production,[85] or marked hypoxia, which leads to fibroblast and collagen degeneration.

Because pressure therapy is a long-term treatment, patient compliance decreases as the duration of therapy increases.

Ligatures

Ligatures may be used for pedunculated keloids in situations in which surgery is either contraindicated or refused by the patient. A 4-0 nonabsorbable suture is tied tightly around the base of the keloid and a new one is applied every few weeks. The sutures gradually cut into and strangulate the keloid, causing it to fall off. Sometimes the patient requires a few days of pain medication (acetaminophen) after the ligature is applied.

Lasers

The use of lasers to treat keloids has had mixed results.[79] The argon laser was the first used for keloid therapy. It seemed to be successful only in early keloids that were undergoing vascular proliferation; however, more recent studies failed to show any improvement of the keloids treated with the argon laser except an improvement in pruritus and other symptoms over several months.

The carbon dioxide laser, when used as monotherapy, has a 40%–90% recurrence rate which, even if combined with postoperative IL corticosteroids, still has high recurrence rates. Its major use today is to debulk large keloids so they can be treated with other modalities.

The neodymium:yttrium–aluminum–garnet (Nd:YAG) 1064-nm laser seems to affect collagen metabolism; it was selectively inhibited without affecting fibroblast viability or DNA replication.[86] A 3-year follow-up of two of these patients revealed softening, size reduction, and normalization of color, but due to such a small patient sample, these results cannot be extrapolated to a large population of keloid patients. Another study reported improvement of keloids in 16 out of 17 patients treated with the Nd:YAG laser.[87] Unfortunately, no significant follow-up was discussed.

The 585-nm pulse-dye laser has been used to successfully treat sternostomy scars.[88] There was a significant decrease in scar height, pruritus and erythema in most of the laser-treated patients. The results persisted for at least 6 months. Combining IL triamcinolone with the pulse-dye laser increased the effectiveness of keloid therapy.

Silicone Gel-Sheeting

Silicone gel-sheeting is a soft, gel-like covering used to treat keloids. Its mechanism of action appears to be a combination of hydration and occlusion. In addition, transforming growth factor beta-2 may be downregulated when exposed to silicone. Nonsilicone gel dressings showed similar success. The younger the keloid and the patient, the better the response. Children like it because the gel-sheeting is painless. It usually takes 6–12 months of therapy to achieve the best results, but most patients become noncompliant after several months of therapy because of its duration and the inconvenience of cutting and placing the silicone gel-sheeting onto the keloid. To prevent maceration and secondary infection of the covered skin, the gel-sheeting should be worn 22–23 hours a day and removed once daily for cleaning the site and making sure that air gets to the covered site. Most of the sheets last 2–3 weeks and then start degrading.

SKIN DISEASES WITH UNUSUAL PRESENTATIONS IN BLACKS

ATOPIC DERMATITIS

Atopic dermatitis presents with pruritic, scaly, erythematous plaques. In blacks it may present with follicular papules. This seems to be especially common in black children.[89] There appears to be increased follicular response or reactivity in black skin. This is seen in the follicular accentuation of many diseases such as atopic dermatitis, pityriasis rosea, and sarcoidosis.

The distribution involves the extensor surfaces and face in children and flexural accentuation in adolescents and adults. It appears to improve with age and is associated with asthma and allergic rhinitis. Significant postinflammatory hypopigmentation and hyperpigmentation are also seen more commonly in blacks.[89] Many etiologic agents have been identified. Among these are xerosis, foods, change in temperature, dust, and pollen. Treatment includes patient education, proper skin care techniques, topical steroids, antihistamines, and avoidance of mentioned etiologic agents (see also Chapter 2).

Pityriasis Rosea

Pityriasis rosea is a common dermatosis that is preceded by a herald patch, followed by oval, scaly lesions with the typical "collarette of scale." These occur in a Christmas-tree distribution. In blacks, these lesions appear more papular and vesicular.[56] There may also be follicular accentuation, and pityriasis rosea tends to occur in a more inverse distribution (face, neck, axilla, lower abdomen) in blacks as compared to the more truncal distribution that occurs in other skin types. Pityriasis rosea recurs twice as often in blacks (6%) compared with whites (2%–3%).[90] It is usually self-limiting, resolving in an average of 6–9 weeks. It tends to be pruritic, and topical steroids may be used for treatment. Ultraviolet B light therapy may be used in severe cases. This disease tends to resolve with postinflammatory hyperpigmentation in blacks. Administration of intramuscular corticosteroids early in the course of the disease may prevent the postinflammatory hyperpigmentation from becoming marked.

Secondary Syphilis

The differential diagnosis of annular dermatoses of the face includes syphilis, seborrheic dermatoses, and sarcoidosis. The annular form of secondary syphilis is almost exclusively found in blacks.[20] Coin-shaped annular lesions on the face are commonly referred to as "nickels and dimes." There is a predilection for the nose, mouth, nostrils, ears, and eyes (Figure 17.7). Follicular patterns have also been described more commonly in blacks.[90,91] Hyperkeratotic lesions, known as lues cornee, on the palms and soles may also occur.[92]

Sarcoidosis

Sarcoidosis is a granulomatous disease that affects blacks more severely and with greater frequency than other races. In the United States, it occurs in 10–14 per 100,000 whites and 35.5–64 per 100,000 blacks.[93] It has also been shown that black women between the ages of 30 and 39 years have the highest incidence, with 107 per 100,000.[93] The cutaneous presentation of sarcoidosis is protean. Cutaneous findings occur in 25% of cases. Papular sarcoidosis is the most common cutaneous presentation in blacks.[94] Lesions are waxy, red-brown papules, sometimes surrounded by an area of hypopigmentation. These are usually found periorbitally, perinasally, and on the nasolabial folds. Hypopigmented macules and annular lesions are also commonly seen in blacks. There are numerous presentations of cutaneous sarcoidosis, including morpheaform, ulcerative, verrucous, lichenoid, ichthyosiform, scarring and nonscarring alopecia, and hypopigmented lesions. Edematous, violaceous plaques around the nose, lips, and cheeks known as lupus pernio are not usually seen in blacks.[94] Lupus pernio can be very disfiguring and indicates involvement of the respiratory system (Figure 17.1).

There are numerous nonspecific lesions of sarcoidosis, the hallmark of which is erythema nodosum. This presents as tender, nonspecific subcutaneous nodules usually located on the anterior surface of the lower legs. This may be associated with constitutional symptoms. Erythema nodosum is less commonly seen as a presenting sign of sarcoidosis in blacks (2%) compared with whites (13%–31%).[95] There are numerous treatment options including topical, intralesional and systemic corticosteroids, antimalarials, methotrexate, allopurinol, and thalidomide (see also Chapter 7).

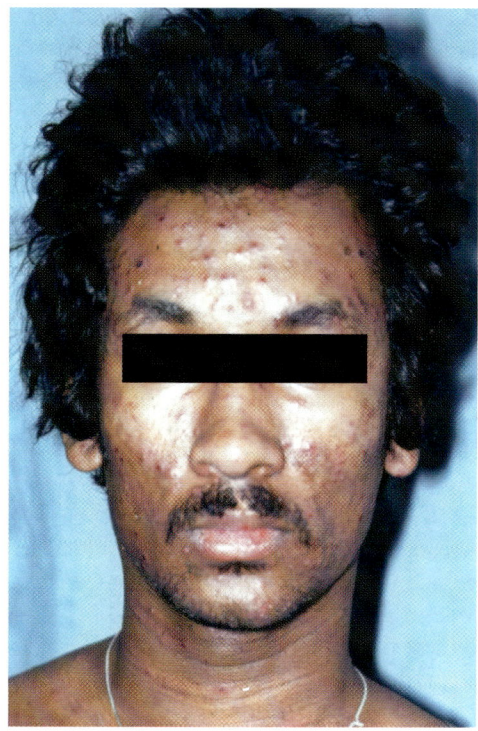

FIGURE 17.7 Papular lesions of secondary syphilis in an Afro-Caribbean.

DISCOID LUPUS ERYTHEMATOSUS

Discoid lupus erythematosus is a form of cutaneous lupus that presents as erythematous, hyperkeratotic, scaly plaques on sun-exposed areas. It is usually seen in young adults, with women affected twice as frequently as men. There may be scale involving the follicular opening in affected plaques. When the edges of these plaques are pulled back, the undersurface may look like that of carpet tacking (carpet-tack sign). Lesions are found on the scalp and areas of the face. In blacks, the conchal bowl of the ears is a common location. The lesions may heal with scarring and hypopigmentation. Squamous cell carcinoma may result in long-standing, nonhealing lesions.[96]

Approximately 95% of patients with discoid lupus erythematosus have disease confined to the skin.[97] Fever may be the first indication of progression to systemic involvement. Evaluation to exclude systemic lupus erythematous should be performed as a baseline in patients diagnosed with discoid lupus erythematosus. Sunscreen use and sun avoidance is critical. Other options include high-potency topical steroids and intralesional corticosteroids. First-line systemic therapy consists of antimalarials. Prednisone, dapsone, thalidomide, and methotrexate can also be used for extensive or disfiguring cutaneous disease (see also Chapter 7).

SYSTEMIC LUPUS ERYTHEMATOSUS

The diagnosis of systemic lupus erythematosus is made by fulfilling the American Rheumatism Association's criteria, which include discoid lupus erythematosus, malar erythema, serositis, nonerosive arthritis, photosensitivity, nephropathy, central nervous system disorder, nephropathy, hematologic disorder, oral ulcers, immunologic disorder, and positive antinuclear antibody. Cutaneous manifestations include the classic malar or butterfly erythematous eruption. Bullous lesions, vascular lesions (telangiectasias, petechiae, and erythema), mucous membrane lesions, and leg ulcers are also seen.

Systemic manifestations include arthralgia, thrombosis, renal involvement, myocarditis, and central nervous system disorders. Blacks appear to have more pronounced systemic involvement than whites. Discoid lesions, nephritis, pneumonitis, and hypocomplementemia have been noted to be more common in blacks.[98] Photosensitivity has been shown to be less commonly seen in blacks, probably because of protection against ultraviolet light by increased melanin in the skin.[99]

The antinuclear antibody test is positive in approximately 95% of patients with SLE.[100] Treatment depends on the severity of the disease. Mild forms may be treated with bed rest and salicylates. As with discoid lupus erythematosus, sunscreen use and sun avoidance are important. More severe cases may be treated with antimalarials, corticosteroids, and immunosuppressive agents (cyclophosphamide, azathioprine, methotrexate) for a steroid-sparing effect (see also Chapter 7).

SCLERODERMA

Scleroderma is defined as sclerosis or hardening of the skin and extracutaneous manifestations. There is a localized and a diffuse form. Both are characterized by smooth, hard areas that appear to be bound down or immobile. Morphea is not common in blacks.[98] Systemic sclerosis or scleroderma, however, does appear to occur with some frequency in blacks. Both hypopigmentation and hyperpigmentation occur in patients with scleroderma. Perifollicular macular hypopigmentation (salt-and-pepper hypopigmentation) is commonly observed on the arms, forearms, trunk, and hands of black patients with scleroderma.[98]

The antinuclear antibody test is positive in greater than 90% of patients with scleroderma.[101] The antinucleolar pattern is considered to be most specific for scleroderma. The anticentromere autoantibody is commonly seen in patients with the CREST variant (calcinosis, Raynaud's phenomenon, esophageal dysmotility, sclerodactyly, telangiectasia) of systemic sclerosis, which is associated with a better prognosis.[102] AntiScl-70 or antitopoisomere I is associated with generalized cutaneous and systemic disease and may indicate a poor prognosis.[103] Reveille et al. performed a study to elucidate the demographic and racial differences in scleroderma-associated antibodies.[103] They discovered that blacks have a lower frequency of anticentromere antibody (4%) than whites (36%). It was also shown that antitopoisomerase I antibodies occurred in 37% of blacks compared to 17% of whites. These data suggest that blacks who have scleroderma are associated with a poor prognosis, as they are more likely than their white counterparts to test positive for the antitopoisomerase antibody.

Treatment options for scleroderma are disappointing. Physical therapy is important as well as massage, warmth, avoidance from trauma, exposure to cold, and smoking avoidance (see also Chapter 7).

SKIN CANCER IN THE BLACK RACES

A more complete review of this subject is presented in Chapter 8.

MELANOMA

Melanoma has not been well documented in blacks. It consists of 1%–3% of all skin cancers. The rate of melanoma in the United States from 1987 to 1988 was 0.9 per 100,000. In whites it is estimated to be 10.9 per 100,000.[104] In blacks and other ethnic groups (Japanese, Hispanics, and Native Americans), it has been found to occur in an acral distribution known as acral lentiginious melanoma. It commonly occurs on the foot in blacks, with 60% having plantar and subungual lesions.[105] This may present as a black macule with irregular borders. The proximal nail fold at the end of a pigmented streak (Hutchinson's sign) may be present. Acral lentiginous melanoma has been reported to have a poor prognosis. The 5-year survival has been reported to be less than

50%.[106] Melanoma in blacks may be more aggressive with a poorer prognosis than in other populations.[96]

BASAL CELL CARCINOMA

Basal cell carcinoma is the most common skin carcinoma in the white population. It is seen much less commonly in blacks because the darker skin pigmentation in blacks allows for greater UVB protection. Blacks with darker pigmentation appear to have a decreased incidence of basal cell carcinoma compared with blacks with lighter pigmentation of skin, as outlined in the Howard University Series.[96] The pigmented type of basal cell carcinoma appears to be more commonly seen in blacks and Asians.[96] Basal cell carcinoma is commonly seen in non-sun-exposed areas of the body, as seen in whites.

SQUAMOUS CELL CARCINOMA

This is the most common type of skin cancer observed in blacks, seen in approximately 33% of one population.[96] It appears to involve non-sun-exposed areas, whereas in whites it involves sun-exposed areas. Squamous cell carcinoma tends to arise in scars, burns, chronic ulcers, infections, and albinism. The mortality rate has been reported to be 29%.[93]

MYCOSIS FUNGOIDES

Mycosis fungoides is a neoplasm of malignant T cells. Over the past few years, there has been increasing evidence that the hypopigmented form is more common in the non-white population.[107] The clinical course of mycosis fungoides appears to be more aggressive in blacks.[96] Some patients have a chronic, eczematous dermatitis for years preceding the diagnosis of mycosis fungoides. This does not appear to be the case, however, for the hypopigmented variant. The risk factors for presenting with the hypopigmented form of mycosis fungoides and the epidemiologic data in blacks have not been clearly defined.

DERMATOFIBROSARCOMA PROTUBERANS

This represents a rare tumor that is sometimes misdiagnosed as a keloid, cyst, or scar in black patients. It presents as firm, erythematous nodules or plaques, usually occurring on the trunk. Dermatofibrosarcoma protuberans is a low-grade tumor that appears to be more common in blacks. It represented approximately 12% of the cases of skin cancer in blacks in the Howard University series.[96] Histologically, pigmented laden cells known as Bednar tumors have been shown to occur more commonly in persons with pigment-laden skin.[99] Treatment consists of surgical removal via the Mohs' technique.

REFERENCES

1. Szabo G, Gerald AB, Pathak MA. Racial differences in the fate of melanosomes in human epidermis. *Nature* 222: 1081, 1969.
2. La Ruche G, Cesarini JP. Histology and physiology of black skin. *Ann Dermatol Venereol* 119(8): 567–574, 1992.
3. Rienertson RP, Wheatley VR. Studies on the chemical composition of human epidermal lipids. *J Invest Dermatol* 32: 49, 1959.
4. Weigand DA, Haygood C, Gaylor JR. Cell layers and density of Negro and Caucasian stratum corneum. *J Invest Dermatol* 62: 563, 1974.
5. Pochi P, Strauss JS. Sebaceous gland activity in black skin. *Dermatol Clin* 6: 349, 1988.

6. Khumalo NP, Doe PT, Dawber RP, Ferguson DJ. What is normal black African hair? A light and scanning electron-microscopic study. *J Am Acad Dermatol* 43: 5, 2000.
7. McMichael AJ, Jackson S. Issues in dermatologic health care delivery in minority populations. *Dermatol Clin* 18: 229–233, 2000.
8. Friedman LC, Bruce S, Weinberg AD, et al. Early detection of skin cancer: racial/ethnic differences in behaviors and attitudes. *J Cancer Educ* 9(2): 105–110, 1994.
9. Powe BD. Cancer fatalism among African-Americans: a review of the literature. *Nurs Outlook*; 46: 18–21, 1996.
10. Webb JA, Friedman LC, Bruce SB, et al. Demographic, psychosocial and objective risk factors related to perceived risk of skin cancer. *J Cancer Educ* 11: 174–177, 1996.
11. Eisenberg DM, Davis RB, Ettner SL, et al. Trends in alternative medicine use in the United States, 1990–1997: results of a follow-up national survey. *JAMA* 280: 1569–1575, 1998.
12. Davis K, Lillie-Blanton M, Lons B, et al. Health care for black Americans: the public sector role. *Milbank Q* 65: 213–247, 1987.
13. Owens SA, Maeyens E, Weary PE. Patients' opinion regarding direct access to dermatologic specialty care. *J Am Acad Dermatol* 36: 250–256, 1997.
14. McMichael AJ. Diagnosis and treatment of cutaneous disorders in African-American patients. *Curr Probl Dermatol* 100: 93–126, 1998.
15. Robinson KD, Kimmel EA, Yasko JM. Reaching out to the African-American community through innovative strategies. *Oncol Nurs Forum* 22: 1383–1391, 1995.
16. James WD, Carter JM, Rodman OG. Pigmentary demarcation lines: a population survey. *J Am Acad Dermatol* 16: 584–590, 1987.
17. Archard HO, Stanley HR. Leukoderma of the oral mucosa: comments on article. *J Am Dent Assoc* 86: 300–301, 1973.
18. White G. Normal skin changes in the black patient. In: Johnson B, Ronald M, White G (Eds) *Ethnic Skin: Medical and Surgical*. Mosby, 1998; 32–40.
19. Odom RB, James WD, Berger TG. Seborrheic dermatitis, psoriasis, recalcitrant palmoplantar eruptions, pustular dermatitis, and erythroderma. In: *Andrew's Diseases of the Skin: Clinical Dermatology*, 9th ed. Philadelphia: Saunders, 2000; 214–218.
20. Mclaurin C. Unusual patterns of common dermatoses in blacks. *Cutis* 32: 352–360, 1983.
21. Martin AG, Kobayashi GS. Yeast infections: candidiasis, pityriasis (tinea) versicolor. In: Freedberg IM, Eisen AZ, Wolff K, Austen KF, Goldsmith CA, Katz SI, Fitzpatrick TB (Eds) *Fitzpatrick's Dermatology in General Medicine*, 5th ed. New York: McGraw-Hill, 1999; 2368–2370.
22. Aljabre SH, Alzayir AA, Abdulghani M, Osman OO. Pigmentary changes of tinea versicolor in dark-skinned patients. *Int J Dermatol* 40: 273–275, 2001.
23. Engasser PG, Maibach HI. Cosmetics and skin care in dermatological practice. In: Freedberg IM, Eisen AZ, Wolff K, Austen KF, Goldsmith CA, Katz SI, Fitzpatrick TB (Eds) *Fitzpatrick's Dermatology in General Medicine*, 5th ed. New York: McGraw-Hill, 1999; 2779.
24. Corbett JF. Hair coloring. *Clin Dermatol* 6: 93–101, 1988.
25. DeLeo VA, Taylor SC, Belsito DV, et al. The effect of race and ethnicity on patch test results. *J Am Acad Dermatol* 46(Suppl): 107–112, 2002.
26. Dawber R. Hair: its structure and response to cosmetic preparations. *Clin Dermatol* 14: 105–112, 1996.
27. Olsen EA. Hair disorders. In: Freedberg IM, Eisen AZ, Wolff K, Austen KF, Goldsmith CA, Katz SI, Fitzpatrick TB (Eds) *Fitzpatrick's Dermatology in General Medicine*, 5th ed. New York: McGraw-Hill, 1999; 732–745.
28. Whiting DA. Structural abnormalities of the hair shaft. *J Am Acad Dermatol* 16: 1–25, 1987.
29. Halder RM. Pseudofolliculits barbae and related disorders. *Dermatol Clin* 6: 407–411, 1988.
30. Alexander AM, Delph WI. Pseudofolliculitis barbae in the military: a medical, administrative, and social problem. *J Natl Med Assoc* 66: 459–469, 1974.
31. Brauner GJ, Flandermeyer KL. Pseudofolliculitis barbae; medical consequences of interracial friction in the U.S. Army. *Cutis* 32: 373–375, 1983.
32. Garcia RL, Henderson R. The adjustable rotary electric razor in the control of pseudofolliculitis barbae. *J Assoc Milit Dermatol* 4: 28, 1978.
33. Alexander AM. Evaluation of foil-guarded shaver in the management of pseudofolliculitis barbae. *Cutis* 27: 534–542, 1981.

34. Brauner GJ, Flandermeyer KL. Pseudofolliculitis 2: treatment. *Int J Dermatol* 16: 520–525, 1977.
35. Steggerda M. Cross section of human hair from four racial groups. *J Hered* 31: 475, 1940.
36. Strauss JS, Kligman AM. Pseudofolliculitis of the beard. *Arch Dermatol* 74: 533–542, 1956.
37. Pinkus H. Chronic scarring pseudofolliculitis of the negro beard. *Arch Dermatol* 47: 782–792, 1943.
38. Greenbaum SC. Folliculitis barbae traumatica. *Arch Dermatol* 32: 237–241, 1935.
39. Brown LA. Pathogenesis and treatment of pseudofolliculitis barbae. *Cutis* 32: 373–375, 1983.
40. Alexander AM. Pseudofolliculitis diatheses. *Arch Dermatol* 109: 729, 1974.
41. Hall JC, Gowtz CS, Bartholome CS, et al. Pseudofolliculitis-revised concepts of diagnosis and treatment: report of three cases in women. *Cutis* 23: 799–800, 1979.
42. Montgomery R. *Dermatopathology*. New York: Harper and Row, 1967.
43. Halder RM. Hair and scalp disorders in blacks. *Cutis* 32: 378–380, 1983.
44. Pinkus H. Mehregen A. *A Guide to Dermatohistopathology*. New York: Appleton-Century Crofts, 1969.
45. Dunn JF. Pseudofollicutis barbae. *Am Fam Physician* 38: 407–412, 1988.
46. Rogers CJ, Glaser PA. Treatment of pseudofolliculitis barbae using the Q-switched Nd:YAG laser with topical carbon suspension. *Dermatol Surg* 26: 737–742, 2000.
47. Cook-Bolden FE, Barba A, Halder RM, Taylor S. Twice daily benzoyl peroxide/clindamycin gel versus placebo in the treatment of pseudofolliculitis barbae. *Cutis* 76(6 Suppl): 18–24, 2004.
48. Halder RM. The role of retinoids in the management of cutaneous conditions in blacks. *J Am Acad Dermatol* 39: S98–S103, 1998.
49. Taylor S. Tazarotene in the treatment of pseudofolliculitis barbae in patients with skin of color: an investigator-masked, split-face, placebo-controlled, parallel-group study. Poster presented at American Academy of Dermatology meeting. July 31–August 4.
50. Perricone NV. Treatment of pseudofolliculitis barbae with topical glycolic acid: a report of 2 studies. *Cutis* 52: 232–235, 1993.
51. Perry PK, Cook-Bolden FE, Rahman Z, et al. Defining pseudofolliculitis barbae in 2001: a review of the literature and current trends. *J Am Acad Dermatol Surg* 26: 737–742, 2000.
52. Crutchfield CE. Treatment of pseudofolliculitis barbae using the Q-switched Nd:YAG laser with topical carbon suspension.
53. Ross EV, Cooke LM, Timko AL, Overstreet KA, et al. Treatment of pseudofolliculitis barbae in skin types IV, V, and VI with a long-pulsed neodynium:yttrium aluminum garnet laser. *J Am Acad Dermatol* 47: 263–270, 2002.
54. Kauvar AN. Treatment of pseudofolliculitis with a pulsed infrared laser. *Arch Dermatol* 136: 1343–1346, 2000.
55. Yamauchi PS, Kelly AP, Lask GP. Treatment of pseudofolliculitis barbae with the diode laser. *J Cutan Ther* 1: 109–111, 1999.
56. Lang PG Jr. Dermatoses in African-Americans. *Dermatol Nurs* 12(2): 87–90, 2000.
57. Halder RM, Young CM. New and emerging therapies for vitiligo. *Dermatol Clin* 1988; 6(3): 79–89, 2000.
58. Johnson BJ. Differences in skin type. In: Johnson B, Ronald M, White G (Eds) *Ethnic Skin: Medical and Surgical*. Mosby, 1998; 3–4.
59. Grimes PE. Melasma. Etiologic and therapeutic considerations. *Arch Dermatol* 131: 1453–1457, 1995.
60. Kimbrough-Green CK, Griffith CE, Finkel LJ, et al. Topical retinoic acid (tretinoin) for melasma in black patients. A vehicle-controlled clinical trial. *Arch Dermatol* 130: 727–733, 1994.
61. Breathnach AS. Melanin hyperpigmentation of skin: melasma, topical treatment with azelaic acid, and other therapies. *Cutis* 57 (Suppl): 36–45, 1996.
62. Halder RM. The role of retinoids in the management of cutaneous conditions in blacks. *J Am Acad Dermatol* 39: S98–S103, 1998.
63. Escarmant P, Zimmerman S, Amar A, et al. The treatment of 783 keloid scars by iridium 192 interstitial irradiation after surgical excision. *Int J Radiat Oncol Biol Phys* 26: 245–251, 1993.
64. Berman B, Flores F. Recurrence rates of excised keloids treated with post-operative triamcinolone acetonide injections or interferon alfa-2b injections. *J Am Acad Dermatol* 137: 755–757, 1997.
65. McCoy BJ, Diegelmann RF, Cohen JK. *In vitro* inhibition of cell growth, collagen synthesis and prolyl hydroxylase activity by triamcinolone acetonide. *Proc Soc Exp Biol Med* 163: 216–222, 1980.
66. Jimenez SA, Freundlich B, Rosenbloom J. Selective inhibition of human diploid fibroblast collagen synthesis by interferons. *J Clin Invest* 74: 1112–1116, 1984.

67. Fitzpatrick RE. Treatment of inflamed hypertrophic scars using intralesional 5-FU. *Dermatol Surg* 25: 224–232, 1999.
68. Berman B, Kaufman J. Pilot study of the effect of postoperative imiquimod 5% cream on the recurrence rate of excised keloids. *J Am Acad Dermatol Venereol* 47 (Suppl): S209–S211, 2002.
69. Bodokh I, Brun P. The treatment of keloids with intralesional bleomycin. *Ann Dermatol Venereol* 123: 791–794, 1996.
70. Kim A, DiCarlo J, Cohen C, et al. Are keloids really "gliloids"? High level expression of gli-1 oncogene in keloids. *J Am Acad Dermatol* 45: 707–711, 2001.
71. Peacock EE. Pharmacologic control of surface scarring in human beings. *Ann Surg* 193: 592–597, 1981.
72. Soderberg T, Hallmans T, Bartholson L. Treatment of keloids and hytrophic scars with adhesive zinc tape. *Scand J Plast Reconstr Surg* 16: 261–266, 1982.
73. De Limpens J. The local treatment of hypertrophic scars and keloids with topical retinoic acid. *Br J Dermatol* 103: 319–323, 1980.
74. Lawrence WT. Treatment of earlobe keloids with surgery plus adjuvant intralesional verapamil and pressure earrings. *Ann Plast Surg* 37: 167–169, 1996.
75. Duncan JL, Thomson AW, Muir LFK. Topical cyclosporin and T-lymphocytes in keloid scars. *Br J Dermatol* 124: 109, 1991.
76. Schorn D, Francis MJD, London M, et al. Skin collagen biosynthesis in patients with rheumatoid arthritis treated with penicillamine. *Scand J Rheumatol* 8: 124, 1979.
77. Unemori EN, Amento EP. Relaxin modulates synthesis and secretion of procollagenase and collagen by human dermal fibroblasts. *J Biochem* 265: 10681–10685, 1990.
78. Darzi MA, Choudii NA, Kaul SK, et al. Evaluation of various methods of treating keloids and hypertrophic scars: a 10-year follow-up study. *Br J Plast Surg* 45: 374, 1992.
79. Kelly AP. Medical and surgical therapies for keloids. *Dermatol Ther* 17: 212–218, 2004.
80. Rusciani L, Rosse G, Bono R. Use of cryotherapy in the treatment of keloids. *J Dermatol Surg Oncol* 19: 529–534, 1993.
81. Ceilley RI, Barin RW. The combined use of cryosurgery and intralesional injections of suspension of fluorinated adrenocorticosteroids for reducing keloids and hypertrophic scars. *J Dermatol Surg Oncol* 5: 54, 1979.
82. Borok TL, Bray M, Sinclair I, et al. Role of ionizing irradiation for 393 keloids. *Int J Radiat Oncol Biol Phys* 15: 836–870, 1998.
83. Hoffman S. Radiotherapy for keloids? *Ann Plast Surg* 9: 205, 1982.
84. Guix B, Henriquez I, Andres A, et al. Treatment of keloids by high-dose-rate brachytherapy: a seven year study. *Int J Radiat Oncol Biol Phys* 50: 167–172, 2001.
85. Baur PS, Larson L, Stacey TR, et al. Burn scar changes associated with pressure. In: Lengacie JJ (Ed) *The Ultrastructure of Collagen*. Springfield: Charles C. Thomas, 1976: 369–376.
86. Abergel RP, Merke CA, Lam TS, et al. Control of connective tissue metabolism by lasers: recent developments and future prospects. *J Am Acad Dermatol* 11: 1142, 1984.
87. Sherman R, Rosenfield H. Experience with the Nd:YAG laser in the treatment of keloidal scars. *Ann Plast Surg* 21: 231–235, 1988.
88. Alster TS, Williams CM. Treat of keloid sternostomy scars with 585 nm flashlamp-pumped laser. *Lancet* 345: 1198–2000, 1995.
89. Mclaurin C. Pediatric dermatology in black patients. *Cutis* 32: 369–371, 1983.
90. Mclaurin C. Unusual patterns of common dermatoses in blacks. *Cutis* 32: 352–360, 1983.
91. Abell E, Marks R, Wilson-Jones E. Secondary syphilis: a clinicopathological review. *Br J Dermatol* 93: 53, 1975.
92. Connolly C, Bikowski J. Syphilis. In: *Dermatological Atlas of Black Skin*. Merit Publishing International, 1998; 73.
93. English JC III, Patel PJ, Greer JE. Sarcoidosis. *J Am Acad Dermatol* 44: 725–743.
94. Minus HR, Grimes PE. Cutaneous manifestations of sarcoidosis in blacks. *Cutis* 32: 361–363, 372, 1983.
95. Caruthers B Jr, Day TB, Minus HR, Young RC. Sarcoidosis: a comparison of cutaneous manifestations with chest radiographic changes. *J Natl Med Assoc* 67(5): 364–367, 1975.

96. Halder RM, Bang KM. Skin cancer in African-Americans in the US. *Dermatol Clin* 6(3): 397–407, 1988.
97. Norton SA, Chesser RS. Sarcoidosis in pseudofolliculitis barbae. *Mil Med* 156: 369–71, 1991.
98. White G. Common diseases in the darker-skinned adult. In Johnson B, Ronald M, White G (Eds) *Ethnic Skin: Medical and Surgical.* Mosby, 1998; 43–120.
99. Odom RB, James WD, Berger TG. Seborrheic dermatitis, psoriasis, recalcitrant palmoplantar eruptions, pustular dermatitis, and erythroderma. In: *Andrew's Diseases of the Skin: Clinical Dermatology*, 9th ed. Philadelphia: Saunders, 2000; 214–218.
100. Odom RB, James WD, Berger TG. Connective tissue diseases. In: *Andrew's Diseases of the Skin: Clinical Dermatology*, 9th ed. Philadelphia: Saunders, 2000; 172–204.
101. Provost TT, Watson R, Simmons-O'Brien E. Significance of the anti Ro(SS-A) antibody in evaluation of patients with cutaneous manifestations of a connective tissue disease. *J Am Acad Dermatol* 32: 49, 1959.
102. Steen VD, Powell DL, Medsger TA Jr. Clinical correlations and prognosis based on serum autoantibodies in patients with systemic sclerosis. *Arthritis Rheum* 31: 196–201, 1988.
103. Reveille JD, Durban E, Goldstein R, et al. Racial differences in the frequencies of scleroderma-related autoantibodies. *Arthritis Rheum* 35(2): 216–218, 1992.
104. Weinstock MA. Epidemiology of melanoma. *Cancer Treat Res* 65: 29–56, 1993.
105. Odom RB, James WD, Berger TG. Melanocytic nevi and neoplasms. In: *Andrew's Diseases of the Skin: Clinical Dermatology*, 9th ed. Philadelphia: Saunders, 2000.
106. Taberi DP, Narurkar B, Moy RL. Skin cancer. In: Johnson B, Ronald M, White G (Eds) *Ethnic Skin: Medical and Surgical.* Mosby, 1998; 8–15.
107. Whitmore SE, Simmons-O'Brien E, Rotter FS. Hypopigmented mycosis fungoides. *Arch Dermatol* 130: 476–480, 1994.

18 Dermatologic Disease in Hispanics/Latinos

Miguel Sanchez

INTRODUCTION

Although routinely merged into a single demographic group, Latinos, in fact, constitute a highly diversified multiracial and intermixed ethnicity of persons from European, African, and Native American ancestries with a variegated spectrum of skin colors.[1] Mestizos, Latinos of European and Native American extraction, and their descendants constitute a majority of the populations of Mexico, and several countries in Central and South America. In contrast, mulattos, Latinos of African and European descent, predominate in Caribbean countries. Notwithstanding differences among subgroups, Latinos are unified by a common language, cultural traditions, historical similarities, and religious beliefs.[1]

The rapid expansion of the Latino population, fueled by an unprecedented ingress of immigration, has already established the United States as the fourth-largest Spanish-speaking country in the world. By the year 2000, the Latino population in this country had catapulted by 58% to 38 million from the 22.4 million recorded in 1990 and, according to U.S. Census projections, in 2050, 25% of the country's population will be Hispanic.[2,3] Currently, Hispanics constitute the largest minority group in the United States.

CULTURAL ASPECTS OF SKIN DISEASE

Success in providing effective health care may hinge on understanding a patient's culture.[4] Typically, the effects of acculturation escalate with each subsequent generation, but offshoot generations of Latinos have continued to embrace and to be influenced by the Hispanic culture's beliefs and values.[4] Notably, acculturation is not necessarily associated with improved health status.[5] The rates of obesity, diabetes, osteoporosis, and cardiovascular disease among Mexican-Americans surge after the native diet is modified by greater consumption of foods high in fats and refined sugars and coupled with a plunge in physical activity. Indeed, recent reports are revising the often-quoted conjectures associated with the "Hispanic Paradox," an observation that despite lower socioeconomic status and impeding barriers to health care, Latinos have favorable health outcomes and lower mortality levels.[5]

Collectively, Latinos trail the general population in income, education, and access to health care insurance. These disparities, in turn, influence their risk of developing disease, reaction to illness, and health promotion practices.[6] Approximately 38% of the Latino population live at a standard below the poverty level. Immigrants often have to settle for low-paying jobs that increase their exposure to occupational and environmental hazards.[7] Barriers to health care among low-income Latinos include language, poverty, lack of insurance, inadequate transportation, fear of deportation, illiteracy, and loss of pay from missed work.[7] Delays in seeking medical care may also result from prevalent pessimistic attitudes (*fatalismo*) and a sense of resigned hopelessness which was immortalized in the once popular song "Que será, será." Fatalismo is kindled by the belief, still held by many devout Latinos, that illness is a punishment for sinful or wrongful thoughts and deeds, which requires resignation to divine intervention, pious bargaining, acts of repentance, and redemption through suffering (*religiosidad*). Also, a culturally sanctioned devotion to the needs of other family members (*familismo*) may prevent patients with home responsibilities from compliance with scheduled appointments.[8]

Latinos regard physicians as authority figures deserving of deference and admiration (*respeto*). Conversely, Latinos expect providers not only to treat them with consideration and respect (*simpatia*) but also to foster an involved, personal relationship (*personalismo*).[9] After a close physician–patient relationship has been established, patients may act toward the physician as a friend or family member bestowing signs of affection and even addressing the physician by the first name (*familiarismo*). Customarily, Latinos expect that a physician will be able to provide them with a diagnosis without lengthy questioning or batteries of tests and that treatments will be rapidly effective in alleviating symptoms.[8]

Central to the factors that shape the concept of health for many Latinos, especially those with lower educational levels, is the belief that wellness is the absence of symptoms. Such a view clashes with attempts to deliver preventive medical care and to reduce the high rates of emergency room use reported in many studies.[6] Treatment may be discontinued as soon as symptoms or clinical findings resolve. Unless such issues are directly addressed, some patients will not fully comply with their therapeutic plan and will disregard the insistence of the medical practitioner to continue treatment or schedule visits.[10] However, lack of compliance also stems from inability to afford treatment or miss work days and other obstacles previously mentioned.[8] A popular opinion is that symptoms originate from internal organic, especially sanguinous, dysfunction. Therefore, some patients may consider evaluation of a skin eruption to be incomplete without blood tests and may prefer injections, which deliver the therapeutic drug internally, to topical medications.[10] On the other hand, considerable apprehension, anxiety, and resistance usually follow prescription of self-administered injections of medications such as insulin or interferon.

In general, Latinos uphold a holistic interpretation of health and disease, which integrates somatic, physiological, psychological, spiritual, moral, social, and metaphysical elements.[10] An inherent factor in understanding Latinos' cultural reaction to illness is the patronage of lay healers, a practice that is nearly always concealed from physicians.[11] One study reported that 51% of Latinos self-treated, 32% sought medical care, and 17% visited folk healers. A survey from Denver found that 29% of 409 Latino patients reported visiting a curandero (healer), including 18.5% of those born in this country.[12] Integrative health care, a relatively new concept in Western medicine, has been practiced for centuries by Latinos who alternate between alternative and allopathic health care.[13] Latino ethnomedicine consisting of use of herbs and botanical remedies remains a popular treatment for a variety of symptoms (Table 18.1).[14] Some Mexicans and Central Americans seek the advise of a curandera(o), a person who practices a synergetic system that integrates Aztec medical and spiritual influences with Christian practices.[12] Curandera subspecialists include sobaderas (masseurs), yerberas (herbalists), and parteras (midwives). Through treatments that include prayer rituals, cleansings with incense, lemon and eggs, aromatic baths, rubbings, and herbs, these lay healers strive to restore health by bringing the body, mind, and spirit into harmony with the environment. Changing with the times, modern curanderismo has evolved to incorporate not only African and Asian influences but also homeopathic treatments and even allopathic medicine.[15] Recommended herbs, oils, candles, and other folk remedies are purchased at specialized neighborhood or Internet stores (*botánicas*).[16] In contrast, patients from some Caribbean countries are more inclined to visit a santero (a), a priest(ess) ordained in santería, a syncretic idolatry that fuses elements from African and Catholic religions. Santeros reputedly heal through rituals, spells, amulets, baths, oils, herbs, and animal sacrifices that procure the intervention of deities (*orishas*) in reversing misfortune and preventing or nullifying the effect of hexes.[17] Although largely underground, the number of santería believers in this country has been reported to be between 500,000 to 5 million.[18] The appeal of both curanderismo and santería rests on their connection with nature

TABLE 18.1
Ethnomedical Treatments of Skin Disease

Condition	Treatment
Acne	Hot pack with crushed rosemary
Abscess	Poultice of oats, milk, honey, and lemon juice
Conjunctivitis	Chamomile drops
Bites	Salt
Burns	Zabila (aloe vera), pork lard, butter, raw onion, toothpaste, egg whites, cooked beans
Calluses	Garlic and honey paste under occlusion
Flushing	Teas of passion flowers (*pasionara*), linden (*tilia*), *zapote blanco* (usually for hypertension)
Insect stings	Crushed garlic in oil
Impetigo	Poultice of bath soap and sugar, Usnea lichen (Spanish moss) tincture
Pruritic eruptions	Corn starch, alcohol rubs, baking soda in water, lemon juice, arnica, oatmeal powder, watermelon shell rubs, frequent baths
Tinea pedis	Urine, garlic powder
Varicella	Tronadora (Trumpet flowers), Damiana
Wounds	Clean with lemon juice, Zabila (aloe vera), raw onions

and stress of emotional and spiritual healing to achieve physical recuperation.[19] Most folk cures are harmless and, at worst, only delay initiation of more effective treatment, but some remedies such as greta and azarcon, which are administered for empacho (gastrointestinal illness) and contain lead, can be harmful.[20]

SKIN DISEASES

The prevalences of skin diseases in the Latino population mirror those within the general population.[21] A comparison of Latino patients with skin diseases treated publicly in a city hospital clinic vs. a private practice showed only minor differences in the frequency of the most frequently encountered diagnoses (Table 18.2).[21] Not surprisingly, eczema and acne were the top diagnoses. The high number of cases in the urban faculty practice group seeking cosmetic care for photoaging reflects the more financially upscale patient population. Except for a handful of diseases that will be discussed, variations in skin disease rates and presentation among Latino subgroups reflect demographic characteristics and customs. The salient distinguishing factor of skin diseases in Latinos is a proclivity to long-lasting, disfiguring pigmentary alteration induced by inflammatory responses, injury, or hormonal effects.[22]

PIGMENTARY DISORDERS

Postinflammatory Hyperpigmentation

Increased pigmentation following cutaneous inflammation is nearly universal among Latinos with IV–VI skin types and is also common in those with lighter olive complexions. Maintenance of constitutive and facultative pigmentation depends on the amount and composition of epidermal melanin, the size of melanosomes, and other unelucidated mechanisms, such as dispersion of melanin.[23] The amount of epidermal melanin in lightly pigmented Mexican skin types is approximately half whereas in the most darkly pigmented African skin types, while Mexican melanosome size trails African and Indian but surpasses Chinese and European.[23]

Hyperpigmentation often develops during active stages of common skin diseases, such as nummular eczema, contact dermatitis, seborrheic dermatitis, acne, tinea, and lichen planus (Figure 18.1).

TABLE 18.2
Dermatologic Diagnoses in Latino Patients

Treated in a Dermatology Private Practice
($n = 1000$)

Acne	20.7%
Eczema/contact dermatitis	19.3%
Photoaging	16.8%
Tinea/onychomycosis	9.9%
Facial melasma	8.2%
Condyloma/warts	7.1%
Hyperpigmentation	6%
Seborrheic keratosis	4.5%
Acrochordons	4.2%
Seborrheic dermatitis	3.2%
Alopecia	2.3%
Psoriasis	0.8%

Treated in a Hospital-Based Clinic ($n = 2000$)

Eczema/contact dermatitis	20.1%
Condyloma/warts	17.5%
Acne	12.3%
Tinea/onychomycosis	9.3%
Pyoderma	8.8%
Hyperpigmentation	7.5%
Seborrheic dermatitis	7.2%
Psoriasis	5.5%
Facial melasma	4.1%
Pruritus	2.3%
Drug eruptions	1.9%
Acrochordons	1.1%

However, most inflammatory dermatological diseases, as well as self-induced (excoriations, rubbing) and accidentally injurious (abrasions, burns) lesions, stimulate melanin synthesis or incontinence. Notably, pigmentation can worsen or arise after the lesions appear to be clinically healed. In darker skin shades, erythema associated with inflammation may be subtle or unapparent. In addition, inflammation that can sustain melanogenesis in pigmented prone skin is pathologically present for weeks after a lesion has visually resolved. For these reasons, continued use of topical anti-inflammatory therapy may need to be continued beyond clinical resolution of lesions and bleaching agents should be administered as soon as progressive pigmentation is observed. Ultraviolet light worsens and perpetuates the pigmentation, so sun protection with clothing and sunblocks is essential. Untreated, pigmentation can persist for several months, especially if there is a dermal component. One of the more baffling challenges for dermatologists is distinguishing among pigmentary disorders. Too often a diagnosis of postinflammatory pigmentation, decisively the predominant cause of pigmented patches, is reached without consideration of other diseases associated with hyperpigmentation, such as drug-induced pigmentation, phototoxic reactions, idiopathic eruptive macular pigmentation, and lichen planus pigmentosus.[24] Conversely, a diagnosis of ashy dermatosis is not uncommonly bestowed on Latino patients with postinflammatory pigmentation or fixed drug reactions with gray-brown colored lesions. A slate-gray color denotes only the presence of melanin deep in the dermis and is not diagnostic of any particular disease in persons with type IV–V skin types.

Dermatologic Disease in Hispanics/Latinos

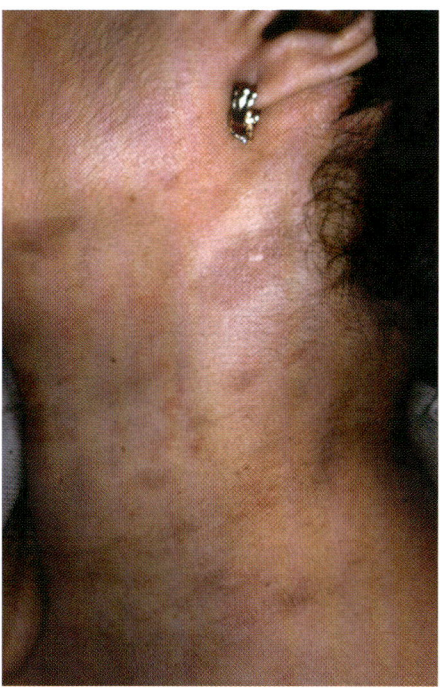

FIGURE 18.1 Brown, well-demarcated patches caused by postinflammatory pigmentation persisting after resolution of an eczematous dermatitis.

Erythema Dyschromicum Perstans

Widely known as ashy dermatosis due to the slate-gray color of the lesions, erythema dyschromicum perstans (EDP) is an acquired cutaneous disease that consists of nonpruritic, oval, polycyclic, irregularly shaped patches of varying sizes that are often symmetrically distributed on the trunk, extremities, and neck (Figures 18.2 and 18.3). The borders of early lesions are faintly erythematous

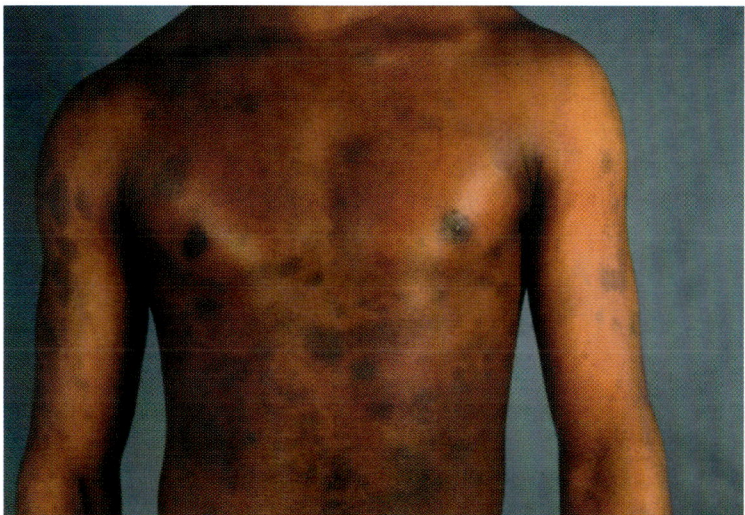

FIGURE 18.2 Ash-colored, polycyclic, irregular, symmetrically distributed patches of varying sizes on the trunk of a man with erythema dyschromicum perstans. Some of the patches still have erythematous borders.

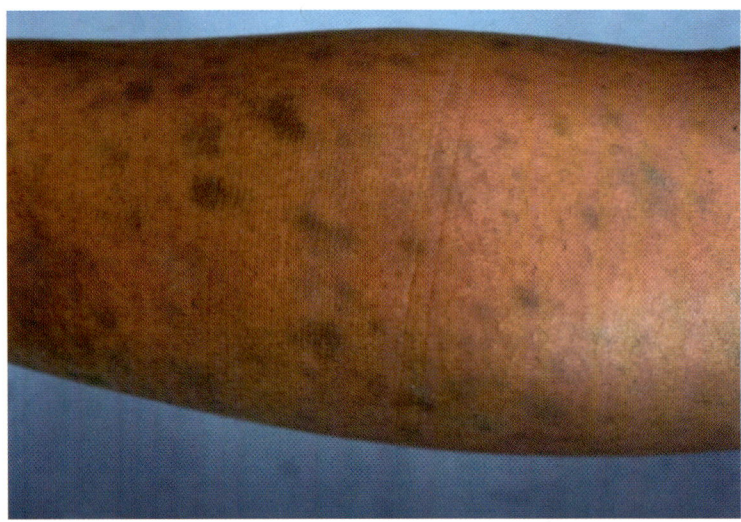

FIGURE 18.3 Discrete gray-brown macules and patches on the forearm of another man with erythema dyschromicum perstans.

and slightly raised features that greatly aid diagnosis. The ash-colored patches persist indefinitely. Contrary to lesions of postinflammatory pigmentation, the patches expand. The diagnosis is facilitated if the histopathologic changes in the border of a plaque are hyperkeratosis, a thinned epidermis, hydropic degeneration of the basal layer, pigment incontinence, and a perivascular lymphohistiocytic infiltrate. Hyperpigmented patches show nondiagnostic changes such as increased pigmentation of the basal layer of the epidermis and a mild perivascular lymphohistiocytic infiltrate with melanophages and pigmentary incontinence in the papillary dermis. Expression of intercellular adhesion molecule-1 HLA-DR in the keratinocyte basal cell layer in affected skin resolves after treatment with clofazimine.[25]

In some cases, EDP may represent a reaction to an ingested or a topically applied chemical, but the vast majority of cases are idiopathic. Contact with the pesticide chlorothalonil was implicated as the cause in Panamanian field workers with positive patch tests.[26] Other reported causes include ingestion of ammonium nitrate, orally administered radiographic contrast media, and an occupationally associated cobalt allergy in one plumber. Some cases presumed to be associated with an intestinal nematode infection resolved after antiparasitic therapy.[27]

The most promising treatment is clofazimine. In one study, seven out of eight patients had good to excellent response. In these patients, clofazimine was initiated at a dose of 100 mg daily in patients who weighed more than 40 kg and 100 mg every other day to those who weighed less. After 3 months, the medication was reduced to 400 mg and 200 mg per week, respectively.[28] Others have reported satisfactory but not curative results with this treatment in early cases. There are sporadic reports of patients responding to corticosteroids administered orally or by intramuscular injection, and this treatment is favored by some Latin American physicians.[27]

Lichen Planus Actinicos

Also known as lichen planus tropicus, lichen planus subtropicus, and summertime actinic lichenoid dermatitis, lichen planus actinicus (Figure 18.4) preferentially affects children and young adults. In Latino patients, this condition is often misdiagnosed as ashy dermatosis, which accounts for the few reported cases in the English medical journals. The lesions develop predominantly but not exclusively on sun-exposed areas during spring and summer and remit in the winter. Lesions can,

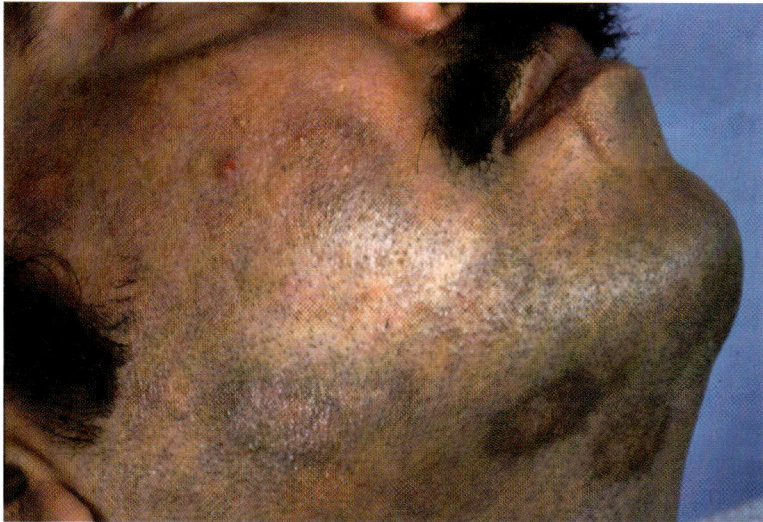

FIGURE 18.4 Annular plaques that become pigmented following exposure to sunlight on the face of a man. The biopsy showed features of lichen planus actinicus.

but do not usually, involve the oral mucosa. Three variants — annular, dyschromic, and pigmented — have been described. The most common presentation is an eruption of erythematous, pigmented, annular plaques. An eruption consisting of discrete and confluent hypopigmented polygonal papules characterizes the dyschromic form. The pigmented type consists of the appearance of hyperpigmented patches that may be diffuse or confined to the face. All variants result in inveterate pigmentation. In addition to the histopathology of lichen planus, there is significant pigment incontinence. Systemic and topical corticosteroids, hydroxychloroquine, and acitretin have been reported to be effective.[29,30]

LICHEN PLANUS PIGMENTOSUS

Lichen planus pigmentosus consists of brownish-black macules or patches, with no active borders predominantly present on the face and intertriginous folds, usually the axillae (Figure 18.5). Idiopathic eruptive macular pigmentation is characterized by asymptomatic brown macules, and occasionally patches, on the trunk, face, neck, and proximal extremities.[31] A key feature is nearly exclusive presence in children and adolescents. It has been suggested that this entity is a pigmented form of pityriasis rosea. Histopathologic changes consist of an intact epidermis with increased pigmentation of the basal layer and a superficial, perivascular lymphohistiocytic infiltrate with melanophages and pigmentary incontinence. The lesions resolve spontaneously over several months to years.[32]

PRURIGO PIGMENTOSA

Prurigo pigmentosa is an idiopathic, recurrent eruption on the back, neck, and chest. The lesions are symmetrically distributed, pruritic, urticarial papules and papulovesicles that resolve with reticulate pigmentation. Spongiosis, ballooning, necrotic keratinocytes, and vacuolar dermoepidermal alteration are characteristic pathologic findings. The infiltrate consists predominantly of neutrophils initially and eosinophils and lymphocytes subsequently. Dapsone or minocycline may be effective.[33]

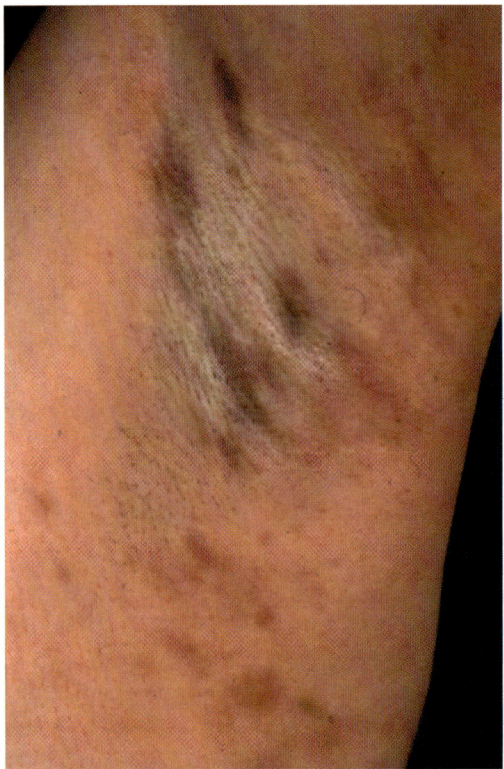

FIGURE 18.5 The axilla is a common area of involvement in lichen planus pigmentosus inversus.

MACULAR AMYLOIDOSIS

The lesions of macular amyloidosis are exceedingly pruritic patches with a characteristically rippled pattern of pigmentation present most commonly on the back and extremities (Figure 18.6). Chronic rubbing results in the development of lichenified plaques (lichen amyloidois). Most cases are sporadic but some are inherited.[34] The amyloid is derived from cytokeratins from epidermal cells that have undergone apoptotic necrosis. Histopathologic changes consist of hyperkeratosis, keratinocyte degeneration, satellite cell necrosis, basal cell destruction, amyloid deposition (best visualized with Congo red stain) in the dermal papillae, and a superficial dermal perivascular lymphohistiocytic infiltrate with melanophages. Topical class I or intralesional corticosteroids remain the treatment of choice. Systemic corticosteroids or cyclosporine may be indicated for widespread cases.

DRUG-INDUCED PIGMENTATION

Drug-induced pigmentation can be caused by a wide variety of medications (Figure 18.7). The most common drugs causing patchy pigmentation of the skin are minocycline and thiazides. Fixed drug eruption is most frequently caused by trimethoprim, acetaminophen, phenolphthalein, barbiturates, ampicillin, aspirin, quinine, chlordiazepoxide, and nonsteroidal anti-inflammatory agents. Photoinduced pigmentation can be caused by amiodarone, phenothiazines, sulfonamides, doxycycline, tetracycline, desipramine, imipramine, thiazides, and phenformin. Pigmentation from antimalarials, clofazimine, busulphan, cyclophosphamide, fluorouracil, and hydroxyurea is diffuse. Bleomycin produces flagellate melanosis (Figure 18.8).

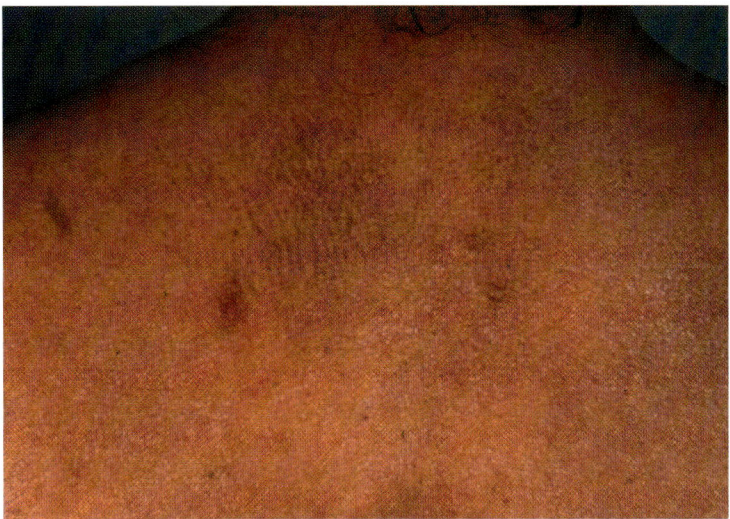

FIGURE 18.6 Upper back of a woman with lichen amyloidosis, showing excoriations and the characteristic rippled pattern of pigmentation.

FIGURE 18.7 In Latinos with darker skin shades, drug eruptions often cause widespread hyperpigmentation.

Melasma

Considering its high prevalence in the Latino population, it is not surprising that melasma is one of the skin conditions for which Latinos seek dermatologic care, even ahead of African-Americans

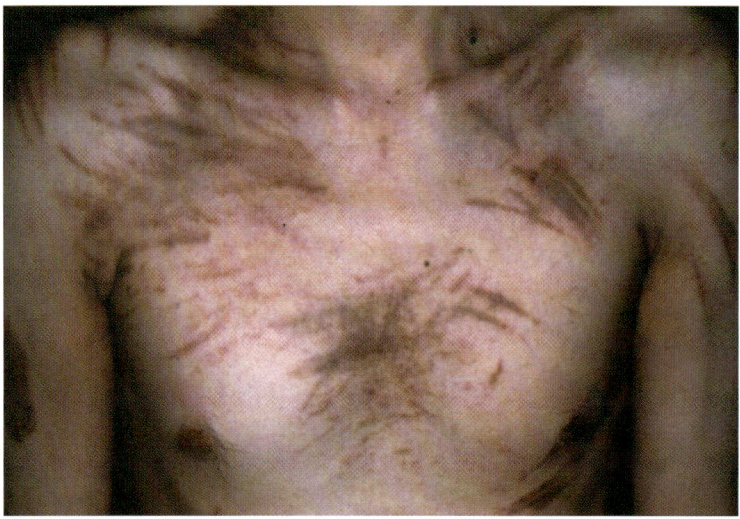

FIGURE 18.8 Flagellate hyperpigmented patches following intravenous administration of bleomycin could be misdiagnosed as self-induced psychocutaneous disorder.

and Asians.[21] As many as half of all Mexican women develop melasma during their pregnancies.[21] Indeed, the affinity for evenly colored complexion has propelled an industry that blankets television programming, web sites, and magazines with ads for over-the-counter creams that promise rapid disappearance of "las manchas" (stains). The most important factors in the development of melasma are pregnancy, oral contraceptives, ultraviolet light exposure, genetic effects, and possibly cosmetic use.[22] The characteristic findings are nearly symmetrical, uniformly irregular, sharply demarcated tan-brown to gray macules and patches on the forehead, nose, cheeks, mustache area and chin (*centrofacial type*), cheeks and nose (*malar type*), or ramus of the mandible (*mandibular type*) (Figures 18.9 and 18.10). Less commonly, lesions also develop on the anterior chest, upper back, and the photoexposed sides of the arms.

The malar and centrofacial clinical variants predominate in all ages, whereas the mandibular type is more common in middle-aged patients. In a study of Puerto Rican women with mandibular melasma, the onset of the pigmentation occurred at an average age of 44 years.[35] Not only is this condition worsened by exposure to ultraviolet light but photodamage also appears to be an important etiologic factor. Patients with mandibular melasma are more prone to having melanophages or

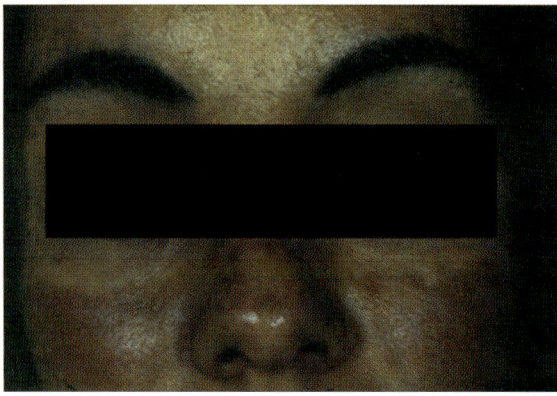

FIGURE 18.9 Symmetrical, sharply demarcated brown patches limited to the bridge of the nose and cheeks in a woman with the malar type of melasma.

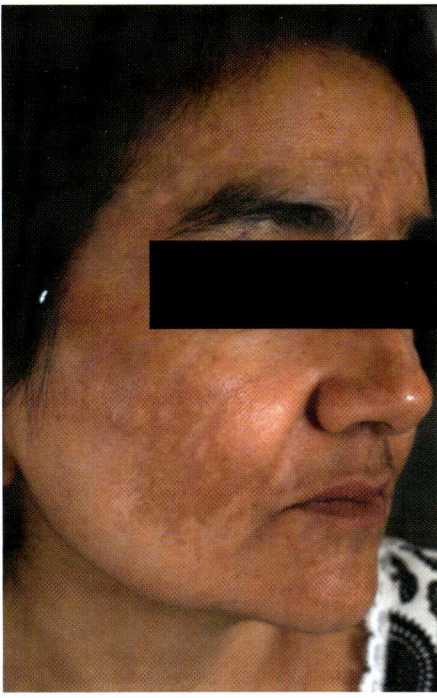

FIGURE 18.10 Diffuse tan-brown patches in a woman with centrofacial melasma, the most common pattern of disease in Latinos.

melanin in the papillary dermis than those with the other two types. As many as 10% of cases occur in men, but they rarely seek medical treatment (Figure 18.11). One study reported higher luteinizing hormone and markedly lower testosterone levels in men with melasma.[36]

The prognosis varies depending on whether the pigmentation is epidermal, dermal, or mixed. For this reason, Wood's light examination and, in some cases, skin biopsy are valuable. Rigorous use of sun blocks that eliminate transepidermal penetration of ultraviolet A and B lights is essential for any therapeutic intervention to succeed. Too often, success is not achieved because patients have not been instructed to protect against sunlight even on cloudy days by wearing hats and applying, at least every 2 hours in the presence of daylight sun blocks with sun protection factor of at least 30 that contain such proven blocking agents as zinc oxide and titanium dioxide.

Conventional treatment for melasma includes elimination of any possible causative factors coupled with use of a sunscreen and hypopigmenting agent, often in combination with other therapies, such as tretinoin, topical corticosteroids, or superficial peeling agents. A reformulated Kligman formula containing 4% hydroquinone, 0.05% tretinoin, and 0.01% fluocinolone acetonide clears more than twice as many melasma patients after 8 weeks as does hydroquinone alone.[37]

Hydroquinone improves pigmentation within weeks, whereas azelaic acid and tretinoin may not produce an effect for approximately 4 months.[38] Pigmentary fading achieved by azelaic acid 20% can be hastened by daily application of 0.05% clobetasol propionate cream.[39] Clobetasol, as a single agent, has been found to improve melasma but results in frequent relapses.

Chemical peels with glycolic acid and trichloroacetic acid, especially when followed by topical corticosteroids, improve pigmentation and enhance the efficacy of other topical agents.[40] Topical corticosteroids are frequently prescribed to prevent potential irritation from other therapeutic agents but also have hypopigmenting effects.

Chemical peels with glycolic acid and trichloroacetic acid, especially when followed by topical corticosteroids, improve pigmentation and enhance the efficacy of other topical agents.[40] Weaker

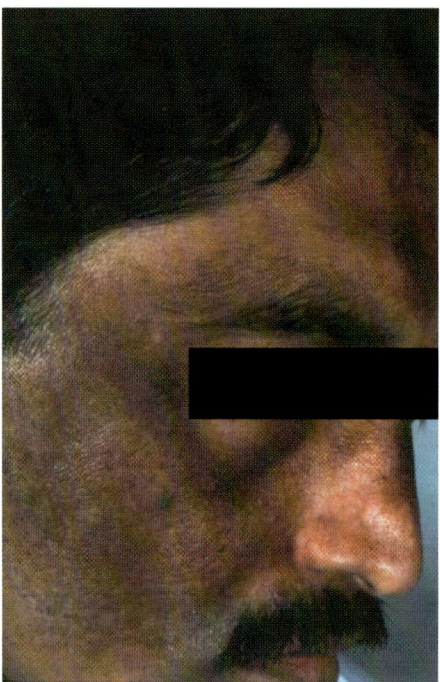

FIGURE 18.11 Melasma is common among Hispanic men with brown skin shades.

concentrations of glycolic acid may not be beneficial in reversing pigmentation, and concentrations of 50%–70% may be necessary to achieve peeling. In a split-faced, prospective trial of 20 Latina women with melasma, 20%–30% glycolic acid peels every 2 weeks did not enhance the effects of hydroquinone in reducing skin pigmentation.[42] Some dermatologists prescribe a steroid cream short term in order to reduce the risk of inducing paradoxical postinflammatory pigmentation.[42] Stronger peels with trichloroacetic acid at 15%–25% concentrations resolved 40% and significantly improved another 50% of localized hyperpigmented lesions on the face and neck.[40] A gel consisting of 50% glycolic acid and 10% kojic acid, on the other hand, is particularly indicated in centrofacial forms of melasma in which the use of a gentle peeling may be sufficient to achieve good cosmetic results without destruction of the skin.[40] A number of lasers have been reported to improve melasma; however, the results are temporary and topical agents need to be continued.[41]

The differential diagnoses of melasma include a number of disorders in which pigmentation of the face or neck are prominent features. These include Riehl's melanosis, poikiloderma of Civatte, erythrosis peribuccale pigmentaire of Brocq, erythromelanosis follicularis, linea fusca, cosmetic hyperpigmentations, and friction melanosis.[43]

Riehl's Melanosis

Riehl's melanosis refers to sudden development of diffuse or patchy facial hyperpigmentation caused by contact dermatitis, usually to sensitizing chemicals in cosmetics or fragrances, including coal tar derivatives, optimal whiteners, musk ambrette, aniline or azo dyes, geranion, hydroxycitronellal, and lemon oil.[43,44] Although infrequently diagnosed, this pigmentary disorder may be the cause of some atypical and treatment recalcitrant cases of melasma and facial pigmentation in Latina women. Brown to slate-gray patches are most pronounced on the forehead and in the zygomatic and temporal regions but may also occur on the chin, nose, and neck of dark-complexioned persons, almost exclusively middle-aged women (Figure 18.12). In some cases, the pattern is reticulate. The absence of marked epidermal edema, erythema, and other characteristic findings of acute contact

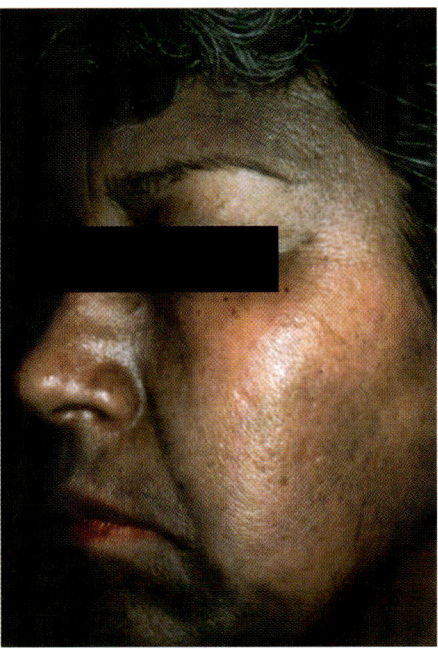

FIGURE 18.12 Discrete and irregular brown to slate-gray patches on the central and lateral aspects of the face of a woman with Riehl's melanosis.

dermatitis has been explained by the low levels of allergens in cosmetics.[44] The contribution of sunlight to this reaction has been long suspected but inconclusively debated. Skin biopsy reveals mild to minimal spongiosis, pigmentary overload of the dermal macrophages, hydropic interface changes leading to melanin incontinence, and a superficial lichenoid mononuclear infiltrate. Patch-testing is often rewardingly positive.[43] The pigmentation clears with time. Topical corticosteroids may be beneficial during the inflammatory stage. Hydroquinone may lighten the lesions if initiated before progression to dermal incontinence occurs.

POIKILODERMA OF CIVATTE

Poikiloderma of Civatte may be a variant of Riehl's melanosis and affects middle-aged to older women with photodamaged skin. The most often implicated cause is photosensitizing chemicals in fragrances and cosmetics, but some cases have an autosomal-dominant genetic pattern with variable penetration. Although lesions on the cheeks may be present in some cases, the predominant findings are on the sides of the neck, where asymptomatic to slightly pruritic, symmetric, reddish-brown reticulate patches appear to be oriented in line with the skin creases. Over time, poikilodermatous changes consisting of telangiectasias and atrophy become prominent and distinguish this entity from berloque dermatitis, a phototoxic reaction to 5-methoxypsoralen (Bergapten) in bergamot oil, a common product in fragrances and perfumes. In this condition brown macules and patches with or without preceding erythema develop along the sides of the neck, usually in a guttate, linear, or pendantlike configuration and less often in other sun-exposed regions impregnated by the fragrance.[43]

ERYTHROMELANOSIS FOLLICULARIS FACEI

Erythromelanosis follicularis facei is a rarely diagnosed disorder characterized by the clinical triad of well-demarcated reddish brown pigmentation, telangiectasias, and follicular plugging on the preauricular and temple areas. The disease has been reported mainly in adolescent men and only a few women.[43] Erythrosis pigmentosa peribuccalis of Brocq is a related disorder seen mainly in women and consists of perioral ringlike reddish-brown pigmentation that may extend to adjacent facial areas.[43]

Linea Fusca

Linea fusca refers to a yellowish-brown band of pigmentation on the upper forehead arching toward the temporal areas. Contact hypersensitivity and photoallergy to facial products, fragrances, and hat materials as well as excessive sun exposure have been proposed as etiologies. Friction melanosis occurs as a result of forceful rubbing of the skin. Circumscribed, glistening, hyperpigmented patches develop in the clavicular zone of young Mexican women as a result of friction from clothing or scrubbing their skin with pads made of sedge.[45] Some patients may purposefully attempt to rub off pigmented blotches, essentially darkening their skin. Histopathologic examination of affected skin shows focal to extensive epidermal necrosis, focal areas of junctional cleavage, and increased melanin deposition within the epidermal basal layer and dermal melanophages.

Arsenical Melanosis

Arsenical melanosis is an early sign of chronic arsenicism and may appear as diffuse dark brown dappling and more frequently as raindrop flecking on any body area, including the palms and soles. This leukoderma may precede the onset of palmoplantar keratosis, and Mee's lines may not be simultaneously present.[46]

Hermansky–Pudlak syndrome

The Hermansky–Pudlak syndrome affects about 1 in 1800 persons in the Northwest of Puerto Rico, possibly making this syndrome the most frequent single-gene disorder on the island. One in every 21 individuals carry the gene and more than 400 Puerto Ricans are affected. These patients are homozygous for 16-base pair (bp) duplication in exon 15 of HPS1, a gene on chromosome 10q23 known to cause the disorder.[73] This clinical manifestation includes tyrosinase-positive oculocutaneous albinism, visual impairment, a platelet dysfunction, and progressive systemic disease. The skin may be creamy white to lightly pigmented (Figure 18.13). Hair color ranges from very light to brown, and eye color varies from blue to brown. Freckling is common. Melanocytic nevi with

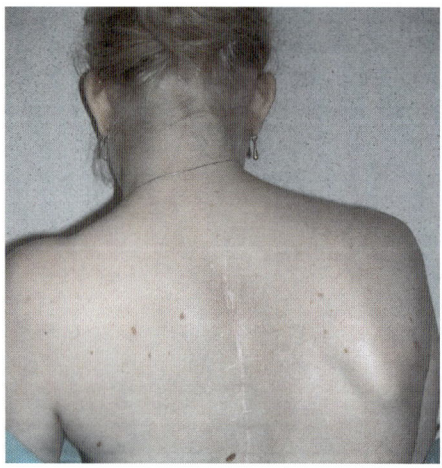

FIGURE 18.13 Puerto Rican woman with the oculocutaneous albinism secondary to the Hermansky–Pudlak syndrome.

dysplastic features, acanthosis nigricans-like lesions in the axilla and neck, and trichomegaly have recently been described.[74] Because platelets have a lower number of dense bodies, they aggregate poorly, leading to bleeding complications. In addition to decreased visual acuity, which in many patients results in legal blindness, ophthalmologic complications include photophobia and strabismus. Accumulation of ceroid lipofuscin in organs can lead to progressive pulmonary fibrosis, inflammatory bowel disease, and granulomatous enteropathic renal disease. The course varies from very mild with few symptoms to severe, disabling, and fatal. Notably, 76% of patients die of causes directly related to the syndrome — half from pulmonary fibrosis and up to 13% from hemorrhagic episodes. Treatment consists of hemostatic agents, such as desmopressin acetate, to diminish the bleeding diathesis and avoidance of aspirin. Many patients exhibit features of solar damage, including multiple freckles, stellate lentigines, actinic keratosis, and basal cell or squamous cell carcinomas.[74] Periodic skin evaluation is important to detect sun-induced cancers and melanomas.

PITYRIASIS ALBA

Although pityriasis alba has been reported to be more common among Caucasians, Latinos are also affected in high numbers. In darker skin types, the lesions are disfiguring. Hypopigmented, 1–4-cm patches with barely perceptible fine scaling involve the face, neck, and shoulders and occasionally the legs, arms, and trunk. Approximately 90% of patients are younger than 12 years of age. The etiology is unknown but the disease has been associated with both atopy and sun exposure. Pityriasis alba is the most common noninfectious disease found in rural Mexicans and was present in 11% of those who reported skin abnormalities. The differential diagnosis, including tinea versicolor, vitiligo, drug-induced leukoderma, and hypopigmented cutaneous T-cell lymphoma, should be excluded histologically.[83] Skin biopsy reveals irregular pigmentation by melanin of the basal layer, follicular plugging and spongiosis, and atrophic sebaceous glands.

IDIOPATHIC GUTTATE HYPOMELANOSIS

This condition is common in fair-to-olive-skinned Latina women with photodamaged skin and evidence of high cumulative levels of ultraviolet light irradiation. In middle age, patients begin to note the scattered, well-demarcated, 1–5-mm, hypopigmented or achromic, quasi-circular macules on the anterior legs and dorsal forearms, invariably when the skin is tanned.[84] The upper back is occasionally involved as well. Men also develop guttate melanosis later in life. The etiology is unclear, but actinic damage is essential. In Latinos, the condition may be a clinical marker that signals increased risk for development of skin cancer. Skin biopsy of a lesion demonstrates basket-weave hyperkeratosis, epidermal atrophy, flat rete ridges, and patchy absence of melanocytes and melanin. There is no consistently effective treatment, and the effect of topical corticosteroids and retinoids is variable. There are scant reports of improvement following dermabrasion and even cryotherapy. Avoidance of further sun tanning is advisable; however, artificial tanning can produce satisfactory camouflage.

ACNE

In the United States, acne outranks only eczema as the most frequent diagnosis for which Latinos visit dermatologists. Neither the incidence nor severity of acne appears to be significantly altered from the general population, although one study reported a higher prevalence of acne in Mexican-American indigent adolescents than in their Caucasian and African-American counterparts.[47] On the other hand, the incidence may be lower in Latinos with native Indian ancestry than in Caucasians. In a cross-sectional study of 2214 Peruvian adolescents, the prevalence of acne varied from 16.33% at 12 years to 71.23% at 17 years.[48] The overall prevalence of acne was lower in Indians (28%) than in Mestizos (43%) or Latino whites (44%).[48] The explanation for this discrepancy in acne rates may be dietary disparities. In a study that has challenged standard concepts of the effect of diet on acne, Aché hunter-gatherers of Paraguay who adhere to traditional diets were found not to develop acne, in contrast to their counterparts who adopted a more glycemic Western diet.[49] The authors postulated that dietary-induced hyperinsulinemia was responsible for the development of acne. Elevated levels of insulin stimulate sebaceous gland activity and follicular keratinization, possibly through enhanced release of insulin growth factor (IGF) and IGF-binding protein, which in turn enhance androgen secretion and interfere with retinoid-signaling pathways.[50]

Culturally sanctioned grooming practices may also contribute to the development of acne. The practice of slicking down the hair with brilliantine and other unguents in the pachuco style has become less popular, but pomade acne is still seen in those who continue to grease their hair. Although many Latina women have adopted lighter cosmetics in response to modern trends, others cling to the use of heavy oil-based makeup to enhance feminine characteristics. Patients with facial pigmentation are particularly inclined to use thick, acnegenic foundations to camouflage their marks. Rather than ban cosmetic use, noncomedogenic brands and camouflage techniques should be recommended to these women. The crucial step in controlling acne-induced pigmentation is the control of acne. Even without bleaching agents, the pigmentation resolves within weeks to months when lesions no longer erupt.

The response to acne treatments is unchanged from the general population; however, specific factors should be taken into consideration in patients with olive to brown skin shades.[51] In this group, acne inflammatory lesions may produce postinflammatory pigmentary changes that are disfiguring and difficult to camouflage (Figure 18.14).[52] The development of these scattered, irregular, pigmented macules has been termed the Polka-dot syndrome[53] and is as, or more, distressing than the presence of acne. Patients may be inclined to pick at their comedones and manually drain their pustules, practices which cause and darken pigmentation and increase the risk of ice pick,

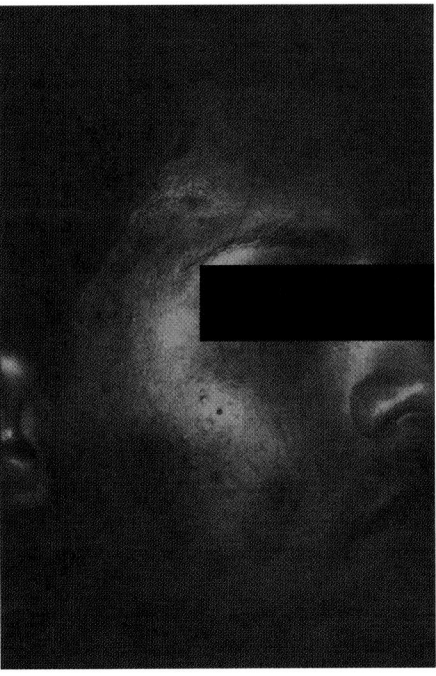

FIGURE 18.14 Inflammatory lesions from acne may produce postinflammatory pigmentary changes that are disfiguring and persistent.

depressed fibrotic, and superficial or deep atrophic scars. These patients usually require systemic treatment with oral antibiotics in addition to topical regimens. Isotretinoin is very effective and should be considered in patients with therapeutically recalcitrant acne, including youngsters whose school performance or socialization is impaired by their reaction to their appearance.

Patients with cystic, cicatricial, or hyperpigmenting acne should not be denied tetracycline antibiotics or isotretinoin; however, it should be remembered that many Latinas are rigid Catholics who would not consider abortion. Therefore, women should be educated about the importance of compliance with contraceptives, the 3% failure rate of oral contraceptives, and, therefore, the need to use more than one method of contraception. Topical preparations that combine more than one medication and decrease the number of applications are preferred.[54] Among topical anti-acne agents, benzoyl peroxide, azelaic acid, and retinoids all possess the added beneficial effect of diminishing pigmentation. Periodic observation for diffuse hypopigmentation, however, is needed. Furthermore, it is important to avoid further hyperpigmentation secondary to irritation and hypersensitivity reactions from topical treatments. Chemical peels with glycolic acid or salicylic acid are effective and well tolerated.[55] Patients should apply noncomedogenic sunblocks as often as needed to block ultraviolet light melanogenesis. Hormonal treatment, although beneficial in chronic cases, may induce or worsen melasma. Because correction of acne scars with the ablative lasers can result in unsightly pigmentation and scarring, the procedure should be limited to physicians with experience in laser surgery in persons with skin of color.[56]

ECZEMA

The incidence of eczema is not known to be increased in Latinos although one study found a significantly higher percentage of Mexican-American adolescents with eczema than Caucasian and African-American adolescents.[47] Notably, eczema and acne were the main health problems found in this group of Latino adolescents. Although there are no studies showing higher rates of atopic dermatitis, the incidence of asthma, another disease associated with atopy, is escalating in Latinos.[57] One study found that 51.2% of Latino asthmatic children were reactive to environmental allergens.[58] As with other inflammatory diseases, hyperpigmentation and hypopigmentation are common sequelae. Therefore, aggressive control of itching to avoid rubbing and scratching is imperative. Pigmentary changes usually resolve over time with good control of the disease, even in patients treated with phototherapy. It is important to assess the use of nonprescription bleaching products, which may be causing allergic or irritant dermatitis.

ACTINIC PRURIGO

Actinic prurigo is an idiopathic, familial photodermatosis that affects the Native Indian and mestizo populations of Mexico and Central and South America. The lesions are polymorphous with intensely pruritic, excoriated, erythematous papules, lichenified plaques, and vesicles present over photoexposed body areas, especially the face, upper chest, hands, and forearms[59] (Figure 18.15). Deep excoriations may heal with scarring. In contrast to polymorphous light eruption, unexposed skin is also affected in about 20% of patients, the disease often persists even during winters, and oral and ocular mucosal involvement occurs in 30%–50% of cases.[60] Ocular features include photophobia, pterygium, pinguecula, hyperemia, Trantas' dots, and hyaline exudates.[61] Most patients have a low minimal erythema response to UVA and also to UVB light. The disease usually starts in childhood in both sexes. Approximately 60% of patients are female.[62] Two thirds of patients have a positive family history of the disease.[62] Many live at altitudes of more than 1000 meters. Human leukocyte antigen (HLA) typing shows the presence of the DR4 allele in approximately 90% of patients, 80% of whom exhibit the rare subtype DRB1*0407.[60,63] The presence of class I antigens

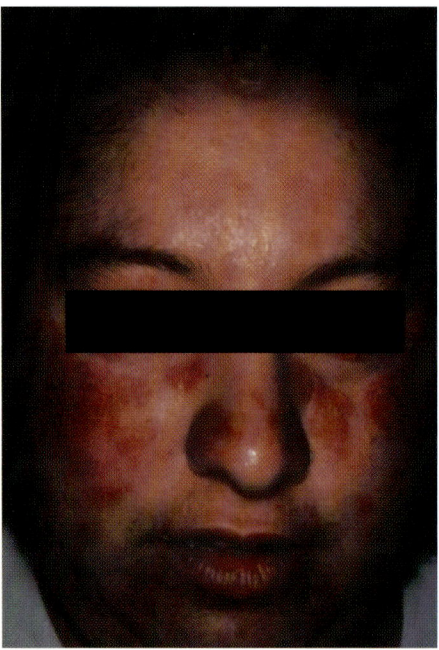

FIGURE 18.15 Erythematous, lichenified, weeping, excoriated papules, plaques, and vesicles with cheilitis and conjunctivitis on the face of a woman with actinic prurigo.

HLA-A28 and HLA-B39 (B16) is also significantly increased compared with normal controls.[63] This pattern is another differentiating feature from polymorphous light eruption. Most subjects have a chronic disease course without spontaneous improvement.[62] The course is milder in those who develop the disease as adults.[64]

Histopathologic examination of affected skin shows epidermal spongiosis, vacuolar degeneration of the basal layer, a superficial (and sometimes deep) perivascular lymphocytic infiltrates, and papillary dermal edema. Marked hyperkeratosis, acanthosis, and elongation of the rete ridges are present in lichenified areas.[65]

The cells in the infiltrate are predominantly helper T lymphocytes admixed with scattered B-cell lymphoid follicles and numerous dermal dendrocytes.[66] Expression of adhesion molecules in the cell infiltrate is increased.[67] Upregulated expression of ICAM-1 can be detected in keratinocytes, which also contain high levels of tumor necrosis factor-alpha and calprotectin.[66] In contrast to normal controls, the number of Langerhans cells in actinic prurigo skin is not significantly altered by ultraviolet irradiation.[67] Presumably, ultraviolet light triggers expression of ICAM-1 and excessive production of tumor necrosis factor-alpha by keratinocytes, whose sustained release in turn promotes an inflammatory reaction that results in deleterious epidermal effects.[66]

The treatment of choice is thalidomide, which at doses ranging from 50 to 200 mg has been effective in practically all patients. The drug is well tolerated and lower doses have been administered to children.[68] Treatment with tetracycline, 500 mg three times daily, together with vitamin E, 100 IU daily, for 6 months relieves the symptoms and skin lesions of many patients.[69] Potent corticosteroids alleviate inflammation and, consequently, itching and may be sufficient in mild cases.[65] The response to psoralen and UVA light (PUVA) or narrow-band UVB phototherapy is variable.[70,71] Treatment with systemic cyclosporine, topical tacrolimus, or topical ascomycin remains investigational. Conjunctival inflammation improves significantly with 2% topical cyclosporine drops.[72]

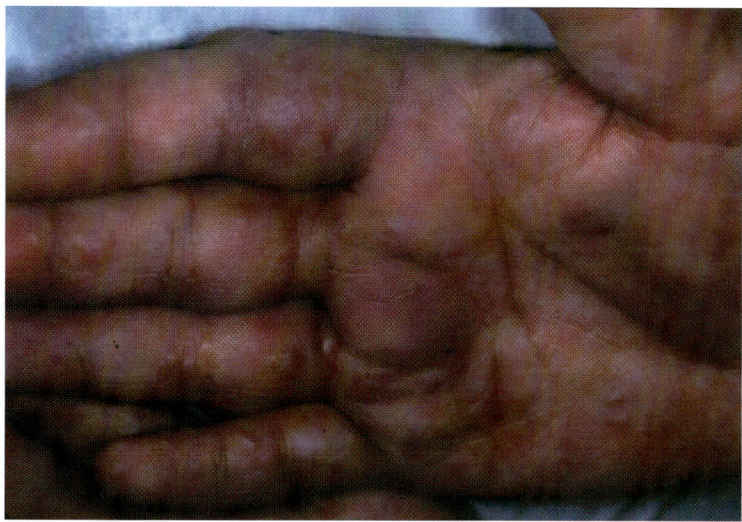

FIGURE 18.16 Painful, edematous, erythematous plaques that developed after cooking with chili peppers.

CAPSAICIN DERMATITIS

Cooks who peel chili peppers may develop erythema and edema on the skin of the hands and fingers, but in contrast to contact dermatitis or dyshidrosis, blisters are not usually present.[75] (Figure 18.16). Depending on the duration of contact, the associated pain ranges from mild to intense and has been described as burnlike, throbbing, or prickling.[76] These symptoms are often delayed and may persist for hours to days. Capsaicin depolarizes nerves, leading to vasodilation, smooth muscle stimulation, and sensory nerve activation.[76] In order to prevent this reaction, patients should be instructed to wear gloves when handling chili peppers. If symptoms develop, hand washing with soap and copious amounts of cold water followed by immersion of the hands in vegetable oil for approximately 1 hour is advisable.[77] Topical anesthetics and high-potency corticosteroids may decrease the pain and erythema.[77]

BALANITIS XEROTICA OBLITERANS

The prevalence of balanitis xerotica obliterans, also known as penile lichen sclerosus, has been reported to be doubled in Latino over Caucasian men.[78] Although this preponderance was only recently recognized, it is not unexpected because this disease is associated with noncircumcision or circumcision after childhood. Another possible contributing factor is the increased rate in Latino men of genital human papilloma virus infection, which has been suggested as a promoter of lichen sclerosus.[79] This chronic, progressive, inflammatory disease of the glans penis may occur at any age but most patients are initially diagnosed during middle age. Initially, one or several discrete erythematous macules or barely elevated papules develop on the glans or prepuce (Figure 18.17). Over time, these lesions grow or coalesce into patches or plaques, which become sclerotic, ivory colored, and atrophic.

A sclerotic white ring at the tip of the prepuce is a common early finding. As a result of trauma, fissures, superficial erosions, blisters, bleeding, and petechiae may develop, particularly when sclerosis is pronounced. In descending frequency of involvement, the frenulum, urethral meatus, sulcus, fossa navicularis, penile shaft, and perianal area may also be affected. Bullous lichen sclerosus is an uncommon variant. With disease progression and development of sclerosis, symptoms

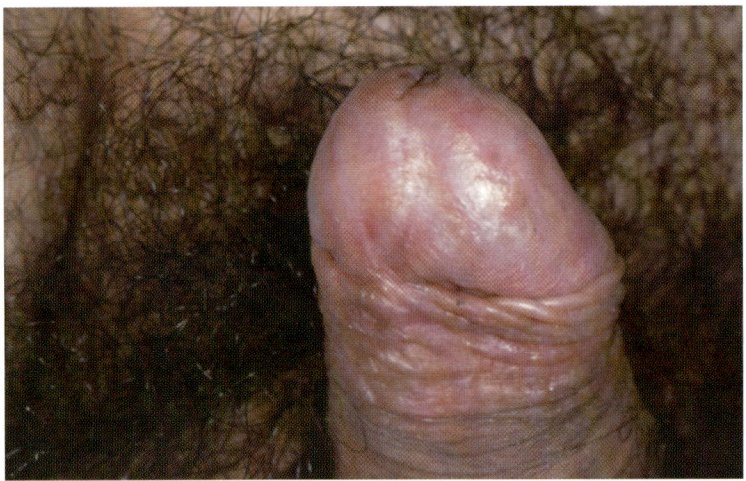

FIGURE 18.17 Mild erythema and hypopigmentation of the glans, coronal sulcus, frenulum and mucosal prepuce of a man with balanitis xerotica obliterans. This disease has devastating effects of many affected Latino men whose perceptions of masculinity are particularly penocentric.

develop and include pruritus, burning, dysuria, dysesthesia, painful erection, reduced urinary flow, and partial urethral stenosis. In late disease, the foreskin will not recoil if retracted (paraphemosis) or will not retract at all (phimosis). In one study, squamous cell carcinoma developed in an average of 17 years in approximately 6% of patients.[80] Histopathologic changes include orthokeratosis, epidermal atrophy, vacuolar degeneration of the basal layer, edema, a superficial infiltrate of lymphocytes and plasma cells, homogenization of collagen, and loss of elastic fibers in the upper dermis.

The treatment of choice is circumcision in uncircumcised men.[81] Alternatives include high-potency topical or intralesionally injected corticosteroids and topical tacrolimus, but topical testosterone has been found to be ineffective. Obliteration of lesions with carbon dioxide or pulse dye lasers has been reported to be beneficial. Reconstructive urologic surgery may be necessary in advanced cases. Acitretin may be needed to halt disease progression in unresponsive cases.

ACANTHOSIS NIGRICANS

In contrast to the 1% prevalence in the general population, acanthosis nigricans is present in 5% of Latinos.[82] The characteristic features are gray-brown to black thickening of the skin, with many small papillomatous elevations and a velvety texture. These changes are most commonly seen on the axillae, back and sides of the neck, and anogenital region and groin and less often on other flexures, the inframammary region, and umbilicus (Figure 18.18). In most Latinos acanthosis nigricans results from insulin resistance associated with diabetes mellitus and obesity. It is important to evaluate patients for the type A (HAIR-AN syndrome) (hyperandrogenemia, insulin resistance, and acanthosis nigricans) syndrome associated with polycystic ovaries, virilization, and elevated plasma testosterone levels. The type B syndrome is associated with acanthosis nigricans, uncontrolled diabetes mellitus, ovarian hyperandrogenism, and autoimmune disease. Histopathologically, there are papillomatosis and hyperkeratosis but only slight, irregular acanthosis and usually no hyperpigmentation. The treatment of type 3 acanthosis nigricans is weight loss and diabetic control. Combinations of salicylic acid, urea, hydroquinone, imidazole antifungal creams, tretinoin 0.1% cream, and corticosteroids have been prescribed with variable degrees of success. Superficial ablation of lesions with trichloroacetic acid peels, cryosurgery, and erbium:YAG or CO_2 laser hastens resolution.

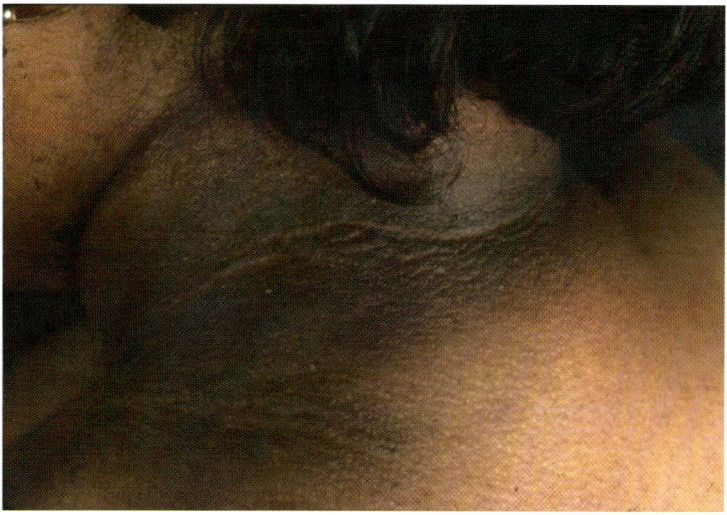

FIGURE 18.18 Acanthosis nigricans is becoming increasingly common as the incidence of obesity and diabetes escalates among Latinos living in the United States.

PRAYER CALLOUSES

Callouses develop on the knees due to repeated pressure and friction from kneeling during prayer (Figure 18.19). Such a practice results in clinical and histopathologic skin thickening and hyperkeratosis.[85] The lesions are often hyperpigmented and do not ulcerate unless traumatized by blunt injury. Callouses findings have become rare since the practice of kneeling during services was abolished by the Catholic Church. However, some highly religious individuals, usually elderly women, continue to kneel during devout prayer, sometimes for hours every day. Intensely pious women may also place corn kernels or similarly hard objects under their knees, believing that mortification better atones for sins. In contrast to Moslems, who develop callouses after praying on their knees with their hands on their forehead, plaques are not present on the forehead of non-Moslem Latinos.[86]

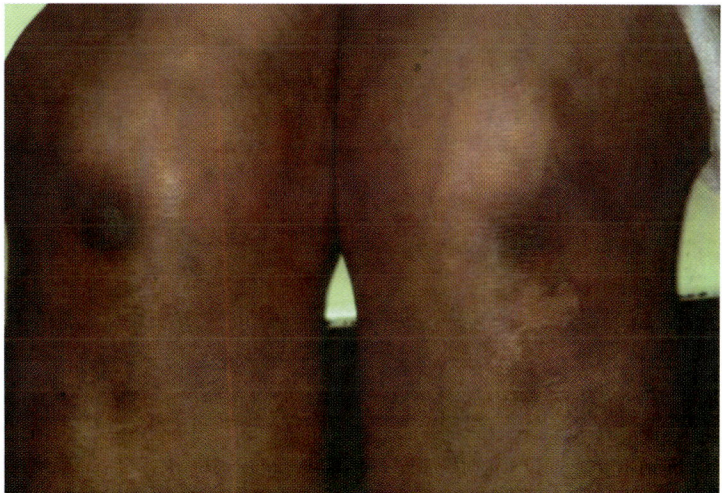

FIGURE 18.19 Round, pigmented, well-demarcated, lichenified, nodular patellar plaques that developed after long sessions of kneeling during prayer.

SKIN CANCER

In addition to high cumulative levels of sunlight, repeated sunburns, and infrequent use of sun protection, environmental factors elevate the risk of cancer in Latinos. The deleterious effects of the ozone layer depletion are being recognized in areas where skin cancer was previously rare. A surveillance study from an ozone-reduced region of Chile demonstrated a 66% increase of skin cancer and a 56% rise in the number of cases of cutaneous malignant melanoma over a 14-year span.[87] Ecologic pollution due to unregulated industrial chemical waste and environmental violations probably account for the increase in skin cancer in certain areas. High relative risks of developing malignant melanoma and soft tissue cancers, as well as stomach, rectal, and renal cancers in men and cervical cancer and lymphomas in women, have been found in Ecuadorian provinces bordering on the Amazon, where extraction of crude oil has dumped billions of gallons of untreated wastes and oils on the land.[88] In several countries of South America, notably in Argentina, Chile, Mexico, Peru, and Bolivia, there are impoverished areas where chronic hydroarsenicism exacerbates oncogenesis. Prolonged ingestion of small amounts of arsenic in contaminated water does not cause acute symptoms but alarmingly high prevalences of cancers of the lung, liver, gastrointestinal tract, bladder, and kidney, in addition to arsenical keratosis, and cutaneous squamous cell carcinomas and basal cell carcinomas have been reported from these regions (Figure 18.20).[89] In the United States, Latinos use sunscreen or conduct skin self-examinations far less often than does the general population.[90,91] Even more educated, suburban Latinos consider themselves to be at average or below average risk, regardless of history of sun exposure, and are less aware of the dangers of melanoma and nonmelanoma skin cancer.[92] In a published survey, Latinos reported that they would be less likely than Caucasians to seek immediate follow-up care for suspicious skin lesions.[93]

BASAL CELL AND SQUAMOUS CELL CARCINOMAS

Compared with that in non-Hispanic whites, the incidence of cutaneous squamous cell carcinomas (SCC) and basal cell carcinomas (BCC) in Latinos is about 11 times lower.[94] The differences in skin shades and susceptibility to the effects of ultraviolet radiation within Latino subpopulations is being recognized.[95] Latinos with light skin shades who grew up in tropical climates often have

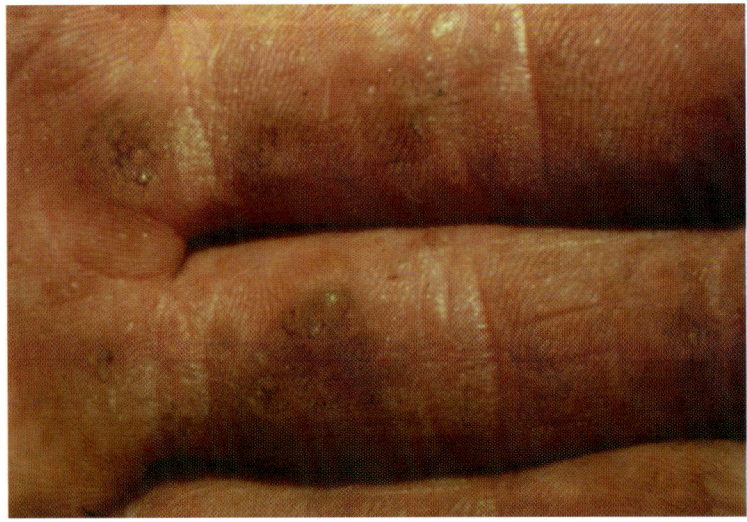

FIGURE 18.20 Multiple, small, yellowish-brown, punctuate, cornlike and verrucous, arsenical keratoses on the ventral surface of the hand.

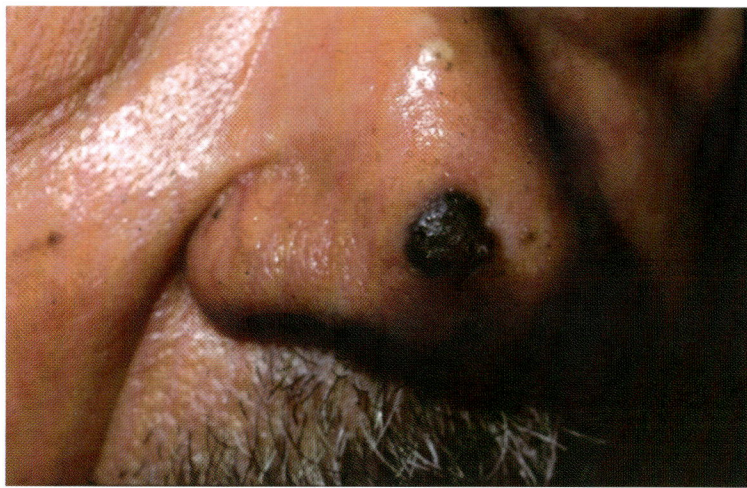

FIGURE 18.21 Pigmented basal cell carcinomas are common in Latinos who rarely seek clinical evaluation of these perceived "lunares" (moles).

signs of photodamaged skin and have high risks for development of both cancers. Furthermore, BCC is being diagnosed with increasing frequency in darker skin types as well. Some studies have reported increased rates of BCC and skin SCC in Latino men, presumably due to greater occupational exposure to ultraviolet light and chemicals,[96] but others have not found gender differences.[94] Although the incidence of BCC has not surged as steeply as in non-Hispanic whites, the number of Latino cases has been steadily increasing.[97] The onset of BCC is earlier than that of SCC in both Latino men and women.[96] BCC is often pigmented and, therefore, more readily overlooked as benign pigmented nevi (Figure 18.21). In a prospective clinico-histopathologic study, biopsies from Latino patients accounted for two thirds of all pigmented BCC but only 11% of nonpigmented BCC.[98] The majority of these neoplasms arise on the face, but according to a large retrospective study, 6% of BCC in Mexicans were located in the extremities or trunk.[99]

Melanoma

The incidence of malignant melanoma among Latinos is 4–6 times lower than in non-Hispanic Caucasians, but the survival prognosis is grimmer. One study found that a diagnosis was established after the development of metastasis in 15% of Latino men but only 6% of Caucasian men with cutaneous melanomas.[100] In 7% of Latinas vs. 4% of non-Hispanic Caucasian women, melanomas were diagnosed in late stages.[100] In a study of 54 cases of melanoma, 70% presented with local stage disease, out of whom 87% survived more than 5 years, whereas 26% presented with metastasis.[101] The prognosis is better among Latino women. Eighty-six percent of them survived for 5 years, compared with 56% of Latino men.[101] Remarkably, survival was better for Latino patients with combined regional and distant disease than for other non-Hispanic groups.[101]

The higher proportions of acral lentiginous melanomas arising in the palms, soles, and subungual regions, as well as mucous membrane melanomas, also contribute to the overall poorer prognosis of melanoma in Latinos (Figure 18.22).[102] The majority of melanomas are located on the trunk, arm, shoulder, leg, and hip in men.[101] Twenty percent are present on the lower extremities.[100] Lentigo maligna melanomas are invariably diagnosed in advanced stages as patients ignore the growth of their lesions (Figure 18.23). In a retrospective study of nine cases of malignant melanoma from Mexico, 88% of melanomas occurred in women, whose mean age was 63 years at the time of diagnosis. Six melanomas were located on the foot, one on the leg, one in the anus, and one on the neck. All tumors were Clark's levels three or higher with a mean tumor thickness of 5.7 mm. Six melanomas were associated with vitiligo and three with leukoderma acquisitum centrifugum.

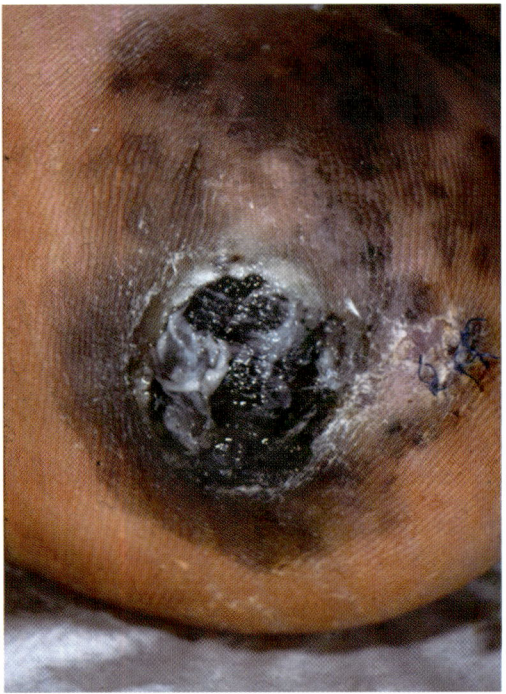

FIGURE 18.22 Acral melanomas are more common in Latinos, and a skin exam should include examination of upper and lower extremities, including nails.

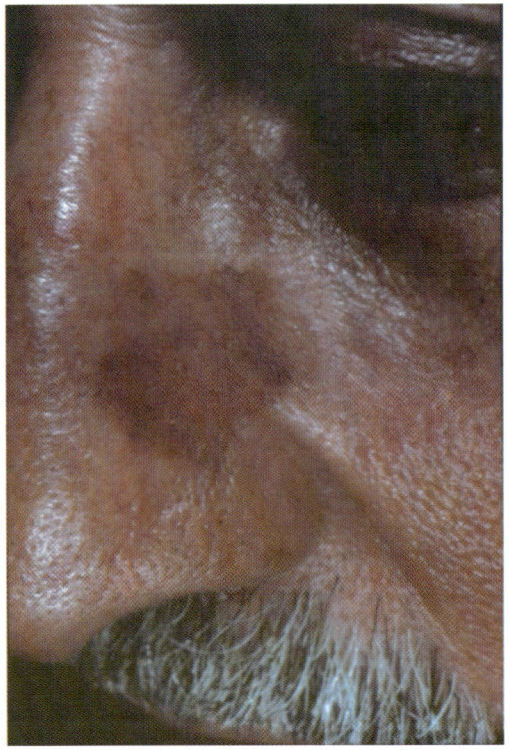

FIGURE 18.23 Latinos usually are not concerned about lentigo maligna melanoma, which is becoming more prevalent in photodamaged elderly individuals, until it becomes nodular or ulcerative.

After noting that eight out of nine cases had no evidence of tumor recurrence following a mean of 55 months after chemotherapy, the authors proposed that patients with depigmentation have a better than expected survival expectancy,[62] a hypothesis that requires further study.

REFERENCES

1. Morales, B. *Handbook of Hispanic Cultures in the United States*. Anthropology Arte Public Press, University of Houston, Houston, TX, 1994.
2. Ramirez, R. U.S. Census Bureau, Ethnic and Hispanic Statistics Branch. Current Population Reports, Series P20-527, The Hispanic Population in the United States: Population.
3. United States Census Bureau. The Population Profile of the United States: 2000. Superintendent of Documents, U.S. Government Printing Office, Washington, DC.
4. Betancourt, J.R., Green, A.R., Carrillo, J.E., et al. Defining cultural competence: a practical framework for addressing racial/ethnic disparities in health and health care. *Public Health Rep*, 118, 293, 2003.
5. Vega, W.A. and Amaro, H. Latino outlook: good health, uncertain prognosis. *Ann Rev Pub Health*, 15, 39, 1994.
6. Majette, G.R. Access to health care: what a difference shades of color make. *Ann Health Law*, 12, 121, 2003.
7. Carrillo, J.E., Trevino, F.M. IV and Coustasse, A. Latino access to health care: the role of insurance, managed care, and institutional barriers. In: Aguirre, M., Molina, C.W., Zambrana, R.E., Bass, J. (Eds.), *Health Issues in the Latino Community*, San Francisco, 2001, pp 55–73.
8. A Provider's Handbook on Culturally Competent Care: Latino Population, prepared by Kaiser Permanente National Diversity Council, Oakland, CA, 1997.
9. Fishman, B.M., Bobo, L., Kosub, K., et al. Cultural issues in serving minority populations: emphasis on Mexican Americans and African Americans. *Am J Med Sci*, 306, 160, 1993.
10. Moy, J.A., McKinley-Grant, L. and Sanchez M. Cultural aspects in the treatment of patients with skin disease. *Dermatol Clin*, 21, 733, 2003.
11. Carballeira, N.P. and Paré-Avila, J. *Latino Values and Implications for Intervention*. Latino Health Institute, Boston, MA, 1997.
12. Padilla, R., Gomez, V., Biggerstaff, S.L., et al. Use of curanderismo in a public health care system. *Arch Intern Med*, 161, 1336, 2001.
13. Murguia, A., Peterson R.A., and Zea, M.C. Use and implications of ethnomedical health care approaches among Central American immigrants. *Health Soc Work*, 28, 43, 2003.
14. Dole, E.J., Rhyne, R.L., Zeilmann, C.A., et al. The influence of ethnicity on use of herbal remedies in elderly Hispanics and non-Hispanic whites. *J Am Pharm Assoc*, 40, 359, 2000.
15. Cushman, L.F., Wade, C., Factor-Litvak, P., et al. Use of complementary and alternative medicine among African-American and Hispanic women in New York City: a pilot study. *J Am Med Womens Assoc*, 54, 193, 1999.
16. Risser, A.L. and Mazur, L.J. Use of folk remedies in a Hispanic population. *Arch Pediatr Adolesc Med*, 149, 978, 1995.
17. Sandoval, M.S. Santería. *J Florida Med Assoc*, 70, 620, 1983.
18. Holloway, J.E. (Ed.). *Africanisms in American Culture*. Indiana University Press, Bloomington, 1990.
19. Musgrave, C.F. Allen, C.E. and Allen, G.J. Spirituality and health for women of color. *Am J Public Health*, 92, 557, 2002.
20. Mikhail, B.I.. Hispanic mothers' beliefs and practices regarding selected children's health problems. *West J Nurs Res*, 16(6), 623, 1994.
21. Sanchez, M. Cutaneous disease in Latinos. *Dermatol Clin*, 21, 689, 2003.
22. Halder, R.M. and Nootheti, P.K. Ethnic skin disorders overview. *J Am Acad Dermatol*, 48, S142, 2003.
23. Alaluf, S., Atkins, D., Barrett, K., et al. Ethnic variation in melanin content and composition in photoexposed and photoprotected human skin. *Pigment Cell Res*, 15, 112, 2002.
24. Pandya, A.G. and Guevara, I.L. Disorders of hyperpigmentation. *Dermatol Clin*, 18, 91, 2000.
25. Baranda, L., Torres-Alvarez, B., Cortes-Franco, R., et al. Involvement of cell adhesion and activation molecules in the pathogenesis of erythema dyschromicum perstans (ashy dermatitis). The effect of clofazimine therapy. *Arch Dermatol*, 133, 325, 1997.

26. Penagos, H., Jimenez, V., Fallas, V., et al. Chlorothalonil, a possible cause of erythema dyschromicum perstans (ashy dermatitis). *Contact Dermatitis*, 35, 214, 1996.
27. Osswald, S.S., Proffer, L.H. and Sartori, C.R. Erythema dyschromicum perstans: a case report and review. *Cutis*, 68, 25, 2001.
28. Piquero-Martin, J., Perez-Alfonzo, R., Abrusci, V., et al. Clinical trial with clofazimine for treating erythema dyschromicum perstans. Evaluation of cell-mediated immunity. *Int J Dermatol*, 28, 198, 1989.
29. Jansen, T., Gambichler, T., von Kobyletzki, L., et al. Lichen planus actinicus treated with acitretin and topical corticosteroids. *Eur Acad Dermatol Venereol*, 16, 174, 2002.
30. Albers, S.E., Glass, L.F. and Fenske, N.A. Lichen planus subtropicus: direct immunofluorescence findings and therapeutic response to hydroxychloroquine. *Int J Dermatol*, 33, 645, 1994.
31. Fernandez Blasco, G., de Unamuno, P. and Armijo, M. Idiopathic eruptive macular pigmentation. *Acta Dermosifiliogr*, 70, 639, 1979.
32. Jang, K.A., Choi, J.H., Sung, K.S., et al. Idiopathic eruptive macular pigmentation: report of 10 cases. *J Am Acad Dermatol*, 44, 351, 2001.
33. Boer, A., Misago, N., Wolter, M., et al. Prurigo pigmentosa: a distinctive inflammatory disease of the skin. *Am J Dermatopathol*, 25, 117, 2003.
34. Lines, R.R. III and Hansen, R.C. A hyperpigmented, rippled eruption in a Hispanic woman. Macular amyloidosis. *Arch Dermatol*, 133, 383, 1997.
35. Mandry Pagan, R. and Sanchez, J.L. Mandibular melasma. *Puerto Rico Health Sci J*, 19, 231, 2000.
36. Sialy, R., Hassan, I., Kaur, I., et al. Melasma in men: a hormonal profile. *J Am Acad Dermatol*, 27, 64, 2000.
37. Taylor, S.C., Torok, H., Jones, T, et al. Efficacy and safety of a new triple-combination agent for the treatment of facial melasma. *Cutis*, 72, 67, 2003.
38. Guevara, I.L. and Pandya, A.G. Melasma treated with hydroquinone, tretinoin, and a fluorinated steroid. *Int J Dermatol*, 40, 212, 2001.
39. Sarkar, R., Bhalla, M. and Kanwar, A.J. A comparative study of 20% azelaic acid cream monotherapy versus a sequential therapy in the treatment of melasma in dark-skinned patients. *Dermatology*, 205, 249, 2002.
40. Cotellessa, C., Peris, K., Onorati, M.T., et al. The use of chemical peelings in the treatment of different cutaneous hyperpigmentations. *Dermatol Surg*, 25, 450, 1999.
41. Nouri, K., Bowes, L., Chartier, T., et al. Combination treatment of melasma with pulsed CO_2 laser followed by Q-switched alexandrite laser: a pilot study. *Dermatol Surg*, 25, 494, 1999.
42. Hurley, M.E., Guevara, I.L., Gonzales, R.M., et al. Efficacy of glycolic acid peels in the treatment of melasma. *Arch Dermatol*, 138, 1578, 2002.
43. Perez-Bernal, A., Munoz-Perez, M.A. and Camacho, F. Management of facial hyperpigmentation. *Am J Clin Dermatol*, 1, 261, 2000.
44. Serrano, G., Pujol, C. and Cuadra, J. Riehl's melanosis: pigmented contact dermatitis caused by fragrances. *J Am Acad Dermatol*, 21, 1057, 1989.
45. Magana-Garcia, M., Carrasco, E., Herrera-Goepfert, R., et al. Hyperpigmentation of the clavicular zone: a variant of friction melanosis. *Int J Dermatol*, 28(2), 119, 1989.
46. Del Razo, L.M., Garcia-Vargas, G.G., Vargas, H., et al. Altered profile of urinary arsenic metabolites in adults with chronic arsenicism. A pilot study. *Arch Toxicol*, 71, 211, 1997.
47. Fitzpatrick, S.B., Fujii, C., Shragg, G.P., et al. Do health care needs of indigent Mexican-American, black, and white adolescents differ? *J Adolesc Health Care*, 11, 128, 1990.
48. Freyre, E.A., Rebaza, R.M., Sami, D.A., et al. The prevalence of facial acne in Peruvian adolescents and its relation to their ethnicity. *J Adolesc Health Care*, 22, 480, 1998.
49. Thiboutot, D.M. and Strauss, J.S. Diet and acne revisited. *Arch Dermatol*, 138, 1591, 2002.
50. Cordain, L., Lindeberg, S., Hurtado, M., et al. Acne vulgaris: a disease of Western civilization. *Arch Dermatol*, 138, 1584, 2002.
51. Taylor, S.C., Cook-Bolden, F., Rahman, Z., et al. Acne vulgaris in skin of color. *J Am Acad Dermatol*, 45, S98, 2002.
52. Taylor, S.C. Cosmetic problems in skin of color. *Skin Pharmacol Appl Skin Physiol*, 12, 139, 1999.
53. Murad, H., Shamban, A.T., Moy, L.S. Polka-dot syndrome: a more descriptive name for a common problem. *Cosmet Dermatol*, 2, 57, 1993.

54. Fernandez-Obregon, A., Davis, M.W. The BEST study: evaluating efficacy by selected demographic subsets. *Cutis,* 71(2 Suppl), 18, 2003.
55. Grimes, P.E. The safety and efficacy of salicylic acid chemical peels in darker racial-ethnic groups. *Dermatol Surg,* 25, 18, 1999.
56. Ruiz-Esparza, J., Barba Gomez, J.M., Gomez de la Torre, O.L., et al. UltraPulse laser skin resurfacing in Hispanic patients. A prospective study of 36 individuals. *Dermatol Surg,* 24, 59, 1998.
57. Lester, L.A., Rich, S.S., Blumenthal, M.N., Togias, A., et al. Ethnic differences in asthma and associated phenotypes: collaborative study on the genetics of asthma. *J Allergy Clin Immunol,* 108(3), 357, 2001.
58. Christiansen, S.C., Martin, S.B., Schleicher, N.C., et al. Exposure and sensitization to environmental allergen of predominantly Hispanic children with asthma in San Diego's inner city. *J Allergy Clin Immunol,* 98, 288, 1996.
59. Lane, P.R., Hogan, D.J., Martel, M.J., et al. Actinic prurigo: clinical features and prognosis. *J Am Acad Dermatol,* 26, 683, 1992.
60. Grabczynska, S.A., McGregor, J.M., Kondeatis, E., et al. Actinic prurigo and polymorphic light eruption: common pathogenesis and the importance of HLA-DR4/DRB1*0407. *Br J Dermatol,* 140, 232, 1999.
61. Magana, M., Mendez, Y., Rodriguez, A., et al. The conjunctivitis of solar (actinic) prurigo. *Pediatr Dermatol,* 17, 432, 2000.
62. Rodriguez-Cuevas, S., Lopez-Chavira, A., Zepeda del Rio, G., et al. Prognostic significance of cutaneous depigmentation in Mexican patients with malignant melanoma. *Arch Med Res,* 29, 155, 1998.
63. Hojyo-Tomoka, T., Granados, J., Vargas-Alarcon, G., et al. Further evidence of the role of HLA-DR4 in the genetic susceptibility to actinic prurigo. *J Am Acad Dermatol,* 36, 935, 1997.
64. Lane, P.R., Murphy, F., Hogan, D.J., et al. Histopathology of actinic prurigo. *Am J Dermatopathol,* 15, 326, 1993.
65. Lane, P.R., Moreland, A.A. and Hogan, D.J. Treatment of actinic prurigo with intermittent short-course topical 0.05% clobetasol 17-propionate. A preliminary report. *Arch Dermatol,* 126, 1211, 1990.
66. Arrese, J.E., Dominguez-Soto, L., Hojyo-Tomoka, M.T., et al. Effectors of inflammation in actinic prurigo. *J Am Acad Dermatol,* 44, 957, 2001.
67. Torres-Alvarez, B., Baranda, L., Fuentes, C., et al. An immunohistochemical study of UV-induced skin lesions in actinic prurigo. Resistance of Langerhans cells to UV light. *Euro J Dermatol,* 8, 24, 1998.
68. Lovell, C.R., Hawk, J.L., Calnan, C.D., et al. Thalidomide in actinic prurigo. *Br J Dermatol,* 108, 467, 1983.
69. Duran, M.M., Ordonez, C.P., Prieto, J.C., et al. Treatment of actinic prurigo in Chimila Indians. *Int J Dermatol,* 35, 413, 1996.
70. Las, D.Y., Youn, J.I., Park, M.H., et al. Actinic prurigo: limited effect of PUVA [Letter]. *Br J Dermatol,* 136, 972, 1997.
71. Collins, P. and Ferguson, J. Narrow-band UVB (TL-01) phototherapy: an effective preventative treatment for the photodermatoses. *Br J Dermatol,* 132, 956, 1995.
72. McCoombes, J.A., Hirst, L.W. and Green, W.R. Use of topical cyclosporin for conjunctival manifestations of actinic prurigo. *Am J Ophthalmol,* 130, 830, 2000.
73. Wildenberg, S.C., Oetting, W.S., Almodovar, C., et al. A gene causing Hermansky–Pudlak syndrome in a Puerto Rican population maps to chromosome 10q2. *Am J Hum Genet,* 57, 755, 1995.
74. Toro, J., Turner, M. and Gahl, W.A. Dermatologic manifestations of Hermansky–Pudlak syndrome in patients with and without a 16-base pair duplication in the HPS1 gene. *Arch Dermatol,* 135, 774, 1999.
75. Burnett, J.W. Capsicum pepper dermatitis. *Cutis,* 534, 1989.
76. Jones, L.A., Tandberg, D. and Troutman, W.G. Household treatment for "chile burns" of the hands. *Clin Toxicol,* 25, 483, 1987.
77. Stoner, J.G. Miscellaneous dermatitis-inducing plants. *Clin Dermatol,* 4, 94, 1986.
78. Kizer, W.S., Prarie, T. and Morey, A.F. Balanitis xerotica obliterans: epidemiologic distribution in an equal access healthcare system. *South Med J,* 96, 9, 2003.
79. Drut, R.M., Gomez, M.A. and Drut, R. Human papillomavirus is present in some cases of childhood penile lichen sclerosus: an *in situ* hybridization and SP-PCR study. *Pediatr Dermatol,* 15, 85, 1998.

80. Nasca, M.R., Innocenzi, D. and Micali, G. Penile cancer among patients with genital lichen sclerosus. *J Am Acad Dermatol*, 41, 911, 1999.
81. Mallon, E., Hawkins, D. and Dinneen, M. Circumcision and genital dermatoses. *Arch Dermatol*, 136, 350, 2000.
82. Burke, J.P, Duggirala, R., Hale, D.E., et al. Genetic basis of acanthosis nigricans in Mexican Americans and its association with phenotypes related to type 2 diabetes. *Hum Genet* 106, 467, 2000.
83. Hay, R.J., Estrada Castanon, R., Alarcon Hernandez, H., et al. Wastage of family income on skin disease in Mexico. *Br Med J*, 309, 848, 1994.
84. Savall, R., Ferrandiz, C., Ferrer, I., et al. Idiopathic guttate hypomelanosis. *Br J Dermatol* 103, 635, 1980.
85. Mishriki, Y.Y. Skin commotion from repetitive devotion. Prayer callus. *Postgrad Med*, 105, 153, 1999.
86. Vollum, D.I. and Azadeh, B. Prayer nodules. *Clin Exp Dermatol*, 4, 39, 1979.
87. Abarca, J.F. and Casiccia, C.C. Skin cancer and ultraviolet-B radiation under the Antarctic ozone hole: Southern Chile, 1987–2000. *Photoderm Photoimmunol Photomed*, 18, 294, 2002.
88. Hurtig, A.K. and San Sebastian, M. Geographical differences in cancer incidence in the Amazon basin of Ecuador in relation to residence near oil fields. *Int J Epidemiol*, 31, 1021, 2002.
89. Grinspan, D. and Biagini, R. Chronic endemic regional hydroarsenicism. The manifestations of arsenic poisoning caused by drinking water. *Medicina Cutanea Ibero-Latino-Americana*, 13, 85, 1985.
90. Hall, H.I., Jones, S.E. and Saraiya, M. Prevalence and correlates of sunscreen use among US high school students. *J School Health*, 71, 453, 2001.
91. Hoegh, H.J., Davis, B.D. and Manthe, A.F. Sun avoidance practices among non-Hispanic white Californians. *Health Educ Behav*, 26, 360, 1999.
92. Pipitone, M., Robinson, J.K., Camara, C., et al. Skin cancer awareness in suburban employees: a Hispanic perspective. *J Am Acad Dermatol*, 47, 118, 2002.
93. Friedman, L.C., Bruce, S., Weinberg, A.D., et al. Early detection of skin cancer: racial/ethnic differences in behaviors and attitudes. *J Cancer Educ*, 9, 105, 1994.
94. Harris, R.B., Griffith, K. and Moon, T.E. Trends in the incidence of nonmelanoma skin cancers in southeastern Arizona, 1985–1996. *J Am Acad Dermatol*, 45, 528, 2001.
95. Zemelman, V., vonBeck, P., Alvarado, O., et al. Sexual dimorphism in skin eye and hair color and the presence of freckles in Chilean teenagers from two socioeconomic strata. *Revista Medica de Chile*, 130, 879, 2002.
96. Shaw, M., Sanguinetti, O., de Kaminsky, A.R., et al. Basal and spinous cell epitheliomas. *Medicina Cutanea Ibero-Latino-Americana*, 3, 471, 1975.
97. Hoy, W.E. Nonmelanoma skin carcinoma in Albuquerque, New Mexico: experience of a major health care provider. *Cancer*, 77, 2489, 1996.
98. Bigler, C., Feldman, J., Hall, E., et al. Pigmented basal cell carcinoma in Hispanics. *J Am Acad Dermatol*, 34, 751, 1996.
99. Maafs, E., De la Barreda, F., Delgado, R., et al. Basal cell carcinoma of trunk and extremities. *Int J Dermatol*, 36, 622, 1997.
100. Cress, R.D. and Holly, E.A. Incidence of cutaneous melanoma among non-Hispanic whites, Hispanics, Asians, and blacks: an analysis of California cancer registry data, 1988–1993. *Cancer Causes & Control*, 8, 246, 1997.
101. Feun, L.G., Raub, W.A. Jr., Duncan, R.C., et al. Melanoma in a southeastern Hispanic population. *Cancer Detect Prev*, 18, 145, 1994.
102. Black, W.C., Goldhahn, R.T. Jr. and Wiggins, C. Melanoma within a southwestern Hispanic population. *Arch Dermatol*, 123, 1331, 1987.

19 Dermatologic Diseases in Native Americans

Willie F. Richardson, Jr. and R. Steven Padilla

BACKGROUND

The diagnosis and treatment of skin diseases in Native Americans represent a unique challenge to the dermatologist. With the increasing population of Native Americans in the United States, from 1.42 million in 1980 to more than 1.9 million in 1990, comes a greater need to understand the biology and pathophysiology of dermatoses in Native American skin.[1] Additionally, a lack of epidemiologic data and clinical trials to guide our diagnostic and therapeutic methods further complicates the challenge. The scant data available was published in the early 20th century and consists primarily of case reports. The unique cultural habits and varied skin pigmentation of Native Americans gives rise to many disease variations. These factors, which alter disease appearance, also alter therapeutic considerations. Our goal is to begin to address some of the more common and unique skin diseases in the Native American population.

For purposes of this text, we will use interchangeably the terms "Native American," "American Indian," and "Indian." Our definition of "Indian" is based on the United States Code Collection Title 25, Chapter 18, General Provisions, section 1603c–d. These terms describe a person who is a member of a tribe, band, or other organized group of Indians, or is an Eskimo or Aleut or other Alaska Native.[2] Within these ethnic groups is a wide range of skin pigmentation. Likewise, not every tribe has the same beliefs, cultural traditions, and practices; therefore, dermatoses common to one tribe may not be prevalent in the next or may be more or less difficult to treat based on their beliefs regarding therapy.

Aside from skin pigmentation in Native Americans, there are several other issues that diminish optimal skin care. One is the lack of appropriate educational materials regarding various dermatoses, including instruction on the importance of photoprotection. The patient's basic understanding of the disease is particularly important in the management of common disorders such as atopic dermatitis, photoexacerbated atopic dermatitis, and hereditary polymorphous light eruption, and the more uncommon dermatoses such as cutaneous malignancies. For Indian people living on the reservation there are few dermatologic services, whereas those who reside in the city have more access to dermatologists. The percentage of Indians living in urban areas has increased from 0.4% in 1900 to more than 50% today.[1] Emigration of Indians off the reservation contributes to disparity of health care resources available.

Our discussion of skin disease in American Indians is based on our experience at the University of New Mexico Department of Dermatology with treating tribes of the Southwest. Our state's Native American population is nine percent, of which the Navajo Reservation in northwestern New Mexico has the largest tribal enrollment.[1] We do not want to generalize our experiences to other tribes but, rather, to only present them as an example of how clinical presentation, diagnostic considerations, and treatment can differ in Native Americans. We hope this information provides a foundation by which clinicians who treat Native Americans will have a better understanding of how cultural practices and pigmentation influence skin disease.

SPECIAL CONSIDERATIONS

In caring for Native American people, one must consider the medicine wheel and the impact that this has on their lives. The medicine wheel has much to teach the Western world, based on the stories that lie within its meaning. The medicine wheel is round, representing the circular sun, moon, earth, seasons, and life. There are four quadrants representing the four directions: the north, the south, the east, and the west. From the north comes wisdom, the place of winter, represented by the color white. From the east quadrant comes the beginning of all, represented by the color red, signifying the Native American race. From the west comes darkness, providing voices of conscience, represented by the color black. Finally, from the south come time and purity, represented by the color yellow, our sun. In all aspects of healing, one must consider the human being as a whole: a balance of mind, body, and spirit in harmony with the universe.[41] It is important to ask of one's spirit and thoughts to show a sense of empathy for the American Indian patient. When the treating physician begins to acknowledge the importance of these elements to Indian people, compliance will come without coercion, and a new level of patient care will be reached.

BASIC SCIENCE OF NATIVE AMERICAN SKIN

Data on the fundamental differences in American Indian skin are nonexistent. However, there is information on the role of pigmentation and its photoprotective action. What is known is that variations exist in the epidermal melanin unit and the shape and distribution of the melanosome.[3]

Empirical data support the notion that variations in skin pigmentation are an evolutionary, environmentally influenced event. Individuals who reside closer to the equator, where the UVR index is highest, have developed greater baseline pigmentation as compared to individuals farther away from the equator.[4] In addition, intermarriage among Native and non-Native Americans has led to greater variation of skin phototypes in the American Indian. Several studies have indicated that the current skin classification system developed by Fitzpatrick may not be ideal for people of color due to the wide range of UVR doses needed to induce erythema or melanogenesis.[4] Taylor proposed the Lancer Ethnicity Scale as a better measure of skin subclassification. This scale was designed to assess response of ethnic skin to various procedures such as chemical peeling and laser resurfacing. She suggested that it would be more beneficial to assess ethnic skin based on its ability to hyperpigment following an inflammatory stimulus.[4]

Current classifications look for differences in the melanocyte number and melanosome distribution. In a study comparing differences in skin biopsy sites among various ethnic groups, including Native Americans, Jimbow et al. found that there was no significant difference in the number of melanocytes and the epidermal melanin unit.[5] There is variation among ethnic and nonethnic populations in the numbers of melanocytes located in various regions of the body and the degree of dendritic cell branching.[5] Based on this information, it is difficult to argue that ethnic skin, based solely on pigmentation, differs physiologically from nonethnic skin. However, the differences resulting in the variation in skin tone can be explained by an understanding of melanosome shape, number, and distribution as well as the interaction of melanocytes with neighboring keratinocytes.

Szabo demonstrated that pigmented ethnic skin has a notable difference in the number and grouping of melanosomes. He noted that with increased skin pigmentation there was a greater number of melanosomes and less tendency of these melanosomes to aggregate as compared to nonethnic lighter skin colors.[4] Melanosome shape in these groups shows a preponderance of elongated melanosomes.[4] Studies that examine the shape and organization of melanosomes in Native American skin are nonexistent; however, one could infer that similar differences in number, shape, and distribution exist in Indian skin.

It is known that melanin provides protection from ultraviolet radiation–induced DNA damage. The lower incidence of photoinduced malignancies in Native Americans can be attributed to the greater degree of constitutive melanosome production that provides a greater degree of photoprotection. The photoprotective role of melanin and the paradoxical increase in the incidence of photoexacerbated dermatoses are unexplained. This lack of true photoprotection infers that there are other mechanisms involved, possibly a soluble mediator within the cytoplasm of keratinocytes or mediators that alter the immune response to light injury.

An important consideration regarding skin disease in Native Americans is the historical influence of population reduction secondary to the wave of immigration that occurred in the early 15th and 16th centuries. This reduction in population gave birth to the concept we know today as the "bottleneck phenomenon." In this setting, genome alleles were selected out of the population in such a way that they were then amplified in the offspring. Although taboos exist, intermarriage among tribal clans caused an amplification of recessive alleles and the emergence of disease-specific entities such as Navajo poikiloderma, Navajo neuropathy, severe combined immunodeficiency, and Athabaskan brainstem dysgenesis. The expression of a recessive allelic gene product appears to contribute to the increased prevalence of certain skin disorders in the Native American populations.[6]

DERMATOSES IN NATIVE AMERICANS: UNIQUE DERMATOSES

HEREDITARY POLYMORPHOUS LIGHT ERUPTION

One of the most well-known dermatoses in Native Americans is hereditary polymorphous light eruption, affecting more than 1% of the population.[7] Some studies cite a prevalence as high as 5% in American Indians and 8% in Indians of Colombia in South America.[8]

The cause is unknown. The disease appears to be autosomal-dominantly inherited with reduced penetrance and more than 75% of patients have first-degree relatives who are also affected.[7] The condition is worsened by both UVA and UVB. Several tribes across North America are reported to be affected, including the Chippewa, Omaha, Winnebag, Ponca, Navajo, and Sioux.[8] Human leukocyte antigen (HLA) associations include B40 and Cw3 in Bogota and A24 and Cw4 in Cree of Saskatchewan.[9] Fusaro and Johnson described a high frequency of DRB1*0407, a subset of DR4, in tribes of North and South American Indians.[8]

Diagnostic considerations include actinic prurigo, though some authors consider hereditary polymorphous light eruption the same disease.

Clinical Presentation

The initial complaint of the patient is that of pruritus following exposure to sunlight, with subsequent development of dermatitis. Everett proposed a classification of clinical presentation based on a study by Lamb et al. that divided clinical lesions into four basic types: plaquelike, contact eczematous, papular and prurigo-like, and erythematous type. Cutaneous plaques are most common, presenting lesions in up to 75% of cases.[10] Patients may have an associated conjunctivitis and cheilitis, especially the pediatric population. The disease will worsen during times of increased ultraviolet radiation intensity, such as the spring and summer, with improvement during the winter months.[10] Disease is distributed in light-exposed areas, sparing those who are adequately protected from UVR.

The mainstay of therapy is broad-spectrum sunscreen usage, providing UVA and UVB protection with at least a sun protection factor (SPF) of 30 and containing an avobenzone. The use of oral beta-carotene may be beneficial, though no controlled trials have been performed.[7] Systemic chloroquine should be reserved for severe cases.[10] Our experience is that topical steroids, broad-spectrum sunscreen, and oral antihistamines provide the patient with relief and improvement in clinical appearance.

NEUTROPENIC POIKILODERMA (FORMERLY KNOWN AS NAVAJO POIKILODERMA)

There have been 20 cases reported to date in various tribes. The inheritance pattern appears to be autosomal recessive. No etiology of the disease has been found to date.[6]

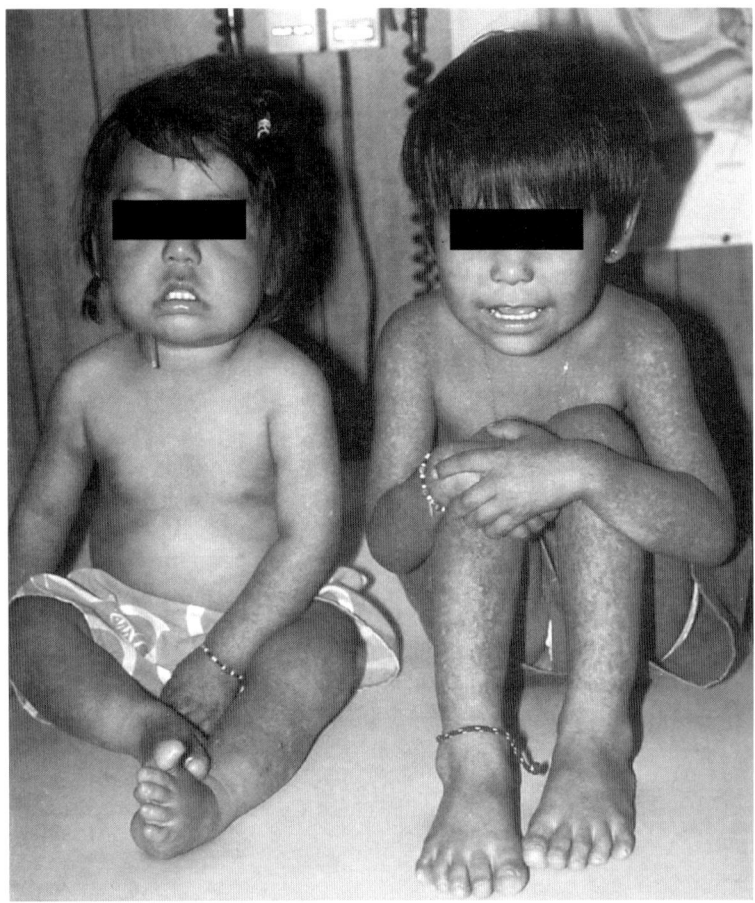

FIGURE 19.1 Two Navajo siblings with neutropenic poikiloderma. The patient on the left demonstrates early findings of erythematous papules on the forearms and early poikilodermatous changes on the upper extremities. The patient on the right demonstrates later findings of significant poikiloderma.

Other poikilodermatous disorders occurring in infancy and childhood include dyskeratosis congenita, congenital telangiectatic erythema (Bloom's syndrome), and poikiloderma congenitale (Rothmund–Thomson syndrome). The absence of an X-linked dominant mode of inheritance and absence of oral and nail lesions exclude dyskeratosis congenita. Absence of an increased number of sister chromatid exchanges should exclude Bloom's syndrome, although patients may be affected by recurrent infections as well. Rothmund–Thomson syndrome will have associated physical exam findings such as warty keratoses of the hands, elbows, knees, and feet.[11]

Patients present during the first year of life, with erythematous papules that enlarge and heal with characteristic findings of poikiloderma: atrophy, telangiectases, and hypo- or hyperpigmentation[6] (Figures 19.1 and 19.2). Sites of predilection tend to be the extremities with associated findings of pachyonychia but no evidence of alopecia or leukoplakia.[6] Growth retardation, short stature, and eczematous dermatitis are common. Abnormalities in levels of lutenizing hormone and antithyroid antibodies have been reported.[12]

No treatment is available at this time other than symptomatic management of dermatitis.

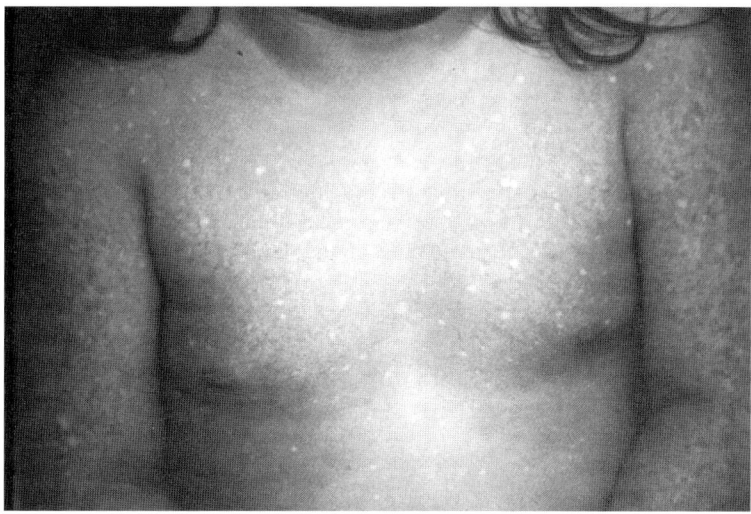

FIGURE 19.2 Neutropenic poikiloderma.

DERMATOSES IN NATIVE AMERICANS: COMMON DERMATOSES

ORAL FOCAL EPITHELIAL HYPERPLASIA (HECK'S DISEASE)

The disease was described in 1961 by John W. Heck, the dental director of the United States Public Health Service Indian Hospital in Gallup, New Mexico. Prevalence of the condition is unknown.[13] The disease is more common in females than males. Onset occurs in childhood, though a subset of Eskimo adults exhibit persistent disease.[13]

Heck's disease is caused by mucosal infection with human papilloma virus strains 13 and 32.[13] Histopathology is consistent with a viral etiology by the demonstration of ballooning degeneration of keratinocytes in the upper stratum spinosum.[13]

Considerations when evaluating affected patients include other causes of white plaques of the mucosa, such as diffuse epithelial hyperplasia seen in individuals who abuse tobacco. Condyloma accuminatum, bite fibroma, mucosal neuroma, verrucca vulgaris, oral white sponge nevus, and hereditary benign intraepithelial dyskeratosis are also diagnostic considerations.[13]

Located on the upper and lower lip, the buccal mucosa, tongue, or gingiva are multiple asymptomatic white papules on a background of normal-appearing mucosa. The papules are soft to palpation in contrast to the firm nature of bite fibroma.[13]

No treatment is needed, as the condition is self-limiting, resolving over several months to a year. Destructive modalities such as cryosurgery, surgical excision, and carbon dioxide laser therapy can be considered.[13]

HEREDITARY BENIGN INTRAEPITHELIAL DYSKERATOSIS

In a recent report, hereditary benign intraepithelial dyskeratosis was described in a small tribe in central North Carolina, the Haliwa-Saponi.[14] The disease appears to be inherited in an autosomal-dominant mode and is due to a duplication of chromosome 4q25.[15]

Considerations include oral white sponge nevus, hereditary mucoepithelial dyskeratosis, and Heck's disease. Patients lack anal and genital psoriasiform dermatitis that may occur with white sponge nevus. There is no involvement of the hair, eyes, nails, and lungs, as may occur with hereditary mucoepithelial dyskeratosis.[16]

The condition presents as a white, spongy plaque involving the lips, ventral surface of the tongue, and floor of the mouth.[14] Associated eye findings include the presence of bilateral white plaques on the cornea, with conjunctival telangiectases described as "red eyes" by Haisley-Royster et al.[14]

No treatment has been reported, though one may consider destructive modalities such as liquid nitrogen or carbon dioxide laser ablation.

ACNE VULGARIS

Prevalence figures in the Native American population are unknown. In our experience, acne vulgaris is common in the Navajo population.

Acne vulgaris may be considered a follicular disorder characterized by abnormal keratinization, sebum overproduction, inflammation, and overgrowth of the normal skin flora *Propionibacterium acne*. Keratinocytes mature as they approach the stratum corneum but maintain their less cohesive properties and do not shed into the follicular ostia. A follicular plug follows with resultant overgrowth of microaerophilic bacteria, the most common being *P. acne*. This coincides with increased production of sebum, secondary inflammation, and resulting follicular destruction.

Few disorders are confused with acne vulgaris. The clinician should give consideration to the diagnosis of acne rosacea in the absence of comedones.

The hallmark primary lesion of acne vulgaris is the comedone, of which there are two types: open and closed. Closed comedones morphologically are white to flesh-colored papules 1–2 mm in diameter. Open comedones are slightly umbilicated, flesh-colored to whitish papules, with central black punctum of similar diameter. The classic distribution of the disease is centrofacial, involving the malar eminences, nasal bridge, forehead and glabella, but may occur anywhere.

Also characteristic is the presence of inflammatory papules and pustules that may be folliculocentric. These papules and pustules may give rise to deep-seated cysts and nodules involving the face, chest, or back. These lesions can be complicated by excoriation, crust, and a seropurulent discharge (Figures 19.3 and 19.4). Progression of the disease may lead to the development of disfiguring nodulocysts that result in scarring.

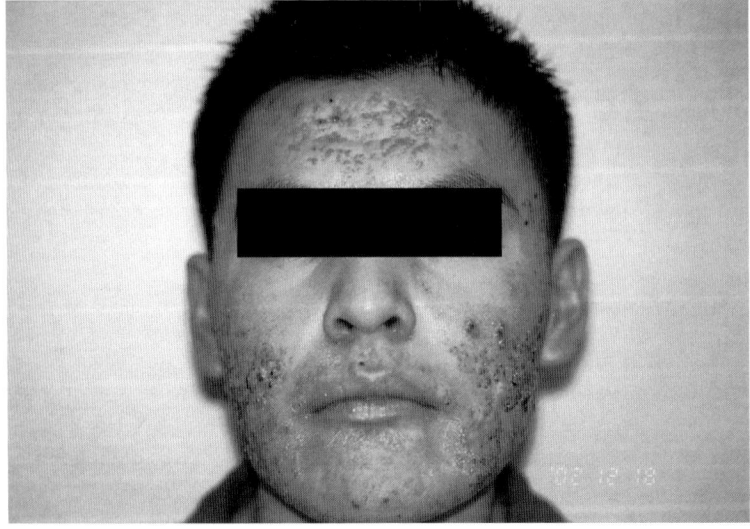

FIGURE 19.3 Eighteen-year-old Navajo male with severe acne vulgaris.

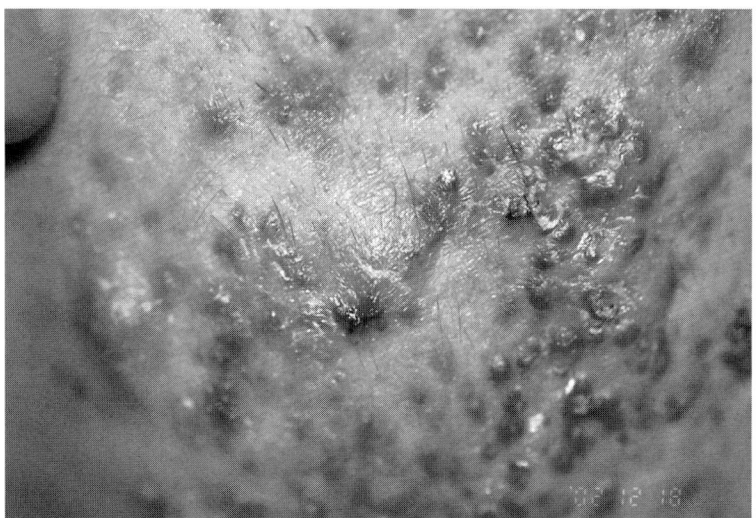

FIGURE 19.4 Erythematous crusted papules and nodules with excoriation.

Initial treatment should focus on the stage and distribution of disease. This initially includes a combination of antibiotics, retinoids, benzoyl peroxide, and salicylic acid preparations. A commonly employed first-line combination includes the use of an oral antibiotic, topical benzoyl peroxide, and a topical retinoid. Another combination for patients who do not tolerate oral antibiotic therapy is the use of a topical antibiotic and benzoyl peroxide with a topical retinoid. The lowest-strength retinoid that provides optimal control with minimal dryness and irritation should be used. Therapies for 3–6 months should be tried before consideration of alternate combinations or additions to therapy. Patients with recalcitrant or severe inflammatory papulopustular or nodulocystic acne should be considered candidates for systemic retinoid therapy.

Treatment of disease is similar to nonethnic skin with few unique considerations. In Native Americans clinicians must consider, as with other dermatoses, the increased likelihood of postinflammatory hyperpigmentation. This may arise secondary to a primary inflammation related to the dermatosis or may be induced by the use of topical agents. Patients must be educated that this is a natural response of their skin and that it should subside over several months.

Scarring from acne is a common problem in Native American patients. This can consist of keloidal scarring on the chest and back and pitted scarring on the face. A family history of scarring acne should be recorded and considered in choosing specific therapy and before institution of systemic retinoid therapy. Early use of such modalities should be incorporated to allow for earlier resolution and the prevention of scarring and emotional distress.

ACNE ROSACEA

Characteristically more common in individuals of Celtic origin, rosacea, when present in Native Americans, has a tendency to be more severe and difficult to manage. The lack of sunscreen usage and the high UV index that exist, in the Southwest are perhaps two reasons for increased prevalence. Further complicating the course of disease are dietary habits, such as the consumption of spicy foods.

The etiology of rosacea is poorly understood. Most evidence points to vascular instability manifesting as a tendency for vessels to dilate early on in the disease and in later stages to remain dilated.[17] Therefore, consideration should be given to the importance of vasomotor control. An increased prevalence of migraine headaches along with a prevalence of rosacea in perimenopausal women further supports this pathogenesis.[18]

It is important to consider other photoexacerbated dermatoses that present with facial erythema, such as systemic lupus erythematosus, and polymorphous light eruptions that present as persistent facial erythema. Systemic causes of facial flushing include carcinoid syndrome and pheochromocytoma.[19] Although many consider acne vulgaris in evaluation of these patients, rosacea characteristically lacks open and closed comedones.

Early on, rosacea may simply manifest as facial redness. Common sites of involvement include the forehead, malar eminences, nasal bridge, postauricular scalp, and V-area of the neck. It may progress to a blanchable, patchy erythema with telangiectases. Many times a history can be elicited that indicates a worsening of the condition with stress, ingestion of hot liquids or alcohol, spicy foods, and exposure to sunlight. In the later stages of disease, it progresses to papules and pustules in a similar distribution.

Chronic untreated rosacea can be extremely disfiguring due to soft-tissue hypertrophy that results in the development of rhinophyma, otophyma, blepharophyma, or gnathophyma.[19] Unfortunately, this stage of disease is commonly the initial presentation of Native American patients to the dermatologist. A delay in therapy with progression to this stage of disease can be attributed to the difficulty in clinically appreciating persistent facial erythema in skin of color.

Management of rosacea can be difficult, depending on patient expectations. The persistent erythema of rosacea is best managed with dietary avoidance of spicy foods and hot liquids, the use of sunscreen with a minimum SPF of 30, and an avobenzone compound. This combination provides adequate UVB and UVA coverage. Oral tetracycline and tetracycline derivatives have been tried, with varying results. In our experience topical antibiotic therapy is of little value, although we have used metronidazole and clindamycin to prevent the progression to papulopustular disease. Other treatments include sulfur-containing lotions, salicylic acid, and azaleic acid preparations, all having varying efficacy.

Special consideration must be given to the patient presenting with soft tissue phymas. Many times this is considered of cosmetic significance with little regard to the emotional disturbance and social implications it carries. Management of hypertrophic disease requires surgical intervention in addition to good medical control.

Atopic Dermatitis

Atopic dermatitis is one of the most common diagnoses in dermatology and primary care clinics and carries a significant degree of morbidity. The disease is estimated to affect 10%–15% of all children.[20] Native American children seem to be especially plagued by the condition, resulting in a population that is challenging to manage due to a lack of understanding of environmental influences.

Several hypotheses on etiology and pathogenesis have been put forth. The most current evidence suggests that atopic dermatitis can be viewed from two different etiologic perspectives: externally and internally induced.[21] The external hypothesis suggests a primary barrier defect resulting in increased transepidermal water loss with resultant tissue dehydration, pruritus, and inflammation. The primary symptom is pruritus.[21] The internal hypothesis emphasizes the role of T-cell-mediated inflammation as the initial event, with subsequent barrier loss and pruritus.[21] Certainly, a combination of the two could play a role in any given population.

An additional component is the role of the IgE response in atopic dermatitis. For decades the increased prevalence of atopic dermatitis in families with an "atopic" background has been noted. Among diseases considered to have an "atopic" component are allergic rhinitis, allergic conjunctivitis, and asthma.

In Native American children diagnosed with atopic dermatitis, we have observed a number of patients whose disease is also worsened by sun exposure. The mechanism of photoexacerbation is unknown, but we commonly observe improvement with sun-protective measures.

When present, the characteristic flexural dermatitis combined with findings of Dennie–Morgan lines and eyelid folds, palmar hyperlinearity, perioral cyanosis, and family history of atopy facilitate diagnosis. Chronic eczema and lichen simplex chronicus may occur with prolonged disease and mechanical irritation. Allergic contact dermatitis and irritant dermatitis may exacerbate the condition and should be considered. An environmental history should be performed to seek out potential allergens or irritants. Hereditary polymorphous light eruption should also be considered.

The classical clinical finding is a poorly demarcated, scaly, erythematous patch or plaque that may be complicated by the secondary findings of excoriation and crusted serosanguinous exudates. The face, neck, and antecubital and popliteal fossa are most often affected. Chronic states present as lichenified plaques. Complaints of pruritus are common as well as a history of worsening with heat and relief with scratching.

Native American patients may have less appreciable erythema. The clinical finding may be as subtle as increased pigmentation. Palpation of the involved areas, however, may elicit appreciable erythema with blanching. A clinical variant, located in the same distribution, is characterized by pruritic, irregularly pigmented patches and plaques. This patchy nature can be associated with the use of topical herbal remedies.

Therapy is directed at controlling inflammation, reducing pruritus, and restoring the epidermal barrier. The choice of topical steroid therapy should be guided by the severity of disease and balanced against side effects such as skin atrophy. To start, we recommend the use of a low-potency steroid. In our experience, the potency of the steroid should be increased slowly and in a stepwise manner. If improvement in the condition is not observed with a Class 5 steroid, one should next employ a Class 4 steroid. In infants, the use of high-potency and ultrapotent corticosteroids should be avoided due to the increased risk of systemic absorption and steroid-induced atrophy. An adequate treatment time period, such as 2–3 weeks, should pass before considering any given steroid class a treatment failure.

Newer therapies in management of atopic dermatitis include the immunomodulators tacrolimus and pimecrolimus. These medications are nonsteroid-containing agents, with their chief actions aimed at the suppression of inflammation. Nonsteroid therapies are free of concern regarding atrophy and may be used in intertrigenous and facial areas of involvement.[22] A common side effect is a burning sensation with application and is more common with tacrolimus.[22]

Thorough education of family members on the importance of emollient therapy is essential to decreasing morbidity associated with the disease and allows for maximal efficacy of steroid therapy. Important in arid environments such as the Southwest United States is the application of emollients to moistened skin. We recommend the avoidance of showers, less frequent bathing, and emollient application immediately after a light towel drying. We use ointment-based emollients to facilitate epidermal rehydration and we avoid the use of soaps and scented bath gels, especially during exacerbations.

Finally, patients should be educated regarding the natural history of the condition and informed that there is no cure for disease, only palliative measures that can keep the disease under control. The recurring nature of the condition, characterized by periods of improvement and exacerbation, should also be described. In our experience with Native American patients, sun protection is encouraged.

DERMATOPHYTE INFECTION

The prevalence of this infection is unknown in Native Americans. We present the dermatophytoses together as fungal infection of the skin, nails, and hair. Exact epidemiologic data in Native Americans are not available, though we have observed more severe disease in this population.

The most commonly isolated fungi belong to one of the following three genuses: trichophyton, microsporum, and epidermophyton. In pediatric populations, tinea capitis is most commonly caused by *Trichophyton tonsurans* or *Microsporum canis*. Tinea cruris is most commonly caused by

Trichophyton rubrum. Tinea pedis tends to be uncommon in pediatric individuals but more common in adults with the most common etiology of *T. rubrum*.

The infection tends to be more common in crowded environments and in individuals with poor personal hygiene. Transmission from inanimate objects, as well as person-to-person transmission, does occur.

The differential diagnosis includes noninfectious etiologies of scaly plaques in the scalp such as seborrheic dermatitis, scalp psoriasis, or tinea amiantacea. The clinical presentation of tinea corporis should prompt the clinician to consider other etiologies of figurate erythema, including granuloma annulare, erythema annulare centrifigum, erythema marginatum, erythema gyratum repens, and erythema chronicum migrans. Granuloma annulare will lack scale with a more infiltrated pattern. The absence of a history of streptococcal disease and underlying malignancy should reduce the likelihood of erythema marginatum and erythema gyratum repens, respectively. Associated clinical findings, negative potassium hydroxide preparation, and negative culture should guide clinical decision-making.

Tinea capitis presents with either a scaly erythematous patch or plaque that is fairly well demarcated. The degree of inflammation varies depending on species involved and is greatest with the genus microsporum. Patients may present with "black dot ringworm," characterized by areas of broken-off hairs and alopecia commonly caused by *T tonsurans*. Favus, a rare diagnosis in America, is characterized by a boggy, inflammatory, scaly plaque and is usually caused by *Trichophyton schonleinii*.

Tinea corporis classically presents as a scaly, erythematous, annular plaque with areas of central clearing distributed on the trunk. In the center of the plaque, there may be folliculocentric erythematous papules. Just beyond the erythematous border is where scrapings for potassium hydroxide preparations and culture should be obtained, as this is where the fungus is located, not centrally. Furthermore, if the patient has vigorously bathed prior to the visit or has applied emollients, scale may not be appreciated and may result in false negative findings on KOH preparation. The degree of pruritus tends to be minimal but, again, depends on the degree of inflammation present, and, is mitigated by the use of topical steroids. Tinea corporis may present as a Majocchi's granuloma, characterized by the presence of a well-demarcated, erythematous, scaly plaque with a central formation of pustules.

Therapy depends on disease being considered, with tinea capitis requiring systemic therapies such as griseofulvin. Hurwitz recommends the following dosage guidelines for micronized griseofulvin:

If less than 2 years of age, 10–20 mg/kg per day
Weight of 30–50 pounds, 10–20 mg/kg per day
Weight of more than 50 pounds, 250–500 mg/day

Ultramicronized griseofulvin is now available, and treatment dosage is approximately reduced by half. Duration of therapy should continue for 6–8 weeks.[23]

Therapy for tinea corporis and dermatophyte infections of regions other than the scalp can generally be managed with topical therapies such as topical clotrimazole, ketoconazole, or terbinafine cream for 4–6 weeks. If patients have tinea pedis, longer courses of therapy for 6–8 weeks may be needed with occasional maintenance use after clearing. Patients should be educated regarding the occurrence of postinflammatory hyperpigmentation and the lack of need for continued treatment when this occurs, as most patients will assume this is the result of the infectious process.

CONGENITAL MELANOCYTIC NEVI, PIGMENTARY ANOMALIES, AND OTHER NEVI

Estimates on the prevalence of congenital nevi such as the Mongolian spot, nevus of Ota, nevus of Ito, and epidermal nevi are not available due to a lack of reporting and the common benign nature of such findings. These diagnoses, however, are known to have increased prevalence in African Americans and Native Americans as well as other patients of ethnic origin.[24]

During embryonic development, neural crest cells migrate to the epidermis and give rise to the melanocyte. If there is migratory arrest, the melanocytes may become trapped within various regions of the dermis. A classic example is the Mongolian spot, characterized histologically by the presence of melanocytes in the lower two thirds of the dermis; melanocytes in the nevus of Ota and nevus of Ito tend to be located in the upper one third of the dermis.[24]

The Mongolian spot and nevi of Ota and Ito belong to a group of disorders referred to as cerulodermas. Given their characteristic location, they are infrequently confused with other diagnoses. Definitive diagnosis is based on histopathology.

The Mongolian spot is characterized by the presence of a blue-brown, hyperpigmented patch, classically located on the lower back and sacral region. The patch may also be located on the extremities or upper back. The patch is classically well demarcated and homogenous in pigmentation.

Nevus of Ota and nevus of Ito vary clinically from the Mongolian spot by a less homogeneous pigmentation and location. Ota's nevus characteristically occurs on the face in the area of the eye and sometimes may be referred to as nevus fuscocaeruleus ophthalmomaxillaris. Ito's nevus has preference for the upper shoulder girdle. Bilateral nevus of Ota has been associated with the presence of an extensive Mongolian spot.[25]

No treatment of Mongolian spot, nevus of Ota, or nevus of Ito is necessary due to the benign nature of the conditions. However, use of topical concealers and cosmetics may be used for facial areas involved.

OTHER NEVI

Epidermal nevi have been treated with a number of different modalities due to their cosmetically disturbing appearance. Destructive measures such as dermabrasion, shave excision, electrodesiccation, and curettage, as well as laser treatment, have been performed in our clinic with some success. However, postinflammatory hyperpigmentation presents a serious risk (Figures 19.5 and 19.6).

PSORIASIS VULGARIS

Estimated prevalence of psoriasis in the general population is only 2%.[26] No prevalence data in Native Americans are currently available.

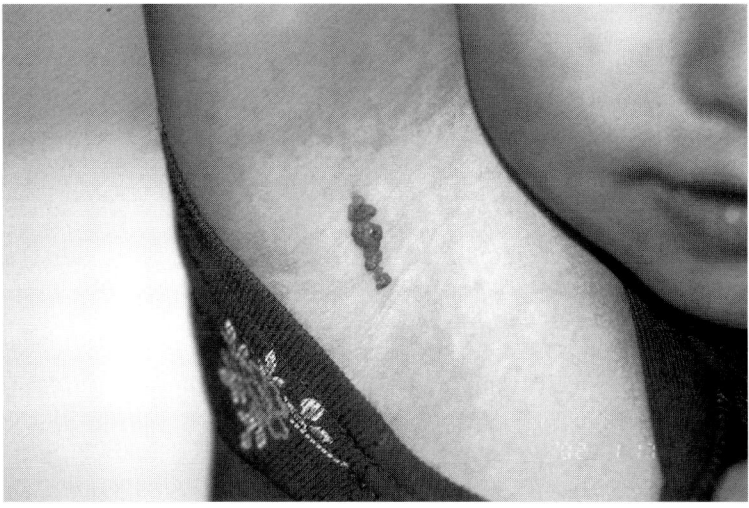

FIGURE 19.5 Epidermal nevus in the axilla of Navajo child.

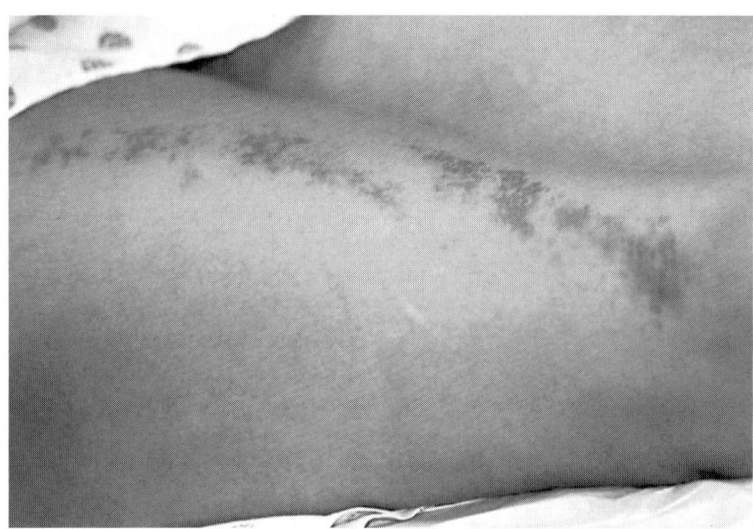

FIGURE 19.6 Inflammatory linear verrucous epidermal nevus, a benign diagnosis, referred for evaluation of malignancy and removal.

The pathogenesis of psoriasis vulgaris has evolved over the years from one of epidermal proliferation to one of immune dysregulation, as can be inferred from the improvement of clinical disease with medications altering these pathways. However, increased epidermal proliferation is the end response, with a reduction in time from 311 to 36 hours according to cell kinetics.[27] The result is increased epidermal cell population in the epidermis.

Psoriasis has been linked to certain HLA haplotypes indicating a genetic role in pathogenesis, including HLA-Cw6, HLA-B17, HLA-B27, and HLA-DR7.[28,29]

Differential Diagnosis

The diagnosis is not difficult in the setting of the classic well-demarcated erythematous plaque with micaceous scale. Other diagnoses to consider include small and large plaque parapsoriasis, eczema, mycosis fungoides, lichen simplex chronicus, pityriasis rubra pilaris, allergic drug dermatitis, and secondary syphilis.

The psoriatic plaque is well demarcated, erythematous, and covered by a fine micaceous scale that, when removed, exhibits punctate areas of bleeding. This phenomenon is known as the Auspitz sign. Pruritus may be associated with the condition. Sites of predilection include the bilateral elbows, umbilicus, sacrum, bilateral knees, and, occasionally, palmar and plantar skin. There is absence of mucosal involvement. Genitalia may be involved as well, and new plaques that may arise in areas of trauma characterize the Koebner phenomenon.

Scalp psoriasis presents differently, arising focally or diffuse, with fine, silvery, scaly erythematous patches and plaques that may not be as well demarcated. Pruritus may be severe here as well, resulting in excoriation and crust.

When examining patients with psoriasis, special attention should be directed at the nail plate and proximal nail fold. Nail-matrix damage leads to nail pits and "oil spots." "Oil spots" are yellow to brown, irregularly shaped macules visible through the nail plate. Disease may be localized to the nails without obvious skin findings.

Traditional therapy has incorporated the use of topical keratolytics, topical steroids, coal tar, anthralin, and retinoids such as tazarotene. Newer agents include topical Vitamin D analogs such as calcipotriene. Phototherapy has long played a role in therapy. Depending on the patient, choices include UVA and narrow-band UVB (311 nm). Other modalities include systemic agents such as methotrexate, cyclosporine, and acitretin. Systemic steroids are best avoided due to the risk of severe life-threatening erythroderma and associated mortality.[30]

SEBORRHEIC DERMATITIS

Seborrheic dermatitis commonly affects 2%–5% of the population with two age peaks, one during infancy and the latter from ages 50 to 80 years.[31] Specific prevalence data in Native Americans do not exist.

Seborrheic dermatitis represents a disorder in which there is hyperproliferation of the epidermis and inflammation resulting in flaking of the skin. In infancy, the disease appears to be related to sebaceous activity, whereas in adults there is no relation to severity of disease.[31] As a result, the distribution is different. There has been an association with inflammation induced by *Pityrosporum ovale*, a yeast, that is considered normal flora of the skin and is found in follicles.[31]

The disease may be idiopathic, associated with drugs, infections, or systemic diseases, or of familial inheritance associated with a C5 deficiency called Lanier's disease in infants. Drugs incriminated include arsenic, gold, cimetidine, methyldopa, and neuroleptics. Seborrheic dermatitis has been associated with acute onset of human immunodeficiency virus infection as well as Parkinson's disease.[31] Other diseases to consider include scalp psoriasis, tinea capitis, tinea corporis, and nummular eczema.

Commonly referred to as "dandruff" when affecting the scalp, the clinical presentation can vary from mild to severe. In its mildest form, it may present with only diffuse, waxy, adherent, fine yellow scale along the base of the hair shaft without scalp involvement. Moderately severe disease involves the scalp with erythema and similar scale. Severe seborrheic dermatitis can present with diffuse, thickened, malodorous, yellow scale that is platelike in adherence to the hair shaft, resulting in matting of the hair. Patients may complain of only mild scalp pruritus or burning.

In adults, facial, paranasal, postauricular, eyebrows, melolabial fold, truncal, axillary, and groin involvement may occur, presenting as erythematous patches that may be characterized by greasy yellow scale. In infants, disease may be more diffuse.

Therapy targets the control of inflammation and the associated organism *P. ovale*. For mild scalp disease, we prescribe a shampoo containing either selenium sulfide or zinc pyrithione. Patients should be instructed to apply the shampoo by massaging it into the scalp, leaving it in contact with the scalp for 5 min before rinsing. This should be repeated at least every other day until the condition is controlled, with twice-weekly maintenance usage. Moderate to severe scalp involvement may require the addition of topical midpotency steroid solutions or foam steroid preparations twice daily.

Non-scalp-involved areas can be treated by topical antifungal creams, such as 2% ketoconazole, to reduce the population of yeast. Adjuvant therapies for more moderate to severe involvement may require the addition of a topical steroid cream. Patients should be educated that the disease process may vary with periods of remission and exacerbation, becoming worse in warmer arid environments. This can be particularly problematic on the reservation, with the use of wood-burning stoves for heating and lack of relative humidity.

LICHEN PLANUS

The general prevalence of lichen planus is estimated at 1%, with no studies to date regarding specific prevalence in Indian people.[32]

Lichen planus is an idiopathic inflammatory dermatosis associated with systemic disorders such as hepatitis C infection, primary biliary cirrhosis, and chronic hepatitis, as well as genetic linkage to HLA B3 and B5.[33] Gold salt therapy has also been commonly associated with disease in some cases.[34] The end result is a T-cell inflammatory infiltrate resulting in epidermal destruction and hyperplasia.

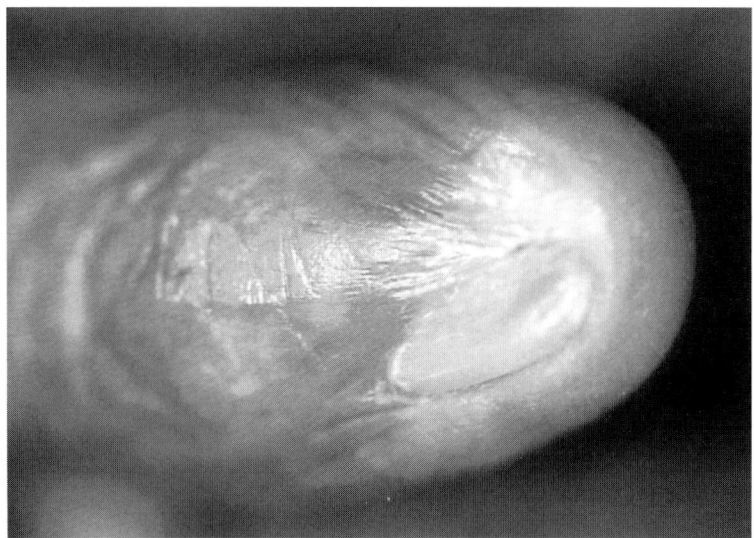

FIGURE 19.7 Fingernail demonstrating pterygium formation in Navajo patient with erosive lichen planus.

Characteristic clinical morphology and location of disease allow for straightforward diagnoses in most cases, whereas other papulosquamous diseases based on location should be ruled out.

Years of anecdotal evidence resulted in characterizing the classic lesion of lichen planus as a planar, pruritic, polygonal, purple papule located around the bilateral ankles and volar wrist. Other areas that may be involved are the buccal region of the oral mucosa, with findings of Wickham's striae, a lacy, netlike, white plaque, or nail involvement with pterygium formation, and points of trauma demonstrating the Koebner phenomenon, or generalization to involve the entire body, typically sparing the face (Figure 19.7). There are many forms of mucous membrane disease. Ulcerative lesions of the mouth should raise the possibility of lichen planus, with aggressive management due to the risk of development of squamous cell carcinoma.[35] Severe erosive disease of the oral mucosa and bilateral feet was observed in a Navajo female in the absence of classic lesions of lichen planus elsewhere (Figures 19.7–19.9).

Management of oral or skin disease is targeted at reduction of the inflammatory response with high to ultrapotent topical steroid ointments. Systemic prednisone at a dosage of 40 mg taken orally may be utilized for immediate relief, with a reduction after the disease improves and the eventual conversion to topical therapy. Patients should be educated that disease may spontaneously improve after 1–2 years, with possibility of recurrence. Aggressive immunosuppressive therapy is generally not required unless severe erosive disease is present. Systemic retinoids, such as isotretinoin, have been used with some success in our practice. Patients should be warned about the occurrence of postinflammatory hyperpigmentation and management, as previously described.

GRANULOMA ANNULARE

Prevalence of granuloma annulare is currently unknown but appears to be more common in children and females.

The etiology and pathogenesis of disease have yet to be elucidated, though there has been an association of generalized disease with diabetes mellitus in approximately 20% of cases.[36] The process involves the presence of a lymphohistiocytic infiltrate in the dermis, resulting in destruction of collagen bundles and necrobiosis of the dermis.

Based on the clinical subtype of disease present, one should consider other causes of figurate erythemas, including erythema annulare centrifigum, erythema marginatum, erythema gyratum repens, erythema chronicum migrans, tinea corporis, and annular lichen planus. Characteristic

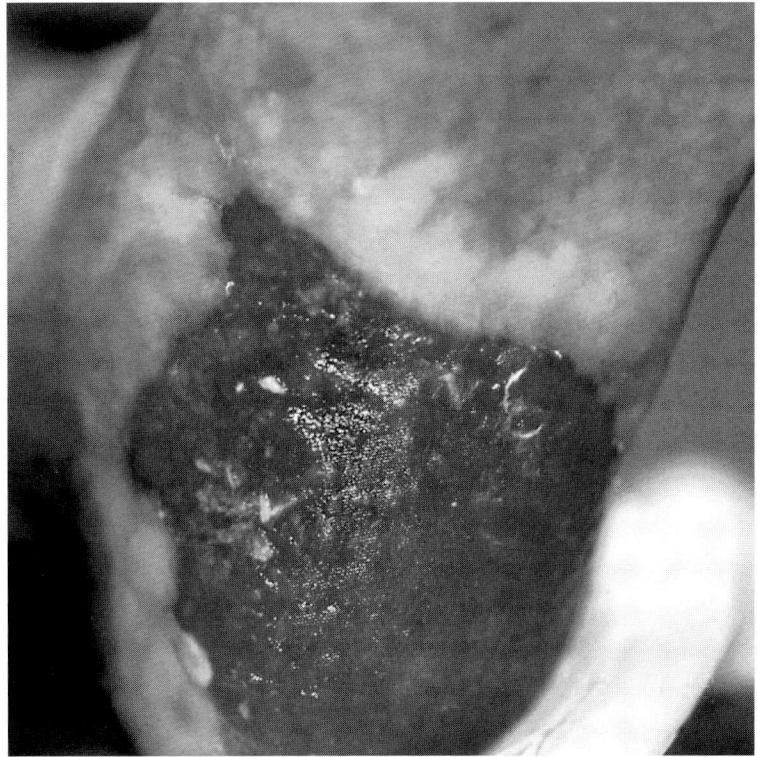

FIGURE 19.8 Erosive lichen planus of the foot.

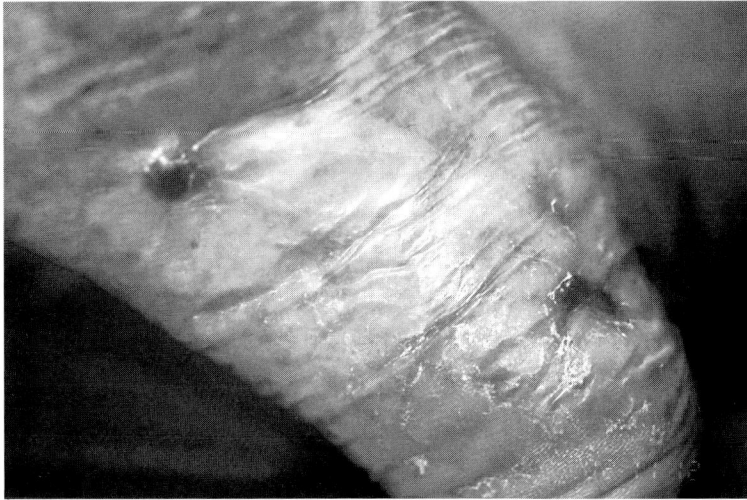

FIGURE 19.9 Healed erosion after high-potency corticosteroids topically for several months.

bilateral disease and an absence of findings on potassium hydroxide in the setting of steroid responsivity should provide a clue to the clinician regarding the diagnosis.

The earliest lesion of granuloma annulare is an isolated, reddish-brown papule that expands with central clearing and may be associated with pruritus. Lesions may enlarge to several centimeters in diameter. Common locations of involvement include the dorsal hands and feet bilaterally;

however, diffuse body involvement may occur. Centrally, there is no atrophy or scale. Arciform and serpigenous forms may occur.

Similar to other inflammatory diseases, therapy is targeted at the reduction of underlying inflammation with use of high to ultrapotent topical steroid therapy until the erythematous component has resolved, with resultant postinflammatory hyperpigmentation. Patients may benefit from the use of occlusion with plastic wrap but should be warned of increased incidence of atrophy with continued use. Systemic prednisone at a dosage of 40 mg taken orally will result in improvement in generalized disease but may unmask underlying diabetes mellitus in genetically prone individuals.[37] Given the high prevalence of diabetes mellitus in Native Americans, it may be prudent to check random serum glucose measurements for possible undiagnosed disease. We have used dapsone therapy 50–100 mg, which offers an alternative systemic therapy with reduced risk of systemic steroid-related side effects. With the use of dapsone, glucose-6-phosphate dehydrogenase levels should be checked initially to avoid hemolytic anemia.

DERMATOSES IN NATIVE AMERICANS: UNCOMMON DERMATOSES

NONMELANOMA SKIN CANCER

The incidence of nonmelanoma skin cancers in Native Americans is not reported. Although the incidence has been very low, Native American people are not exempt from the development of actinic keratoses, squamous cell carcinoma, and basal cell carcinoma.

The clinical morphology is similar to the presentation in nonethnic skin. Wiegand suggested that when basal cell carcinomas arise in Native Americans, they have a tendency to be of the pigmented variation.[7]

Actinic keratoses present as scaly macules or papules on normal or erythematous skin. Sites most affected are regions with significant sun exposure. We have observed the presence of multiple actinic keratoses arising on the face of an elderly Native American female with a significant history of sun exposure, as demonstrated by the prominent photoaging observed on clinical examination (Figures 19.10 and 19.11).

Squamous cell carcinoma may present as scaly erythematous papules, keratotic nodules, or plaques. Secondary findings of ulceration are not uncommon. The distribution, like actinic keratoses, favors sun-exposed regions of the body, including the head, neck, and extremities. The development of basal cell carcinoma, like other nonmelanoma skin cancer, is also influenced by UVR exposure. The early manifestation of the disease is a pearly papule. More advanced disease may present as nodules or tumors.

Treatment of nonmelanoma skin cancers includes a variety of destructive modalities and surgical methods. Electrodesiccation and curettage with three cycles of therapy is reserved for nodular basal cell carcinoma, whereas excision is the treatment of choice for infiltrative basal cell carcinoma and squamous cell carcinoma. It is best to keep in mind that scars will be more apparent in people of color, and patients should be educated that scars do not repigment with time.

MELANOMA

The New Mexico Melanoma Registry found that over a 20-year period, there were 16 cases of melanoma in Native Americans.[38]

The classic clinical presentation of melanoma is characterized by the presence of a darkly colored, irregularly bordered, irregularly shaped macule. Rarely, melanoma may present without pigmentation. The distribution of melanoma in Native Americans reported in a study of 16 cases by Black and Wiggins found a predilection for subungual location, followed by palmoplantar and mucosal locations.[39]

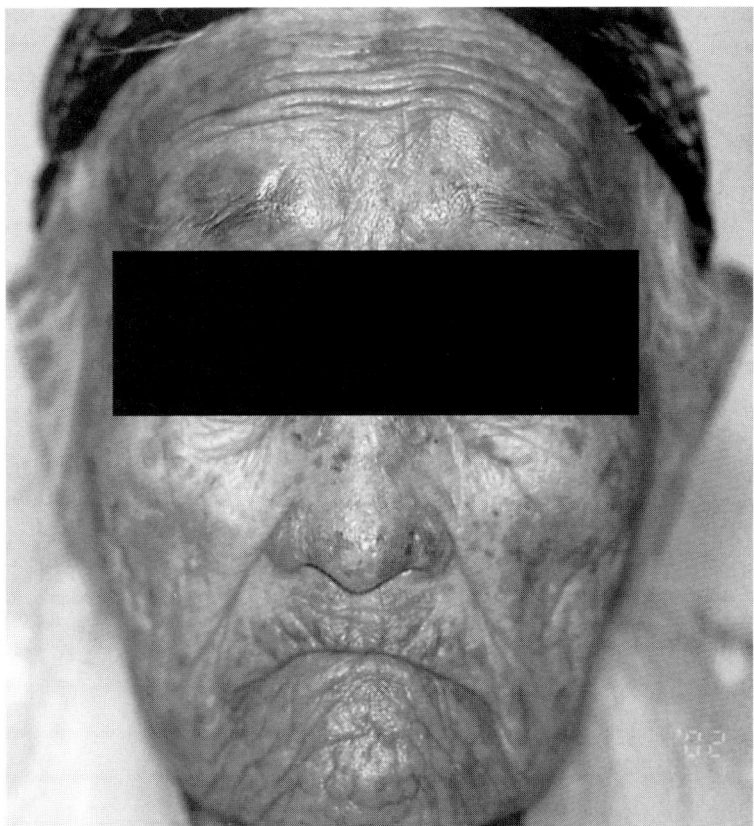

FIGURE 19.10 Elderly Navajo female demonstrating severe photodamage.

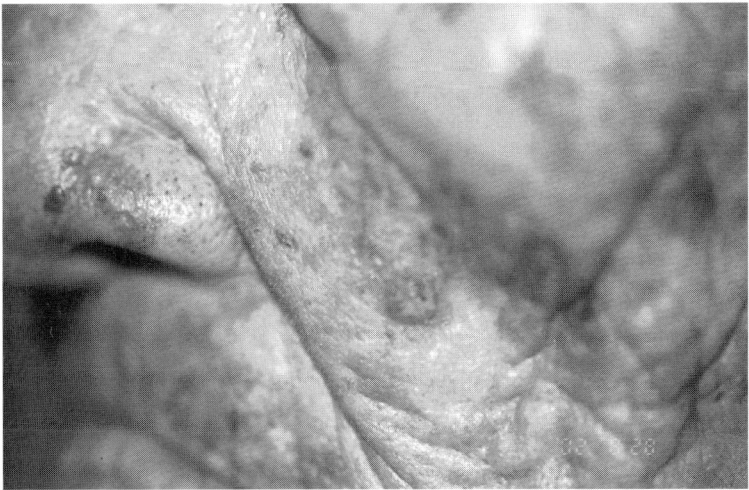

FIGURE 19.11 Actinic keratosis on patient in Figure 19.10.

Treatment of melanoma is surgical excision with adequate margins directed by Breslow's depth of tumor invasion. The current guidelines are as follows: tumors less than 1 mm in depth, excision with 1-cm margins; tumors 2–4 mm in depth may need 2.0–2.5-cm margins based on location on the body.[40] The excision goes to the overlying fascia but does not excise it. Definitive recommendations on the use of sentinel lymph node dissection are not available. This procedure is still considered experimental but may prove to be a very useful prognostic and therapeutic tool.[40]

There are several adjuvant therapies for patients with metastatic disease. These include the use of chemotherapy, immunotherapy, radiation, interferon, interleukins, monoclonal antibodies, and surgical debulking of metastatic disease. The development and implementation of protocols utilizing melanoma vaccines with significant efficacy have yet to be demonstrated.

CONCLUSION

Although dermatoses in Native American people have not been evaluated by controlled studies, we hope that the information presented here will provide insight into how clinical presentation and therapeutics may differ compared to non-Native American patients. The impact of history on the American Indian has molded the prevalence of genetic disease in these people. It is important to remember the history, cultural differences, and beliefs of the people regarding therapeutics in order to provide care in a culturally sensitive manner. Migration to and from the reservation continues to introduce new diseases not previously seen in this population through intermarriage with non-Native Americans. The importance of dermatology in Native American communities will continue to grow as these changes occur.

REFERENCES

1. Thornton, R., Tribal membership requirements and the demography of "old" and "new" Native Americans. *Popul. Res. Policy Rev.*, 16, 33, 1997.
2. United States Code Collection: Title 25, Chapter 18, General Provisions, Section 1603.
3. Alaluf, S., Ethnic variation in melanin content and composition in photoexposed and photoprotected human skin. *Pigment. Cell Res.*, 15, 112, 2002.
4. Taylor, S.C., Skin of color: biology, structure, function, and implications for dermatologic disease. *J. Am. Acad. Dermatol.*, 46, S41, 2002.
5. Jimbow, K. et al., Biology of melanocytes, in *Fitzpatrick's Dermatology in Medicine*, 5th ed., Freedburg, I.M. et al., Eds., McGraw-Hill, New York, 1999, 192.
6. Erickson, R.P., Southwestern Athabaskan (Navajo and Apache) genetic diseases. *Genet. Med.*, 1, 151, 1999.
7. Weigand, D.A., Diseases among Native American people, in *Global Dermatology: Diagnosis and Management According to Geography, Climate, and Culture*, Springer, New York, 1994, 165.
8. Fusaro, R.M. and Johnson, J.A., Hereditary polymorphic light eruption of American Indians: occurrence in non-Indians with polymorphic light eruption. *J. Am. Acad. Dermatol.*, 34, 612, 1996.
9. Hawk, J.L.M. and Norris, P.G., Abnormal responses to ultraviolet radiation: idiopathic, in *Fitzpatrick's Dermatology in Medicine*, 5th ed., Freedburg, I.M. et al., Eds., McGraw-Hill, New York, 1999, 1573.
10. Everett, M.A. et al., Light-sensitive eruptions in American Indians. *Arch. Dermatol.*, 83, 243, 1961.
11. Weedon, D., The lichenoid reaction pattern ("interface dermatitis"), in *Skin Pathology*, 2nd ed., Churchill Livingstone, London, 2002, 31.
12. Clericuzio, C., personal communication, 2002.
13. Cohen, P.R., Herbert, A.A. and Adler-Storthz, K., Focal epithelial hyperplasia: Heck Disease. *Pediatr. Dermatol.*, 10, 245, 1993.
14. Haisley-Royster, C.A. et al., Hereditary benign intraepithelial dyskeratosis: report of two cases with prominent oral lesions, *J. Am. Acad. Dermatol.*, 45, 634, 2001.
15. Allingham, R.R., A duplication in chromosome 4q35 is associated with hereditary benign intraepithelial dyskeratosis, *Am. J. Hum. Genet.*, 68, 491, 2001.
16. Rogers, M., Kourt, G. and Cameron, A., Hereditary mucoepithelial dysplasia. *Pediatr. Dermatol.*, 11, 133, 1994.
17. Bikowski, J.B., Treatment of rosacea with doxycycline monohydrate. *Cutis*, 66, 149, 2000.

18. Wilkin, J.K., Rosacea. *Int. J. Dermatol.,* 22, 393, 1983.
19. Plewig, G. and Jansen, T., Rosacea, in *Fitzpatrick's Dermatology in Medicine*, 5th ed., Freedburg, I.M. et al., Eds., McGraw-Hill, New York, 1999, 785.
20. Hurwitz, S., Eczematous eruptions in childhood, in *Clinical Pediatric Dermatology: A Textbook of Skin Disorders of Childhood and Adolescence,* 2nd ed., Saunders, Philadelphia, 1993, 45.
21. Natalija, N. et al., Dichotomic nature of atopic dermatitis reflected by combined analysis of monocyte immunophenotyping and single nucleotide polymorphisms of the interleukin-4/interleukin-13 receptor gene: the dichotomy of extrinsic and intrinsic atopic dermatitis. *J. Invest. Dermatol.,* 119, 870, 2002.
22. Nghiem, P., Pearson, G. and Langley, R.G., Tacrolimus and pimecrolimus: from clever prokaryotes to inhibiting calcineurin and treating atopic dermatitis. *J. Am. Acad. Dermatol.,* 46, 228, 2002.
23. Hurwitz, S. Skin disorders due to fungi, in *Clinical Pediatric Dermatology: A Textbook of Skin Disorders of Childhood and Adolescence,* 2nd ed., Saunders, Philadelphia, 1993, 372.
24. Elder, D. et al., Benign pigmented lesions and malignant melanoma, in *Lever's Histopathology of the Skin,* 8th ed., Lippincott-Raven, Philadelphia, 1997, 625.
25. Mishima, Y. and Mevorah, B., Nevus Ota and nevus Ito in American Negroes. *J. Invest. Dermatol.,* 36, 133, 1961.
26. Farber, E.M. and Nall, M.L., The natural history of psoriasis in 5600 patients, *Dermatologica,* 148, 118, 1974.
27. Van-Scott, E.J. and Ekel, T.M., Kinetics of hyperplasia in psoriasis. *Arch. Dermatol.* 88, 373, 1963.
28. Henseler, T. and Christophers, E., Psoriasis of early and late onset: characterization of two types of psoriasis vulgaris. *J. Am. Acad. Dermatol.,* 13, 450, 1985.
29. Christophers, E. and Henseler, T., Psoriasis type I and type II as subtypes of nonpustular psoriasis, in *Psoriasis,* 2nd ed., Roenig, H.H. and Maibach, H., Eds., Marcel Dekker, New York, 1990, 15.
30. Drew, G.S., Dermatology. *Primary Care Clin. Office Pract.,* 27, 2000.
31. Plewig, G. and Jansen, T., Seborrheic dermatitis, in *Fitzpatrick's Dermatology in Medicine,* 5th ed., Freedburg, I.M. et al., Eds., McGraw-Hill, New York, 1999, 1482.
32. Braun-Falco, O. et al., Erythemato-papulosquamous diseases, in *Dermatology,* 2nd ed., Springer, Berlin, 1996, 571.
33. Boyd, A.S. and Nelder, K.H., Lichen planus. *J. Am. Acad. Dermatol.,* 25, 593, 1991.
34. Halevy, S. and Shai, A., Lichenoid drug eruptions. *J. Am. Acad. Dermatol.,* 29, 249, 1993.
35. Eisen, D., The clinical features, malignant potential, and systemic associations of oral lichen planus: a study of 723 patients, *J. Am. Acad. Dermatol.,* 46, 207, 2002.
36. Braun-Falco, O. et al., Granulomatous diseases, in *Dermatology,* 2nd ed., Springer, Berlin, 1996, 1379.
37. Huntley, A.C. and Davis, C.A., The cutaneous manifestations of diabetes mellitus. *J. Am. Acad. Dermatol.,* 7, 427, 1982.
38. Black, W.C. et al., The New Mexico Melanoma Registry: a model of a statewide cooperative program. *Am. J. Dermatopathol.,* 9, 10, 1987.
39. Black, W.C. and Wiggins, C., Melanoma among Southwestern American Indians. *Cancer,* 55, 2899, 1985.
40. Kanzler, M.H. and Mraz-Gernhard, S., Primary cutaneous malignant melanoma and its precursor lesions: diagnostic and therapeutic overview. *J. Am. Acad. Dermatol.,* 45, 260, 2001.
41. The medicine wheel. Shadow Woman. 1998. Information available at www.walkingant.com.

Index

Italicized page numbers refer to tables and illustrations.

A

Absorption spectrum chart, 260, *261*
Acanthosis nigricans, 159–160, *160*, 376, *377*
Acetobacter sp., 105
Acne
    conglobata type, 18
    Hispanics/Latinos, 371–373, *372*
    keloidalis nuchae type, 76–77, *77–78*
    laser therapy, 273
    pomade acne, 20
    pseudofolliculitis barbae, *337*, 337–338
    rosacea type, 391–392
    treatment, 21–25
    vulgaris, 17–18, *18–21*, 270, 289–292, 390–391, *390–391*
Acral lentiginous melanoma, 193
Acropustulosis, infancy, 45–46, *46–47*
Actinic prurigo, 301–304, 373–374, *374*
Adapalene, 44–45, 224
Aedes genus, 124
Aeste studies, 35
African-American patients, *see also* Black patients
    acanthosis nigricans, 159
    acne conglobata, 18
    acne keloidalis nuchae, 76–77
    acne vulgaris, 17–18
    allergic contact dermatitis, 72
    atopic dermatitis, 27, 53
    central centrifugal cicatricial alopecia, 80
    chemicals, 85–86
    dermatomyositis, 75, 158
    diabetes mellitus, 158
    dissecting cellulitis, 78
    familial racial periorbital hyperpigmentation, 103
    granulomatous rosacea, 21
    hair care guidelines, *85*
    hair care products, *86*
    hair shaft disorders, 84
    hair structure, 63–64
    hair transplantation, women, 246, 248–251
    heat, 85
    intrinsic skin aging, 198, 200
    Kawasaki disease, 51
    keloids, 12
    lupus erythematosus, 75, 153
    melasma, 101
    Mongolian spot, 43
    nickel contact dermatitis, 54
    psoriasis vulgaris, 68
    renal disease, 164
    sarcoidosis, 83, 147–148
    scleroderma, 150–151
    seborrheic dermatitis, 64–66
    skin cancer, 181–189, *182–188*
    systemic medication reaction, 168
    tinea capitis, 33–38, 72–73
    uncomplicated folliculitis, 76
African patients
    atopic dermatitis, 27
    hair structure, 64
    melasma, 101
    retinoids, 24
    sarcoidosis, 148
    skin cancer, 181–189, *182–188*
Afro-Caribbean patients
    atopic dermatitis, 26–27
    familial racial periorbital hyperpigmentation, 103
    granulomatous rosacea, 21
    skin cancer, 181–189, *182–188*
    tinea capitis, 34
Albinism, 108–109, *110*
Aljabre studies, 334
Allergic contact dermatitis, 12, 72, *73*
Allopurinal, 168–169
Alpha interferon, 59
Alster, Manaloto and, studies, 265
Amiodarone, 168
Ancylostoma spp., 126
Anderson, Battle and, studies, 259
Anthropologic factors, 198, 200, *200*
Antibiotics, 22–23, 77, 225–226, *see also specific type*
Antifungal creams, 57
Antihistamines
    acropustulosis, infancy, 46
    atopic dermatitis, 54
    contact dermatitis, 32
    lichen striatus, 58
    nickel contact dermatitis, 54
    pityriasis rosea, 56
    polymorphous light eruption, 58
Anti-infective therapy, 225–226
Antimalarials, 50
Arabic patients, 31
Aramaki studies, 31
Ara studies, 181–194
Arbutin, 105
Arsenical melanosis, 370
Ascosubramania melanographoides, 132
Ashy dermatosis, 100–101, *101*

Asian patients
    acne vulgaris, 289–292
    actinic prurigo, 301–304
    atopic dermatitis, 26–27, 292–294
    basics, 289, 323
    chronic actinic dermatitis, 319–320
    contact dermatitis, 29–31, 295–299
    cultural medical practices, cause of, 321–323, *323*
    diabetes mellitus, 158
    dyshidrotic eczema, 294–295
    epidermis comparison, *5*
    erythema dyschromicum perstans, 100
    erythropoietic protoporphyria, 320–321
    hair follicles and hair structure, 10
    Hermansky-Pudlak syndrome, 109
    intrinsic skin aging, 198
    Kawasaki disease, 51
    lichen planus, 162
    lupus erythematosus, 155
    melanoma, 314–316
    melasma, 101–102, 307–310
    Mongolian spot, 43, 310–311
    nevus of Ota/nevus of Ito, 311–312
    nonmelanoma skin cancer, 313–314
    nummular dermatitis, 294–295
    Ofuji's disease, 316–318
    pigmented dermatitis, 299–301
    primary cutaneous amyloidosis, 304–307
    prurigo nodularis, 301–304
    prurigo pigmentosa, 301–304
    sarcoidosis, 147
    skin appendages comparison, *9*
    skin cancer, 191–193
    vitiligo, 318–319
    xerosis, 294–295
Asian patients, dermatologic disease
    acne vulgaris, 289–292
    actinic prurigo, 301–304
    atopic dermatitis, 292–294
    basics, 289, 323
    chronic actinic dermatitis, 319–320
    contact dermatitis, 295–299
    cultural medical practices, cause of, 321–323, *323*
    dyshidrotic eczema, 294–295
    erythropoietic protoporphyria, 320–321
    melanoma, 314–316
    melasma, 307–310
    Mongolian spot, 310–311
    nevus of Ota/nevus of Ito, 311–312
    nonmelanoma skin cancer, 313–314
    nummular dermatitis, 294–295
    Ofuji's disease, 316–318
    pigmented dermatitis, 299–301
    primary cutaneous amyloidosis, 304–307
    prurigo nodularis, 301–304
    prurigo pigmentosa, 301–304
    vitiligo, 318–319
    xerosis, 294–295
Aspergillus sp., 105
Aspirin, 53
Atenolol, 168

Atopic dermatitis
    Asian patients, 292–294
    basics, 25–27, *28–30,* 70–71
    Black patients, 347–348
    Native Americans, 392–393
    neonatal and pediatric dermatological diseases, 53–54, *54*
    therapy, 71
Autoimmune disease, 149–158
Autologous minigrafts, 94
Autologous thin Thiersch grafts, 94
Azathioprine, 59, 84
Azelaic acid, 25, 91, 104–105

B

Babel and Baughman studies, 36
Balamuthia mandrillaris infection, 138–139
Balanitis xerotica obliterans, 375–376, *376*
Bartonellosis, 125–126, *126*
Basal cell carcinomas, 189, 192, 351, 378–379, *379*
Battle and Anderson studies, 259
Battle studies, 259–274
Baughman, Babel and, studies, 36
Ben-Gashier studies, 26
Benzoyl peroxide, 22, 225
Berardesca and Maibach studies, 29
Berardesca studies, 4, 29
Berman and Flores studies, 344
Berman and Kaufman studies, 344
Berman studies, 344
Bernard studies, 63
Bernstein studies, 251
Bhawan studies, 222
Biology, stratum corneum, 3–4
Biophysical properties, stratum corneum, 4
Black and Wiggins studies, 400
Black patients, *see also* African-American patients
    allergic contact dermatitis, 12
    atopic dermatitis, 25–26
    contact dermatitis, 28–29
    dermal structure, 8, *8,* 9
    epidermis, 5, *5*
    erythema dyschromicum perstans, 100
    hair follicles and hair structure, 10–11
    hair transplantation, women, 251–255, *252*
    irritation, 12
    keratinocytes, 6
    melanocytes, 6–7
    nails, 11
    photoaging, 214–216, *215*
    racial differences, *9,* 13
    skin appendages, *9*
    sweat glands and sebaceous glands, 9
Black patients, dermatologic disease
    atopic dermatitis, 347–348
    basal cell carcinoma, 351
    common diseases, *333,* 333–347
    contact dermatitis, 334
    cultural issues, 331–332

    dermatofibrosarcoma protuberans, 351
    dermatosis papulosa nigra, 340–341, *341*
    discoid lupus erythematosus, 349
    hair structure, 331
    keloids, 342–347, *343*
    melanoma, 350–351
    melasma, 341–342
    mycosis fungoides, 351
    normal variants, 332–333
    pigment disorders, 341–342, *342*
    pityriasis rosea, 348
    pseudofolliculitis barbae, 335–340
    sarcoidosis, *334,* 348
    scleroderma, 350
    seborrheic dermatitis, 333, *334*
    secondary syphilis, 348, *349*
    skin cancer, 350–351
    skin structure, 331
    squamous cell carcinoma, 351
    systemic lupus erythematosus, 349–350
    tinea versicolor, 334
    trichorrhexis nodosa, 334–335
    unusual presentations, 347–350
    vitiligo, 341, *342*
Bleach, hair, 280, *see also* Color, hair
Bleaching agents, skin, 218, *see also* Brighteners
Bleomycin, 344
Blepharoplasty, 204
Body image and body-contouring procedures, 240–241, *see also* Cosmetic and dermatologic surgery
Bonis studies, 270
Botulinum toxin, 233, *235*
Bovine collagen, 161, *see also* Collagen
Bowen's disease, 184–185, 192–193
Braiding, *see* Plaiting
Breathnach studies, 342
Bridgeman-Shah studies, 147–169
Brighteners, 281–282, *282, see also* Bleaching agents, skin
Bronson studies, 35
Brooks studies, 17–38
Brown, Pierce and, studies, 238
Bulengo-Ransby studies, 86
Bump Fighter razor, 338
Burns studies, 236

C

Caballero studies, 17–38
Calcipotriene, 69
Callen and Kasteler studies, 75
Callender studies, 63–88, 245–255
Cantharidin, 44
Capsaicin, 165, 375, *375*
Carbon dioxide lasers, 77, 265, *see also* Laser therapy
Carlisle, Montagna and, studies, 214
Carrion's disease, 125–126, *126*
Caucasian patients, racial differences
    acanthosis nigricans, 159
    acne keloidalis nuchae, 77
    acne vulgaris, 17

    atopic dermatitis, 25–27
    contact dermatitis, 28, 30–31
    dermal structure, 7–8, *8,* 9
    epidermis, 5, *5*
    hair follicles and hair structure, 10–11, 63–64
    irritation, 12
    keratinocytes, 6
    lupus erythematosus, 155
    melanocytes, 6–7
    Mongolian spot, 43
    morphology comparison, 200
    nails, 107
    palmoplantar racial difference, 107
    photoaging, 216
    psoriasis vulgaris, 69
    racial differences, 13
    sarcoidosis, 147
    scleroderma, 150
    skin appendages, *9*
    stratum corneum, 3–4
    sweat glands and sebaceous glands, 9
    systemic medication reaction, 168–169
    tinea capitis, 34
CCCA, *see* Central centrifugal cicatricial alopecia (CCCA)
CCLE, *see* Chronic cutaneous lupus erythematosus (CCLE)
Central American patients, 100
Central centrifugal cicatricial alopecia (CCCA), 80–83, *81–83,* 249–254, *251, 253*
Chagas disease, 122–124, *123*
Chan studies, 264
Chemical peels
    basics, 25
    cosmetic and dermatologic surgery, 234–238
    hyperpigmentation, 98, 106
    photoaging, 218
    pseudofolliculitis barbae, 339–340
Chemicals, hair and scalp disorders, 85–88, *87*
Child studies, 26
Chinese medicine, *see* Traditional Chinese medicine
Chlorambucil, 84
Chromomycosis, 132–133, *138*
Chronic actinic dermatitis, 319–320
Chronic cutaneous lupus erythematosus (CCLE), 75
Chronic infective lymphocytic psoriform dermatitis, 139
Chui studies, 263
Chung studies, 213–214
Cladosporium carrionii, 132
Clindamycin, 22, 225, *see also* Antibiotics
Clinical manifestations
    acne vulgaris, 289–290, *290–291*
    actinic prurigo, 302–303
    atopic dermatitis, *293,* 293–294
    chronic actinic dermatitis, 319
    contact dermatitis, 296–297, *296–297*
    dyshidrotic eczema, 294, *295*
    erythropoietic protoporphyria, 320–321, *321*
    melanoma, 315, *315*
    melasma, 307–309, *308–309*
    Mongolian spot, 310–311, *311*
    nevus of Ota/nevus of Ito, 312, *312*
    nonmelanoma skin cancer, 313, *313–314*

nummular dermatitis, 294, *295*
Ofuji's disease, 316–317, *316–317*
pigmented dermatitis, 300, *300*
primary cutaneous amyloidosis, 305–306, *305–306*
prurigo nodularis, 302–303
prurigo pigmentosa, 302–303
sarcoidosis, 148
vitiligo, 318, *318*
Xerosis, 294, *295*
Clinical presentations
    atopic dermatitis, 53–54, *54*
    erythema, 53, *53*
    lichen planus, 58–59, *59*
    lichen striatus, 58, *58*
    neurofibromatosis 1, 59, *60*
    nickel contact dermatitis, 54, *55*
    pityriasis rosea, 55–56, *56–57*
    polymorphous light eruption, 58
    seborrheic dermatitis, 55, *56*
    tinea versicolor, 56–57, *57*
Clobetasol ointment/gel, 344
Clotrimazole, 57
Cochliomyia hominivorax, 130
Cohen, Vargo and, studies, 36
Coin rubbing, 322–323, *323*
Colchicine, 345
Collagen, 7–8, 161, 240, *see also* Keloids
Colophony allergy, 298
Color, hair, 280, 334
Color cosmetics, *284,* 284–285
Combination therapy, 22, 106
Common diseases
    acne conglobata, 18
    acne vulgaris, 17–18, *18–21*
    antibiotics, 22–23
    atopic dermatitis, 25–27, *28–30*
    azelaic acid, 25
    benzoyl peroxide, 22
    Black patients, *333,* 333–347
    chemical peels, 25
    contact dermatitis, 28–33
    dermatitis, 25–33
    follicular occlusion triad, 19
    hydroquinone, 24–25
    microdermabrasion, 25
    Native Americans, 389–400
    oral contraceptives, 24
    pomade acne, 20
    retinoids, 23–24, *24*
    rosacea, 20–21, *22–23*
    tinea capitis, *33,* 33–38
Communication, 255
Conditioners, 66, 280–281
Congenital melanocytic nevi, 394–395
Contact dermatitis
    Asian patients, 295–299
    basics, 28–33
    Black patients, 334
    hair and scalp disorders, 71–72
    pathophysiology, 297–299
Contact irritants, pathophysiology, 299

Corticosteroids
    acne keloidalis nuchae, 77
    acropustulosis, infancy, 46
    atopic dermatitis, 71
    basics, 226–227
    central centrifugal cicatricial alopecia, 83
    combination therapy, 106
    contact dermatitis, 32
    dyspigmentation, 44
    hypopigmented mycosis fungoides, 50
    lichen planus, 59
    lichen striatus, 58
    lupus erythematosus, 50
    neonatal lupus erythematosus, 51
    nickel contact dermatitis, 54
    pigmentary disorders, 103
    pityriasis rosea, 56
    polymorphous light eruption, 58
    psoriasis vulgaris, 69
    sarcoidosis, 83
    seborrheic dermatitis, 66
Cosmetic and dermatologic surgery, *see also* Rejuvenation procedures
    basics, 233
    body image and body-contouring procedures, 240–241
    botulinum toxin, 233, *235*
    chemical peels, 234–238
    collagen, 240
    deep peels, 238
    glycolic acid, 236, *236*
    hyaluronic acid, 240
    hydroxylapatite, 240
    injectable filling agents, 238–240, *240*
    Jessner's solution, 237–238
    medium peels, 238
    microdermabrasion, 238, *239*
    peeling agents and protocol, 234–236
    salicylic acid, 236–237, *237*
    trichloroacetic acid, 237
    tumescent liposuction, 241
Cosmetics
    basics, 277
    color, *284,* 284–285
    hyperpigmentation, 98
    hypopigmentation, 99
    piebaldism, 108
    vitiligo, 94
Cradle cap, 65
Cryoglobulinemia, 163
Cryosurgery, 346
Cultural issues, *see also* Traditional Chinese medicine
    Asian patients, 321–323, *323*
    Black patients, 331–332
    Hispanic and Latino patients, 357–359, *359*
Cupping, 323, *324*
Curls (permanent wave), 279–280
Cutaneous appendages, *9,* 9–11
Cutaneous *Balamuthia mandrillaris* infection, 138–139
Cutaneous larva currens, 127
Cutaneous larva migrans, 126–127, *127*
Cutaneous manifestations, systemic disease

acanthosis nigricans, 159–160, *160*
autoimmune disease, 149–158
basics, 147, 169
cryoglobulinemia, 163
dermatomyositis, 157–158
dermopathy, 159
diabetes mellitus, 158–162
diabetic bullae, 161–162
endocrine disease, 158–162
foot ulcers, 160, *161*
hematologic disease, 158
hepatic disease, 162–163
hepatitis C, 163
Hermansky-Pudlak syndrome, 158
Kyrle's disease, 164, *165*
lichen planus, 162
lupus erythematosus, 151–157, *154–156*
medication reactions, systemic, 165–169, *166–167*
necrobiosis lipoidica diabeticorum, 160–161
pruritus, 163–165
renal disease, 164–165
sarcoidosis, 147–149, *148–152*
scleroderma, 149–151, *152–153*
waxy skin, 159
Cyclophosphamide, 84
Cyclosporine, 32, 59, 161, 345
Cysticercosis, 120–121
Cyst-type disorders, 75–79
Czernielewski studies, 224

D

Dapsone, 59
Decreased incidence, 60
Deep peels, 238, *see also* Chemical peels
De la Guardia, Mario, 278
DeLeo studies, 334
Dematiaceous fungi, 132
Dengue fever, 124
Depigmentation, 93–95
Depilatories, 281
Dermal structure, skin and hair, 7–9
Dermatitis, 25–33, *see also specific type*
Dermatobia hominis, 129–130
Dermatofibrosarcoma protuberans, 185, 351
Dermatologic disease, Asians
  acne vulgaris, 289–292
  actinic prurigo, 301–304
  atopic dermatitis, 292–294
  basics, 289, 323
  chronic actinic dermatitis, 319–320
  contact dermatitis, 295–299
  cultural medical practices, cause of, 321–323, *323*
  dyshidrotic eczema, 294–295
  erythropoietic protoporphyria, 320–321
  melanoma, 314–316
  melasma, 307–310
  Mongolian spot, 310–311
  nevus of Ota/nevus of Ito, 311–312
  nonmelanoma skin cancer, 313–314
  nummular dermatitis, 294–295
  Ofuji's disease, 316–318
  pigmented dermatitis, 299–301
  primary cutaneous amyloidosis, 304–307
  prurigo nodularis, 301–304
  prurigo pigmentosa, 301–304
  vitiligo, 318–319
  xerosis, 294–295
Dermatologic disease, Blacks
  atopic dermatitis, 347–348
  basal cell carcinoma, 351
  common diseases, *333,* 333–347
  contact dermatitis, 334
  cultural issues, 331–332
  dermatofibrosarcoma protuberans, 351
  dermatosis papulosa nigra, 340–341, *341*
  discoid lupus erythematosus, 349
  hair structure, 331
  keloids, 342–347, *343*
  melanoma, 350–351
  melasma, 341–342
  mycosis fungoides, 351
  normal variants, 332–333
  pigment disorders, 341–342, *342*
  pityriasis rosea, 348
  pseudofolliculitis barbae, 335–340
  sarcoidosis, *334,* 348
  scleroderma, 350
  seborrheic dermatitis, 333, *334*
  secondary syphilis, 348, *349*
  skin cancer, 350–351
  skin structure, 331
  squamous cell carcinoma, 351
  systemic lupus erythematosus, 349–350
  tinea versicolor, 334
  trichorrhexis nodosa, 334–335
  unusual presentations, 347–350
  vitiligo, 341, *342*
Dermatologic disease, Hispanics and Latinos
  acanthosis nigricans, 376, *377*
  acne, 371–373, *372*
  actinic prurigo, 373–374, *374*
  arsenical melanosis, 370
  balanitis xerotica obliterans, 375–376, *376*
  basal cell carcinomas, 378–379, *379*
  basics, 357, 359, *360*
  capsaicin dermatitis, 375, *375*
  cultural aspects, 357–359, *359*
  drug-induced pigmentation, 364, *365–366*
  eczema, 373
  erythema dyschromicum perstans, 361–362, *361–362*
  erythromelanosis follicularis facei, 369–370
  Hermansky-Pudlak syndrome, *370,* 370–371
  idiopathic guttate hypomelanosis, 371
  lichen planas actinicos, 362–363, *363*
  lichen planas pigmentosus, 363, *364*
  linea fusca, 370
  macular amyloidosis, 364, *365*
  melanoma, 379, *380,* 381
  melasma, 365–368, *366–368*
  pigmentary disorders, 359–371

pityriasis alba, 371
poikiloderma of Civatte, 369
postinflammatory hyperpigmentation, 359–360, *361*
prayer callouses, 377, *377*
prurigo pigmentosa, 363
Riehl's melanosis, 368–369, *369*
skin cancer, *378,* 378–381
skin diseases, 359, *360*
squamous cell carcinomas, 378–379, *379*
Dermatologic disease, Native Americans
    acne rosacea, 391–392
    acne vulgaris, 390–391, *390–391*
    atopic dermatitis, 392–393
    basics, 386–387, 402
    common dermatoses, 389–400
    congenital melanocytic nevi, 394–395
    considerations, 386
    dermatophyte infection, 393–394
    granuloma annulare, 398–400
    Heck's disease, 389
    hereditary benign intraepithelial dyskeratosis, 389–390
    hereditary polymorphous light eruption, 387
    historical perspectives, 385
    lichen planus, 397–398, *398–399*
    melanoma, 400–402
    Navajo poikiloderma, 387–388, *388–389*
    neutropenic poikiloderma, 387–388, *388–389*
    nevi, various types, 394–395, *395–396*
    nonmelanoma skin cancer, 400, *401*
    oral focal epithelial hyperplasia, 389
    pigmentary anomalies, 394–395
    psoriasis vulgaris, 395–397
    seborrheic dermatitis, 397
    uncommon dermatoses, 400, 402
    unique dermatoses, 387–388
Dermatomyositis, 75, 157–158
Dermatophyte infection, 393–394
Dermatosis papulosa nigra, 340–341, *341*
Dermatosis papulosis nigra, 266–267
Dermopathy, 159
Diabetes mellitus, 158–162
Diabetic bullae, 161–162
Dicarboxylic acid, *see* Azelaic acid
Discoid lupus erythematosus, 349
Dissecting cellulitis, 78–79, *79*
D-penicillamine, 345
Drug-induced pigmentation, 364, *365–366*
Drying agents, 85–88, *87*
Dunwell and Rose studies, 25
Dyshidrotic eczema, 294–295
Dyspigmentation, 44–45, *45–46*

E

East Indian patients
    familial racial periorbital hyperpigmentation, 103
    keloids, 12
    photoaging, *212–213,* 212–214
Eczema, 373
Electrolysis, 339
Elias studies, 4
Endocrine disease, 158–162
Endoscopic brow lifting, 204
Epidermal structure, skin and hair, 5, *5*
Epogen administration, 165
Erythema, 53, *53*
Erythema dyschromicum perstans
    Hispanics and Latinos, 361–362, *361–362*
    pigmentary disorders, 100–101, *101*
Erythromelanosis follicularis facei, 369–370
Erythromycin, 22, 56, 225, *see also* Antibiotics
Erythropoietic protoporphyria, 320–321
Ethiopian patients, 101
Ethnomedical treatments, 358, *359*
Excision, 77, 345–346
Exophiala spp., 132
Exophila spp., 116

F

FACE, *see* Facial Afro-Caribbean childhood eruption (FACE) syndrome
Facial Afro-Caribbean childhood eruption (FACE) syndrome, 21
Facial characteristics, 198, 200, *200*
Facial fat transfer, 204, *206*
Familial racial periorbital hyperpigmentation, 103
Figueroa studies, 37
Filipino patients, 51
Firooz studies, 31
Fisher studies, 12
Fitzpatrick and Szabo studies, 6
Fitzpatrick's skin types, 25, 234
Fitzpatrick studies, 310
Flaking-type disorders, 64–75
Flores, Berman and, studies, 344
Fluconazole, 57, 74
Flurandrenolide tape, 334, 344
5-Flurouracil therapy, 344
Follicular occlusion triad, 19
Folliculitis, uncomplicated, 76
Folliculitis decalvans, 76
Fonsecaea spp., 132
Foot ulcers, diabetic, 160, *161*
Foy studies, 30
Fragrance-mix, 298, 301
Franbourg studies, 64
Fusaro and Johnson studies, 387

G

Gaylor, Weigand and, studies, 28
Gean studies, 29
Genetic diseases, 107–109
George studies, 66
Gladstone, Migliori and, studies, 200
Glucocorticoid, 83
Glycolic acid, 236, *236*

GM-CSF, *see* Granulocyte-monocyte colony stimulating factor (GM-CSF)
Gnathostomiasis, *128,* 128–129
Goh studies, 213, 289–323
Goldman, Leon, 259
Gout, 168
Grafts, hair transplantation, 251–254, *see also* Skin grafts
Granular cell tumors, 187–188
Granulocyte-monocyte colony stimulating factor (GM-CSF), 161
Granuloma annulare, 398–400
Granulomatous rosacea, 21
Greenbaum, Rubin and, studies, 218
Greenbaum studies, 336
Griffiths studies, 213, 310
Grimes studies, 25, 221–228, 233–241
Griseofulvin, 38, 74, 394

H

Hair
    characteristics, 277
    loss, 80–84
    permanent waves, 279–280
    relaxers, 71–72, 83, 85–86, 278–279, *279*
    removal, 270–273, *271–273*
    structure, racial differences, 10
    acne keloidalis nuchae, 76–78, *77–78*Hair and scalp disorders
    allergic contact dermatitis, 72, *73*
    atopic dermatitis, 70–71
    basics, 63–64, *64,* 88
    central centrifugal cicatricial alopecia, 80–83, *81–83*
    chemicals, 85–88, *87*
    contact dermatitis, 71–72
    cyst-type disorders, 75–79
    dermatomyositis, 75
    dissecting cellulitis, *78–79, 79*
    drying agents, 85–88, *87*
    flaking-type disorders, 64–75
    folliculitis decalvans, 76
    hair loss, 80–84
    hair shaft disorders, 84–88
    heat, 85
    inflammatory-type disorders, 64–79
    irritant contact dermatitis, 71–72, *72*
    lupus erythematosus, 74–75
    psoriasis vulgaris, 67–70, *70–71*
    pustule-type disorders, 75–79
    sarcoidosis, 83–84, *84*
    scarring hair loss, 80–84
    seborrheic dermatitis, 64–67, *65*
    tinea capitis, 72–74, *73–74*
    traction alopecia, 80, *81*
    trichorrhexis nodosa, 84, *85–86*
    uncomplicated folliculitis, 76
Hair care products
    basics, 277
    bleach, 280
    central centrifugal cicatricial alopecia, 83
    color, 280, 334
    curls, 279–280
    depilatories, 281
    hair characteristics, 277
    permanent waves, 279–280
    relaxers, hair, 71–72, 83, 85–86, 278–279, *279*
    shampoos, conditioners, styling products, 35, 280–281
    thermal reconditioning, 279–280
    thioglycolates, 279–280
Hair follicles, 5, 10
Hair glue, 72
Hair rollers, 80
Hair shaft disorders, 84–88
Hair structure, 331
Hair transplantation
    African-American women, 248–251
    basics, 245–246, 255
    Black women, 251–255, *252*
    central centrifugal cicatricial alopecia, 249–254, *251, 253*
    communication, 255
    larger grafts, 251–254, *253*
    physician-patient communication, 255
    racial variations, morphology, 246–248, *247*
    scarring reduction, 254, *254–255*
    traction alopecia, 249, *249–250*
Haisley-Royster studies, 390
Hakozaki studies, 225
Halder and Nootheti studies, 26
Halder studies
    alopecia, 248
    common dermatological diseases, 17–38
    dermatologic disease, Blacks, 331–351
    photoaging, 211–219
    pigmentary disorders, 91–109
    postinflammatory hyperpigmentation, 266
    skin cancer, 181–194
Hall studies, 283
Hanifin and Rajka studies, 26–27
Hansen's disease, 133–135, *134–135*
Harris studies, 197–206
Hashimoto, Kumakiri and, studies, 306
Hay studies, 34
Headington studies, 251
Heat, 85
Heck's disease, 389
Hematologic disease, 158
Hepatic disease, 162–163
Hepatitis, 118, *119,* 163
Hereditary benign intraepithelial dyskeratosis, 389–390
Hereditary polymorphous light eruption, 387
Hermansky-Pudlak syndrome
    cutaneous manifestations, 158
    Hispanics and Latinos, *370,* 370–371
    pigmentary disorders, 108–109, *110*
Hicks studies, 29
Hispanic patients, *see also* Latino patients
    acne vulgaris, 17–18
    atopic dermatitis, 27
    dermal structure, 9
    dermis racial differences, 8

diabetes mellitus, 158
Kawasaki disease, 51
Mongolian spot, 43
photoaging, 216
renal disease, 164
scleroderma, 149–151
skin cancer, 189–191, *190–191*
Hispanic patients, dermatologic disease
    acanthosis nigricans, 376, *377*
    acne, 371–373, *372*
    actinic prurigo, 373–374, *374*
    arsenical melanosis, 370
    balanitis xerotica obliterans, 375–376, *376*
    basal cell carcinomas, 378–379, *379*
    basics, 357, 359, *360*
    capsaicin dermatitis, 375, *375*
    cultural aspects, 357–359, *359*
    drug-induced pigmentation, 364, *365–366*
    eczema, 373
    erythema dyschromicum perstans, 361–362, *361–362*
    erythromelanosis follicularis facei, 369–370
    Hermansky-Pudlak syndrome, *370,* 370–371
    idiopathic guttate hypomelanosis, 371
    lichen planas actinicos, 362–363, *363*
    lichen planas pigmentosus, 363, *364*
    linea fusca, 370
    macular amyloidosis, 364, *365*
    melanoma, 379, *380,* 381
    melasma, 365–368, *366–368*
    pigmentary disorders, 359–371
    pityriasis alba, 371
    poikiloderma of Civatte, 369
    postinflammatory hyperpigmentation, 359–360, *361*
    prayer callouses, 377, *377*
    prurigo pigmentosa, 363
    Riehl's melanosis, 368–369, *369*
    skin cancer, *378,* 378–381
    skin diseases, 359, *360*
    squamous cell carcinomas, 378–379, *379*
Histology
    acne vulgaris, 291
    acropustulosis, infancy, 46
    actinic prurigo, 304
    atopic dermatitis, 54, 294
    chronic actinic dermatitis, 319
    dyshidrotic eczema, 295
    erythropoietic protoporphyria, 321
    hypopigmented mycosis fungoides, 50
    Kawasaki disease, 51, 53
    lichen planus, 59
    lichen striatus, 58
    lupus erythematosus, 50
    melanoma, 315
    melasma, 309
    Mongolian spot, 43, 311
    necrobiosis lipoidica diabeticorum, 161
    neonatal lupus erythematosus, 51
    neurofibromatosis 1 (NF 1), 59
    nevus of Ota/nevus of Ito, 312
    nonmelanoma skin cancer, 314
    nummular dermatitis, 295
    Ofuji's disease, 317
    pigmented dermatitis, 301
    pityriasis rosea, 56
    polymorphous light eruption, 58
    primary cutaneous amyloidosis, 306
    prurigo nodularis, 304
    prurigo pigmentosa, 304
    sarcoidosis, 147
    scleroderma, 150
    tinea versicolor, 57
    traction folliculitis, 48
    vitiligo, 318
    Xerosis, 295
Historical perspectives, 385
HIV disease, 65
Hobbs studies, 259–274
Holloway studies, 277–285
Ho studies, 263
HPV, *see* Human papilloma virus (HPV)
Hsu studies, 31
Human papilloma virus (HPV), *118*
Hyaluronic acid, 240
Hydralazine, 168
Hydroquinone
    basics, 104, 227–228
    combination therapy, 106
    common dermatological diseases, 24–25
    hyperpigmentation, 98
Hydroxychloroquine, 59, 84
Hydroxylapatite, 240
Hyperpigmentation, 99–103
Hypertrophic scars, 254, 269
Hypopigmentation disorders, 91–93
Hypopigmented mycosis fungoides, 49–50

I

Idiopathic guttate hypomelanosis, *92,* 92–93, 371
IL verapamil, 345
Imiquimod therapy, 344
Immunomodulators, 71, 228
Immunosuppressive therapy, 50
Incidence
    acne vulgaris, 289
    actinic prurigo, 301
    atopic dermatitis, 292
    chronic actinic dermatitis, 319
    contact dermatitis, 295–296
    dyshidrotic eczema, 294
    erythropoietic protoporphyria, 320
    melanoma, 314–315
    melasma, 307
    neonatal and pediatric dermatological diseases, 43–53, 60
    nevus of Ota/nevus of Ito, 311
    nonmelanoma skin cancer, 313
    nummular dermatitis, 294
    Ofuji's disease, 316
    pigmented dermatitis, 299–300
    primary cutaneous amyloidosis, 305

prurigo nodularis, 301
prurigo pigmentosa, 301
vitiligo, 318
Xerosis, 294
Infectious diseases
  Bartonellosis, 125–126, *126*
  basics, 115
  Carrion's disease, 125–126, *126*
  Chagas disease, 122–124, *123*
  chromomycosis, 132–133, *138*
  chronic infective lymphocytic psoriaform dermatitis, 139
  cutaneous *Balamuthia mandrillaris* infection, 138–139
  cutaneous larva currens, 127
  cutaneous larva migrans, 126–127, *127*
  cysticercosis, 120–121
  Dengue fever, 124
  gnathostomiasis, *128,* 128–129
  Hansen's disease, 133–135, *134–135*
  hepatitis, 118, *119*
  human papilloma virus, 117, *118*
  leishmaniasis, 130–132, *131*
  lymphatic filariasis, 139–140
  Mycobaterium infection, *121,* 121–122
  myiasis, 129–130, *130*
  onchocerciasis, 119–120
  Paederus dermatitis, 124–125
  paracoccidioidomycosis, 136–137
  rhinoscleroma, 136
  South American blastomycosis, 136–137
  sporotrichosis, 137–138, *138*
  superficial fungal infections, 115–117, *116–117*
  syphilis, 119, *120*
Inflammatory-type disorders, 64–79
Injectable filling agents, 238–240, *240*
Intense pulse light systems, 264, *see also* Laser therapy
Interferon therapy, 344
International Study of Asthma and Allergies in Childhood (ISAAC) study, 25, 31
Intravenous immunoglobulin (IVIG), 53
Intrinsic skin aging
  African-American morphology, 198, 200
  anthropologic considerations, 198, 200, *200*
  Asian morphology, 198
  basics, 197, *199,* 206
  ethnic considerations, 202–204
  facial characteristics, 198, 200, *200*
  Latino morphology, 198
  lower face, 203–204
  midface, 202–203, *203*
  morphological facial aging, 200–201, *201*
  rejuvenation procedures, 204–206, *205–208*
  upper face, 202
Irritant contact dermatitis, 71–72, *72*
Irritation, 12
ISAAC, *see* International Study of Asthma and Allergies in Childhood (ISAAC) study
Isotretinoin, 24, 78
Ito studies, 312
Itraconazole, 38, 74
IVIG, *see* Intravenous immunoglobulin (IVIG)

J

Jackson studies, 233–241
Janumpally studies, 26
Jessner's solution, 237–238
Jimbow studies, 386
Johnson, Fusaro and, studies, 387
Johnson, George, 278

K

Kang studies, 223–224
Kaposi's sarcoma, 186
Kasteler, Callen and, studies, 75
Kaufman, Berman and, studies, 344
Kawasaki disease, 51, *52,* 53
Kelly studies, 331–351
Keloids
  Black patients, 342–347, *343*
  dissecting cellulitis, 78
  laser therapy, 269
  medical therapies, 343–345
  physical modalities therapies, 346–347
  prevention, 254, *254–255*
  radiation therapies, 346
  scars, racial differences, 11–12
  surgical therapies, 345–346
Keratinocytes, 6
Ketoconazole, 38, 57, 65
Khumale studies, 331
Kikuchi studies, 313
Kimbrough-Green studies, 342
Kim studies, 344
Klebsiella rhinoscleromatis, 136
Klein studies, 241
Kligman, Kotrajaras and, studies, 212
Kligman, Strauss and, studies, 335–336, 338
Kligman and Willis studies, 103, 310
Kligman studies, 222
Kojic acid, 98, 105
Kompaore studies, 4
Kotrajaras and Kligman studies, 212
Kumakiri and Hashimoto studies, 306
Kwon studies, 214
Kyrle's disease, 164, *165*

L

Lamb studies, 387
Larva currens, 127
Larva migrans, 126–127
Laser therapy
  acne keloidalis nuchae, 77, 273
  acne vulgaris, 270
  basics, 259–262, *261,* 274
  dermatosis papulosis nigra, 266–267
  disorders, common, 265–270
  dissecting cellulitis, 79
  familial racial periorbital hyperpigmentation, 103

hair removal, 270–273, *271–273*
hyperpigmentation, 98, 106
hypertrophic scars, 269
intense pulse light systems, 264
keloids, 269, 347
lentigines, 266
light sources, 262–264
melasma, 106, 265–266
nevus of Ota/nevus of Ito, 106, 267
newer applications, 270
nonablative lasers, 273–274
pigmented lesions, 264–265
postinflammatory hyperpigmentation, 266
pseudofolliculitis barbae, 340
psoriasis vulgaris, 269–270
tattoos, 267–269, *268*
types of lasers, 262–265
vascular lasers, 262–264
vitiligo, 94, 270
Latino patients, 101, 198, *see also* Hispanic patients
Latino patients, dermatologic disease
  acanthosis nigricans, 376, *377*
  acne, 371–373, *372*
  actinic prurigo, 373–374, *374*
  arsenical melanosis, 370
  balanitis xerotica obliterans, 375–376, *376*
  basal cell carcinomas, 378–379, *379*
  basics, 357, 359, *360*
  capsaicin dermatitis, 375, *375*
  cultural aspects, 357–359, *359*
  drug-induced pigmentation, 364, *365–366*
  eczema, 373
  erythema dyschromicum perstans, 361–362, *361–362*
  erythromelanosis follicularis facei, 369–370
  Hermansky-Pudlak syndrome, *370*, 370–371
  idiopathic guttate hypomelanosis, 371
  lichen planas actinicos, 362–363, *363*
  lichen planas pigmentosus, 363, *364*
  linea fusca, 370
  macular amyloidosis, 364, *365*
  melanoma, 379, *380*, 381
  melasma, 365–368, *366–368*
  pigmentary disorders, 359–371
  pityriasis alba, 371
  poikiloderma of Civatte, 369
  postinflammatory hyperpigmentation, 359–360, *361*
  prayer callouses, 377, *377*
  prurigo pigmentosa, 363
  Riehl's melanosis, 368–369, *369*
  skin cancer, *378*, 378–381
  skin diseases, 359, *360*
  squamous cell carcinomas, 378–379, *379*
Laude studies, 34, 37
Lee studies, 27, 289–323
Leg veins, 263
Leishmaniasis, 130–132, *131*
Lentigines, 266
Le studies, 198
Lichen planus
  cutaneous manifestations, 162
  Hispanics and Latinos, 362–363, *363–364*

Native Americans, 397–398, *398–399*
neonatal and pediatric dermatological diseases, 58–59, *59*
Lichen striatus, 58, *58*
Licorice extract, 105
Ligatures, 347
Lighteners, 281–282, *282*
Light sources, 262–264, *see also* Laser therapy
Light therapy, 33, *see also* Laser therapy
Lim and Tham studies, 236
Lim studies, 289–323
Lindelof studies, 10
Linea fusca, 370
Linea nigra, 100
Liquid nitrogen, 44
Liver transplants, 163
Lobato studies, 35
LoPresti studies, 81
Lower-eyelid surgery, 204
Lower face, aging, 203–204
Lupus erythematosus
  cutaneous manifestations, 151–157, *154–156*
  hair and scalp disorders, 74–75
  neonatal and pediatric dermatological diseases, 50–51, *50–51*
Lutzomyia sand flies, 131
Lymphatic filariasis, 139–140
Lymphocytic psoriaform dermatitis, chronic infective, 139

M

Macular amyloidosis, 364, *365*
Maibach, Berardesca and, studies, 29
Maiman studies, 259
Malassezia furfur, 65, 91
Manaloto and Alster studies, 265
Manifestations, *see* Clinical manifestations
Marshal studies, 28
Mar studies, 292
McMichael studies, 63–88
Medication reactions, systemic, 165–169, *166–167*, 298
Mediterranean patients, 162
Medium peels, 238, *see also* Chemical peels
Melanin granule dispersion, 24
Melanoctyes, skin and hair, 6–7
Melanoctye transplantation, 95
Melanoma
  Asian patients, 314–316
  Black patients, 350–351
  Hispanics and Latinos, 379, *380*, 381
  Native Americans, 400–402
Melasma
  Asian patients, 307–310
  Black patients, 341–342
  Hispanics and Latinos, 365–368, *366–368*
  laser therapy, 265–266
  pigmentary disorders, 101–103, *102–103*
Merkel cell carcinoma, 189, 193
Methotrexate, 84, 344–345
Methyldopa, 168

Index

Miconazole, 57
Microcystic adnexal carcinoma, 187
Microdermabrasion
    basics, 25
    cosmetic and dermatologic surgery, 238, *239*
    hyperpigmentation, 106
    photoaging, 218
Microsporum spp., 34, 37, 48, 74, 91, 116, 393
Midface, aging, 202–203, *203*
Migliori and Gladstone studies, 200
Minoxidil, 72, 80
Mongolian spot, 43, *44,* 310–311
Monobenzone, 104
Monotherapy, acne, 22
Montagna and Carlisle studies, 214
Morphology
    African-American morphology, 198, 200
    Asian morphology, 198
    epidermis, 5
    facial aging, 200–201, *201*
    hair follicles, 11
    hair transplantation, 246–248
    Latino morphology, 198
    mast cells, 13
Moxibustion, 323
Mycobaterium spp., *121,* 121–122, 133
Mycosis fungoides, 186, 351
Myiasis, 129–130, *130*

N

N-acetyl-4-cysteaminylphenol (NCAP), 104
Nails, 11, 107
NAMCS, *see* National Ambulatory Medical Care Survey (NAMCS)
Nandedkar studies, 91–109
National Ambulatory Medical Care Survey (NAMCS), 73
Native American patients
    diabetes mellitus, 158
    Mongolian spot, 43
    skin cancer, 193
Native American patients, dermatologic disease
    acne rosacea, 391–392
    acne vulgaris, 390–391, *390–391*
    atopic dermatitis, 392–393
    basics, 386–387, 402
    common dermatoses, 389–400
    congenital melanocytic nevi, 394–395
    considerations, 386
    dermatophyte infection, 393–394
    granuloma annulare, 398–400
    Heck's disease, 389
    hereditary benign intraepithelial dyskeratosis, 389–390
    hereditary polymorphous light eruption, 387
    historical perspectives, 385
    lichen planus, 397–398, *398–399*
    melanoma, 400–402
    Navajo poikiloderma, 387–388, *388–389*
    neutropenic poikiloderma, 387–388, *388–389*
    nevi, various types, 394–395, *395–396*
    nonmelanoma skin cancer, 400, *401*
    oral focal epithelial hyperplasia, 389
    pigmentary anomalies, 394–395
    psoriasis vulgaris, 395–397
    seborrheic dermatitis, 397
    uncommon dermatoses, 400, 402
    unique dermatoses, 387–388
Navajo poikiloderma, 387–388, *388–389*
NCAP, *see* N-acetyl-4-cysteaminylphenol (NCAP)
Nd:YAG lasers, 263–269, *see also* Laser therapy
Neal studies, 91–109
Neame studies, 26
Necrobiosis lipoidica diabeticorum, 160–161
Negishi studies, 264
Neonatal and pediatric dermatological diseases
    acropustulosis, infancy, 45–46, *46–47*
    atopic dermatitis, 53–54, *54*
    clinical presentations, 53–59
    decreased incidence, 60
    dyspigmentation, 44–45, *45–46*
    erythema, 53, *53*
    hypopigmented mycosis fungoides, 49–50
    incidence, 43–53, 60
    Kawasaki disease, 51, *52,* 53
    lichen planus, 58–59, *59*
    lichen striatus, 58, *58*
    lupus erythematosus, 50–51, *50–51*
    Mongolian spots, 43, *44*
    neonatal lupus erythematosus, 50–51, *51*
    neurofibromatosis 1 (NF 1), 59, *60*
    nickel contact dermatitis, 54, *55*
    pityriasis rosea, 55–56, *56–57*
    polymorphous light eruption, 58
    seborrheic dermatitis, 55, *56*
    tinea capitis, 48–49, *49*
    tinea versicolor, 56–57, *57*
    traction folliculitis and/or alopecia, 47–48, *47–48*
    transient neonatal pustular melanosis, 43, *44*
Neonatal lupus erythematosus, 50–51, *51*
Neurofibromatosis 1 (NF 1), 59, *60*
Neutropenic poikiloderma, 387–388, *388–389*
Nevi, various types, 394–395, *395–396*
Nevus of Ota/nevus of Ito
    Asian patients, 192, 311–312
    laser therapy, 107, 267
    pigmentation disorders, 107, *108*
NF 1, *see* Neurofibromatosis 1 (NF 1)
Niacinamide, 161, 224–225
Nickel contact dermatitis, 54, *55,* 298
Nitrogen mustard, 50
Nonablative lasers, 273–274, *see also* Laser therapy
Nonmelanoma skin cancer
    Asian patients, 192, 313–314
    Native Americans, 400, *401*
    Puerto Rican patients, 190
Nootheti, Halder and, studies, 26
Nootheti studies, 331–351
Nouri studies, 265
Nummular dermatitis, 294–295

O

Obasi studies, 67
Ofuji's disease, 316–318
Onchocerciasis, 119–120
Oral contraceptives, 24
Oral focal epithelial hyperplasia, 389
Orentreich, Norman, 251
Oresajo studies, 3–13
Osmundsen studies, 299

P

Pacific Island patients, 102, 158
Padilla studies, 385–402
Paederus dermatitis, 124–125
Pakaistani patients, 103
Palmoplantar racial difference, 107
Paracoccidioidomycosis, 136–137
Para-phenylenediamine (PPD), 298
Pathak studies, 309–310
Pathophysiology
    acne vulgaris, 291
    actinic prurigo, 304
    atopic dermatitis, 294
    contact dermatitis, 297–299
    dyshidrotic eczema, 295
    erythropoietic protoporphyria, 321
    melanoma, 315
    melasma, 309–310
    Mongolian spot, 311
    nonmelanoma skin cancer, 314
    nummular dermatitis, 295
    Ofuji's disease, 317
    pigmented dermatitis, 301
    primary cutaneous amyloidosis, 306
    prurigo nodularis, 304
    prurigo pigmentosa, 304
    vitiligo, 318
    Xerosis, 295
Pediatric diseases, *see* Neonatal and pediatric dermatological diseases
Peeling agents and protocol, 234–236, *see also* Chemical peels
Penicillum sp., 105
Penile lichen sclerosus, *see* Balanitis xerotica obliterans
Pentoxifylline (Trental), 345
Percutaneous midface life, 205, *208*
Permanent waves, 279–280
Personal care products
    basics, 277, 285
    color cosmetics, *284*, 284–285
    hair care, 277–281, *279*
    hair color, 280, 334
    skin care, 281–284, *282*
Pessa studies, 203
Pharmacological agents
    adapalene, 224
    antibiotics, 225–226
    anti-infective therapy, 225–226
    basics, 221
    benzoyl peroxide, 225
    corticosteroids, 226–227
    hydroquinone, 227–228
    immunomodulators, 228
    niacinamide, 224–225
    retinoids, 222–224
    retinol, 224
    systemic antibiotics, 225–226
    tazarotene, 223–224
    tretinoin, 221–222
    vitamin C, 227
Phenolic agents, 104
Phialophora verrucosa, 132
Photoaging
    basics, 211, 216–217
    Black patients, 214–216, *215*
    bleaching agents, 218
    chemical peels, 218
    East Indian patients, *212–213*, 212–214
    Hispanics, 216
    microdermabrasion, 218
    photorejuvenation, 218–219
    retinoids, 217–218
    Southeast Indian patients, *212–213*, 212–214
    systemic retinoid therapy, 218
    therapy, 217–219
    tretinoin, 217–218
Photocontact dermatitis, 298
Photorejuventation, 218–219, *see also* Rejuvenation procedures
Physician-patient communication, 255
Piebaldism, 107–108
Piedra hortae, 117
Pierce and Brown studies, 238
Pigmentary anomalies, 394–395
Pigmentary disorders
    albinism, 108–109, *110*
    arbutin, 105
    ashy dermatosis, 100–101, *101*
    azelaic acid, 104–105
    basics, 91
    combination therapy, 106
    corticosteroids, 103
    depigmentation, 93–95
    erythema dyschromicum perstans, 100–101, *101*
    familial racial periorbital hyperpigmentation, 103
    genetic diseases, 107–109
    Hermansky-Pudlak syndrome, 108–109, *110*
    Hispanics and Latinos, 359–371
    hyperpigmentation, 99–103
    hypopigmentation disorders, 91–93
    idiopathic guttate hypomelanosis, *92*, 92–93
    kohic acid, 105
    licorice extract, 105
    linea nigra, 100
    management, 103–107
    melasma, 101–103, *102–103*
    nails, 107
    nevus of Ota/nevus of Ito, 107, *108*
    palmoplantar racial difference, 107

Index

phenolic agents, 104
piebaldism, 107–108
pigmented nevi, 107
pityriasis alba, 92
pityriasis versicolor, 91–92
postinflammatory hyperpigmentation and hypopigmentation, 95–99, *98–100*
retinoids, 105–106
tacrolimus, 106
tars, 106
vitiligo, 93–95, *93–97*
Pigmented dermatitis, 299–301
Pigmented lesions, 264–265
Pigmented nevi, 107
Pillai studies, 3–13
Pimecrolimus, 69, 71
Pinkus studies, 335
Pityriasis alba, 92, 371
Pityriasis rosea, 55–56, *56–57*, 348
Pityriasis versicolor, 91–92
Pityrosporum spp., 56, 65, 91–92, 104, 397
Plaiting, 35, 80
Pochi and Strauss studies, 331
Poikiloderma of Civatte, 369
Polymorphous light eruption, 58
Polynesian patients, 12, 51
Pomade acne, 20
Pomeranz studies, 36
Pony tails, 80
Port wine stains, 262
Postinflammatory hyperpigmentation and hypopigmentation
Hispanic and Latinos, 359–360, *361*
laser therapy, 266
pigmentary disorders, 95–99, *98–100*
PPD, *see* Para-phenylenediamine (PPD)
Presentations, *see* Clinical presentationsPrayer callouses, 377, *377*
Preservatives, 298
Pressure, 346–347
Prevalence
acne vulgaris, 289
actinic prurigo, 301
atopic dermatitis, 292
chronic actinic dermatitis, 319
contact dermatitis, 295–296
dyshidrotic eczema, 294
erythropoietic protoporphyria, 320
melanoma, 314–315
melasma, 307
nevus of Ota/nevus of Ito, 311
nonmelanoma skin cancer, 313
nummular dermatitis, 294
Ofuji's disease, 316
pigmented dermatitis, 299–300
primary cutaneous amyloidosis, 305
prurigo nodularis, 301
prurigo pigmentosa, 301
vitiligo, 318
Xerosis, 294
Primary cutaneous amyloidosis, 304–307

Primary excision, 345–346
Propionibacterium acnes, 23, 225, 270, 291–292
Prurigo nodularis, 301–304
Prurigo pigmentosa, 301–304, 363
Pruritus, 32, 163–165
Pseudofolliculitis barbae, 335–340
Pseudo-Hutchinson's sign, 107
Pseudomonas aeuroginosa, 124
Psoralen UVA (PUVA)
hypopigmentation, 99
hypopigmented mycosis fungoides, 50
lichen planus, 59
necrobiosis lipoidica diabeticorum, 161
piebaldism, 108
vitiligo, 94
Psoralen UVA using natural sunlight (PUVASOL), 94
Psoriasis vulgaris
basics, 67–68, *70–71*
laser therapy, 269–270
Native Americans, 395–397
therapy, 68–70
Ptotic malar fat, 204–205
Public health issues, 193–194
Puerto Rican patients
Hermansky-Pudlak syndrome, 109
nonmelanoma skin cancer, 190
tinea capitis, 34
Pustule-type disorders, 75–79
PUVA, *see* Psoralen UVA (PUVA)
PUVASOL, *see* Psoralen UVA using natural sunlight (PUVASOL)

Q

Q-switched lasers, 264–268, *see also* Laser therapy

R

Racial differences, *see also specific disorder or race*
allergic contact dermatitis, 12
dermal structure, 7–9
epidermis, 5, *5*
hair morphology, 246–248, *247*
hair structure, 10, 277
hair transplant surgery, 251, *252*
irritation, 12
keloid scars, 11–12
melanoctyes, 6–7
nails, 11
scarring, 11–12
skin immunological responses, 13
stratum corneum, skin and hair, 3–4
Rajka, Hanifin and, studies, 26–27
Reconditioning, thermal, 279–280
Rehydrating skin, 32
Rejuvenation procedures, 204–206, *205–208*, *see also* Cosmetic and dermatologic surgery; Photorejuvenation
Relaxers, hair

central centrifugal cicatricial alopecia, 83
chemicals, 85–86
contact dermatitis, 71–72
hair care products, 278–279, *279*
Relaxin, 345
Renal disease, 164–165
Retinoids
   basics, 222–224
   common dermatological diseases, 23–24, *24*
   hyperpigmentation, 98
   lichen planus, 59
   necrobiosis lipoidica diabeticorum, 161
   photoaging, 217–218
   pigmentary disorders, 105–106
Retinol, 224
Reveille studies, 350
Rhinocladiella aquaspersa, 132
Rhinoscleroma, 136
Richardson studies, 385–402
Richards studies, 3–13, 211–219
Riehl's melanosis, 368–369, *369*
Ringworm, *see* Tinea capitis
Roberts studies, 331–351
Robinson studies, 29, 31
Rosacea, 20–21, *22–23*
Rose, Dunwell and, studies, 25
Ross studies, 340
Rubber chemical allergies, 298
Rubin and Greenbaum studies, 218

S

Salicylic acid
   chemical peels and microdermabrasion, 25
   cosmetic and dermatologic surgery, 236–237, *237*
   psoriasis vulgaris, 69
   seborrheic dermatitis, 65
Sanchez studies, 115–140, 216, 310, 357–381
Sarcoidosis
   Black patients, *334,* 348
   cutaneous manifestations, 147–149, *148–152*
   hair and scalp disorders, 83–84, *84*
Saripalli studies, 147–169
Scalp and hair disorders
   acne keloidalis nuchae, 76–78, *77–78*
   allergic contact dermatitis, 72, *73*
   atopic dermatitis, 70–71
   basics, 63–64, *64,* 88
   central centrifugal cicatricial alopecia, 80–83, *81–83*
   chemicals, 85–88, *87*
   contact dermatitis, 71–72
   cyst-type disorders, 75–79
   dermatomyositis, 75
   differential diagnosis, *64*
   dissecting cellulitis, 78–79, *79*
   drying agents, 85–88, *87*
   flaking-type disorders, 64–75
   folliculitis decalvans, 76
   hair loss, 80–84
   hair shaft disorders, 84–88

   heat, 85
   inflammatory-type disorders, 64–79
   irritant contact dermatitis, 71–72, *72*
   lupus erythematosus, 74–75
   psoriasis vulgaris, 67–70, *70–71*
   pustule-type disorders, 75–79
   sarcoidosis, 83–84, *84*
   scarring hair loss, 80–84
   seborrheic dermatitis, 64–67, *65*
   tinea capitis, 72–74, *73–74*
   traction alopecia, 80, *81*
   trichorrhexis nodosa, 84, *85–86*
   uncomplicated folliculitis, 76
Scalp ringworm, *see* Tinea capitis
Scarring
   hair loss, 80–84
   racial differences, 11–12
   reduction, hair transplantation, 254, *254–255*
Schawlow, Townes and, studies, 259
Scleroderma, 149–151, *152–153,* 350
Sebaceous glands, 9
Seborrheic dermatitis
   basics, 64–65, *65*
   Black patients, 333, *334*
   Native Americans, 397
   neonatal and pediatric dermatological diseases, 55, *56*
   nickel contact dermatitis, 55
   therapy, 65–67, *66–67*
Secondary syphilis, 348, *349*
Selenium sulfide, 57, 65
Shampoos
   atopic dermatitis, 71
   hair care products, 280–281
   psoriasis vulgaris, 68–70
   seborrheic dermatitis, 65
Sharma studies, 35, 74
Silicone gel-sheeting, 347
Silverberg studies, 36–37, 65, 73
Skin and hair, structure and function
   allergic contact dermatitis, 12
   basics, 3–11
   Black patients, 331
   cutaneous appendages, *9,* 9–11
   dermal structure, 7–9
   epidermal structure, 5, *5*
   hair follicles and hair structure, 10
   irritation, 12
   keloid scars, 11–12
   melanoctye biology, 6–7
   nails, 11
   scarring, 11–12
   sebaceous glands and sweat glands, 9
   skin immunological responses, 13
   stratum corneum biology, 3–4
Skin cancer
   African-American patients, 181–189, *182–188*
   African patients, 181–189, *182–188*
   Afro-Caribbean patients, 181–189, *182–188*
   Asians, 191–193
   basics, 181
   Black patients, 350–351

Hispanics, 189–191, *190–191, 378,* 378–381
Latinos, *378,* 378–381
Native Americans, 193
public health issues, 193–194
Skin care, 281–285, *282–283*
Skin diseases, *see specific disorder*
Skin grafts, 94, 99, 108
Skin immunological responses, 13
Sladden studies, 26
South African Black patients, 12, 148
South American blastomycosis, 136–137
South Asian patients
 diabetes mellitus, 158
 familial racial periorbital hyperpigmentation, 103
 scleroderma, 150
 systemic medication reaction, 168
Southeast Indian patients, *212–213,* 212–214
Sperling studies, 63, 82, 248
Spitz nevus, 192
Sporotrichosis, 137–138, *138*
Squamous cell carcinomas, 192, 351, 378–379, *379*
Steroids
 acne keloidalis nuchae, 77
 dermatomyositis, 158
 hypopigmentation, 99
 keloids, 343–344
 necrobiosis lipoidica diabeticorum, 161
 vitiligo, 94
Stratum corneum, skin and hair, 3–4
Strauss, Pochi and, studies, 331
Strauss and Kligman studies, 335–336, 338
Streptomyces tsukubaensis, 106
Strongyloides stercoralis, 127, 139
Styling products, 35, 280–281
Submandibular liposuction, 205
Sueki studies, 13
Sugino studies, 4
Sun avoidance, 50–51
Sunscreens
 dermatomyositis, 158
 polymorphous light eruption, 58
 public health issues, 193
 racial differences, 217
 skin care, 282–284, *283*
Superficial fungal infections, 115–117, *116–117*
Surgical therapies, 339–340, *see also* Therapies
Sutter and Turley studies, 200
Sweat glands, 9
Swee studies, 279
Swlerenga studies, 198
Syphilis, 119, *120*
Systemic lupus erythematosus, 349–350
Systemic medications
 antibiotics, 225–226
 reactions, 165–169, 298
 retinoid therapy, 218
Szabo, Fitzpatrick and, studies, 6
Szabo studies, 386

T

Tacrolimus
 atopic dermatitis, 71
 contact dermatitis, 32–33
 keloids, 344
 pigmentary disorders, 106
 psoriasis vulgaris, 69
 vitiligo, 94
Taenia solium, 120–121
Takahasi, Watanabe and, studies, 312
Tanghetti studies, 223
Tang studies, 289–323
Tan studies, 289–323
Tars, 65, 69, 106
Tattoos, 267–269, *268*
Taylor studies, 24, 386
Tazarotene, 69, 223–224
Terbinafine, 38, 74
Tham, Lim and, studies, 236
Therapies, *see also* Treatments
 acne vulgaris, 291–292
 actinic prurigo, 304
 atopic dermatitis, 294
 chronic actinic dermatitis, 319–320
 contact dermatitis, 299
 dyshidrotic eczema, 295
 erythropoietic protoporphyria, 321
 melanoma, 316
 melasma, 310
 Mongolian spot, 311
 nevus of Ota/nevus of Ito, 312
 nonmelanoma skin cancer, 314
 nummular dermatitis, 295
 photoaging, 217–219
 pigmented dermatitis, 301
 primary cutaneous amyloidosis, 306–307
 prurigo nodularis, 304
 prurigo pigmentosa, 304
 vitiligo, 319
 xerosis, 295
Thermal reconditioning, 279–280
Thibaut studies, 11
Thioglycolates, 86, 279–280
Tinea capitis
 basics, *33,* 33–38, 72–74, *73–74*
 neonatal and pediatric dermatological diseases, 48–49, *49*
Tinea versicolor, 56–57, *57,* 334
Topical agents, *see specific agent*
Townes and Schawlow studies, 259
Traction alopecia, 80, *80,* 249, *249–250*
Traction folliculitis and/or alopecia, 47–48, *47–48*
Traction hair styling, 35
Traditional Chinese medicine, 296, 298, 321–323, *see also* Cultural issues
Transient neonatal pustular melanosis, 43, *44*
Treadwell studies, 43–60
Treatments
 acropustulosis, infancy, 46
 atopic dermatitis, 54

dermatomyositis, 158
hyperpigmentation, 98
hypopigmented mycosis fungoides, 50
Kawasaki disease, 53
lichen planus, 59
lichen striatus, 58
lupus erythematosus, 50, 156–157
Mongolian spot, 43
neonatal lupus erythematosus, 51
neurofibromatosis 1 (NF 1), 59
Ofuji's disease, 317
piebaldism, 108
pityriasis rosea, 56
polymorphous light eruption, 58
pseudofolliculitis barbae, *334, 336,* 338–340
renal disease, 164–165
sarcoidosis, 149
scleroderma, 151
seborrheic dermatitis, 55
tinea capitis, 48–49
tinea versicolor, 57
traction folliculitis, 48
vitiligo, 94–95
Trental, 345
Trepanema pallidum, 119
Tretinoin
    basics, 105–106, 221–222
    combination therapy, 106
    dyspigmentation, 44
    photoaging, 217–218
Trichloroacetic acid, 237
Trichophyton spp., 34–37, 48, 74, 116, 393–394
Trichorrhexis nodosa, 84, *85–86,* 334–335
Trichosporon, 116
Trypanosoma cruzi, 122
Tsai studies, 238
Tse studies, 267
Tumescent liposuction, 241
Turley, Sutter and, studies, 200

U

Ultraviolet light therapy, 33, *see also specific UV rays*
Uncommon, unique, and unusual dermatoses and presentations
    Black patients, 347–350
    Native Americans, 387–388, 400, 402
Uncomplicated folliculitis, 76
Upper face, aging, 202
Urea, 69
UVA protection, 50–51
UVB treatment
    hypopigmentation, 99
    hypopigmented mycosis fungoides, 50
    lichen planus, 59

piebaldism, 108
polymorphous light eruption, 58
renal disease, 164
vitiligo, 94

V

Vargo and Cohen studies, 36
Vascular lasers, 262–264, *see also* Laser therapy
Venenum bufonis, 298
Vitamin C, 227
Vitiligo
    Asian patients, 318–319
    basics, 93–95, *93–97*
    Black patients, 341, *342*
    laser therapy, 270
Voorhees, Wilkins and, studies, 17

W

Waardenburg syndrome, 108
Watanabe and Takahasi studies, 312
Waxy skin, 159
Weaves, hair, 80
Weigand and Gaylor studies, 28
Weigand studies, 28
White skin, *see* Caucasian patients, racial differences
Wiegand studies, 400
Wiggins, Black and, studies, 400
Wilkins and Voorhees studies, 17–38
Williams studies, 26, 31
Willis, Kligman and, studies, 103, 310
Women, 248–255, 337
Woolf syndrome, 108
Wuchereria bancrofti, 139–140

X

Xerosis, 294–295

Y

Yin/yang, 321–322
Yohimbine, 168

Z

Zelickson studies, 273
Zhu studies, 224
Zinc, 78, 345
Zinc pyrithione, 72